Essentials of
Plastic Surgery

A UT Southwestern Medical Center Handbook

Essentials of
Plastic Surgery

A UT Southwestern Medical Center Handbook

Edited by

JEFFREY E. JANIS, MD

Assistant Professor, Department of Plastic Surgery,
University of Texas Southwestern Medical Center;
Chief of Plastic Surgery, Parkland Health and Hospital System;
Co-Director, Plastic Surgery Residency Program,
University of Texas Southwestern Medical Center,
Dallas, Texas

With Illustrations by
Jennifer N. Gentry, MA, CMI

Quality Medical Publishing, Inc.
St. Louis, Missouri
2007

Cover art: Picasso, Pablo (1881-1973) © Artist Rights Society (ARS), NY. Girl Before a Mirror. 1932. Oil on Canvas, 64 x 51¼". Gift of Mrs. Simon Guggenheim. (2.1938). The Museum of Modern Art, New York, NY, USA. Digital Image © The Museum of Modern Art/Licensed by SCALA/Art Resource, NY. © Estate of Pablo Picasso/ARS, New York.

Printed in Italy

This book presents current scientific information and opinion pertinent to medical professionals. It does not provide advice concerning specific diagnosis and treatment of individual cases and is not intended for use by the layperson. Medical knowledge is constantly changing. As new information becomes available, changes in treatment, procedures, equipment, and the use of drugs become necessary. The editor/author/contributors and the publisher have, as far as it is possible, taken care to ensure that the information given in this text is accurate and up to date. However, readers are strongly advised to confirm that the information, especially with regard to drug usage, complies with the latest legislation and standards of practice. The authors and publisher will not be responsible for any errors or liable for actions taken as a result of information or opinions expressed in this book.

The publisher has made every effort to trace the copyright holders for borrowed material. If any have been inadvertently overlooked, we will be pleased to make the necessary arrangements at the first opportunity.

PUBLISHER: Karen Berger
EDITOR: Michelle Berger
ASSISTANT EDITOR: Linda Stagg
PROJECT MANAGER: Keith Roberts
DIRECTOR OF EDITING: Suzanne Wakefield
DIRECTOR OF PRODUCTION AND MANUFACTURING: Carolyn Garrison Reich
PRODUCTION: Carol Stonebraker; Sandra Hanley
COVER DESIGN: Amanda Yarberry Behr
GRAPHICS TECHNICIAN: Brett Stone
ADDITIONAL MEDICAL ILLUSTRATION: Bradley Powell

Quality Medical Publishing, Inc.
2248 Welsch Industrial Court
St. Louis, Missouri 63146
Telephone: 1-314-878-7808
Web site: *http://www.qmp.com*

LIBRARY OF CONGRESS CATALOGING-IN-PUBLICATION DATA

Essentials of plastic surgery: A UT Southwestern Medical Center handbook / edited by Jeffrey E. Janis.
    p. ; cm.
  Includes bibliographical references and index.
  ISBN 1-57626-208-1 (pbk.)
  1. Surgery, Plastic—Handbooks, manuals, etc.   I. Janis, Jeffrey E.
  [DNLM: 1. Reconstructive Surgical Procedures—Outlines.
 WO 18.2 E78 2006]
 RD118.E87 2006
 617.9′5—dc22

2006012504

QM/LG/LG
5 4 3 2 1

Contributors

George Broughton II, MD, PhD, Colonel, MC, US Army
Chief, Department of Plastic and Reconstructive Surgery, Landstuhl Regional Medical Center, Landstuhl, Germany

John L. Burns, MD
Clinical Instructor, Department of Plastic Surgery, University of Texas Southwestern Medical Center; Associate, Department of Plastic Surgery, Dallas Plastic Surgery Institute, Dallas, Texas

David S. Chang, MD
Chief Resident, Division of Plastic Surgery, University of California–San Francisco, San Francisco, California

Melissa A. Crosby, MD
Assistant Professor, Department of Plastic and Reconstructive Surgery, M.D. Anderson Cancer Center, Houston, Texas

Michael E. Decherd, MD
Private Practice, San Antonio, Texas

C. Alejandra Garcia, MD
Surgery Resident, Department of Plastic Surgery, University of Texas Southwestern Medical Center, Dallas, Texas

Ashkan Ghavami, MD
Chief Resident, Department of Plastic Surgery, University of Texas Southwestern Medical Center, Dallas, Texas

Amanda A. Gosman, MD
Assistant Professor, Director of Pediatric Plastic Surgery, Department of Surgery, Division of Plastic Surgery, University of California–San Diego School of Medicine, San Diego, California

Bishr Hijazi, MD
Hand and Microsurgery Fellow, Department of Plastic Surgery, University of Texas Southwestern Medical Center, Dallas, Texas

John E. Hoopman, CMLSO
Certified Medical Laser Safety Officer, Department of Environmental Health and Safety, University of Texas Southwestern Medical Center, Dallas, Texas

Jeffrey E. Janis, MD
Assistant Professor, Department of Plastic Surgery, University of Texas Southwestern Medical Center; Chief of Plastic Surgery, Parkland Health and Hospital System; Co-Director, Plastic Surgery Residency Program, University of Texas Southwestern Medical Center, Dallas, Texas

Rohit K. Khosla, MD
Chief Resident, Department of Plastic Surgery, University of Texas Southwestern Medical Center, Dallas, Texas

Danielle M. LeBlanc, MD
Private Practice, Fort Worth, Texas

Jason E. Leedy, MD
Private Practice, Mayfield Heights, Ohio

Joshua A. Lemmon, MD
Hand and Microsurgery Fellow, Department of Orthopaedics and Department of Plastic and Reconstructive Surgery, University of Pittsburgh, Pittsburgh, Pennsylvania

David W. Mathes, MD
Assistant Professor of Surgery, Division of Plastic and Reconstructive Surgery, University of Washington, Seattle, Washington

Ricardo A. Meade, MD
Aesthetic Surgery Fellow and Assistant Faculty
Instructor, Department of Plastic Surgery,
University of Texas Southwestern Medical
Center, Dallas, Texas

Blake A. Morrison, MD
Clinical Instructor, Department of Plastic
Surgery, University of Texas Southwestern
Medical Center; Attending Hand Surgeon,
Department of Surgery, Presbyterian Hospital of
Dallas, Dallas Texas

Scott W. Mosser, MD
Private Practice, San Francisco, California

Sacha I. Obaid, MD
Craniofacial Fellow, Institute of Reconstructive
Plastic Surgery, New York University Medical
Center, New York, New York

Thornwell Hay Parker III, MD
Chief Resident, Department of Plastic Surgery,
University of Texas Southwestern, Dallas, Texas

Jason K. Potter, MD, DDS
Attending Surgeon, Department of Plastic
Surgery, Legacy Emanuel Hospital and Health
Center; Clinical Instructor, Department of Oral
and Maxillofacial Surgery, Oregon Health
Sciences University, Portland, Oregon

Edward M. Reece, MD, MS
Resident, Department of Plastic Surgery,
University of Texas Southwestern Medical
Center, Dallas, Texas

Jose L. Rios, MD
Private Practice, Dermatology and Plastic
Surgery Associates, SC, Frankfurt, Joliet,
Naperville, Illinois

Michel Saint-Cyr, MD, FRCS(C)
Assistant Professor, Department of Plastic
Surgery, University of Texas Southwestern
Medical Center, Dallas, Texas

Holly P. Smith, BFA
Medical Photographer, Department of Plastic
Surgery, University of Texas Southwestern
Medical Center, Dallas, Texas

Sumeet S. Teotia, MD
Private Practice, Charlotte Plastic Surgery PA,
Charlotte; Clinical Assistant Professor, Division
of Plastic and Reconstructive Surgery and
Surgery of the Hand, University of North
Carolina, Chapel Hill, North Carolina

Dawn D. Wells, PA-C
Physician Assistant, Department of
Dermatology, Grapevine Dermatology,
Grapevine, Texas

Foreword

Essentials in Plastic Surgery: A UT Southwestern Medical Center Handbook, edited by Dr. Jeffrey E. Janis, represents the next generation of plastic surgery education. It is a welcome addition to the numerous reviews and manuals currently available, because it elevates this genre to the next level with its systematic, algorithmic approach and the many special features that permeate its pages.

This unique handbook provides an important foundation for current and future plastic surgeons. It is a concise resource for medical students and residents interested in learning the core content of plastic surgery, as well as for practicing plastic surgeons who are keeping current with the ever-evolving field of plastic surgery. Although it is more than 900 pages long, it is surprisingly compact and able to fit conveniently into a lab coat pocket for ready reference. The information is organized in an outline format with many visual aids, helpful tips, and key points, making it easy to locate important information quickly. It is an ideal companion for any student of plastic surgery regardless of his or her level of training. It includes the entire gamut of plastic surgery, from the basic principles of wound healing to refinements in the use of lasers, massive-weight-loss surgery, and to the tremendous advances in reconstructive and aesthetic cosmetic surgery.

It is with great pride that I write this foreword for *Essentials in Plastic Surgery.* This book is an outgrowth of the ideals and the emphasis on high-quality education and academic excellence that typifies the UT Southwestern Medical Center training program in plastic surgery. Dr. Janis is an outstanding example of the talent and creativity that has been fostered in the program's rich environment. He and his contributors, many of whom are former residents or fellows at UT Southwestern Medical Center, have put together a valuable publication that will assist others in their training and professional growth.

This book provides insight into the complexities and uniqueness of plastic surgery as a specialty. Dr. Janis and his contributors have capsulized this field into a truly superb handbook. Each page provides pearls to be learned that can be incorporated easily into your practice. This book will fill a void for practicing plastic surgeons who want to stay current with advances in plastic surgery. Furthermore, as we enter the era of Maintenance of Certification (MOC), I can think of no other summary text of the state of the art of plastic surgery that provides such ready access in a unique outline format. Dr. Janis and his coauthors should be congratulated for this tremendous educational tool.

Rod J. Rohrich, MD
Professor and Chairman
Crystal Charity Ball Distinguished Chair in Plastic Surgery
Betty and Warren Woodward Chair in Plastic and Reconstructive Surgery
Department of Plastic Surgery
University of Texas Southwestern Medical Center
Dallas, Texas

Preface

The idea for this book originated with one of my best friends and colleagues, Jose Rios, during a conversation we had in 2003 while sitting at his kitchen table. At the time he was relying on the skeleton notes he had assembled on a broad variety of plastic surgery topics, and he was lamenting the fact that there was no true "handbook of plastic surgery" available for use as a "quick and dirty" reference. That conversation was the catalyst and inspiration for developing this handbook. My goal was to produce a handbook of exceptional quality that would cover the entire breadth of plastic surgery in a portable, clear, and concise format. Equally important, it had to be up-to-date and contain useful and digestible "high impact" information. Although the original target audience was to be students, residents, and fellows, in its final form it should benefit anyone seeking a grounding in plastic surgery, including those studying for in-service exams, written and oral boards, and even the recertification exam that is mandatory every 10 years.

This handbook is **not** meant to be an exhaustive shelf reference on the entirety of plastic surgery. Rather, it is intended to convey the "essentials" and provide a valuable plastic surgery foundation. It contains 88 chapters divided into 7 parts: Fundamentals and Basics; Skin and Soft Tissue; Head and Neck; Breast; Trunk and Lower Extremity; Hand, Wrist, and Upper Extremity; and Aesthetic Surgery. For the most part, the chapters were written by current and former residents and fellows from the Department of Plastic Surgery at the University of Texas Southwestern Medical Center in Dallas. All authors took time and care to ensure their chapters are complete and understandable.

As a recent resident and lifelong student, I feel that I have a good grasp of the key ingredients that make a handbook useful. I have tried to incorporate those elements into this publication. First and foremost, it was important that this handbook fit easily into the pocket of a lab coat. To this end we selected a size and number of pages to ensure a comfortable fit, even going so far as to measure out the dimensions of coat pockets. To convey the information without ambiguity, we used a consistent, bullet-point outline format with numerous figures, diagrams, and tables. A second color was added to enhance the presentation of information. Each chapter also incorporates Tips, providing additional insights and practical advice not always available in textbooks or articles. Each chapter concludes with Key Points, which provide the reader a quick source of information and refresher for the essential points highlighted in the chapter. Finally, references enable the reader to go to the source material for more in-depth reading on any given subject. In summary, this book has been purposefully designed to be the "complete" handbook: ergonomic, navigable, and definitive.

To bring the entire project to the next level, the content of the handbook is being made available in an electronic format for laptops and desktops, as well as for Palm Pilots and Pocket PCs.

It is my hope that this book will find a comfortable place in the pockets of students and practitioners alike, and that its worn corners and highlighted, tattered pages will be a testament to its ultimate utility.

Jeffrey E. Janis, MD

Acknowledgments

Books do not happen in isolation, and this one is no exception. There are many individuals who contributed their efforts and support to this project.

First, a special acknowledgment is due Jose Rios, a former fellow resident and lifelong friend, who had the original idea that led to this book's development.

I would also like to acknowledge my mentor and chairman, Rod Rohrich, for his guidance, wisdom, and encouragement, which have been invaluable to me throughout my career. His premier program at UT Southwestern Medical Center in Dallas, of which I am a proud graduate, is a testament to his efforts to train the next generation of leaders in plastic surgery.

Sincere and special thanks are also due the contributors to this handbook, many of whom are present and former residents of this program, and all of them are friends. The quality of this publication is largely from their efforts and their willingness to work and rework their manuscripts until they achieved the quality and clarity reflected in these chapters.

I would also like to recognize Karen Berger and her incredible staff at Quality Medical Publishing, who deserve my deepest gratitude for their expertise and professionalism, and for making this dream become a reality.

Grateful acknowledgment also goes to Teresa Endsley for her invaluable organizational skills and assistance.

To my family, an unpayable debt of gratitude is owed for their unconditional love and support, and the encouragement that only they can give.

Finally, and most important, I would like to thank my wife, Dawn, for her love, support, patience, and understanding during the time it took to put this book together. This publication simply could not have been done without her.

Contents

PART VII ◆ AESTHETIC SURGERY

PART I

Fundamentals and Basics

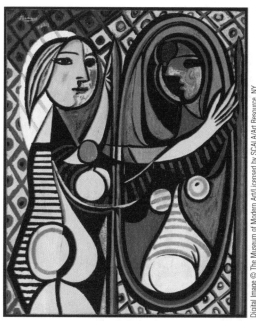

1. Basic Principles of Wounds

Thornwell Hay Parker III
Jeffrey E. Janis

Part I: Wound Healing

Thornwell Hay Parker III

THREE PHASES OF WOUND HEALING[1,2]

- Inflammatory phase (days 1 to 6)
- Fibroproliferative phase (day 4 to week 3)
- Maturation/remodeling phase (week 3 to 1 year)

INFLAMMATORY PHASE (DAYS 1 TO 6)
- **Vasoconstriction:** Constriction of injured vessels for 5-10 minutes following injury
- **Coagulation:** Clot formed by platelets and fibrin (end product of coagulation cascade)
- **Vasodilation and increased permeability:** Mediated by histamine, serotonin (from platelets), and nitrous oxide (from endothelial cells)
- **Chemotaxis:** Signaled by platelet products (from alpha granules), coagulation cascade, complement activation (C5a), tissue products, and bacterial products
- **Cell migration**
  - Margination: Increased adhesion to vessel walls
  - Diapedesis: Movement through vessel wall
  - Fibrin: Creates initial matrix for cell migration
- **Cellular response**
  - Neutrophils: 24-48 hours—produce inflammatory products and phagocytosis, not critical to wound healing
  - Macrophages: 48-96 hours—become dominant cell population (until fibroblast proliferation), most critical to wound healing—orchestrate growth factors
  - Lymphocytes: 5-7 days—role poorly defined, possible regulation of collagenase and extracellular matrix (ECM) remodeling

FIBROPROLIFERATIVE PHASE (DAY 4 TO WEEK 3)
- **Matrix formation**
  - Fibroblasts: Move into wound days 2-3, dominant cell at 7 days, high rate of collagen synthesis from day 5 to week 3
  - Glycosaminoglycan (GAG) production
    - Hyaluronic acid first
    - Then chondroitin-4 sulfate, dermatan sulfate, and heparin sulfate
    - Followed by collagen production (see later)
  - Tensile strength begins to increase at days 4-5

- **Angiogenesis:** Increased vascularity—vascular endothelial growth factor (VEGF)/nitrous oxide
- **Epithelialization** (see later)

MATURATION/REMODELING PHASE (WEEK 3 TO 1 YEAR)

- After 3-5 weeks an equilibrium is reached between collagen breakdown and synthesis, subsequently no net change in quantity
- Increased collagen organization and stronger crosslinks
- Type I collagen replacement of type III collagen, restoring normal **4:1** ratio
- Decrease in GAGs, water content, vascularity, and cellular population
- **Peak tensile strength at 60 days—80% preinjury strength**

COLLAGEN PRODUCTION

- Collagen composed of three polypeptides wound together into a helix
- High concentration of **hydroxyproline** and **hydroxylysine** amino acids (only found in collagen, elastin, and complement C1q)
- More than 20 types of collagen based on amino acid sequences
  Type I: Most abundant (90% of body collagen)—dominant in skin, tendon, and bone
  Type II: Cornea and hyaline cartilage
  Type III: Vessel and bowel walls, uterus, and skin (type I/type III ratio is 4:1 in skin)
  Type IV: Basement membrane only
- Collagenase activation: Parathyroid hormone, adrenal corticosteroids, and colchicines
- Collagenase inhibition: Serum α-2 macroglobulin, cysteine, and progesterone

GROWTH FACTORS

- **Platelet-derived growth factor (PDGF):** From platelets, macrophages, and keratinocytes—chemotaxis, other wound healing
- **Interleukin-1 (IL-1)** and **tumor necrosis factor (TNF-α):** From neutrophils—fibroblast and collagen up and down regulation
- **Transforming growth factor (TGF-β):** From macrophages and platelets—collagen production, remodeling, epithelialization, chemotaxis
- **VEGF:** From keratinocytes and platelets—angiogenesis
- **Epidermal growth factor (EGF), fibroblastic growth factors (FGFs), insulinlike growth factor (IGF), keratinocyte growth factors (KGFs):** Epithelialization

EPITHELIALIZATION

- **Mobilization:** Loss of contact inhibition—cells at edge of wound or in appendages (in partial thickness wounds) flatten and break contact (integrins) with neighboring cells.
- **Migration:** Cells move across wound until meeting cells from other side, then contact inhibition reestablished.
- **Mitosis:** As cells at edge are migrating, basal cells further back from the wound edge proliferate to support cell numbers needed to bridge wound.

- **Differentiation:** Reestablishment of epithelial layers are from basal layer to stratum corneum after migration ceases.

CONTRACTION

- Myofibroblast: Specialized fibroblast with contractile cytoplasmic microfilaments and distinct cellular adhesion structures (desmosomes and maculae adherens)
  - Dispersed throughout granulating wound, act in concert to contract entire wound bed
  - Appear day 3, are maximal at day 10-21, and disappear as contraction is complete
- *Less contraction when more dermis is present in wound, just as full-thickness skin grafts have less secondary contraction than split-thickness grafts*

TYPES OF WOUND HEALING

- **Primary:** Closed within hours of creation by reapproximating edges of wound
- **Secondary:** Wound allowed to heal on its own by contraction and epithelialization
- **Delayed primary:** Subacute or chronic wound converted to acute wound by sharp debridement, then closed primarily; healing comparable to primary closure

FACTORS AFFECTING WOUND HEALING

GENETIC
- **Predisposition to hypertrophic or keloid scarring**
- **Hereditary conditions causing slow healing**
  - Typically abnormalities in collagen and elastin production and breakdown that may increase skin laxity, fragility, and inelasticity
  - May cause systemic problems (e.g., aneurysms)
  - Examples:
    - Pseudoxanthoma elasticum (increased collagen breakdown)
    - Cutis hyperelastica (i.e., Ehlers-Danlos syndrome, abnormal collagen crosslinking)
    - Progeria
    - Werner's syndrome
    - Epidermolysis bullosa
- **Skin type:** Pigmentation (Fitzpatrick type), elasticity, thickness, sebaceous quality, and location (e.g., shoulder, sternum, earlobe)
- **Age:** Affects rate of healing

SYSTEMIC HEALTH
- **Comorbidities**
  - Diabetes
  - Atherosclerotic disease
  - Renal failure
  - Immunodeficiency

- **Nutritional deficiencies**
  - Vitamins (e.g., vitamin C, zinc, copper, iron) (see below)
  - Caloric
  - Protein (follow albumin, prealbumin, transferin, or haptoglobin)

VITAMINS

> TIP: Supplements typically only help when deficiencies exist.

- **Vitamin A:** Reverses effects of steroids
  - 25,000 IU by mouth once per day increases tensile strength, or 200,000 IU topical every 8 hours increases epithelialization.
- **Vitamin C:** Important for collagen synthesis
  - Deficiency leads to scurvy: Immature fibroblast, deficient collagen synthesis, capillary hemorrhage, decreased tensile strength.
- **Vitamin E:** Antioxidant, stabilizes membranes
  - Large doses inhibit healing, but unproven to reduce scarring.
- **Zinc:** Cofactor for many enzymes
  - Deficiency causes impaired epithelial and fibroblast proliferation.

DRUGS
- **Smoking:** Increases vasoconstriction (nicotine—also with nicotine gum); increases carboxyhemoglobin and decreases oxygen delivery (carbon monoxide)
- **Steroids:** Impair wound healing
- **Antineoplastic agents:** Decrease fibroblast proliferation and wound contraction
  - Few or no adverse effects if administration delayed for 10-14 days after wound closure
- **Antiinflammatory medicine:** Decreases collagen synthesis by 45%
- **Lathyrogens:** Prevent cross-linking of collagen, decreasing tensile strength
  - β-aminopropionitrile (BAPN): Product of ground peas and d-penicillamine
  - Possible therapeutic use for decreasing scar tissue

LOCAL WOUND FACTORS
- **Oxygen delivery**

> TIP: The most common cause of failure to heal and wound infection is poor oxygen delivery associated with various disease states and local conditions (microvascular disease).

  - Atherosclerosis, Raynaud's disease, scleroderma
  - Adequate cardiac output, distal perfusion, oxygen delivery (hematocrit, oxygen dissociation curve)
  - Hyperbaric oxygen: Increases angiogenesis and new fibroblasts
- **Infection**
  - Clinical infection ($>10^5$): Decreases oxygen tension, lowers pH, increases collagenase activity, retards epithelialization and angiogenesis, prolongs inflammation and edema
- **Chronic wound**
  - Metalloproteases abundant, promote extracellular matrix turnover, slow wound healing

- Debridement of chronic wound: Removes excess granulation tissue and metalloproteases, transforms it to an acute wound state, and expedites healing
- **Denervation**
  - Aggressive pressure sores caused by high rate of collagenase activity and loss of protective mechanisms (e.g., diabetic neuropathy or spinal cord injury).
- **Radiation therapy**
  - Causes stasis/occlusion of small vessels, damages fibroblasts, chronic damage to nuclei
- **Moisture**
  - Speeds epithelialization
- **Warmth**
  - Increased tensile strength (better perfusion)
- **Free radicals**
  - Reactive oxygen species increased by ischemia, reperfusion, inflammation, radiation, vitamin deficiencies, and chemical agents

SCARRING (Table 1-1)

- **Hypertrophic scars (HTS)**
  - Scar elevated but within borders of original scar; more common than keloids (5%-15% of wounds)
    - ▶ Predisposition to areas of tension, flexor surfaces
    - ▶ Less recurrence following excision and adjuvant therapy

Table 1-1 *Comparison of Abnormal Scars*

	Keloid	Hypertrophic Scar	Widely Spread Scar
Genetics	Significant familial predilection	Low familial incidence	Not inherited
Race	Blacks more than Caucasians	Low racial incidence	Not related to race
Sex	Females more than males	Equal sex ratio	Unknown
Age	Most common 10-30 years	Any age, but mostly less than 20 years	Any age
Borders	Outgrows wound borders	Remains within wound borders	Wide, flat, often depressed
Natural history	Appears months after injury, rarely subsides	Appears soon after injury, subsides with time	Appears within 6 months of injury
Location	Mostly face, earlobes, anterior chest	Across flexor surfaces	Arms, legs, and abdomen
Etiologic factors	Possible autoimmune phenomenon	Tension and timing of closure	Tension and mobility of edges
Treatment	Intralesional steroids, excision, compression therapy, silicone gel sheeting, radiation therapy, and others; often worse after surgery alone	Same as for keloids, but outcomes usually more successful	Scar excision/layered closure

- **Keloid scars**
  - Grow outside original wound borders
  - May occur with deep injuries (less common than HTS)
    - ▸ Genetic and endocrine influences (increased growth in puberty and pregnancy)
    - ▸ Rarely regress and more resistant to excision and therapy
    - ▸ Histology similar for both HTS and keloid scars, differentiation usually based on clinical findings
- **Widened scars**
  - Wide and depressed from wound tension and mobility during maturation phase
- **Scar management**
- **Fetal healing**
  - Potentially scarless healing
  - Higher concentrations of type III collagen and hyaluronic acid, no inflammation, no angiogenesis, relative hypoxia

Part II: General Management of Complex Wounds

Jeffrey E. Janis

GENERAL POINTS

ALGORITHMIC APPROACH
- Thorough and comprehensive patient evaluation
- Examination and evaluation of the wound
- Lab tests and imaging
- Assessment, plan, and execution

HISTORY
- Age
- General health
- Presence of comorbidities
- Prewound functional and ambulatory capacity
- Associated factors that influence wound healing
  - Diabetes mellitus
  - End-stage renal disease
  - Cardiac disease
  - Peripheral vascular disease
  - Tobacco use
  - Vasculitis
  - Malnutrition
  - Steroid therapy

- Radiation
- Mobility impairment

PHYSICAL EXAMINATION
- **Assessment of vascular system**
  - Palpable pulses
  - Temperature
  - Hair growth
  - Skin changes
- **Assessment of neurosensory system**
  - Reflexes
  - Two-point discrimination/vibratory testing (128 Hz)

WOUND EVALUATION
- **Wound history**
  - Circumstances surrounding the injury
  - History of wound healing problems
  - Chronicity
  - Previous diagnostics
  - Previous treatments
- **Components of wound evaluation**
  - Location (helps determine underlying causes)
    - Pressure
    - Vascular insufficiency
  - Size
    - Length
    - Width
    - Depth
    - Area
  - Extent of defect
    - Skin
    - Subcutaneous tissue
    - Muscle, tendon, nerve
    - Bone
- **Condition of surrounding tissue and wound margins**
  - Color
  - Pigmentation
  - Inflammation/induration
  - Satellite lesions
  - Edema
- **Condition of wound bed**
  - Odor
  - Necrosis
  - Granulation tissue
  - Exposed structures
  - Fibrin
  - Exudate
  - Eschar

- Foreign bodies
- Inflammation/infection
- Tunneling/sinuses

LABORATORY STUDIES
- **Complete blood count (CBC)**
  - Elevated white-cell count? Left shift?
  - Hemoglobin/hematocrit with indices
  - Correctable forms of anemia
- **Blood urine nitrogen (BUN)/creatinine**
  - Assessment of renal function and hydration status
- **Glucose/hemoglobin A$_1$C**
  - Assessment of hyperglycemia and its trend
  - Normal A$_1$C <6.0
- **Albumin and prealbumin**
  - **Albumin** (t$_{1/2}$ = ~20 days)
    - ▶ Mild malnutrition if 2.8-3.5 g/dl
    - ▶ Moderate malnutrition if 2.1-2.7 g/dl
    - ▶ Severe malnutrition if less than 2.1 g/dl
  - **Prealbumin** (t$_{1/2}$ = ~3 days)
    - ▶ Rule of fives
      - ◆ Normal: Greater than 15 mg/dl
      - ◆ Mild deficiency: Less than 15 mg/dl
      - ◆ Moderate deficiency: Less than 10 mg/dl
      - ◆ Severe deficiency: Less than 5 mg/dl
- **Erythrocyte sedimentation rate/C-reactive protein (ESR/CRP)**
  - Nonspecific inflammatory markers
  - Obtain baseline
  - Subsequent measurements to help follow potential recurrence of osteomyelitis

IMAGING
- **Plain films**
  - Fractures
  - Foreign bodies
  - Osteomyelitis
- **CT scan**
  - Abscess
  - Extent of wound
  - Tracking/tunneling
- **MRI/MRA**
  - Osteomyelitis
  - Assessment of vascular status
- **Angiography**
  - Assessment of vascular status

DIAGNOSTIC TESTS
- **Handheld Doppler**
- **Ankle-brachial index**
  - Greater than 1.2: Noncompressible (calcified)
  - 0.9-1.2: Normal
  - 0.5-0.9: Mixed arterial/venous disease
  - Less than 0.5: Critical stenosis
  - Less than 0.2: Ischemic gangrene likely
- **Transcutaneous oxygen tension (TcPo$_2$)**
  - Evaluation of response to oxygen administration as a surrogate marker for reversible hypoxia
  - Greater than 40 mm Hg: Normal
  - Less than 30 mm Hg: Abnormal
- **Cultures**
  - Identification of specific microorganisms and sensitivities
- **Biopsy**
  - Vasculitis
  - Marjolin's ulcer/malignancy
  - Pyogenic granulomas

ASSESSMENT
- Working diagnosis
- Set treatment goals
- Define monitoring parameters

PLAN (RECONSTRUCTIVE LADDER)
- Do nothing
- Debride/dressing changes/VAC
- Primary closure
- Skin graft
- Local flap
- Regional flap
- Free tissue transfer

CONSIDERATIONS
- Functional impact
- Durability
- Individualize treatment to the patient (socioeconomic impact)
  - Does the patient need to minimize hospital stay, decrease the need for staged procedures, or get back to work quickly?
- Appearance
- Make sure solution not more complicated than problem

KEY POINTS

- ✔ The three stages of wound healing are inflammatory phase (macrophage most important), fibroproliferative phase, and maturation phase.
- ✔ Peak tensile strength occurs at 42-60 days (80% of original strength).
- ✔ Epithelialization is initiated by loss of contact inhibition.
- ✔ The amount of dermis present is inversely proportional to the amount of secondary contraction (i.e., more dermis equates to less secondary contraction).
- ✔ Vitamin A is used to reverse detrimental effects of steroids on wound healing.
- ✔ Hypertrophic scars and keloids have a similar histology and are distinguished clinically; both have high recurrence unless combined modalities are used.

REFERENCES

1. Broughton G, Rohrich RJ. Wounds and scars. Sel Read Plast Surg 10:7, 2005.
2. Glat P, Longaker M. Wound healing. In Aston SJ, Beasley RW, Thorne CHM, et al, eds. Grabb and Smith's Plastic Surgery, 5th ed. Philadelphia: Lippincott-Raven, 1997.
3. Michelle P, Hardesty R. Basic techniques and principles in plastic surgery. In Aston SJ, Beasley RW, Thorne CHM, et al, eds. Grabb and Smith's Plastic Surgery, 5th ed. Philadelphia: Lippincott-Raven, 1997.

2. Sutures and Needles

Scott W. Mosser

QUALITIES OF SUTURE MATERIALS: THE ESSENTIAL VOCABULARY[1]

PERMANENCE: ABSORBABLE VERSUS NONABSORBABLE
- **Absorbable**
  - Lose at least 50% of their strength in 4 weeks
  - Eventually are completely absorbed
  - Absorption process and inflammation
    - *Hydrolytic process*
      - Enzyme-mediated
      - Process for synthetic suture absorption
      - Minimal inflammation
    - *Proteolytic process*
      - Cellular inflammation-mediated
      - Sutures of natural origin (e.g., gut, from beef or sheep intestine)
      - More inflammation leads to more scarring around the suture site
- **Nonabsorbable**
  - Even nonabsorbable natural filaments (e.g., silk and cotton) induce a cell-mediated reaction until the suture becomes encapsulated.

CONFIGURATION
- **Monofilament** or **multifilament** (twisted or braided)
  - Monofilament sutures slide through tissue with less friction and have less capillary action but more memory than multifilament sutures.

> TIP: Gut sutures do not fit into either category but behave more like monofilament sutures.

KNOT SECURITY
The force necessary to cause a knot to slip
- Knot security is proportional to the coefficient of friction and the ability of the suture to stretch.
- More knot security means fewer throws necessary to tie a reliable knot.
- Braided sutures (e.g., silk, Vicryl®) have excellent knot security.
- Monofilaments (e.g., Prolene®, nylon) have less security.

ELASTICITY
The tendency of a suture to return to its original length after stretching
- Elastic sutures stretch in edematous wounds, then return to their original size while maintaining tension.
- Inelastic sutures (e.g., steel) cut through edematous tissues instead of forgiving the added tension.

MEMORY
Tendency of a suture material to return to its original shape (similar to stiffness)
- Sutures with more memory are less pliable, more difficult to handle.
- More memory leads to less knot security.

FLUID ABSORPTION AND CAPILLARITY
Fluid absorption is the amount of fluid retained by a suture.
Capillarity is the tendency of fluid to travel along the suture.
- Capillarity is thought to correlate with adhesion and harboring of bacteria.

COST
- Cost includes both the suture material and the needle.
- Sutures attached to *precision needles* (which are sharper and made of high-grade alloys) are more expensive than sutures with standard needles.

VISIBILITY
- Dyeing aids in visibility during placement and removal.
- Braided sutures are usually visible even if undyed, because they become saturated with blood intraoperatively.

TIP: The United States Pharmacopoeia (USP) rating system is often used.[2]

- Diameters are given in #-0 values based on USP breaking strength rating, not the width of the suture.
- Two different sutures with the same number can have different diameters (e.g., a 3-0 stainless steel suture is thinner than a 3-0 silk suture but has the same breaking strength).

NEEDLE CONFIGURATIONS[3,4]

POINT CONFIGURATION (Fig. 2-1)
- **Cutting needles**
  - Cutting needles have sharp edges that run the length of the needle tip and are better at penetrating tough tissues.
  - Skin and dermis are sutured with cutting needles.
  - **Conventional versus reverse cutting needles**
    - *Conventional cutting* needles have a sharp edge on the inner side of the curve. This creates a weak point on the tract where the suture can cut through the skin.
    - *Reverse cutting* needles have a flat surface on the interior of the curve and are preferable for skin closure.
- **Taper needles**
  - Taper needles have a sharp tip but no sharp edge.
  - Tissue spreads around the needle instead of being cut by it.
  - Suture material is less likely to cut through tissue if the tract is made with a taper needle.
  - Taper needles are typically used for tendon and deep tissue closure.

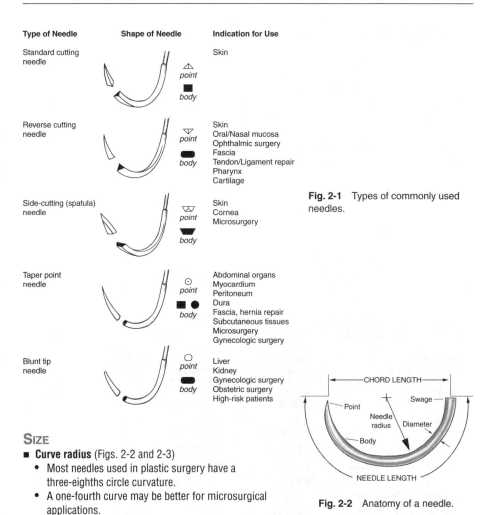

Type of Needle	Shape of Needle	Indication for Use
Standard cutting needle	point / body	Skin
Reverse cutting needle	point / body	Skin Oral/Nasal mucosa Ophthalmic surgery Fascia Tendon/Ligament repair Pharynx Cartilage
Side-cutting (spatula) needle	point / body	Skin Cornea Microsurgery
Taper point needle	point / body	Abdominal organs Myocardium Peritoneum Dura Fascia, hernia repair Subcutaneous tissues Microsurgery Gynecologic surgery
Blunt tip needle	point / body	Liver Kidney Gynecologic surgery Obstetric surgery High-risk patients

Fig. 2-1   Types of commonly used needles.

Fig. 2-2   Anatomy of a needle.

Size

- **Curve radius** (Figs. 2-2 and 2-3)
  - Most needles used in plastic surgery have a three-eighths circle curvature.
  - A one-fourth curve may be better for microsurgical applications.
- **Length**
- **Diameter**
  - The diameter of a needle is determined by the balance between material strength and the smallest diameter possible for the required suture size.
  - Some wound geometries require a semicircle needle to facilitate tissue handling.

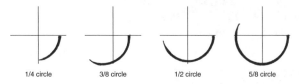

1/4 circle   3/8 circle   1/2 circle   5/8 circle

Fig. 2-3   Curvature of a needle.

FACTORS THAT GUIDE SUTURE CHOICE (Tables 2-1 and 2-2)

ABSORBABLE VERSUS NONABSORBABLE

- Rapidly absorbing suture can be used for layers closed under *minimal tension* (e.g., gut suture to close mucosa or skin after deep sutures are placed).
- Absorbable sutures that maintain strength for 4-6 weeks are used for closures under *short-term* tension (e.g., Vicryl or PDS to close fascia and subcutaneous tissue).
- Considerable *long-term* tension requires permanent sutures (e.g., Nylon, polypropylene, or polyester for bone anchoring, ligament, and tendon repair).
- Choose an absorbable suture that loses strength comparable to the timing of wound strength recovery (Fig. 2-4).

CALIBER

- Caliber is largely dictated by the strength of suture needed.
- Choose the smallest caliber suture that provides sufficient strength.

TYPE OF TISSUE AND NEEDLE CHOICE

- Generally, use permanent sutures on taper needles for fascia, tendon, or cartilage under tension.
- Use absorbable sutures on cutting needles for subcutaneous, dermis, and skin closures.

Table 2-1 *Qualities of Absorbable Sutures[3,5]*

Composition (Proprietary Name)	Approximate Time to 50% Original Strength	Configuration	Absorption Method (Reactivity)	Memory
Plain gut*	5-6 days (unpredictable)	Natural monofilament	Cell-mediated (high)	Low
Chromic gut*	14 days (unpredictable)	Natural monofilament	Cell-mediated (high)	Low
Polyglytone 6211 (Caprosyn†)‡	5-7 days	Monofilament	Hydrolytic (low)	Medium
Poliglecaprone 25 (Monocryl¶)‡	7-10 days	Monofilament	Hydrolytic (low)	Medium
Glycolide, dioxanone, and trimethylene carbonate polyester (Biosyn†)‡	2-3 weeks	Monofilament	Hydrolytic (low)	Medium
Glycolide/lactide copolymer (Vicryl,¶ Polysorb†)‡	2-3 weeks	Braided	Hydrolytic (low)	Low
Polyglycolic acid (Dexon II†)‡	2-3 weeks	Braided	Hydrolytic (low)	Low
Polyglyconate (Maxon†)‡	4 weeks	Monofilament	Hydrolytic (low)	High
Polydioxanone (PDS II¶)‡	4 weeks	Monofilament	Hydrolytic (low)	High

*Animal source.
†US Surgical Corporation.
‡Synthetic.
¶Ethicon.

Table 2-2 *Qualities of Nonabsorbable Sutures*[3,5]

Composition (Proprietary Name)	Configuration	Reactivity	Memory/Handling
Cotton	Twisted multifilament	High	−/Good
Silk	Braided	High	−/Good
Nylon			
Monofilament (Ethilon,*Dermalon,† Monosoft†)	Monofilament	Low	+/Fair
Braided (Nurolon,* Surgilon†)	Braided	Moderate	−/Good
Polypropylene (Prolene,* Surgipro†)	Monofilament	Low	++/Poor
Polybutester (Novafil†)	Monofilament	Low	+/Fair
Polyester			
Uncoated (Mersilene*)	Braided	Moderate	−/Good
Coated (Ethibond,* Surgidac,† Ti-Cron†)	Braided	Moderate	−/Good
Stainless steel	Monofilament	Low	++/Poor

*Ethicon.
†US Surgical Corporation.

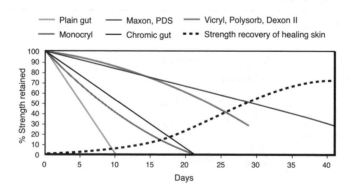

Fig. 2-4 Suture absorption and wound strength recovery. After a procedure, skin strength can be expected to regain 5% of its original strength within a week, nearly 50% within 4 weeks, and 80% within 6 weeks of skin closure. Even after collagen maturation is complete (6 months to 1 year postoperatively), a wound will only regain 80% of its original strength. (Modified from Levenson SM, Geever EF, Crowley LV, et al. The Healing of Rat Skin Wounds. Ann Surg 161:293-308, 1965.)

WOUND CONTAMINATION AND INFLAMMATION

> TIP: Monofilament sutures should be used for contaminated and infected wounds to prevent harboring bacteria in the suture material.

- Wound infection accelerates the process of suture absorption.

PATIENT FACTORS
- Patient reliability, age, and overall wound-healing capability affect how long the sutures must maintain closure tension.

> TIP: In thin patients, buried knot configurations with braided, absorbable suture will prevent palpability of sutures after surgery.

MICROSUTURES AND NEEDLES (see Chapter 5)
- Suture choice depends on vessel or structure size.
  - 8-0 is used for large (4 mm) vessels (e.g., radial and ulnar arteries).
  - 9-0 is used for 3-4 mm vessels (e.g., internal mammary, dorsalis pedis, and posterior tibial arteries).
  - 10-0 is used for 1-2 mm structures (e.g., digital arteries and nerves).
  - 11-0 is used for very small (<1 mm) vessels, such as those in children and infants.
- Microsutures behave similarly in their tying and memory characteristics at these diameters.
- Sutures are nearly always *monofilament synthetic* (e.g., nylon or polypropylene).

SUTURE REMOVAL

TIMING OF SUTURE REMOVAL (Table 2-3)

Table 2-3   *Recommended Timing of Suture Removal by Location*

Bodily Area	Days to Removal
Eyelid	3-5
Face	5-7
Lip	5-7
Hand/foot	10-14
Trunk	7-10
Breast	7-10

POTENTIAL COMPLICATION: RAILROAD TRACK SCAR (Fig. 2-5)
A "railroad track" scar is the formation of punctate scars and parallel rows of scar beneath them.
- The *punctate component* of the scars results from delayed suture removal.
  - Epithelial cells that abut a skin suture form a cylindrical cuff and grow downward along the suture.
  - The cells continue to develop after suture removal and keratinize the length of the suture tract, resulting in inflammation and punctate scar formation.

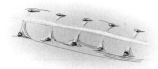

Fig. 2-5   Railroad track scar deformity.

- *Parallel rows* result from pressure necrosis of the skin and subcutaneous tissue beneath the external suture. This can be prevented by tying sutures loose enough to allow for postoperative edema.

OTHER CLOSURE MATERIALS

STAINLESS STEEL STAPLES
- Nonreactive, but inelastic and offer inaccurate epidermal approximation
- Least ischemic method of closure

CYANOACRYLATE
- Rapid and effective for well-aligned wounds under no tension
- Imprecise edge approximation
- Does not support significant skin edge tension during healing

---

KEY POINTS
- ✔ In a contaminated wound, monofilament suture should be used.
- ✔ Tissue under significant long-term tension should be closed with permanent suture only.
- ✔ Choose an absorbable suture that loses strength comparable to the timing of wound strength recovery.[6]
- ✔ Of the absorbable sutures available for skin closure, only fast-absorbing plain gut is absorbed in time to prevent punctate scar formation.
- ✔ To avoid *railroad track scars,* sutures in the skin layer should be removed promptly. Therefore the final skin layer should not be closed under tension, and a gaping skin wound should be approximated first with deep sutures.

REFERENCES

1. Friedman J, Mosser SW. Closure material. In Evans G, ed. Operative Plastic Surgery. New York: McGraw-Hill, 2000.
2. United States Pharmacopeia, vol 25. Rockville, MD: United States Pharmacopeia, 2002.
3. Ethicon. Wound Closure Manual. Somerville, NJ: Ethicon, 2004.
4. Nahai F, Sherman R, eds. Needles in plastic surgery. Roundtables Plast Surg. 1(1):Whole issue, 2003.
5. US Surgical, 2004. Available at *www.ussurgical.com.*
6. Levenson SM, Geever EF, Crowley LV, et al. The healing of rat skin wounds. Ann Surg 161:293-308, 1965.

3. Basics of Flaps

Amanda A. Gosman

DEFINITION

A flap is a unit of tissue that maintains its own blood supply while being transferred from a donor site to a recipient site.

CLASSIFICATION

- Most flaps can be classified according to **three principles:**
  1. Method of movement
  2. Vascularity
  3. Tissue composition

> TIP: The intrinsic vascularity of a flap is the most critical determinant of successful transfer and is therefore the most clinically valid method of classification.

METHOD OF MOVEMENT
- **Local flaps:** Used to close defects adjacent to the donor site
  - **Advancement flaps:** *Slid directly forward into a defect by stretching the skin, without rotation or lateral movement* (Fig. 3-1)
    - Single-pedicle advancement
    - Double-pedicle advancement
    - V-Y advancement (Fig. 3-2)
  - **Rotation flaps:** *Semicircular—rotated about a pivot point into the defect to be closed* (Fig. 3-3)
    - Donor site can be closed primarily or with a skin graft.
    - To facilitate rotation, the base can be back-cut at the pivot point or a triangle of skin (Burow's triangle) can be removed external to the pivot point.
  - **Transposition flaps:** *Rotated laterally about a pivot point into an immediately adjacent defect*
    - Effective length of the flap becomes shorter the farther the flap is rotated, therefore the flap must be designed longer than the defect to be covered, otherwise a back-cut may be necessary (Fig. 3-4).

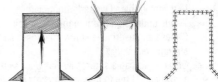

Fig. 3-1 Rectangular advancement flap.

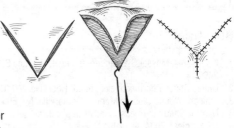

Fig. 3-2 V-Y advancement flap.

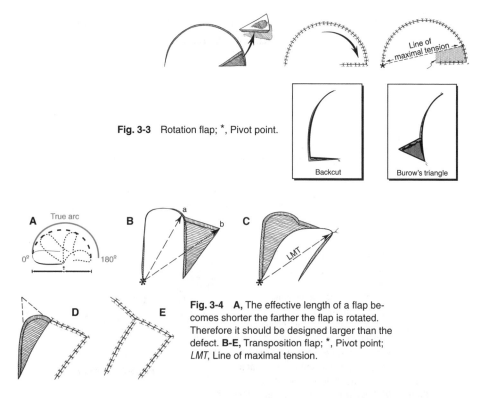

Fig. 3-3 Rotation flap; *, Pivot point.

Backcut

Burow's triangle

A True arc 0° 180° **B** a b **C** LMT **D** **E**

Fig. 3-4 A, The effective length of a flap becomes shorter the farther the flap is rotated. Therefore it should be designed larger than the defect. **B-E,** Transposition flap; *, Pivot point; *LMT*, Line of maximal tension.

▶ Donor site can be closed by skin graft, direct suture, or secondary flap (e.g., bilobed flap) (Fig. 3-5).
▶ **Z-plasty** is a variation of the transposition flap in which two adjacent triangular flaps are reversed.
  ◆ The three limbs of the Z must be of equal length, and the two lateral-limb to central-limb angles should be equivalent.
  ◆ *Gain in length is related to the angles between the central and lateral limbs* (Table 3-1).

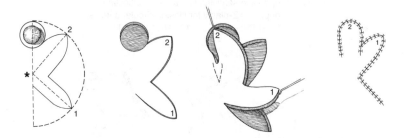

Fig. 3-5 Bilobed flap; *, Pivot point.

Table 3-1 *Theoretical Gain in Length of the Central Limb With Various Angles in Z-Plasty*

Angle of Each Lateral Limb of Z-Plasty (Degrees)	Theoretical Gain in Length of Central Limb (%)
30	25
45	50
60	75
75	100
90	120

From Rohrich RJ, Zbar RI. A simplified algorithm for the use of Z-plasty. Plast Reconstr Surg 103:1513, 1999.

TIP: The 60-degree Z-plasty is most effective because it lengthens the central limb without placing too much tension laterally (Fig. 3-6).

---

* Gain in central limb length is estimated to be 55%-84% of predicted and varies with local skin tension.[1]
* Multiple Z-plasties can be designed in series, but the geometry of one large Z-plasty is more effective for achieving skin lengthening.[2]
* Curvilinear modification of the Z-plasty using double opposing semicircular flaps can close circular defects[3] (Fig. 3-7).

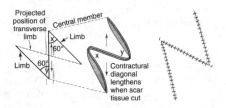

Fig. 3-6 Z-plasty.

▸ **Rhomboid (Limberg) flap** is a variation of the transposition flap in which the longitudinal axis of the rhomboid excision parallels the line of minimal skin tension.
* Rhomboid defect must have 60- and 120-degree angles (Fig. 3-8).
* Technique can be expanded to create a double or triple rhomboid flap.
▸ **Dufourmentel flap** is similar to the rhomboid flap but can be drawn with angles up to 90 degrees.

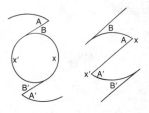

Fig. 3-7 Double opposing semicircular flaps. (From Keser A, Sensöz O, Mengi AS. Double opposing semicircular flap: A modification of opposing Z-plasty for closing circular defects. Plast Reconstr Surg 102:1001, 1998.)

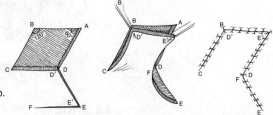

Fig. 3-8 Rhomboid (Limberg) flap.

- **Interpolation flaps:** *Rotate on a pivot point into a defect that is near* but not adjacent to *the donor site—flap pedicle must pass over or under intervening tissue.* Examples:
  - ▶ Deltopectoral (Bakamjian) flap
  - ▶ Island flaps such as the Littler neurovascular digital pulp flap (Fig. 3-9)

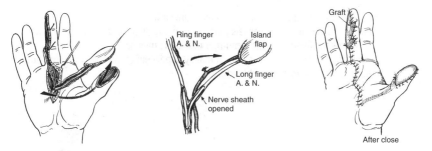

Fig. 3-9 Neurovascular island flap (Littler) is a type of interpolation flap. (From Daniel RK, Kerrigan CL. Principles and physiology of skin flap surgery. In McCarthy JG, ed. Plastic Surgery, vol 1. Philadelphia: Saunders, 1990, p 305.)

- **Distant flaps:** Donor and recipient sites not close to one another
  - Direct flaps can be used when the donor site can be approximated to the defect. Examples:
    - ▶ Thenar flap
    - ▶ Cross-leg flap
    - ▶ Groin flap
  - When the two sites cannot be approximated, tubed flaps or microvascular free tissue transfers are indicated.
    - ▶ *Tubed flaps* are pedicled flaps that can be "walked" to the recipient site, in multiple stages, from a distant location. For example, a pedicled groin flap can be transferred to the forearm, and then later it can be divided and transferred to a recipient site on the face. The lateral edges of the flap are sutured together to create a tube and decrease the risk of infection and the amount of raw surface exposed.
    - ▶ *Free tissue transfer* moves a unit of tissue that has a pedicle consisting of a feeding artery and a draining vein. The pedicle is anastomosed to an artery and vein at the recipient site to reestablish blood flow to the unit of tissue.

VASCULARITY

- **Vascular anatomy of the skin** (Fig. 3-10)
  - Taylor and Palmer[4] propose two theories of blood supply to tissues.

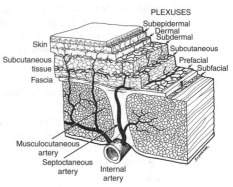

Fig. 3-10 Cutaneous circulation. (From Daniel RK, Kerrigan CL. Principles and physiology of skin flap surgery. In McCarthy JG, ed. Plastic Surgery, vol 1. Philadelphia: Saunders, 1990, p 305.)

1. **Angiosome:** *A composite unit of skin with its underlying deep tissue supplied by a source artery*
   * Taylor and Palmer[4] described **40 angiosomes** (Fig. 3-11) that are linked to one other by either "true" anastomotic arteries of similar caliber or reduced-caliber "choke" anastomotic vessels.[5] Choke vessels can potentially dilate to the caliber of a true anastomosis after surgical delay or with a decrease in sympathetic tone.
   * Routes by which integument is supplied by source artery
     - *Direct* route encompasses vessels that are primarily directed toward the skin, whether they follow the intermuscular septum or pierce the muscle.
     - *Indirect* route constitutes vessels that mainly supply either muscle or another deep tissue and only secondarily supply the skin.

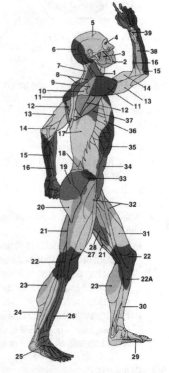

Fig. 3-11   The angiosomes of the source arteries of the body. *1*, Thyroid; *2*, facial; *3*, buccal internal maxillary; *4*, ophthalmic; *5*, superficial temporal; *6*, occipital; *7*, deep cervical; *8*, transverse cervical; *9*, acromiothoracic; *10*, suprascapular; *11*, posterior circumflex humeral; *12*, circumflex scapular; *13*, profunda brachii; *14*, brachial; *15*, ulnar; *16*, radial; *17*, posterior intercostals; *18*, lumbar; *19*, superior gluteal; *20*, inferior gluteal; *21*, profunda femoris; *22*, popliteal; *22A*, descending geniculate saphenous; *23*, sural; *24*, peroneal; *25*, lateral plantar; *26*, anterior tibial; *27*, lateral femoral circumflex; *28*, adductor profunda; *29*, medial plantar; *30*, posterior tibial; *31*, superficial femoral; *32*, common femoral; *33*, deep circumflex iliac; *34*, deep inferior epigastric; *35*, internal thoracic; *36*, lateral thoracic; *37*, thoracodorsal; *38*, posterior interosseous; *39*, anterior interosseous.

2. **Fasciocutaneous plexus:** *A communicating network of the subfascial, intrafascial, suprafascial, subcutaneous, and subdermal vascular plexuses fed by different configurations of inflow vessels.*
   * Architecture of this network varies according to anatomic region, but it extends throughout the body as a continuous system encompassing the dermal, subdermal, superficial, and deep adipofascial layers.
   * Nakajima et al[6] identified six vessel types that perforate the deep fascia to supply the fasciocutaneous plexus (Fig. 3-12).
   * Two systems for venous drainage of skin[7]:
     - Valvular superficial and deep cutaneous veins parallel the course of adjacent arteries.
     - Avalvular oscillating veins permit bidirectional flow between adjacent venous territories.
     - *Anastomotic connections between the two systems permit flow reversal in distally based flaps.*

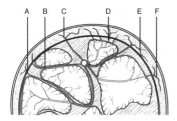

Fig. 3-12 The six distinctive deep fascia perforators. A separate type of fasciocutaneous flap may be named for each different perforator. *A,* Direct cutaneous branch of a muscular vessel; *B,* septocutaneous perforator; *C,* direct cutaneous; *D,* musculocutaneous perforator; *E,* direct septocutaneous; *F,* perforating cutaneous branch of a muscular vessel.

■ **Cutaneous flaps**
- McGregor and Morgan[8] categorized flaps as *random* or *axial.*
  ▶ **Random flaps** are based off the subdermal plexus and are traditionally limited to 3:1 length-to-width ratios.
  ▶ **Axial pattern flaps** contain a specific direct cutaneous artery within the longitudinal axis of the flap.
  ▶ **Reverse axial pattern flaps** (reverse-flow flaps) are based on distal vessels after division of the proximal blood supply.
  ▶ **Island flap** is an axial pattern flap that is raised on a pedicle devoid of skin to facilitate distant transfer.
- Nakajima et al[6] classified skin flaps into five types based on vascularization (not tissue composition):
  1. Cutaneous (equivalent to an axial flap)
  2. Fasciocutaneous
  3. Adipofascial
  4. Septocutaneous
  5. Musculocutaneous
- All skin flaps are based on the *fasciocutaneous plexus,* which is supplied from perforating vessels that penetrate the deep fascia either directly or indirectly. On the basis of this vascularity all skin flaps generally can be classified as fasciocutaneous flaps.
- Skin flaps can be classified simply and accurately as a *direct* or an *indirect* perforator flap[9] (Fig. 3-13).
  ▶ *Direct perforators* pierce the deep fascia without having traversed any deeper structures.
  ▶ *Indirect perforators* pass through deeper tissues, usually muscle or septum, before entering the deep fascia.

■ **Perforator flaps**
- Consist of skin or subcutaneous fat supplied by isolated perforator vessel (or vessels).
- May pass from their source vessel origin either through or between the deep tissues
- Classified into three categories based on the three different kinds of perforator vessels[10] (Fig. 3-14).
  ▶ *Indirect muscle perforator:* Musculocutaneous perforator flap

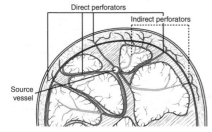

Fig. 3-13 The distinct deep fascial perforators of Nakajima can be considered more simply to be either *direct* or *indirect* perforators. These perforators all arise from the same source vessel, but only *indirect* perforators *(dotted lines)* first course through some other intermediary tissue (here depicted as muscle), before piercing the deep fascia.

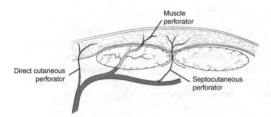

Fig. 3-14 Different types of direct and indirect perforator vessels with regard to their surgical importance: Direct perforator perforating the deep fascia only, indirect muscle perforator traveling through muscle before piercing the deep fascia, and indirect septal perforator traveling through the intermuscular septum before piercing the deep fascia.

> ▸ *Indirect septal perforator:* Septocutaneous perforator flap
> ▸ *Direct cutaneous perforator:* Direct cutaneous perforator flap

- **Perforator flaps are named for their nutrient vessel** (e.g., deep inferior epigastric perforator [DIEP] flap) **except in areas where multiple perforator flaps can be raised from a single vessel, then the flap is named for its anatomic region or muscle** (e.g., anterolateral thigh [ALT] flap).
- **Advantages of perforator flaps[11]**
  - ▸ Numerous potential donor sites
  - ▸ Often able to incorporate muscle, fat, and bone into the flap design
  - ▸ Preserve muscle function
  - ▸ Minimal donor site morbidity
  - ▸ Reduced postoperative recovery time and pain medication requirements
  - ▸ Versatility of size and thickness
- **Disadvantages of perforator flaps[11-17]**
  - ▸ Tedious pedicle dissection
  - ▸ Variation in perforator anatomy and size
  - ▸ Increased risk of fat necrosis compared with musculocutaneous flaps

■ **Neurocutaneous and venocutaneous flaps**
Skin flaps based off of the perforating arteries accompanying cutaneous nerves and veins[18]
- Run in the deep adipofascial layer of the skin[19]
- Are sensate (neurocutaneous flaps)
- Commonly used as pedicled flaps for coverage of local or regional extremity defects
- Examples:
  - ▸ Sural nerve
  - ▸ Saphenous vein flap

■ **Venous flaps**
Skin flaps supplied through a venous pedicle
- Thatte and Thatte[20] classify venous flaps into three groups (Fig. 3-15).
    Type I is an unipedicled venous flap, or a pure venous flap with a single cephalad vein as the only vascular conduit.

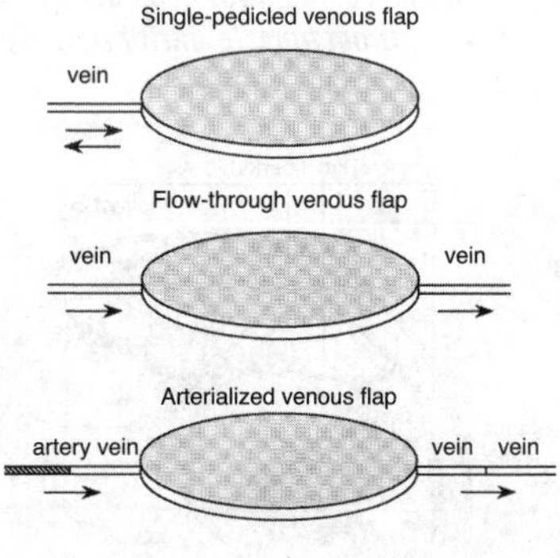

Single-pedicled venous flap

vein

Flow-through venous flap

vein   vein

Fig. 3-15 Three types of venous flaps. (From Inoue G, Suzuki K. Arterialized venous flap for treating multiple skin defects of the hand. Plast Reconstr Surg 91:299-302; discussion 303-306, 1993.)

Arterialized venous flap

artery vein   vein   vein

Type II venous flaps are bipedicled "flow through" flaps with afferent and efferent veins exhibiting flow from caudal to cephalad.

Type III venous flaps are arterialized through a proximal arteriovenous anastomosis and drained by a distal vein.

- The mechanism of venous flap perfusion is still not completely understood and has been attributed to a number of factors, including[21]:
  - ▶ Plasmatic imbibition
  - ▶ Perfusion pressure
  - ▶ Sites of arteriovenous anastomosis
  - ▶ Perivenous arterial networks
  - ▶ Vein-to-vein interconnections
  - ▶ Circumvention of venous valves
- **Advantages of venous flaps**[22-25]
  - ▶ Minimal donor site morbidity requiring only the sacrifice of a vein and no artery
  - ▶ Long and very thin
  - ▶ Anatomically constant pedicle (e.g., saphenous vein)
  - ▶ Fast and expedient flap elevation
- **Disadvantages of venous flaps**
  - ▶ Poorly understood physiology
  - ▶ Unpredictable survival, making clinical application controversial

TISSUE COMPOSITION
- **Fascial and fasciocutaneous flap**

Fasciocutaneous flaps are created by elevating skin with its underlying deep fascia
- **Fasciocutaneous flaps:** Supplied by the fasciocutaneous plexus

> TIP: Including the deep fascia is not necessary for flap survival, although some authors advocate its preservation to protect the suprafascial portion of the fasciocutaneous plexus.

- **Fascial and adipofascial flaps:** Created by elevating the deep fascia with or without subcutaneous adipose tissue without the overlying skin component
- Mathes[26] classified fasciocutaneous flaps as those supplied by:
  - ▶ Direct cutaneous pedicle
  - ▶ Septocutaneous pedicle
  - ▶ Musculocutaneous pedicle
- Can be used as pedicled flaps for coverage of local, regional, and distant defects, or as free tissue transfer flaps
- **Advantages of fascial and fasciocutaneous flaps**
  - ▶ Preservation of muscle
  - ▶ Thin and pliable
  - ▶ Amenable to tissue expansion
  - ▶ Can incorporate sensory nerves
- **Disadvantages of fascial and fasciocutaneous flaps**
  - ▶ Donor site morbidity (may require skin graft)
  - ▶ Less resistant to infection than muscle flaps

- **Muscle and musculocutaneous flaps**
  - Muscle flaps can be transferred as pedicled flaps or free tissue transfer based on their dominant vascular pedicle.
  - Musculocutaneous flaps are composites of skin and underlying muscle supplied by a dominant vascular pedicle.
  - Musculocutaneous flaps are primarily used for breast, head and neck, and pressure sore reconstruction.
  - Muscle flaps are indicated for coverage of infected, radiated, or traumatic wounds.
  - **Musculocutaneous versus fasciocutaneous flaps:**
    - Musculocutaneous and fasciocutaneous flaps demonstrate a marked increase in blood flow to all levels of tissue after elevation.[27]
    - The decrease in bacterial concentration is significantly greater in wounds covered with musculocutaneous flaps than in those covered with fasciocutaneous flaps (10^4 versus 10^2).[27]
    - Musculocutaneous flaps exhibit more collagen deposition than fasciocutaneous flaps.[28]
  - **Mathes and Nahai**[29] developed a classification of muscles based on their circulatory patterns (Fig. 3-16).

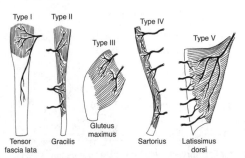

Type I   Type II   Type III   Type IV   Type V

Tensor fascia lata   Gracilis   Gluteus maximus   Sartorius   Latissimus dorsi

Fig. 3-16   Patterns of vascular anatomy. *Type I,* one vascular pedicle; *type II,* dominant pedicle(s) and minor pedicle(s); *type III,* two dominant pedicles; *type IV,* segmental vascular pedicles; *type V,* one dominant pedicle and secondary segmental pedicles. (From Mathes SJ, Nahai F. Classification of the vascular anatomy of muscles: Experimental and clinical correlation. Plast Reconstr Surg 67:177, 1981.)

  - Types I, III, and V muscle flaps have the most reliable vascularity.
  - Type II and IV muscle flaps are less reliable because the vascular pedicle to distal muscle must be divided to achieve adequate arc of rotation.
  - **Advantages of muscle and musculocutaneous flaps**
    - Potential to obliterate dead space with vascularized tissue
    - Increased resistance to infection
  - **Disadvantages of muscle and musculocutaneous flaps**
    - Functional deficit at the donor site
    - Flap bulk
- **Vascularized bone flaps**
  - Vascularized bone flaps can be transferred in a pedicled or free fashion based on their nutrient vessels.
  - **Advantages of vascularized bone flaps compared with bone grafts**
    - Can be used to reconstruct large bony defects
    - Undergo primary bony healing
    - Withstand radiation and implantation
    - Can be transferred as a composite with other tissue types (e.g., scapular flap and free toe transfers)
  - Most commonly transferred vascularized bone flaps:
    - Fibula (peroneal artery)

▸ Iliac crest (deep circumflex iliac artery)
▸ Radius (radial artery)
■ **Visceral flaps**
  • The omentum, colon, and jejunum can be transferred as visceral flaps based on their dominant pedicles or vascular arcades.
  • Intestinal flaps are primarily useful in pharyngoesophageal reconstruction.
  • The omentum is a versatile flap that can be tailored to many different defects.
■ **Innervated flaps**
  Functional muscle flaps and sensory flaps can be created by inclusion of the appropriate motor or sensory nerve for coaptation at the recipient site after flap transfer.
  • To restore muscle function after transfer, the original tension and length/width ratio of the fibers need to be recreated during inset.
  • The gracilis, latissimus, and serratus muscles are frequently used for functional muscle transfers.
  • Many flaps can be modified to include a sensory nerve for creating a sensory flap.
■ **Compound and Composite Flaps**
  • *Compound flaps:* Contain diverse tissue components such as bone, skin, fascia, and muscle that are incorporated into an interrelated unit to allow single-stage reconstruction of complex defects.
  • Classified into two groups based on vascularization[30] (Fig. 3-17)
    1. *Compound flap with solitary vascularization* is a composite flap that incorporates multiple tissue components dependent on a single vascular supply.
    2. *Compound flaps of mixed vascularization* are further subdivided into siamese flaps, conjoint flaps, and sequential flaps.

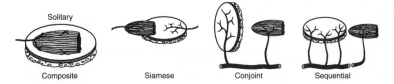

Fig. 3-17 Compound flaps can be classified based on solitary or combined vascularity. (From Hallock GG. Simplified nomenclature for compound flaps. Plast Reconstr Surg 105:1465, 2000.)

■ **Prefabricated flaps**
  Prefabrication is a two-stage technique in which a flap is surgically altered by partial elevation, structural manipulation, and incorporation of other tissue layers in the first stage to create a specialized composite flap.
  • The altered flap is allowed to heal, and transfer is delayed for the second stage.
  • Prefabrication is useful for nasal reconstruction where skin grafts and cartilage can be used to reconstruct lining and framework in a forehead or free radial forearm flap.
  • Prefabrication also can be used to create a vascular pedicle for a flap subsequent to transfer by transposing an adjacent artery and vein into the area of flap design. This technique is named *prelamination* and is unreliable.

FLAP PHYSIOLOGY

REGULATION OF BLOOD FLOW TO SKIN
■ Systemic and local factors regulate cutaneous blood flow at the level of microcirculation.[31]

- **Systemic control**
  - **Neural regulation**
    - ▸ Regulation occurs primarily through <u>sympathetic adrenergic fibers.</u>
      - ✦ Alpha-adrenergic receptors induce vasoconstriction, and beta-adrenergic receptors induce vasodilatation.
      - ✦ Sympathetic adrenergic fibers maintain basal tone of vascular smooth muscle at the arteriovenous anastomoses, arterioles, and arteries.
    - ▸ Cholinergic fibers initiate bradykinin release, which contributes to vasodilation.
  - **Humoral regulation**
    - ▸ **Mediators of vasoconstriction**
      - ✦ Epinephrine
      - ✦ Norepinephrine
      - ✦ Serotonin
      - ✦ Thromboxane A_2
      - ✦ Prostaglandin F_2-α
    - ▸ **Mediators of vasodilation**
      - ✦ Bradykinin
      - ✦ Histamine
      - ✦ Prostaglandin-E_1
- **Local control (autoregulation)**
  - **Metabolic factors** (act primarily as vasodilators)
    - ▸ Hypercapnia
    - ▸ Hypoxia
    - ▸ Acidosis
    - ▸ Hyperkalemia
  - **Physical factors**
    - ▸ Myogenic reflex triggers vasoconstriction in response to distention of isolated cutaneous vessels and maintains capillary flow at a constant level independent of arterial pressure.
    - ▸ Local hypothermia (which acts directly on the smooth muscle in vessel walls) decreases flow.
    - ▸ Increased blood viscosity (hematocrit >45%) decreases flow.
- **Differences in blood flow regulation for skin and muscle** (Table 3-2).

Table 3-2   *Differences in Blood Flow Regulation for Skin and Muscle*

	Skin	Muscle
Neuronal Control		
Sympathetic vasoconstriction	Most important	Less important
Humoral Control		
Epinephrine	Vasoconstriction	Vasodilation
Metabolic Factors		
Autoregulation	Important	Most important
Physical Factors		
Temperature	Important	Not important
Myogenic tone	Less important	More important

FLAP TRANSFER
- **The elevation of a skin flap results in changes that disrupt the equilibrium of homeostasis, including:**
  - Loss of sympathetic innervation
  - Ischemia
    - ▶ Change from aerobic to anaerobic metabolism
    - ▶ Increased lactate production
    - ▶ Increased levels of superoxide radicals
    - ▶ Changes in blood viscosity and clotting
- ***Ischemia-induced reperfusion injury (IIRI):*** Direct cytotoxic injury results from the accumulation of oxygen-derived free radicals during flap ischemia. After reperfusion, the free radicals are attacked by free radical scavengers, causing further injury to the cells.
  - The transition from normal reperfusion and reperfusion injury differs according to tissue type.
  - Skin and bone can usually tolerate ischemia for up to 3 hours, but muscle and intestinal mucosa are much less tolerant.[32]

FLAP DELAY

The surgical interruption of a portion of the blood supply to a flap at a preliminary stage before transfer
- **Purpose:** To increase the surviving length of a flap or to improve the circulation of a flap and diminish the insult of transfer.
- **Two theories**
  1. The delay conditions tissue to ischemia, allowing it to survive on less nutrient blood flow than normally needed.
  2. The delay improves or increases vascularity through the dilation of choke vessels connecting adjacent vascular territories.
- Contribution to flap survival is likely to be a combination of both mechanisms acting to a greater or lesser extent at various times during surgical delay of a flap.
- **Five mechanisms of delay**
  1. Sympathectomy
  2. Vascular reorganization
  3. Reactive hyperemia
  4. Acclimatization to hypoxia
  5. Nonspecific inflammatory reaction
- **Timing of delay**
  - Flaps can be divided as early as the third day after delay in animal models; however, the clinical delay period should be lengthened to suit specific anatomy, expected flap viability, and characteristics of the recipient site.
- Most flaps can be divided safely at **10 days to 3 weeks.**
- Tissue expansion is a form of delay that has similar histologic features to incisional delay.

FLAP CHOICE[33]

- The goals of surgical reconstruction are the preservation and restoration of form and function while minimizing morbidity.
- The optimal reconstructive solution can be designed through a systematic analysis of:
  - Wound defect

- Medical and functional status of the patient
- Available reconstructive options

DEFECT ANALYSIS

- **Location**
- **Size and surface area** of wound after adequate debridement
- **Tissue components missing or exposed in defect** (e.g., skin, hair, mucosa, subcutaneous tissue, muscle, vessels, nerves, cartilage, bone)
  - Which components need to be replaced?
  - Which components can feasibly be replaced?
- **Vascular status of wound**
  - Presence of vascular disease
  - Evaluation of zone of injury (trauma)
  - Adequate microcirculation to support grafts or local flaps
  - Suitable recipient vessels available for free tissue transfer
  - Previous radiation
  - Previous surgery or trauma
- **Infection and bacteriology of wound**
- **Future management concerns** (e.g., need for postoperative radiation, future surgical needs)

PATIENT FACTORS

- Reconstructing wounds that are not life threatening is secondary to treating any vital organ system dysfunction.
- Conditions that influence the safety and success of reconstructive options:
  - Diabetes
  - Peripheral vascular disease
  - Hypertension
  - Obesity
  - Hematologic disorders
  - Immunosuppression
  - Pulmonary dysfunction
  - Tobacco use
- Functional status, lifestyle, and rehabilitative capacity of the patient also require consideration.
- Complex reconstruction may be questionable in a patient with a limited life expectancy or with central nervous system dysfunction.
- The sacrifice of specific muscles for flap coverage impacts individuals differently depending on other disabilities present (e.g., paraplegia) or their occupation and lifestyle (e.g., professional athlete versus accountant).

RECONSTRUCTIVE OPTIONS

- **Reconstructive ladder** (Fig. 3-18)
  - A dated but useful paradigm that organizes reconstructive solutions in order of complexity
  - Systematic consideration of the most simple to the most complex solution

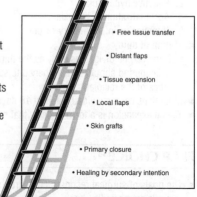

- Free tissue transfer
- Distant flaps
- Tissue expansion
- Local flaps
- Skin grafts
- Primary closure
- Healing by secondary intention

Fig. 3-18   Reconstructive ladder.

- ▶ Healing by secondary intention
- ▶ Direct closure
- ▶ Skin graft
- ▶ Local flap
- ▶ Regional flap
- ▶ Distant flap
- ▶ Free tissue transfer
- ■ In the current era of microvascular proficiency, free tissue transfer is no longer a last resort, and complex solutions often yield superior results to the simpler options.
- ■ The use of tissue expansion, prefabrication, and composite flaps enables surgeons to optimize the balance between donor site preservation and restoration of defect form and function.

FLAP SURVIVAL

PHYSICAL FACTORS
- ■ Physical factors that have experimentally demonstrated a survival advantage include[34-36]:
  - • Maintenance of a moist environment along flap edges
  - • Avoidance of local hypothermia

PHARMACOLOGIC FACTORS
- ■ **Anticoagulants**
  - • **Dextran**
    - ▶ Originally designed as a volume expander
    - ▶ Effects:
      - ◆ Decreased platelet adhesiveness and procoagulant activity
      - ◆ Inhibition of platelet aggregation
      - ◆ Increased bleeding time
      - ◆ Decreased blood viscosity
    - ▶ Has been shown to improve short-term microcirculatory patency[37-39]
    - ▶ Associated with significant systemic morbidity including:
      - ◆ Anaphylaxis
      - ◆ Pulmonary edema
      - ◆ Cardiac complications
      - ◆ Adult respiratory distress syndrome
      - ◆ Renal failure
    - ▶ Routine use in free tissue transfer is discouraged[40,41]
  - • **Heparin**
    - ▶ Anticoagulant
    - ▶ Acts in conjunction with antithrombin III to inhibit thrombosis by inactivation of factor X
    - ▶ More effective at preventing venous thrombosis than arterial thrombosis
    - ▶ Both unfractionated and low molecular weight heparin (LMWH) improve microcirculatory perfusion, but only LMWH has been shown to improve anastomotic patency while minimizing hemorrhage.[42]
  - • **Thrombolytic agents**
    - ▶ Stimulates the conversion of plasminogen to plasmin, which acts to cleave fibrin within a thrombus

- ▸ **First generation agents**
  - ✦ Streptokinase
  - ✦ Urokinase
- ▸ **Second generation agents**
  - ✦ Tissue plasminogen activator (t-PA)
  - ✦ Acylated plasminogen-streptokinase activator complex (APSAC)
- ▸ Have been effective in salvaging flaps after microvascular thrombosis[43,44]
- • **Medicinal leeches** *(Hirudo medicinalis)*
  - ▸ Exert their effect by injecting hirudin at the site of bite.
    - ✦ *Hirudin:* A naturally occurring anticoagulant that inhibits the conversion of fibrin to fibrinogen, but unlike heparin does not require antithrombin-III for activation
  - ▸ Also secrete[45]:
    - ✦ Hyaluronidase: Facilitates spread of the anticoagulant within the tissues.
    - ✦ A vasodilator: Contributes to prolonged bleeding (up to 48 hours).
  - ▸ Mechanical effect of creating physical channels through which venous drainage can occur
  - ▸ Risks:
    - ✦ Bacterial infection from the gram-negative rod *Aeromonas hydrophila*
    - ✦ Anaphylaxis
    - ✦ Persistent bleeding
    - ✦ Excessive scarring
  - ▸ Use of antibiotic prophylaxis against *Aeromonas hydrophila* recommended
    - ✦ Fluoroquinolones
    - ✦ Resistance to amoxicillin/clavulanate and all generations of cephalosporins reported
- ■ **Vasodilators**
  - • **Calcium-channel blockers**
    - ▸ Act on the vascular smooth muscles to cause vasodilation
    - ▸ Increased flap survival in experimental models after topical and intravenous administration
    - ▸ No clinical evidence to support use
  - • **Topical nitroglycerin**
    - ▸ A potent vasodilator with a greater effect on venous circulation than on arterial vessels
    - ▸ Improved survival of axial flaps reported from treatment with transdermal nitroglycerin[46]
  - • **Topical lidocaine and pentobarbital**
    - ▸ Inhibit endothelium-dependent relaxation on the vascular smooth muscle[47]
    - ▸ Have demonstrated effective resolution of mechanically induced vasospasm
- ■ **Antiinflammatory agents**
  - • **Steroids**
    - ▸ Increased flap survival in some experimental models, but no evidence to support clinical use of corticosteroids to enhance flap viability
  - • **Aspirin (ASA)**
    - ▸ Aspirin acetylates the enzyme cyclooxygenase, thereby decreasing the synthesis of thromboxane A_2 (TxA_2), a potent vasoconstrictor in platelets, and prostacyclin (PGI_2), a potent vasodilator in vessel walls.
    - ▸ At low doses the effect of aspirin is selective, and only the cyclooxygenase system in platelets is inhibited, blocking the formation of thromboxane.
    - ▸ Experimentally, preoperative aspirin decreases thrombus formation at venous anastomoses and improves capillary perfusion in the microcirculation.[48]

▸ Studies demonstrate increased early anastomotic patency, but there is no difference from controls after 24 hours to 1 week.[32]

▸ There is no empiric support in the literature for using aspirin postoperatively.[32]

■ **Nicotine**

  • Acute exposure of human skin vasculature to nicotine is associated with amplification of norepinephrine-induced skin vasoconstriction and impairment of endothelium-dependent skin vasorelaxation.[49]

FLAP MONITORING

■ Strict evaluation of flap perfusion is essential to prevent, recognize, and treat complications.

■ **Venous insufficiency is the most common cause of flap failure.**

■ The failure rate of free tissue transfer is reported to be less than 5%. However, the incidence of pedicle thrombosis is higher than the failure rate reflects, because the salvage rate after pedicle thrombosis ranges from 36% to 70%.[44]

■ Because of more successful salvage within the first 24 hours after initial surgery, hourly monitoring is recommended for the first 24 hours and then every 4 hours for 48 hours.[50]

SUBJECTIVE AND PHYSICAL CRITERIA

■ **Clinical observation remains the most effective method of flap monitoring.**

  • Subjective evaluation of flap viability by color, capillary blanching, and warmth can be unreliable.[51]

  • Bleeding from a stab wound is the most accurate clinical test.

  • Clinical signs can be used to differentiate venous from arterial insufficiency in flaps (Table 3-3).

■ **Temperature monitoring is a simple technique that can be accomplished by measuring surface temperature and differential thermometry.**

  • Surface temperature is clinically useful for monitoring extrinsic complications but is an inadequate indicator of intrinsic flap failure.

  • Differential thermometry is useful for monitoring vascular patency in buried free tissue transfers in which a temperature gradient exceeding **3° C** is considered significant.[51]

Table 3-3 *Signs of Arterial Occlusion and Venous Congestion*

	Arterial Occlusion	Venous Congestion
Skin color	Pale, mottled, bluish, or white	Cyanotic, bluish, or dusky
Capillary refill	Sluggish	Brisker than normal
Tissue turgor	Prune-like; turgor decreased	Tense, swollen; turgor increased
Dermal bleeding	Scant amount of dark blood or serum	Rapid bleeding of dark blood
Temperature	Cool	Cool

Adams JF, Lassen LF. Leech therapy for venous congestion following myocutaneous pectoralis flap reconstruction. ORL Head Neck Nurs 13:12, 1995.

VITAL DYE MEASUREMENTS

■ Fluorescein is reported to be better than 70% accurate as an indicator of the circulatory status of a flap.[52]

  • Fluorescein is usually given in a bolus injection of 500 to 1000 mg (15 mg/kg).

- After waiting 20-30 minutes, the extent of dye staining in tissues that are adequately perfused can be seen with a Wood's lamp.

PHOTOELECTRIC ASSESSMENT[53]

- **Two types of Doppler instruments are currently in clinical use**
  1. *Ultrasound Doppler* uses reflected sound to pick up pulsatile vessels.
  2. *Laser Doppler* measures the frequency shift of light and therefore has limited penetration (1.5 mm).
- **Advantages of Doppler probing**
  - High reliability (approaching 100% 24 hours after flap transfer)
  - Continuous monitoring by a noninvasive technique
- **Disadvantages of Doppler probing**
  - Not quantitative
  - Obtains information from a single site
  - Sensitive to movement of the subject
  - Limited accuracy below the critical threshold at which tissue necrosis is guaranteed

METABOLIC

- *Transcutaneous oxygen tension* measures the partial-pressure of oxygen and has been shown to be an accurate predictor of the effectiveness of the delay procedure.[54]
- *Photoplethysmography* is a technique that measures fluid volume by detecting variations in infrared light absorption by the skin.
  - A *pulse oximeter* displays photoplethysmographic waveforms and measures light absorption to derive oxygen saturation of arterial hemoglobin.
  - This method has been inaccurate and disappointing when applied in a clinical setting.[51]

KEY POINTS

✔ Vascularity is the most valid method of flap classification because it is the most critical determinant of successful flap transfer.

✔ The *fasciocutaneous plexus* is an intercommunicating network between the deep fascia and the dermis fed by different configurations of deep fascial perforators.

✔ All skin and fascial flaps are supplied by the *fasciocutaneous plexus*. Inclusion of the deep fascia is not required for the survival of cutaneous or fasciocutaneous flaps.

✔ Anastomotic connections between valvular veins (venae comitantes) and avalvular oscillating veins permit reversal of flow in distally based flaps.

✔ Musculocutaneous flaps exhibit more collagen deposition and are more resistant to infection than fasciocutaneous flaps.

✔ Muscle flaps with a segmental vascular pattern (type IV) have the most limited arc of rotation and are the least reliable for transfer (e.g., the sartorius muscle).

✔ The sympathetic nervous system is the most important factor for regulating blood flow to the skin.

✔ Metabolic autoregulation plays a more important role for regulating blood flow to muscle because it has a higher metabolic demand than skin.

✔ Venous insufficiency is the most common cause of flap failure.

✔ Clinical observation is the most effective method of flap monitoring.

REFERENCES

1. Furnas DW, Fischer GW. The Z-plasty: Biomechanics and mathematics. Br J Plast Surg 24:144, 1971.
2. Seyhan A. A V-shaped ruler to detect the largest transposable Z-plasty [letter]. Plast Reconstr Surg 101:870, 1994.
3. Keser A, Sensoz O, Mengi AS. Double opposing semicircular flap: A modification of opposing Z-plasty for closing circular defects. Plast Reconstr Surg 102:1001, 1998.
4. Taylor GI, Palmer JH. The vascular territories (angiosomes) of the body: Experimental study and clinical applications. Br J Plast Surg 40:113, 1987.
5. Taylor G. The blood supply to the skin. In Aston SJ, Beasley RW, Thorne CH, et al, eds. Grabb and Smith's Plastic Surgery, 5th ed. Philadelphia: Lippincott, 1997, p 47.
6. Nakajima H, Fujino T, Adachi S. A new concept of vascular supply to the skin and classification of skin flaps according to their vascularization. Ann Plast Surg 16:1, 1986.
7. Taylor GI, Caddy CM, Watterson PA, et al. The venous territories (venosomes) of the human body: Experimental study and clinical implications. Plast Reconstr Surg 86:185, 1990.
8. McGregor IA, Morgan G. Axial and random pattern flaps. Br J Plast Surg 26:202, 1973.
9. Hallock G. Direct and indirect perforator flaps: The history and the controversy. Plast Reconstr Surg 111:855, 2003.
10. Blondeel PN, Van Landuyt K, Hamdi M, et al. Perforator flap terminology: Update 2002. Clin Plast Surg 30:343, 2003.
11. Geddes CR, Morris SF, Neligan PC. Perforator flaps: Evolution, classification, and applications. Ann Plast Surg 50:90, 2003.
12. Nahabedian MY, Momen B, Galdino G, et al. Breast reconstruction with the free TRAM or DIEP flap: Patient selection, choice of flap, and outcome. Plast Reconstr Surg 110:466, 2002.
13. Celik N, Wei FC, Lin CH, et al. Technique and strategy in anterolateral thigh perforator flap surgery, based on an analysis of 15 complete and partial failures in 439 cases. Plast Reconstr Surg 109:2211, 2002.
14. Chen HC, Tang YB. Anterolateral thigh flap: An ideal soft tissue flap. Clin Plast Surg 30:383, 2003.
15. Kimata Y, Uchiyama K, Ebihara S, et al. Anatomic variations and technical problems of the anterolateral thigh flap: A report of 74 cases. Plast Reconstr Surg 102:1517, 1998.
16. Craigie JE, Allen RJ, DellaCroce FJ, et al. Autogenous breast reconstruction with the deep inferior epigastric perforator flap. Clin Plast Surg 30:359, 2003.
17. Kroll SS. Fat necrosis in free transverse rectus abdominis myocutaneous and deep inferior epigastric perforator flaps. Plast Reconstr Surg 106:576, 2000.
18. Masquelet AC, Romana MC, Wolf G. Skin island flaps supplied by the vascular axis of the sensitive superficial nerves: Anatomic study and clinical experience in the leg. Plast Reconstr Surg 89:1115, 1992.
19. Nakajima H, Imanishi N, Fukuzumi S, et al. Accompanying arteries of the cutaneous veins and cutaneous nerves in the extremities: Anatomical study and a concept of the venoadipofascial and/or neuroadipofascial pedicled fasciocutaneous flap. Plast Reconstr Surg 102:779, 1998.
20. Thatte MR, Thatte RL. Venous flaps. Plast Reconstr Surg 91:747, 1993.
21. Thornton JT, Gosman AA. Skin grafts and skin substitutes and principles of flaps. Sel Read Plast Surg 10(1), 2004.
22. De Lorenzi F, van der Hulst R, den Dunnen WFA, et al. Arterialized venous free flaps for soft-tissue reconstruction of digits: A 40-case series. J Reconstr Microsurg 18:569, 2002.
23. Koshima I, Soeda S, Nakayama Y, et al. An arterialised venous flap using the long saphenous vein. Br J Plast Surg 44:23, 1991.
24. Inoue G, Suzuki K. Arterialized venous flap for treating multiple skin defects of the hand. Plast Reconstr Surg 91:299, 1993.
25. Lee W. Discussion of "Arterialized venous flap for treating multiple skin defects of the hand," by G. Inoue and K. Suzuki. Plast Reconstr Surg 91:303, 1993.
26. Mathes SJ. Clinical Applications for Muscle and Musculocutaneous Flaps. St Louis: Mosby, 1981.
27. Gosain A, Chang N, Mathes S, et al. A study of the relationship between blood flow and bacterial innoculation in musculocutaneous and fasciocutaneous flaps. Plast Reconstr Surg 86:1152, 1990.

28. Calderon W, Chang N, Mathes SJ. Comparison of the effect of bacterial inoculation in musculocutaneous and fasciocutaneous flaps. Plast Reconstr Surg 77:785, 1986.
29. Mathes SJ, Nahai F. Classification of the vascular anatomy of muscles: Experimental and clinical correlation. Plast Reconstr Surg 67:177, 1981.
30. Hallock G. Simplified nomenclature for compound flaps. Plast Reconstr Surg 105:1465, 2000.
31. Daniel RK, Kerrigan CL. Skin flaps: An anatomical and hemodynamic approach. Clin Plast Surg 6:181, 1979.
32. Carroll WR, Esclamado RM. Ischemia/reperfusion injury in microvascular surgery. Head Neck 22:700, 2000.
33. Hoopes JE. Pedicle flaps: An overview. In Hoopes JE, Krizek TJ, eds. Symposium on Basic Science in Plastic Surgery. St Louis: Mosby, 1976, p 241.
34. Sasaki A, Fukuda O, Soeda S. Attempts to increase the surviving length in skin flaps by a moist environment. Plast Reconstr Surg 64:526, 1979.
35. McGrath M. How topical dressings salvage "questionable" flaps: Experimental study. Plast Reconstr Surg 67:653, 1981.
36. Awwad AM, White RJ, Webster MH, et al. The effect of temperature on blood flow in island and free skin flaps: An experimental study. Br J Plast Surg 36:373, 1983.
37. Rothkopf DM, Chu B, Bern S, et al. The effect of dextran on microvascular thrombosis in an experimental rabbit model. Plast Reconstr Surg 92:511, 1993.
38. Zhang B, Wieslander JB. Improvement of patency in small veins following dextran and/or low-molecular-weight heparin treatment. Plast Reconstr Surg 94:352, 1994.
39. Salemark L, Knudsen F, Dougan P. The effect of dextran 40 on patency following severe trauma in small arteries and veins. Br J Plast Surg 48:121, 1995.
40. Hein KD, Wechsler M, Schwartzstein RM, et al. The adult respiratory distress syndrome after dextran infusion as an antithrombotic agent in free TRAM flap breast reconstruction. Plast Reconstr Surg 103:1706, 1999.
41. Brooks D, Okeefe P, Buncke HJ. Dextran-induced acute renal failure after microvascular muscle transplantation. Plast Reconstr Surg 108:2057, 2001.
42. Ritter EF, Cronan JC, Rudner AM, et al. Improved microsurgical anastomotic patency with low molecular weight heparin. J Reconstr Microsurg 14:331, 1998.
43. Serletti JM, Moran SL, Orlando GS, et al. Urokinase protocol for free-flap salvage following prolonged venous thrombosis. Plast Reconstr Surg 102:1947, 1998.
44. Yii NW, Evans GR, Miller MJ, et al. Thrombolytic therapy: What is its role in free flap salvage? Ann Plast Surg 46:601, 2001.
45. Soucacos PN, Beris AE, Malizos KN, et al. The use of medicinal leeches, Hirudo medicinalis, to restore venous circulation in trauma and reconstructive surgery. Int Angiol 13:251, 1994.
46. Rohrich RJ, Cherry GW, Spira M. Enhancement of skin-flap survival using nitroglycerin ointment. Plast Reconstr Surg 73:943, 1984.
47. Wadstrom J, Gerdin B. Modulatory effects of topically administered lidocaine and pentobarbital on traumatic vasospasm in the rabbit ear artery. Br J Plast Surg 44:341, 1991.
48. Peter FW, Franken RJ, Wang WZ, et al. Effect of low dose aspirin on thrombus formation at arterial and venous microanastomoses and on the tissue microcirculation. Plast Reconstr Surg 99:1112, 1997.
49. Black CE, Huang N, Neligan PC, et al. Effect of nicotine on vasoconstrictor and vasodilator responses in human skin vasculature. Am J Physiol Regul Integr Comp Physiol 281:R1097, 2001.
50. Brown JS, Devine JC, Magennis P, et al. Factors that influence the outcome of salvage in free tissue transfer. Br J Oral Maxillofac Surg 41:16, 2003.
51. Daniel RK, Kerrigan CL. Principles and physiology of skin flap surgery. In McCarthy JG, ed. Plastic Surgery, vol 1. Philadelphia: Saunders, 1990.
52. Lange K, Boyd LJ. The use of fluorescein to determine the adequacy of the circulation. Med Clin North Am 26:943, 1942.
53. Hallock GG, Altobelli JA. Assessment of TRAM flap perfusion using laser Doppler flowmetry: An adjunct to microvascular augmentation. Ann Plast Surg 29:122, 1992.
54. Tsur H, Orenstein A, Mazkereth R. The use of transcutaneous oxygen pressure measurement in flap surgery. Ann Plast Surg 8:510, 1982.

4. Tissue Expansion

Joshua A. Lemmon

PHYSIOLOGY

STRUCTURAL COMPONENTS OF SKIN
- **Collagen**
  - Predominant protein of the dermis
  - Synthesized by fibroblasts
  - Bundled in fibrils and fibers
  - Aligned in a wavy, convoluted state
- **Elastin**
  - Skin protein
  - Synthesized by fibroblasts
  - Bundled in fibers finer than collagen
  - Arranged in a loose network that assists in returning collagen to its resting state
  - Permits skin recoil
  - Can fragment with excessive deformational force
- **Ground substance**
  - Occupies the interstices within the collagen-elastin matrix
  - A proteoglycan is a core protein linked to the glycosaminoglycans—these proteoglycans compose the ground substance
  - Can bind large amounts of water, forming a viscous hydrated gel
  - Serves as a lubricant

VISCOELASTIC PROPERTIES OF SKIN
- **Creep**

Skin and soft tissue permanently elongate when subjected to an external force because of creep.
  - **Mechanical creep:** Occurs when tissue is *acutely* stretched
    - ▶ Collagen fibers straighten and realign parallel to one another and with the vector of force.
    - ▶ Elastic fibers microfragment.
    - ▶ Water is displaced from the ground substance.
    - ▶ Adjacent tissue is recruited into the expanded field.

TIP: Mechanical creep is the basis of intraoperative tissue expansion for acute wound closure.

  - **Biologic creep:** Occurs when tissue is *chronically* stretched
    - ▶ Cellular growth and tissue regeneration is initiated.
    - ▶ Stretch-induced signal transduction pathways lead to increased production of collagen, angiogenesis, fibroblast mitosis, and epidermal proliferation.
    - ▶ Multiple molecular cascades involving growth factors and protein kinases have been discovered that are initiated by mechanical force.[1]

- **Stress relaxation**
The force required to maintain tissue elongation decreases over time.
  - A corollary of creep, not a separate process

HISTOLOGY[2-4]

Predictable changes occur to the layers of the skin and soft tissue in response to tissue expansion.

EPIDERMIS
- Mitotic activity increases.
- Thickens through hyperkeratosis and acanthosis.
- Intercellular spaces narrow.
- Normalizes after 6 months.[5]

DERMIS
- Thins
- Fibroblasts increase in number.
- Myofibroblasts present in greater number.
- Sweat glands and hair follicles become further apart.
- Thickness returns to normal 2 years following expansion.

MUSCLE
- Decreases in thickness and mass.
- There is no loss of function.
- Myofibril and myofilament arrangement becomes disorganized.

FAT
- Extremely sensitive to mechanical force.
- 30%-50% of the adipocytes are lost.
- Subcutaneous fat layer thins.
- Fat loss is permanent in expanded tissue.

CAPSULE
- Forms around the expander within days
- Composed of elongated fibroblasts and few myofibroblasts within a layer of thick collagen bundles oriented parallel to the surface of the expander

VASCULARITY
- Angiogenesis occurs rapidly in expanded soft tissue.
- Highest density of vessels is found at junction of capsule and host tissue.
- Connections form between these vessels and the vessels within the overlying dermis.

> TIP: Flaps raised on expanded skin have an improved survival compared with flaps raised on nonexpanded skin because of the increased vascularity.[6-8]

TYPES OF EXPANDERS

BASIC DESIGN
- Inflatable silicone elastomer reservoir

FILLING PORTAL
- **Remote filling port**
  - Connected to the reservoir with tubing
  - Usually placed in the subcutaneous tissue where it can be located percutaneously
  - Can also be placed externally to obviate the need for skin puncture
- **Integrated**
  - Incorporated into the reservoir itself
  - Subcutaneous tunneling and separate port site not necessary, but carries the risk of inadvertent expander puncture

SHAPE
- Available in many shapes and can be custom designed
- Amount of tissue expanded in vivo only a fraction of that expected by mathematical calculation
- Expander geometry influences the amount of surface area gained[9]:
  - **Round expander:** 25% of calcuated tissue expansion
  - **Crescent expander:** 32% of calculated tissue expansion
  - **Rectangular expander:** 38% of calculated tissue expansion

CONTOUR
- Many expanders possess rigid backs, permitting directional expansion.
- Others are designed to expand in nonconcentric, differential fashion to impart a certain contour to the expanded pocket (as in breast reconstruction).

PERMANENT EXPANDERS[10]
- Used for breast reconstruction
- Possess two compartments
  - *Outer compartment:* Filled with silicone gel
  - *Inner compartment:* Saline-filled reservoir connected to a remote fill port
- Port intended to be removed when expansion complete
- Designed to remain in position permanently

OSMOTIC SELF-INFLATING EXPANDERS
- Contain hypertonic sodium chloride crystals and fill by osmosis
- Rarely used and largely experimental

ADVANTAGES OF TISSUE EXPANSION

- Larger defects can be closed than by using local flaps alone.
  - Expansion usually used for simple advancement flaps, but some prefer transposition flaps[12]
  - May also be used in preparation for expanded axial, myocutaneous, or fasciocutaneous flaps
- Donor tissue is adjacent tissue and shares similar color, texture, thickness, sensation, and hair-bearing characteristics.

- Primary closure is often an option, thus limiting donor site morbidity.
- Scar location can be manipulated.
- Expanded tissue can be expanded repeatedly.
- Methods are reliable.

DISADVANTAGES OF TISSUE EXPANSION

- Multiple operations (at least two) are required.
- Reconstruction is delayed until expansion is complete.
- Multiple outpatient visits are required.
- A temporary dramatic aesthetic deformity exists during expansion process.
- Tissue expansion risks complications (e.g., exposure or infection).

TECHNIQUE

CHOICE OF EXPANDER
- **Size**
  - Base diameter of expander should be 2 to 2.5 times the diameter of the defect to be covered.[9,11]

TIP: Volume is a minor issue because most expanders can be overfilled many times their listed volume.

- **Shape**
  - Mostly depends on location
  - Rectangular expanders well suited to long, narrow extremities
  - Circular shapes excellent for the breast
  - Crescent shapes often used in the scalp
- **Number**
  - May use multiple expanders for a single defect
  - Depends on availability of adjacent tissue

INCISION
- Made perpendicular to the direction of expansion (long axis of the expander) to avoid tension across the incision
- May also be made in existing incisional scars or at the edge of the defect to be excised so that the scar can be removed at the time of reconstruction (Fig. 4-1)

Fig. 4-1 The access incision may be placed at the margin of the defect. (Although this is not the "preferable" incision, it is probably the one most often used.)

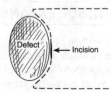
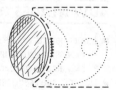

POCKET
- Suprafascial, submuscular, or subgaleal depending on location
- Must be large enough to allow expander to lie flat without creases, but not so large that it allows migration or excessive movement of the expander
- Hemostasis and meticulous dissection essential for preserving overlying vascularity

EXPANSION PROCESS
- Expansion usually started within 2-3 weeks of expander placement and takes 6-12 weeks to complete
- 23 gauge (or smaller) needle or Huber needle used to access the filling port
- Expander filled until patient senses discomfort or the overlying skin blanches
- Frequency
  - Expansion can be repeated after 3-4 days, but is usually done weekly to facilitate scheduled clinic visits.
  - Rapid expansion can be associated with higher extrusion rates.
- Completion
  - Expansion is complete when enough soft tissue is available to cover the defect.
  - Determining when expansion is complete can be a difficult clinical decision.

TIP: The amount of tissue available for advancement is equal to the circumference minus the base width of the expander.[3,9]

RECONSTRUCTION
- Undertaken when expander inflated to desired volume
  - **Expanded circumference (dome length) minus the base diameter of the expander estimates the amount of tissue available for a simple advancement flap (Fig. 4-2)**
- When placed before excising a defect (scar, nevi, etc.), the incision is made at the junction of defect and expanded tissue.
- Capsule
  - May be scored perpendicular to the direction of advancement to increased flap mobilization
  - May also be completely excised

TIP: Remember, the capsule is highly vascular and capsulectomy or scoring can compromise the vascularity of the overlying skin.[13]

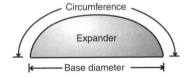

Circumference – Base diameter = Tissue available

Fig. 4-2   Amount of tissue available equals circumference minus base diameter.

CLINICAL APPLICATIONS

HEAD AND NECK

- **Scalp**
  - Defects involving up to **50%** of the scalp can be reconstructed with tissue expansion without significant thinning of the remaining hair.[14]
  - Expanders with remote filling ports are placed in the subgaleal plane.
  - Multiple expansions and combinations of rotation and advancement flaps are used.
  - Applications:
    - Male pattern baldness
    - Traumatic defects
    - Burn alopecia
    - Congenital nevi
    - Skin malignancy reconstruction
- **Facial defects**
  - Reconstruction can be accomplished with adjacent tissue for a precise match in color, thickness, texture, and hair-bearing qualities.
  - The final scar may be placed in the most camouflaged location.
- **Ear**
  - Postauricular skin can be expanded before reconstruction of congenital and acquired auricular deformities.[15,16]
  - Thin, non–hair-bearing skin may be draped over the reconstructed cartilage framework.
- **Nose**
  - Forehead tissue expanders can be placed before using forehead flaps for nasal reconstruction.
    - Flap dimensions are increased, which allows for primary closure of the donor site.
    - Authors argue that expanded forehead flaps are not ideal and that the donor site is best left to heal by secondary intention.[17]

TRUNK

- **Breast**
  - Tissue expanders are most commonly used for immediate and delayed breast reconstruction.
  - An expander with an integrated filling port is most often used.
  - More information is found in Chapter 43.
- **Giant congenital melanocytic nevi**
  - Tissue expansion is indicated for large lesions involving the back, abdomen, and chest that cannot be serially excised in three stages or fewer.[18]
  - Allows for excision of nevus and resurfacing with normal skin of appropriate color and texture.
- **Abdominal wall reconstruction**
  - Skin grafting is often performed in the management of complex abdominal wounds following trauma, infection, and dehiscence of midline incisions.
  - Tissue expansion allows for excision of the grafted skin and coverage with vascularized and innervated local tissue.

- For reconstructing large myofascial defects, expanders can be placed between the external and internal oblique muscles.
  - ▸ After expansion, component separation allows primary closure of defects that involve more than 50% of the abdominal surface area.[19,20]

EXTREMITIES

- **Multiple uses**
  - Permits excision of lesions: Nevi, postburn contractures
  - Preexpansion of extremity donor sites for skin grafting or fasciocutaneous flaps
  - Allows for improvement of donor site defects: Scar reconstruction, skin graft donor sites, contour deformities

TIP: Extremity tissue expansion has been associated with higher levels of complications.[21-23]

COMPLICATIONS

MINOR COMPLICATIONS

- Pain
- Scar widening
- Transient neuropraxia
- Temporary body contour distortion

MAJOR COMPLICATIONS

- Exposure
- Infection
- Hematoma
- Expander deflation
- Skin ischemia and necrosis

RISK FACTORS ASSOCIATED WITH HIGHER COMPLICATION RATES

- Children, especially under age 7
- Use in the extremities: Lower extremities associated with more complications than upper extremities
- Burn reconstruction

TIP: An exposed expander can be salvaged and expansion resumed in some cases.[23]

KEY POINTS

✔ Tissue expansion takes advantage of the viscoelastic properties of the skin, specifically creep and stress relaxation.

✔ The epidermis is the only layer to thicken in response to tissue expansion. The other layers become thinner.

✔ Rectangular expanders give the most skin expansion (relative to what is mathematically expected) of all shapes of expanders.

✔ The base diameter of the expander should be 2.5 times the diameter of the defect to be covered.

✔ The access incision should be placed at the margin of the defect.

✔ Wait 2 weeks after placement of the expander to begin expansion, which can then be carried out every week.

✔ The amount of tissue available for advancement equals the circumference minus the base width of the expander.

✔ Up to 50% of the scalp can be reconstructed using tissue expansion.

REFERENCES

1. Takei T, Mills I, Arai K, et al. Molecular basis for tissue expansion: Clinical implications for the surgeon. Plast Reconstr Surg 102:247-258, 1998.
2. Johnson TM, Lowe L, Brown MD, et al. Histology and physiology of tissue expansion. J Dermatol Surg Oncol 19:1074-1078, 1993.
3. Malata CM, Williams NW, Sharpe DT. Tissue expansion: An overview. J Wound Care 4:37-44, 1995.
4. Austad ED, Pasyk KA, McClatchey KD, et al. Histomorphologic evaluation of guinea pig skin and soft tissue after controlled tissue expansion. Plast Reconstr Surg 70:704-710, 1982.
5 Olenius M, Johansson O. Variations in epidermal thickness in expanded human breast skin. Scand J Plast Reconstr Hand Surg 29:15-20, 1995.
6. Cherry GW, Austad E, Pasyk K, et al. Increased survival and vascularity of random-pattern skin flaps elevated in controlled, expanded skin. Plast Reconstr Surg 72:680-687, 1983.
7. Sasaki GH, Pang CY. Pathophysiology of skin flaps raised on expanded pig skin. Plast Reconstr Surg 74:59-67, 1984.
8. Saxby PJ. Survival of island flaps after tissue expansion: A pig model. Plast Reconstr Surg 81:30-34, 1988.
9. van Rappard JH, Molenaar J, van Doorn K, et al. Surface-area increase in tissue expansion. Plast Reconstr Surg 82:833-837, 1988.
10. Becker H. Breast reconstruction using an inflatable breast implant with detachable reservoir. Plast Reconstr Surg 73:678-683, 1984.
11. Wilhelmi BJ, Blackwell SJ, Mancoll JS, et al. Creep vs. stretch: A review of the viscoelastic properties of skin. Ann Plast Surg 41:215-219, 1998.
12. Joss GS, Zoltie N, Chapman P. Tissue expansion technique and the transposition flap. Brit J Plast Surg 43:328-333, 1990.
13. Manders EK, Schenden MJ, Furrey JA, et al. Soft-tissue expansion: Concepts and complications. Plast Reconstr Surg 74:493-507, 1984.
14. MacLennan SE, Corcoran JF, Neale HW. Tissue expansion in head and neck burn reconstruction. Clin Plast Surg 27:121-132, 2000.
15. Hata Y, Hosokawa K, Yano K, et al. Correction of congenital microtia using the tissue expander. Plast Reconstr Surg 84:741-751, 1989.

16. Sasaki GH. Tissue expansion in reconstruction of acquired auricular defects. Clin Plast Surg 17:327-338, 1990.
17. Burget GC. Axial paramedian forehead flap. In Strauch B, ed. Grabb's Encyclopedia of Flaps. Philadelphia: Lippincott, 1998, pp 203-212.
18. Ameja JS, Gosain AK. Giant congenital melanocytic nevi of the trunk and an algorithm for treatment. J Craniofac Surg 16:886-893, 2005.
19. Byrd HS, Hobar PC. Abdominal wall expansion in congenital defects. Plast Reconstr Surg 84:347-352, 1989.
20. Jacobsen WM, Petty PM, Bite U, et al. Massive abdominal-wall hernia reconstruction with expanded external/internal oblique and transversalis musculofascia. Plast Reconstr Surg 100:326-335, 1997.
21. Antonyshyn O, Gruss JS, Mackinnon SE, et al. Complications of soft tissue expansion. Brit J Plast Surg 41:239-250, 1988.
22. Hallock GG. Extremity tissue expansion. Orthop Rev 16:606-611, 1987.
23. Pandya AN, Vadodaria S, Coleman DJ. Tissue expansion in the limbs: A comparative analysis of limb and non-limb sites. Brit J Plast Surg 55:302-306, 2002.

5. Basics of Microsurgery

David S. Chang
Jeffrey E. Janis

INDICATIONS FOR MICROSURGICAL RECONSTRUCTION

HIGHEST LEVEL ON RECONSTRUCTIVE LADDER
- Consider for covering difficult wounds (e.g., reconstruction after cancer extirpation, covering open fractures) when more simple or local options for wound coverage are unavailable
- Possible to transplant composite tissue (e.g., skin, subcutaneous tissue, fascia, muscle) to distant sites

OTHER INDICATIONS
- Hand and digit replantation or reconstruction
- Functional muscle transfer
- Vascularized bone and nerve grafts

POTENTIAL CONTRAINDICATIONS

In general, there are no *absolute* contraindications to microsurgical reconstruction
- **Age:** Extremes of age alone are not a contraindication.
- **Systemic disease:** There are no absolute contraindications to microsurgical reconstruction. However, the patient must be able to tolerate prolonged general anaesthesia.
- **Smoking:** Free flaps do not have greater flap loss, so not an absolute contraindication, but smokers have approximately 50% greater chance of wound healing complications.[1]

CAUTION: Smoking after digital replantation is associated with 80%-90% failure rate.[2] Patients must be counseled before replanting.

- **Preoperative radiation:** Not a contraindication. Free flaps have similar failure rates in irradiated and nonirradiated tissue.[3]

> TIP: Great care should be exercised when working with irradiated vessels. Dissection should be limited, the finest caliber suture and needle should be used, and the needle should be passed from inside out when possible to avoid separation of the vessel layers.

EQUIPMENT AND INSTRUMENTS[5]

- **Magnification**
  - Ocular loupes at least 3.5× for dissection, at least 4.0× can also be used for anastomosis of vessels smaller than 1 mm
  - Microscope: 200 mm focal length with 6× to 40× for anastomosis

- Double-headed system for two surgeons
- Useful to have monitor set up for teaching purposes if scope has video output
- **Forceps**
  - #2 through #5 jeweler's forceps
  - Round or flat handles
  - 4-6 inches long
- **Scissors**
  - Fine tipped, spring handled
  - Serrated straight and curved
  - Used for dissecting and trimming vessels
- **Vessel dilator**
  - Smooth, fine tipped
  - Can be used to gently dilate vessel to relieve spasm or correct size mismatch
- **Needle holder:** Curved or straight, nonlocking; some prefer to use jeweler's forceps
- **Microvascular clamps**
  - Single clamps of various sizes and adjustable double clamps for tension-free approximation of vessel ends
  - Closing pressure less than 30 g/mm^2 avoids trauma to endothelium
- **Background**
  - MicroMat (PMT Corp, Chanhassen, MN) or other thin sheet of plastic in a color that maximizes contrast of suture and tissue (e.g., light blue or yellow)
- **Irrigation**
  - 3 ml syringe with 27-gauge angiocath or blunt-tip needle
  - Heparinized saline (100 U/ml)[6]
  - Topical papaverine: Calcium channel blocker, used to stop vasospasm
  - 4% lidocaine: Can also stop vasospasm
- **Other equipment**
  - Cellulose sponges (Weck-Cel® spears [Medtronic, Jacksonville, FL] or half-inch cottonoids) to blot blood from field
  - Bipolar electrocautery: Useful for vessels smaller than 1 mm
  - Hemoclips: For vessels larger than 1 mm
  - "Bird bath": Specimen cup filled with heparinized saline and gauze to clean instruments
  - Merocel® (Medtronic) (moistened with saline) used to clear debris from instruments

SUTURE AND NEEDLES

NOTE: There is no ideal suture and needle.

- Suture is typically monofilament nylon or polypropylene in sizes from 8-0 to 11-0 depending on size of vessel (Table 5-1).

MICRONEEDLE (Fig. 5-1)

- Diameter: 75 to 135 microns
- Shape: Three-eighths circle or one-half circle
- Size of needle diameter determines size of suture hole

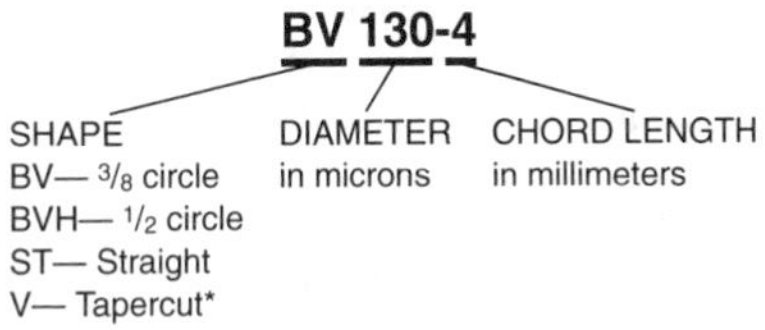

BV 130-4

SHAPE	DIAMETER	CHORD LENGTH
BV— 3/8 circle	in microns	in millimeters
BVH— 1/2 circle		
ST— Straight		
V— Tapercut*		

Fig. 5-1 Nomenclature of a microsuture needle.

- Length: Circumference of needle (distance from swage to point along the curve of the needle)
- Radius: Distance from center of circle to needle
- Chord length: Distance from swage to point in straight line
- Swage: Where needle is attached to suture

Table 5-1 *Commonly Used Sutures and Needles*

Suture	Needle	Typical Vessels
8-0	BV130-5	Radial, ulnar, anterior tibial, or peroneal
9-0	BV100-4	Dorsalis pedis, posterior tibial
10-0	BV75-3	Digital vessels
11-0	BV50-3	Children

PLANNING

- Discuss plan with anaesthesiologist; avoid placing IVs in flap harvest sites (e.g., free radial forearm flaps).
- Prep widely: Anticipate need for skin graft and include donor site in preparations.
- Scrub nurse should have instruments on Mayo stand next to operative field.
- Surgeon posture and position are essential to avoid fatigue and tremor.
  - Feet flat on floor; hips, knees, and elbows at right angles; back straight
  - Support hands and forearms with stacks of towels
- Caffeine: Routine consumption of caffeine should not have adverse effects; therefore drink your normal amount.[7,8]
- Exposure is critical: Use self-retaining retractors and keep operative field dry.

TIP: Elastic Stay Hooks (Lone Star Medical, Stafford, TX) clamped to drapes work well as retractors.

The MicroMat suction background can help keep the operative field dry.

It is useful to mark donor vessels with methylene blue or a marking pen before dividing pedicle to avoid twisting vessels at anastomosis.

TECHNICAL CONSIDERATIONS[9,10]

- Keep vessels moist.
- Avoid traumatizing vessels, only grasp adventitia.
- Tension-free anastomosis is critical for patency; mobilize donor pedicle and recipient vessels from their native beds.

VESSEL PREPARATION (Fig. 5-2)
- Cut back to healthy vessel if ends are traumatized.
- If traumatic wound, choose vessels outside zone of injury.

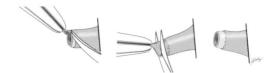

Fig. 5-2 Proper vessel preparation.

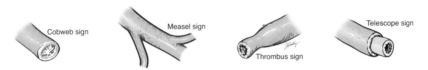

Fig. 5-3 Signs of microvascular trauma.

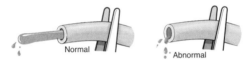

Fig. 5-4 Spurt test.

- Prepare vessels by dissecting 2-5 mm of adventitia from vessel end.
- Watch for signs of microvascular trauma (Fig. 5-3).

TIP: Always remember to check your inflow before performing the microvascular anastomosis ("spurt test") (Fig. 5-4).

- Flush artery and vein with heparinized saline.
- Always release arterial clamp to test inflow before anastomosis.

ESTABLISHING ANASTOMOSIS

TIP: Start with the more difficult anastomosis (e.g., if artery is deep to vein, do arterial anastomosis first).

- Needles should enter vessel at 90 degrees, full thickness, and follow curve of needle.
- Tie all knots square (usually three throws) and place precisely. If microscope has video output, it is useful to set up monitor for teaching purposes and for scrub nurse to follow case.
- Sutures should completely coapt the vessel edges, because exposure of the vascular endothelium can promote platelet aggregation and subsequent thrombus.

TIP: Cut one limb of suture long to use as a handle.

- Flush vessels with heparinized saline solution before tying last stitch to check for placement of "back wall" sutures.
- Number of stitches:
  - Size of vessel determines number of stitches.
  - More sutures yield more foreign bodies and therefore are not necessarily better.
  - Use minimal number to approximate vessel, but a leaking anastomosis can promote hematoma formation and subsequent extrinsic compression of the vessel.

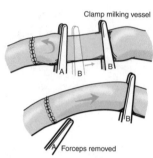

Clamp milking vessel

Forceps removed

Fig. 5-5   Strip test to check vessel patency.

COMPLETION OF ANASTOMOSIS

- Release distal clamp first and watch for backflow through anastomosis.
- **Strip test:** Gently grasp vessel distal to anastomosis with two forceps; gently milk blood distally so vessel is collapsed between the two forceps; release proximal forceps; blood should fill collapsed vessel if anastomosis is patent (Fig. 5-5).
- Clip or sew any bleeding side branches.

ANASTOMOTIC TECHNIQUES

END-TO-END

- **Halving technique** (Fig. 5-6)
  - First two sutures are placed 180 degrees apart beginning with midpoint of back wall.
  - Vessel is then rotated 90 degrees in either direction to place sutures between the first two sutures by halving the distance between.
- **Triangulation technique**
  - Place three sutures 120 degrees apart.
  - Vessel is rotated to place sutures between the first three sutures, spacing appropriately.
- **Back wall up technique**
  - Place interrupted sutures beginning at midpoint of back wall.
  - Sutures are placed up one side then the other.
  - Technique is useful when working in a cavity.

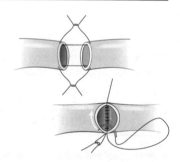

Fig. 5-6   End-to-end anastomosis (halving technique).

END-TO-SIDE

- Useful for size discrepancy or to preserve in-line flow and distal perfusion
- Patency equivalent to end-to-end
- Ideal angle of entry between 30 and 75 degrees
- Ideal 2:1 ratio of anastomosis to vessel diameter (Fig. 5-7)
- Arteriotomy is key step (three suggested techniques) (Fig. 5-8)
  - Use No. 11 blade or eye knife to make initial arteriotomy, then cut out ellipse with scissors.
  - Can place single microsuture full-thickness, tent up vessel, and cut out ellipse with curved serrated microscissors to create arteriotomy.
  - Use 2.5 mm vascular punch.

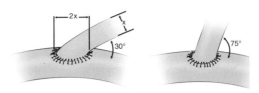

Fig. 5-7 Ideal characteristics of an end-to-side anastomosis.

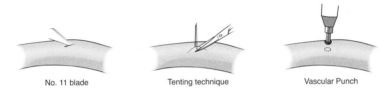

No. 11 blade   Tenting technique   Vascular Punch

Fig. 5-8 Methods of performing an arteriotomy.

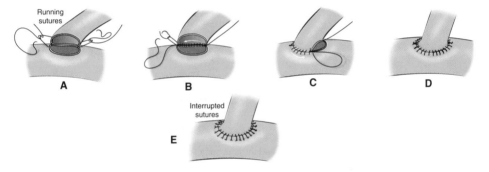

Fig. 5-9 End-to-side anastomosis. **A-D,** Running suture technique. **E,** Interrupted sutures.

- Interrupted sutures
  - Place first sutures 180 degrees apart, then front wall and back wall.
- Running sutures
  - Place interrupted sutures at toe and heel, leave long, and run in opposite directions (Fig. 5-9).

VEIN GRAFTS

> TIP: Excessive tension can compromise anastomosis; consider a vein graft any time there is
> tension.

- Vein grafts are useful to span a gap in either arterial or venous anastomosis.
- Donor sites are volar wrist or forearm and dorsum of foot.
- Mark top of vein before completing harvest to avoid twisting.
- Vein grafts have similar patency as arterial grafts.

> TIP: Always mark direction of flow before completing vein harvest to preserve antegrade orientation (e.g., flow toward the clip).

OVERCOMING SIZE DISCREPANCY (Fig. 5-10)
- Vein graft
- End-to-side anastomosis
- Sleeving technique
  - Similar patency if proximal vessel is telescoped into distal vessel
- Triangular wedge cut out of larger vessel to cone down and anastomose to smaller vessel
- Also can use spatulation
- Microvascular coupling devices (Fig. 5-11)
  - Ring devices used to create anastomosis
  - Similar healing as conventional suturing[11]
  - Most useful for end-to-end venous anastomoses
  - Less flexibility in creating anastomosis, limited by size of device

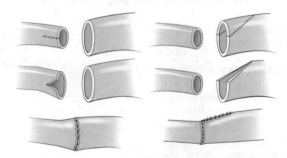

Fig. 5-10 Size discrepancies can be handled through spatulation or longitudinal wedge resection.

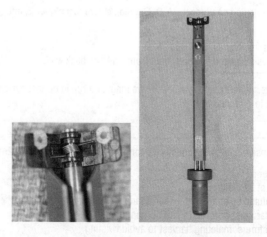

Fig. 5-11 Microvascular coupler.

POSTOPERATIVE CARE[12]

MONITORING ANASTOMOSIS
- **Clinical exam**
  - Assess color, capillary refill, bleeding from cut edges, tissue turgor, and temperature.
  - Flap or digit should be warm and pink with capillary refill in 2 seconds or less.
  - *Venous congestion:* Flap appears purple or blue and swollen, with rapid capillary refill.
  - *Arterial insufficiency:* Flap may appear pale, cool, and flaccid; lack of capillary refill.
  - If unsure, prick with 22-gauge needle and assess bleeding; blood should be bright red.
  - Assess for arterial or venous Doppler signals in the flap using a handheld probe.

> TIP: Doppler imaging is not always reliable because surrounding vessels can also transmit.

  - When in doubt return to the OR.
- **Venous Doppler**
  - Implantable Doppler probe around venous anastomosis can alert to problem before clinical signs.
  - Place Doppler before insetting flap to alert of potential flow issues during inset.
  - If the signal goes down, do not hesitate to return patient to the OR immediately.
  - 100% salvage rate has been reported using implantable Doppler.
- **Thermography**[13,14]
  - Thermography is a simple way of monitoring flap perfusion by measuring skin surface temperature using a thermocouple.
  - Both arterial and venous occlusion cause skin temperature to drop.
  - Acland[13] found temperatures above 32° C to be good, 32°-30° C is marginal, and less than 30° C indicates a problem.
  - Surface temperature can change with changes in ambient or body temperature, therefore relative changes are more important.
  - A relative change in temperature of more than **1.8° C** has a sensitivity of 98%, and a specificity of 99% for vascular compromise.
  - Thermography is not accurate for intraoral flaps because the closed environment of the mouth does not allow heat loss.

FLAP FAILURE

- Success rates greater than 90% in experienced hands
- **Flap salvage:** Time to restoration of perfusion is critical
  - Take change in appearance or Doppler signal seriously.
  - Take down dressings at bedside to relieve any potential constricting effect.
  - Sutures can be removed to relieve pressure.
  - Prompt return to OR can save a flap.
- **No-reflow phenomenon**
  - Potential source of flap failure despite patent anastomosis
  - Thought to be caused by endothelial swelling, platelet aggregation, and leaky capillaries, ultimately resulting in poor tissue perfusion
  - Reversible at 4-8 hours, irreversible after 12 hours

USE OF ANTICOAGULANTS IN MICROSURGERY

ASPIRIN
- Aspirin inhibits platelet aggregation through inhibition of cyclooxygenase.
- Lower doses (81 and 325 mg) inhibit thromboxane, but not prostacyclin.[15]
- Dose per rectum is given preoperatively or immediately postoperatively, then continue daily for 2-4 weeks.
- There have been no randomized controlled trials showing improved patency for microsurgery with aspirin, but its use has become standard practice.

HEPARIN
- Binds antithrombin III, inducing conformational change and accelerating inhibition of thrombin and factor Xa
- No evidence that systemic heparinization increases anastomotic patency, but does increase risk for postoperative bleeding and hematoma[16,17]
- Systemic anticoagulation with heparin only advocated if intraoperative clot appears at anastomosis or anastomosis is revised[18]
  - Keep partial thromboplastin time 1.5 to 2 times control
  - Continue 5-7 days postoperatively

10% DEXTRAN 40[19]
- Low molecular weight polysaccharide
- Exact mechanism unknown, but has the following effects:
  - Volume expansion
  - Inactivates von Willebrand's factor
  - Imparts negative charge on platelets
  - Fibrinolytic effects
- Use is controversial: Used by some routinely and by others only for anastomotic complications
- Evidence that routine use increases complications without increasing patency rates[20]
- Test dose given first to check for allergic reaction (<5 ml of 10% solution of Dextran 40) followed by infusion of 25 ml/hr for 3-5 days
- Adverse effects: Anaphylaxis (1:70,000), pulmonary edema, and nephrotoxicity

MICRONEURAL REPAIR

See also Chapter 68.

GENERAL PRINCIPLES OF REPAIR
- Assess preoperative function.
- Nerves are coapted without tension.
- Use interposition graft if there is tension.
- None of the repair types are superior to the others.

TYPES OF REPAIR
- **Epineurial**
  - Standard for small nerves
  - 10-0 or 11-0 suture

- Fascicles lined up and trimmed to avoid buckling of fibers
- Suture passes through epineurium only (two to three sutures)
- 180-degree technique

■ **Perineurial (fascicular)**
- Technically more difficult
- Individual fascicles lined up and sutured
- Theoretically improves coaptation of fascicles, but no superior results

■ **Grouped fascicular**
- Distinct fascicular groups sutured together at inner epineurial level
- Can be used for larger nerves at level where specific branches can be identified

NERVE GRAFTS AND CONDUITS[21]
■ Used if gap or excessive tension is present
■ Common donor nerves: Sural nerve, lateral or medial antebrachial cutaneous nerve
■ Vein grafts and polyglycolic acid nerve tubes can be used for sensory nerve defects up to 3 cm with results comparable to nerve grafts[22-25]

KEY POINTS

✔ There are no absolute contraindications to microsurgical reconstruction.
✔ Surgeon comfort and exposure of the working field are essential for successful microsurgery.
✔ Tension-free anastomoses of vessels and coaptation of nerves are critical.
✔ Monitoring devices are helpful postoperatively, but should not supplant a good clinical examination.
✔ If you are concerned about the patency of an anastomosis, do not hesitate to take the patient back to the OR—timely reexploration can save a flap.

REFERENCES

1. Reus WF, Colen LB, Straker DJ. Tobacco smoking and complications in elective microsurgery. Plast Reconstr Surg 89:490-494, 1992.
2. Chang LD, Buncke G, Slezak S, et al. Cigarette smoking, plastic surgery, and microsurgery. J Reconstr Microsurg 12:467-474, 1996.
3. Bengtson BP, Schusterman MA, Baldwin BJ, et al. Influence of prior radiotherapy on the development of postoperative complications and success of free tissue transfers in head and neck cancer reconstruction. Am J of Surg 166:326-330, 1993.
4. Guelinckx PJ, Boeckx WD, Fossion E, et al. Scanning electron microscopy of irradiated recipient blood vessels in head and neck free flaps. Plast Reconstr Surg 74:217-226, 1984.
5. Acland RD. Instrumentation for Microsurgery. Orthop Clin North Am 8:281-294, 1973.
6. Cox GW, Runnels S, Hsu HS, et al. A comparison of heparinised saline irrigation solutions in a model of microvascular thrombosis. Br J Plast Surg 45:345-348, 1992.
7. Arnold RW, Springer DT, Engel WK, et al. The effect of wrist rest, caffeine, and oral timolol on the hand steadiness of ophthalmologists. Ann Ophthalmol 25:250-253, 1993.
8. Pederson WC, Sanders WE. Principles of microsurgery. In Green DP, Hotchkiss RN, Pederson WC, eds. Green's Operative Hand Surgery, 4th ed. Philadelphia: Churchill Livingstone, 1999, p 1094-1110.

9. Weiss DD, Pribaz JJ. Microsurgery. In Achauer BM, ed. Plastic Surgery, Indications, Operations, and Outcomes. St Louis: Mosby, 2000, p 163.
10. Shenaq SM, Sharma SK. Principles of microvascular surgery. In Aston SJ, ed. Grabb and Smith's Plastic Surgery. Philadelphia: Lippincott-Raven,1997, p 73.
11. Gilbert RW, Ragnarsson R, Berggren A, et al. Strength of microvascular anastomosis: Comparison between the unilink anastomotic system and sutures. Microsurgery 10:40-46, 1989.
12. Buncke HJ, et al: Monitoring. In Buncke HJ, ed. Microsurgery: Transplantation-Replantation. Philadelphia: Lea & Febiger, 1991.
13. Acland RD. Experience in monitoring the circulation in free-flap transfers. Plast Reconstr Surg 68:554-555, 1981.
14. Khouri RK, Shaw WW. Monitoring of free flaps with surface temperature recordings: Is it reliable? Plast Reconstr Surg 68:495-553, 1981.
15. Weksler BB, Pett SB, Alonso D, et al. Differential inhibition by aspirin of vascular and platelet prostaglandin synthesis in atherosclerotic patients. N Engl J Med 308:800-805, 1983.
16. Pugh CM, Dennis RH II, Massac EA. Evaluation of intraoperative anticoagulants in microvascular free-flap surgery. J Natl Med Assoc 88:655-657, 1996.
17. Kroll SS, Miller MJ, Reece GP, et al. Anticoagulants and hematomas in free flap surgery. Plast Reconstr Surg 96:643-647, 1995.
18. Conrad MH, Adams WP Jr. Pharmacologic optimization of microsurgery in the new millennium. Plast Reconstr Surg 108:2088-2096, 2001.
19. Jallali N. Dextrans in microsurgery. Microsurgery 23:78-80, 2003.
20. Disa JJ, Polvora VP, Pusic AL, et al. Dextran-related complications in head and neck microsurgery: Do the benefits outweigh the risks? A prospective randomized analysis. Plast Reconstr Surg 112:1534-1539, 2003.
21. Walton RL, Brown RE, Matory WE Jr, et al. Autogenous vein graft repair of digital nerve defects in the finger: A retrospective clinical study. Plast Reconstr Surg 84:944-949, 1989.
22. Wang H, Lineaweaver WC. Nerve conduits for nerve reconstruction. Op Tech Plast Reconstr Surg 9:59-66, 2003.
23. Chiu DT, Strauch B. A prospective clinical evaluation of autogenous vein grafts used as a nerve conduit for distal sensory nerve defects of 3 cm or less. Plast Reconstr Surg 86:928-934, 1990.
24. Mackinnon SE, Dellon AL. Clinical nerve reconstruction with a bioabsorbable polyglycolic acid tube. Plast Reconstr Surg 85:419-424, 1990.
25. Weber RA, Breidenbach WC, Brown RE, et al. A randomized prospective study of polyglycolic acid conduits for digital nerve reconstruction in humans. Plast Reconstr Surg 106:1036-1045, 2000.

6. Biomaterials

Jason K. Potter

DEFINITION

Biomaterials are naturally occurring and synthetic materials that are used to replace, reconstruct, or augment tissues in the human body.

CHOOSING A BIOMATERIAL

- *Permanence* is the most important clinical aspect of an implanted material.
- The long-term biocompatibility of a material is a function of the dynamic relationship between the host and implant.
- Permanence is achieved when there is harmony among host, chemical, and mechanical factors.
- The interaction between host and implant commonly is not ideal, and various biologic reactions may be observed.

IDEAL PROPERTIES FOR GENERIC BIOMATERIAL

Chemically inert	Sterilizable
Biocompatible	Easy handling
Nonallergenic	Ability to stabilize
Noncarcinogenic	Radiopaque
Cost effective	

BIOLOGIC REACTION TO FOREIGN BODY

Immediate inflammation with early rejection
Delayed rejection
Fibrous encapsulation
Incomplete encapsulation with ongoing cellular reaction
Slow resorption
Incorporation

CLASSIFICATION OF BIOMATERIALS

Autograft: Living tissue derived from the host.
Allograft: Nonliving tissue derived from same species donor (e.g., cadaver).
Xenograft: Nonliving tissue derived from different species donor (e.g., bovine, porcine).
Alloplast: Implant derived from synthetic material.

AUTOGRAFTS

ADVANTAGES
- Gold standard to which all biomaterials are compared because of their tolerance and incorporation in the host

DISADVANTAGES
- Require a second operative site
- Require increased operative time to harvest
- Increase patient morbidity
- Limited quantity
- Resorb to a variable amount over time

TYPES
- **Bone**
  - **Sources**
    - Calvarium
    - Iliac crest
    - Rib
    - Tibia
    - Radius
    - Mandible
  - **Advantages**
    - Relative resistance to infection
    - Incorporation by the host into new bone
    - Lack of host response against the graft
  - **Disadvantages**
    - Donor site morbidity
    - Variable graft resorption
    - Limited ability to contour some types of bone
  - **Resorption/remodeling**
    - All free bone grafts undergo some degree of resorption and remodeling.
    - Cortical grafts maintain their volume significantly better than cancellous grafts regardless of embryologic origin.[1]
    - Fixation of bone grafts has been shown to reduce graft resorption when grafts are placed under mobile tissues.[2]
- **Cartilage**
  - Infection and resorption of autogenous cartilage grafts are rare.[3]
  - Histologic studies have demonstrated the survival of chondrocytes within normal matrix and a general absence of fibrous ingrowth and resorption of the graft.[2,4-7]
  - It has been postulated that cartilage grafts calcify with time.[8]
  - **Main Sources**
    - Cartilaginous nasal septum
    - Conchal cartilage
    - Rib

TIP: Autogenous cartilage grafts are frequently used for soft tissue augmentation and nasal and ear reconstruction.

- **Advantages**
  - ▶ Ease of harvest
  - ▶ Flexibility
  - ▶ Limited donor site morbidity
- **Disadvantages**
  - ▶ Donor site morbidity
  - ▶ Tendency to warp[4,9,10]

ALLOGRAFTS

- Allogenic materials (allografts, homografts) and xenografts do **not** contain living cells.
- They are processed by various methods to reduce antigenicity.
- They may possess osteoinductive and/or osteoconductive properties.
- These materials become incorporated into host tissues by providing a structural framework for ingrowth of host tissues.
- They do not require a second operative site.
  - Require less operative time
  - Abundant

Caution: Xenografts possess more antigenic potential than do homografts, which are used less frequently.

Before placement of xenografts, the surgeon should inquire about previous use of xenografts in the patient, because delayed hypersensitivity reactions have been reported.[11]

- Despite meticulous sterilization techniques, the risk of infectious disease transmission remains the most worrisome disadvantage of allogenic materials.
- Variable resorption is common.

LYOPHILIZED FASCIA
- **Two major sources**
  1. Lyophilized dura
  2. Lyophilized tensor fascia lata
- Resorption rates for lyophilized fascia are reported to be up to 10% of the original graft volume.[12]
- *Lyophilized tissues carry the risk of transmitting infectious disease.*
  - Creutzfeldt-Jakob disease has been reported with a case of lyophilized dura implantation.[13]

HOMOLOGOUS BONE
- Provides a scaffold for new bone formation and has the same working properties of autogenous bone
- Slower to become incorporated and revascularized than autogenous bone[14]
- Low incidence of complications reported for maxillofacial applications, according to some studies[15]
- Supplied in many forms including whole bone cribs

HOMOLOGOUS CARTILAGE
- Has been shown to undergo ossification and calcification with time[4,16]
- Greater tendency to undergo resorption and replacement with fibrous tissue than autogenous cartilage[3-6]
- Reported to have increased rates of infection compared with autologous cartilage[3]

ALLODERM® (LifeCell Corporation, Branchburg, NJ)
- **Homologous dermis**
- Cadaveric human dermis is processed to remove all cellular elements, leaving only the collagen dermal framework.
- The host response to AlloDerm is minimal because there are no antigenic cells remaining.
- The material is incorporated into the host tissue.
- Resorption is variable.

SURGISIS® (Cook Surgical, Bloomington, IN)
- Produced from **porcine small intestine submucosa**
- Provides an acellular matrix that is purported to allow tissue ingrowth and therefore is incorporated into the host
- Used for fascia replacement
- No good clinical data available to assess effectiveness

INTEGRA® (Integra NeuroSciences, Plainsboro, NJ)
- *Bilayered dermal regenerate template used for skin replacement*
  - The top layer is **silicone.**
    - ▸ It provides temporary epidermal coverage.
    - ▸ It controls fluid loss.
    - ▸ It imparts strength and mechanical protection to the matrix.
  - The bottom layer is a **collagen/glycosaminoglycan matrix.**
    - ▸ It promotes cellular ingrowth to create a dermal regenerate.
  - Silicone layer is removed after approximately 21-28 days, and dermal regenerate is covered with a split thickness skin graft.
- **Advantages**
  - Creation of a new dermis that allows reconstruction of pliable skin
  - Reconstruction of large defects
  - Can be placed over exposed tendon
- **Disadvantage**
  - Very expensive

ALLOPLASTIC MATERIALS

ADVANTAGES
- Off-the-shelf availability
- Lack of donor site morbidity

DISADVANTAGES

- They are foreign bodies.
- All elicit some degree of host reaction to the material.
- They are expensive.

NONRESORBABLE ALLOPLASTS

- **Metals**
  - **Types**
    - ▶ Stainless steel
    - ▶ Vitallium alloy
    - ▶ Titanium alloys (most commonly used)
      - ✦ Available as plates, screws, mesh, and custom implants
      - ✦ **Advantages**
        - Ten times stronger than bone
        - Easy to bend
        - Extremely well tolerated by the host
      - ✦ **Disadvantages**
        - Low fatigue tolerance—failure may develop from cyclic loading of implant
- **High-density porous polyethylene** (MEDPOR®; Porex Surgical, College Park, GA)
  - High-density polyethylene (HDPE) is a pure polyethylene implant.
  - It is processed specifically to include and control pore size.
    - ▶ Pore size is engineered to range from 100 to 200 μm with more than 50% larger than 150 μm.[17]
    - ▶ Pore size has been demonstrated to directly influence the rate and amount of bony and fibro-vascular ingrowth into the implant.[18]
  - HDPE is available in many different shapes.

TIP: The material should be soaked in an antibiotic solution before placement.

  - It is easily and reliably stabilized with screws.[18]
  - **Advantages**
    - ▶ Highly biocompatible
    - ▶ Insoluble in tissue fluids
    - ▶ Does not resorb or degenerate
    - ▶ Incites minimal surrounding soft tissue reaction
    - ▶ Possesses high-tensile strength
  - **Disadvantages**
    - ▶ Not radiodense—its position cannot be easily determined on immediately postoperative CT scans
    - ▶ Cost
- **Hydroxyapatite** (BoneSource®; Stryker Corp., Portage, MI)
  - Hydroxyapatite (HA) [$Ca_{10}(PO4)_6(OH)_2$] is a calcium phosphate salt that is a major constituent of bone.
  - Several forms are available for reconstruction of the facial skeleton.
    - ▶ **Dense HA** is produced synthetically through high-pressure compaction of calcium phosphate crystals that are then sintered (fused) into a solid form.
    - ▶ **Porous HA** can be produced synthetically or naturally. Various pore sizes may be engineered into synthetically produced material.

- ▸ A "natural" HA can be produced by heating marine coral at elevated pressures in the presence of aqueous phosphate solutions. This causes a chemical substitution of calcium phosphate for calcium carbonate in the preexisting porous skeleton of the coral.
- **Advantages**
  - ▸ Highly biocompatible
  - ▸ Causes minimal inflammatory reaction in surrounding tissues
  - ▸ Produces a strong mechanical bond with host bone
  - ▸ Allows ingrowth of host tissue, providing a scaffold for bone repair
  - ▸ Demonstrates limited resorption[19]
  - ▸ Off the shelf
  - ▸ Favorable infection rate of 2.7% for craniofacial reconstruction[20]
- **Disadvantages**
  - ▸ Brittle
  - ▸ Difficult to shape/carve intraoperatively
- **Silicone**
  - Refers to a group of polymers based on the element silicon
  - May be produced as oils, gels, or elastomers (rubbers)
    - ▸ The physical state is determined by the degree of chemical cross-linking.
    - ▸ Cross-linking occurs between vinyl and hydrogen groups on silicon atoms.
    - ▸ Silicone oils are straight chains of polydimethylsiloxane (PDMS) without cross-linking that are insoluble in water. PDMS remains in liquid form indefinitely.
    - ▸ Silicone gels consist of cross-linked PDMS chains of various degrees with variable amounts of PDMS liquid.
  - Classified as a **medical device,** meaning that silicone does not achieve its primary intended purpose by chemical action or through its metabolism
  - **Advantages**
    - ▸ Thermal and oxidative stability
    - ▸ Chemical and biologic inertness
    - ▸ Hydrophobic nature
    - ▸ Sterilization capability
  - **Disadvantages**
    - ▸ It becomes encapsulated, not incorporated.
    - ▸ There are unsubstantiated concerns for silicone-linked illnesses.
- **Expanded polytetrafluoroethylene** (ePTFE)
  - GOR-TEX® (WL Gore & Associates, Flagstaff, AZ), SoftForm® (Tissue Technologies Inc, San Francisco, CA), UltraSoft® (Tissue Technologies Inc), and Advanta® (Atrium Medical Corp, Hudson, NH)
  - **Advantages**
    - ▸ Available in sheets, tubes, or strands
    - ▸ Nonresorbable
    - ▸ Porosities allow some degree of tissue ingrowth
    - ▸ Various applications including soft tissue augmentation and fascial replacement
  - **Disadvantages**
    - ▸ Soft tissue augmentation: Palpability, extrusion alters lip movement
    - ▸ Fascia replacement: Minimal tissue ingrowth results in weak adherence between ePTFE and abdominal wall

RESORBABLE ALLOPLASTS
- **Polylactide (PLLA) derivatives**

TIP: Advocates believe PLLA systems perform comparably to metal fixation systems.

- **Advantages**
  - ▸ Complete resorption, preventing growth interference or late complication
  - ▸ No long-term/life-long risk of complications characteristic of nonresorbable alloplasts
- **Disadvantages**
  - ▸ Less precise conformation to osseous structures than metal alloys
  - ▸ Instrumentation requires tapping all screw holes
- *LactoSorb*® (Walter Lorenz Surgical, Jacksonville, FL) is a biodegradable copolymer of polylactic and polyglycolic acids that has been in use clinically for more than 10 years.
  - ▸ Degrades within 9-15 months
  - ▸ Good results throughout the craniofacial skeleton[21-23]

■ **Polyglactin 910**®
- Known as the suture material Vicryl®
- Resorbable, synthetic material composed of lactide and glycolide
- Both film and mesh forms available

TIP: Vicryl mesh is frequently used for temporary abdominal wall repair.

■ **Gelatin Film**
- Bioabsorbable sheeting material manufactured from denatured collagen
- Clear, nonporous, 0.075 mm thick
- Brittle when dry but pliable when wet
- Suggested for the repair of small orbital floor defects (<5 mm) or as an interpositional material between the periorbital tissues and reconstructive plates or mesh[24]
- **Advantages**
  - ▸ Entirely absorbed within 2-3 months[24]
- **Disadvantages**
  - ▸ Brittle
  - ▸ Poor mechanical properties to reconstruct true orbital defects

KEY POINTS

- ✔ Autografts have the best tolerance and host incorporation profile but suffer from a variable amount of resorption over time and the need for a secondary operative (donor) site.
- ✔ Cortical bone grafts have greater initial strength than cancellous bone grafts, although cancellous grafts are revascularized more quickly.
- ✔ Delayed hypersensitivity has been reported with xenografts.
- ✔ Integra bilaminate neodermis can be used to successfully bridge over exposed bone, cartilage, and tendon without overlying periosteum, perichondrium, and paratenon, as long as the wound bed is healthy.
- ✔ High-density porous polyethylene (MEDPOR) is incorporated into host tissues by fibrovascular tissue and bony ingrowth, which also makes it difficult to remove.
- ✔ Resorbable alloplasts are very useful in the pediatric population.

REFERENCES

1. Ozaki W, Buchman SR. Volume maintenance of onlay grafts in the craniofacial skeleton: Microarchitecture versus embryologic origin. Plast Reconstr Surg 102:291-299, 1998.
2. Lin KY, Bartlett SP, Yaremchuk MJ, et al. The effect of rigid fixation on the survival of onlay bone grafts: An experimental study. Plast Reconstr Surg 86:449-456, 1990.
3. Vuyk HD, Adamson PA. Biomaterials in rhinoplasty. Clin Otolaryngol Allied Sci 23:209-217, 1998.
4. Peer LA. The fate of living and dead cartilage transplanted in humans. Surg Gynecol Obstet 68:603-610, 1939.
5. Peer LA. Diced cartilage grafts. Arch Otolaryngol 38:156, 1943.
6. Peer LA. Cartilage grafting. Br J Plast Surg 7:250-262, 1954.
7. Ballantyne DL, Rees TD, Seidman I. Silicone fluid: Response to massive subcutaneous injections of dimethylpolysiloxane fluid in animals. Plast Reconstr Surg 36:330-338, 1965.
8. Werther JR. Not seeing eye to eye about septal grafts for orbital fractures [letter]. J Oral Maxillofac Surg 56:906-907, 1998.
9. Converse JM, Smith B. Reconstruction of the floor of the orbit by bone grafts. Arch Ophthalmol 44:1-21, 1950.
10. Antonyshyn O, Gruss JS, Galbraith DJ, et al. Complex orbital fractures: A critical analysis of immediate bone graft reconstruction. Ann Plast Surg 22:220-233, 1989.
11. Waite PD, Clanton JT. Orbital floor reconstruction with lyophilized dura. J Oral Maxillofac Surg 46:727-730, 1988.
12. Celikoz B, Duman H, Selmanpakoglu N. Reconstruction of the orbital floor with lyophilized tensor fascia lata. J Oral Maxillofac Surg 55:240-244, 1997.
13. Prichard J, Thadani V, Kalb R, et al. Leads from the MMWR. Rapidly progressive dementia in a patient who received a cadaveric dura mater graft. JAMA 257:1036-1037, 1987.
14. Ellis E. Biology of Bone Grafting: An Overview. Selected Readings Oral Maxillofacial Surgery. San Francisco: Guild for Scientific Advancement in Oral and Maxillofacial Surgery, 1991.
15. Ellis E III, Sinn DP. Use of homologous bone in maxillofacial surgery. J Oral Maxillofac Surg 51:1181-1193, 1993.
16. Chen JM, Zingg M, Laedrach K, et al. Early surgical intervention for orbital floor fractures. A clinical evaluation of lyophilized dura and cartilage reconstruction. J Oral Maxillofac Surg 50:935-941, 1992.
17. Romano JJ, Iliff NT, Manson PN. Use of Medpor porous polyethylene implants in 140 patients with facial fractures. J Craniofac Surg 4:142-147, 1993.
18. Haug RH, Kimberly D, Bradick JP. A comparison of microscrew and suture fixation of porous high-density polyethylene orbital floor implants. J Oral Maxillofac Surg 51:1217-1220, 1993.
19. Holmes RE, Hagler HK. Porous hydroxyapatite as a bone graft substitute on cranial reconstruction: A histometric study. Plast Reconstr Surg 81:662-671, 1988.
20. Rubin JP, Yaremchuk MJ. Complications and toxicities of implantable biomaterials used in facial reconstructive and aesthetic surgery: A comprehensive review of the literature. Plast Reconstr Surg 100:1336-1353, 1997.
21. Enislidis G, Pichorner S, Kainberger F, et al. Lactosorb panel and screws for repair of large orbital floor defects. J Craniomaxillofac Surg 25:316-321, 1997.
22. Ahn DK, Sims CD, Randolph MA, et al. Craniofacial skeletal fixation using biodegradable plates and cyanoacrylate glue. Plast Reconstr Surg 99:1508-1515, 1997.
23. Eppley BL, Sadove AM, Havlik RJ. Resorbable plate fixation in pediatric craniofacial surgery. Plast Reconstr Surg 100:1-7, 1997.
24. Mermer RW, Orban RE. Repair of orbital floor fractures with absorbable gelatin film. J Craniomaxillofac Trauma 1:30-34, 1995.

7. Lasers in Plastic Surgery

John E. Hoopman

DEFINITION[1]

LASER is an acronym for Light Amplification by Stimulated Emission of Radiation. Energy is created by stimulation of atoms within a medium.

LASER PHYSICS[1]

- **Laser device components**
  - Lasing medium
  - Pump source
  - Mirrors (reflect and multiply photonic energy)
- **Laser light "characteristics"**
  - Coherent (in phase)
  - Monochromatic (one color)
  - Collimated (tight formation)
- **Lasing medium**
  - Each medium releases a wavelength specific to that medium.
- **Measurements**
  - Wavelengths measured in nanometers (nm), or billionths of a meter
  - Laser energies
    - ▸ Watt-seconds or Joules
      - ✦ Concentrations of energies measured in Joules(J)/cm^2
  - Electromagnetic spectrum
    - ▸ Ultraviolet (UV): 200-400 nm
    - ▸ Visible: 400-755 nm
    - ▸ Near-infrafred (IR): 755-1400 nm
    - ▸ Mid-IR: 1400-20,000 nm
- **Characteristics of laser energy**
  - Reflects: Light reflects off shiny surfaces (safety hazard)
  - Absorbs: Ideal—energies transferred, work
  - Transmits: Light passes through a pane of glass with no effect
  - Scatters: Light passes through a glass of milk with little effect
- **Energy delivery modes**
  - Continuous wave: A continuous flow of energy
  - Pulsed: Bursts of energy with specific intervals of microseconds
  - Q-Switched: Extremely high bursts of energy with short intervals in the nanosecond and picosecond ranges

LASER SAFETY[2]

EYE PROTECTION

- Lasers are rated by the amount of ocular damage they can cause.
- Medical lasers are all class IV, and **eye protection is mandatory.**
  - **Optical density (OD)** is the inverse base 10 log that represents the amount of energy transmitted through protective lenses.
    - An OD of 1 equals $\frac{1}{10}$, and an OD of 4 equals $\frac{1}{10,000}$.
    - An OD of 4 or more is recommended for most laser wavelengths.
  - UV and IR lasers can cause corneal damage.
  - Visible and near IR lasers can cause retinal damage.
- Laser-specific signs must be posted at all entrances to a treatment room.
  - Signs must indicate that a laser procedure is in progress and eye protection is required.
  - The wavelength and power of the laser being used must be listed on the signs.
- The four walls of the treatment area are the *nominal hazard zone.*
  - All persons within the nominal hazard zone must adhere to all safety precautions.
- Laser-specific eye protection for the patient must isolate the entire orbit from laser radiation.
- All windows must have an opaque covering corresponding to the wavelength being used, and additional safety eyewear must be placed at the entrance to the room.

FIRE SAFETY

- Prepare patients with nonflammable solutions, and use nonflammable anaesthetics.
- Surround the treatment area with wet towels in case of accidental ignition of other materials.
- Never wear jewelry or leave reflective instruments in the treatment area.

SMOKE PLUMES

- Smoke plumes have been known to contain carbonized tissue, blood, and viruses.
- Use a smoke evacuator with HEPA-quality filters.
- Wear laser-quality masks with 0.1 μm particulate filtration.
- Treat smoke evacuation tubing and filters as biohazard waste.

TISSUE EFFECTS[3]

SELECTIVE PHOTOTHERMOLYSIS

- Damage is determined by **wavelength, power, spot size,** and **pulse time.**
- Laser energies are absorbed by specific **chromophores** within tissue.
  - Laser pulses must be the correct duration to deposit enough energy in the target tissues before they can cool.
  - As soon as the target is heated, it begins to dissipate heat through conduction.
  - The amount of absorption in selected chromophores determines the amount of energy necessary to achieve the desired clinical effect.
- The exposure time, or **pulse width,** is determined by the size and location of the target.
- **Thermal relaxation time (TRT)** is the time for target chromophores to release at least 64% of the energy absorbed to surrounding tissue (cool down to one time constant of tissue heating, or 36%).
  - Exceeding the TRT results in no effect, a need for more energy, or a potential for damaging surrounding tissues as a result of excessive heat.

- **Ideal pulse time (IPT)** is the amount of time within the TRT to selectively absorb energies in target chromophores while protecting surrounding tissues.

TIP: The IPT is usually best at half the TRT.

- **Thermal effects**
  - Once light is absorbed in the selected tissue it is converted to **heat.**
  - Different energies result in different therapeutic effects, such as wound healing, coagulation, or vaporization.

LASER APPLICATIONS

VASCULAR LESIONS[1]
- **Laser therapy objectives**
  - Raise blood temperature to more than 70° C
  - Damage intima/internal lining
  - Contract type I collagen surrounding vessel
  - Achieve flow stasis
- **Common wavelengths** (for hemoglobin and oxyhemoglobin)
  - Potassium titanyl phosphate (KTP): 532 nm
  - Pulsed dye: 585 nm
  - Neodymium: yttrium aluminum garnett (Nd:YAG): 1064 nm
- **KTP (532 nm)**
  - Solid state laser
  - 1064 nm Nd:YAG wavelength sent through a frequency doubling crystal, KTP halves the wavelength to 532 nm.
  - Slightly more shallow penetration than pulsed dye
  - Better selection of pulse widths
  - High absorption in blood
  - Ideal for treatment of rosacea, port wine stains, and telangiectasia up to 1 mm
  - Minimal purpura when used properly
- **Pulsed dye (585-600 nm)**
  - Commonly used for rosacea and port wine stains: 20 to 100 μm
  - Particular wavelength achieved by exciting dye with a flashlamp
  - High absorption in blood at short pulse width results in purpuric response, which resolves in 7-10 days
  - 0.5-1.0 mm depth of penetration at 585 nm
- **Nd:YAG (1064 nm)**
  - Sees target chromophores in shades of gray in the near IR
  - Absorbed in darkest target at the selected pulse-width (size)
  - Uses higher energies (3-15 times more) than visible wavelengths
  - Deepest penetrating laser—up to 8 mm in tissue
  - Ideal for treatment of rosacea, port wine stains, telangiectasia, and venulectasia—100 μm to 2 mm

PIGMENTED SKIN LESIONS[1]

- Examples: Solar lentigines, café au lait, and nevus of Ota
- Target chromophore of **melanin**
  - Effective absorption of melanin spans the visible spectrum.
  - Longer wavelengths isolate melanin absorption from hemoglobin and are desirable for pigmented lesions.
- KTP (532 nm), ruby (694 nm), alexandrite (755 nm), both Q-switched and pulsed modes
- Intense pulsed light (IPL) with a range of 400-1400 nm may be most commonly used
- Energy absorbed in melanin, which is fragmented and naturally exfoliated

HAIR REDUCTION[1]

- **Melanin** is the primary chromophore targeted in laser hair reduction.
  - Hyperpigmentation and hypopigmentation are potential side effects with visible wavelengths and darker skin types.
- Multiple treatments are required depending on growth cycles at the treatment site.
- Follicles must be treated while in the **anagen** cycle.
- No plucking, tweezing, or waxing one month before treatment.
- **Common lasers**
  - Alexandrite (755 nm)
  - Diode (810 nm, 900 nm)
  - Nd:YAG (1064 nm)
  - Intense pulsed light (400-1400 nm)
- Nd:YAG (1064 nm) is the safest for darker skin types.

TATTOO REMOVAL[1]

- Q-switched laser energy penetrates to the level of the upper papillary dermis and selectively targets ink particles by color.
- Shock waves fragment the ink into pieces that can be cleared by phagocytosis.
- Four to eight treatments may be necessary for resolution depending on type, location, and color of the tattoo.
- Allow 8 to 12 week treatment intervals.
- **Treatment guidelines:**
  - Dark inks (black, blue, and brown): 1064 nm
  - Red inks (orange, purple, red): 532 nm
  - Green inks (green): 650 nm

> TIP: The largest spot size that produces sufficient energies should be used for best treatment results.

NONABLATIVE RESURFACING[4]

- Wavelength ranges from 532 to 1540 nm
- Goal is to deposit heat to create a wound-healing response in the dermal and epidermal layers *without creating traumatic wound*
- Stimulates collagen synthesis
- Reduces appearance of fine wrinkles (20% to 30% reduction according to some studies)

ABLATIVE RESURFACING[4]

■ **Histologic effects**
- *Induced thermal injury* removing layers of the epidermis and dermis with resultant wound healing
- Reepithelialization through proliferation of keratincytes
- Increased collagen synthesis
- Skin contraction caused by shrinkage of type I collagen

■ **Carbon dioxide (CO_2) laser**
- Gas laser: 10,600 nm
- Chromophore is **water**
- Pulsed or continuous modes
- Improvement of both fine and deep wrinkles
- Side effects: Prolonged erythema, hypopigmentation, and hyperpigmentation
- 10,600 nm (CO_2) laser is the longest wavelength laser used in medicine and therefore has the highest inherent thermal effect
- Ablation threshold approximately 5.0 J/cm^2

■ **Erbium: yttrium aluminum garnet (Er:YAG) laser**
- Solid state laser: 2940 nm
- Chromophore is **water** (highest)
- Ablation independent of thermal damage
- Can be used on areas of very thin skin, such as tip of nose and neck
- Can add thermal effect by using subablative pulse of energy following ablative pulses
- Ablation threshold approximately 0.7 J/cm^2
- Laser of choice for microlaser peel and deeper resurfacing

KEY POINTS

✔ Laser light is coherent, monochromatic, and collimated.
✔ The absorption of laser energy lends to the desired (or undesired) effect.
✔ The ideal pulse time is usually half the thermal relaxation time.
✔ The pulsed dye laser is most commonly used in the treatment of port wine stains and rosacea.
✔ The Nd:YAG laser is most commonly used in the treatment of spider veins.
✔ Hair follicles must be treated while they are in the anagen (active) phase.
✔ Different tattoo pigments require different lasers and wavelengths for sucessful treatment.

REFERENCES

1. Hoopman JE. Lasers in Medicine. Dallas: University of Texas Southwestern Medical Center, 2000.
2. Safe use of lasers in healthcare facilities, ANSI Z136.3, Washington DC: American National Standards Institute, 2005.
3 Goldman MP, Fitzpatrick RE. Cutaneous Laser Surgery: The Art and Science of Selective Photothermolysis, 2nd ed. St Louis: Mosby, 1999.
4. Kenkel JM. Personal communication. University of Texas Southwestern Medical Center, Department of Plastic Surgery. Dallas.

8. Anaesthesia

George Broughton II*

LOCAL ANAESTHETICS[1-3]

- **Chemistry:** An aromatic moiety connected to a substituted amine through an ester or an amide linkage (Fig. 8-1)

Ester bond: $R-\langle\rangle-C-O-CH_2-R'$ Amide bond: (structure with CH_3, CH_3, $NH-C-R$)

Fig. 8-1 Two different bonds of local anaesthetics.

MECHANISM OF ACTION

- Local anaesthetics block conduction in nerves by impairing propagation of the action potential in axons.
  - No effect on the resting or threshold potential
  - Act at a specific receptor site, (e.g., **sodium channel**)
  - Stability enhanced by adjusting pH of solutions

CLINICAL CHARACTERISTICS

- Differential blockade of nerve fibers—myelinated and smaller nerves are most affected.
- Sequence of clinical anaesthesia is reflected in the involved nerves (Table 8-1).
  - Vasodilation (nerve B)
  - Loss of pain and temperature sensation (nerves A-δ and C)
  - Loss of pressure sensation (nerve A-β)
  - Loss of motor function (nerve A-α)

CLASSES[3,4,6,7] (Table 8-2)

- **Amino-esters**
  - Metabolism by pseudocholinesterase creates short plasma half-life.
  - Product of metabolism includes **para-aminobenzoic acid (PABA),** which is associated with **hypersensitivity** in some people.
  - Examples: Procaine (Novocaine), cocaine, benzocaine, chloroprocaine, and tetracaine (Pontocaine)

---

*The opinions or assertions contained herein are the private views of the author and are not to be construed as official or as reflecting the views of the Department of the Army or the Department of Defense.

Table 8-1 *Classification and Physiologic Characteristics of Nerve Fibers* [4,5]

Nerve Type	Function	Myelin	Diameter (μm)	Conduction Speed (m/sec)
A-α	Motor	Heavy	12-20	70-120
A-β	Touch/pressure	Heavy	5-12	30-70
A-γ	Proprioception/motor tone	Moderate	5-12	30-70
A-δ	Pain/temperature	Moderate	1-4	12-30
B	Preganglionic autonomic (sympathetic)	Light	1-3	14.8
C	Pain/temperature	None	0.5-1	1.2

Table 8-2 *Commonly Available Local Anaesthetics* [5]

Name	Concentration (%)	Onset (min)	Duration (hr)	Maximum Dose (mg/kg)
Ester Class				
Procaine (Novocaine)	1, 2, 10	2-5	0.25-1	7
Chloroprocaine (Nesacaine)	1, 2, 3	6-12	0.5	N/A
Amide Class				
Lidocaine (Xylocaine)	0.5, 1, 1.5, 2	<2	0.5-1	4-5
Lidocaine + epinephrine	0.5, 1, 1.5, 2	<2	2-6	7
Mepivacaine (Carbocaine)	1, 1.5, 2, 3	3-5	0.75-1.5	N/A
Bupivacaine* (Marcaine)	0.25, 0.5, 0.75	5	2-4	2
Bupivacaine + epinephrine	0.25, 0.5, 0.75, 1	0.5	3-7	3
Ropivacaine (Naropin)	0.2, 0.5, 0.75, 1	1-15	2-6	2.5

*Bupivacaine is not approved by the FDA for use in children less than 12 years of age.

■ **Amino-amides**

TIP: Amino-amides have the letter "i" in the prefix.

- Metabolized in the liver
- Elimination half-life: 2-3 hours
- True allergy rare
- Examples: L*i*docaine (Xylocaine), bup*i*vacaine (Marcaine), mep*i*vacaine (Carbocaine), pr*i*locaine (Citanest), et*i*docaine (Duranest), d*i*bucaine, rop*i*vacaine (Naropin)

MIXING (COMPOUNDING)[8]

- Toxicity of a mixture is no greater than that of its individual components.
- Lidocaine (fast acting with short duration) and bupivacaine (longer acting) are a common mixture.
- Mixtures of ester- and amide-type local anaesthetics benefit from different modes of elimination.

EPINEPHRINE[9-11]

TIP: Local anaesthetics that contain epinephrine have red labels or red text.

- **Advantages**
  - Causes vasoconstriction
  - Increases duration of action
  - Decreases bleeding
- **Disadvantages**
  - Increases myocardial irritability
  - May cause tachycardia, hypertension, and arrhythmias
  - Use cautiously in patients with known cardiac disease
- **Concentrations used**
  - Commonly used concentrations are 1:100,000 and 1:200,000 (or 1 mg/100 ml or 1 mg/200 ml, respectively).

CAUTION: Concentrations of epinephrine of 1:200,000 or more are detrimental to survival of delayed skin flaps.[9]

- **Contraindications**
  - **Absolute**
    - ▸ Do not use in penis.
    - ▸ Do not use in any skin flap with limited perfusion.
    - ▸ Do not use in hand when disease processes potentially involve the digital vessels at the base of the proximal phalanx (e.g., infection or trauma).
  - **Relative** _(use cautiously)_
    - ▸ Hypertension (can worsen)
    - ▸ Diabetes (limited cutaneous perfusion may become severely compromised)
    - ▸ Heart disease (myocardium sensitivity to epinephrine may precipitate ischemia, infarct, or both)
    - ▸ Thyrotoxicosis (epinephrine could trigger a thyroid storm)
    - ▸ Certain concomitant uses of drugs
  - **Drug interactions:** The following drug interactions are unlikely with the small volume of local anaesthetics used in most cutaneous surgery; however, these interactions, although rare, have been reported. If larger doses of local anaesthetics with epinephrine are used, caution is indicated in the presence of these drugs.
    - ▸ **MAO inhibitors** may cause a hypertensive crisis when epinephrine is used, because a pool of available endogenous catecholamines is created.
    - ▸ **β-Adrenergic blocking agents** have been reported to cause a serious hypertension-bradycardia crisis in rare instances because of interaction with epinephrine.

EPINEPHRINE USE ON DIGITS[12]
- Small amounts of local anaesthetics with dilute epinephrine are probably safe for digital infiltration or blocks.
- Use dilute solutions such as 1:200,000 or less.
- Do not perform a circumferential block of the digits.
- Block preferentially at the level of the metacarpal heads rather than the digit.
- Use small needles to avoid injuring the vessels.
- Avoid postoperative hot soaks.
- Buffer the anaesthetic to avoid acidic solutions.
- Bandages should not be constrictive or excessively tight.
- Patients should be followed regarding prolonged ischemia, which could require reversal with phentolamine injections or nitroglycerin ointment.
- Avoid using epinephrine in patients with vasospastic, thrombotic, or extreme medical conditions.

TOXICITY[4,13,14]
- **Local hypersensitivity**
  - **Not a toxic effect**
  - Most common *adverse* effect
  - Symptoms: Erythema, urticaria, edema, and dermatitis
- **Central nervous system (CNS)**
  - Prodromal symptoms
    - ▸ Light-headedness, dizziness
    - ▸ Metallic taste in mouth
    - ▸ **Circumoral numbness**
    - ▸ **Tinnitus**
  - Severe toxicity
    - ▸ Grand mal **seizures**
    - ▸ Unconsciousness
- **Cardiovascular**
  - **Bupivacaine** has the greatest cardiac toxicity, especially after inadvertent intravascular injection.
  - Ropivacaine was developed as a long-acting local anaesthetic with less cardiac toxicity.
  - Toxicity varies with agent and the health of the patient's heart.
  - Symptoms:
    - ▸ Hypotension
    - ▸ Tachyarrhythmias or bradyarrhythmias
    - ▸ Ventricular fibrillation
    - ▸ Cardiovascular collapse
- **Idiosyncratic**
  - Pseudocholinesterase deficiency increases the toxicity of esters
  - Anaphylaxis in patients with hypersensitivity to esters (PABA)
  - Liver disease increases toxicity of amides
  - Toxicity because of epinephrine

PREVENTION OF TOXICITY
- Avoid excessive doses.
- Avoid intravascular injection.
- Avoid rapid absorption by adding epinephrine whenever possible.

TIPS: To avoid toxicity, consult the following checklist.
- Always calculate a maximum allowable dosage by weight.
- Mix two anaesthetics to increase volume for administration but also decrease the total individual local anaesthetic given.
- Dilute lidocaine with saline.
- Use solutions with epinephrine whenever possible to increase the maximum allowable dosage.
- Always aspirate before injecting to confirm the needle tip is not intravascular.

MANAGEMENT OF TOXICITY (Table 8-3)

- *Give no more anaesthetic!*
- **CNS**
  - Toxicity is exacerbated by hypercarbia. Treat with hyperventilation and give supplemental oxygen.
  - If the seizure does not terminate, administer intravenously diazepam (Valium) at 0.1 mg/kg or thiopental at 2 mg/kg.
- **Cardiovascular**
  - Hypotension: Administer fluids.
  - Treat arrhythmias according to advanced cardiac life support protocols, except avoid giving more lidocaine.
- **Hypersensitivity reactions**
  - Treat as for anaphylaxis.

Table 8-3 *Treatment of Local Anaesthetic Problems*[5]

Signs and Symptoms	Problem	Treatment
Rash, redness of skin, itchiness, hives, and swelling; later signs: bronchoconstriction, asthmatic breathing, hypotension, and syncope	Allergic reaction	1. Ensure airway patency 2. Administer oxygen 3. Diphenhydramine (Benadryl) 50 mg IV 4. IV fluids for hypotension 5. Vasopressors 6. Bronchodilators
Headache, increased heart rate, increased blood pressure, palpitations, apprehension, sweating, tremors	Reaction to epinephrine	1. Ensure airway patency 2. Administer oxygen 3. Continue to monitor for potential cardiovascular problems
Numbness of the tongue, blurred vision, tinnitus, dizziness, drowsiness, confusion; later signs: Loss of consciousness, tonic-clonic convulsions, CNS depression, respiratory depression, cardiac/respiratory arrest	Toxic overdose	1. Ensure airway patency 2. Administer oxygen 3. Diazepam 50 mg IV 4. Succinylcholine 0.1-0.2 mg/kg IVP followed by intubation 5. If CNS signs, then hyperventilate to bring PCO_2 to 30 mm Hg

TECHNIQUES OF LOCAL AND REGIONAL ANAESTHESIA[3,5,15,16]

> TIP: You can take the sting out of local anaesthetics by adding 1 ml of sodium bicarbonate for
> every 9 ml of local anaesthetic.

- **Peripheral nerve blockade**
  - **Percutaneous infiltration**
    - ▸ Most commonly used for minor surgeries and for suturing lacerations.
    - ▸ Anaesthetic agents are not as effective in the presence of infection. Infected tissues are acidic
      as a result of inflammation, which causes local anaesthetics to largely exist in a charged
      cationic state, thus limiting diffusion across nerve cell membranes.
    - ▸ Local anaesthetics diffuse easily when in a free, uncharged base form.
  - **Nerve block**
    - ▸ Injection of anaesthetic in proximity to a peripheral nerve
    - ▸ Includes digital blocks and rib blocks
- **Intravenous regional anaesthesia**
  - Performed by anaesthesia personnel
  - Injection of a local anaesthetic solution in proximity to a nerve plexus (e.g., brachial)—large
    volumes required
  - **Bier block**
    - ▸ Anaesthetic is injected into a vein of a limb under a <u>double</u> tourniquet.
    - ▸ The anaesthetic persists as long as the tourniquet is inflated (maximum 2 hours).
    - ▸ The tourniquet can safely be deflated after 30 to 45 minutes.
    - ▸ The technique is especially useful for forearm and hand operations.

> TIP: Watch for systemic signs and symptoms of toxicity with Bier blocks that are caused by a
> faulty tourniquet.

- **Central nerve blockade**
  - **Epidural anaesthesia**
    - ▸ Local anaesthetic injected into epidural space
    - ▸ Requires **larger volumes** of anaesthetic
    - ▸ Usually performed as a continuous technique using a catheter
    - ▸ Intended to block sensory functions, not necessarily motor functions
    - ▸ Used extensively in obstetrics
  - **Spinal (intrathecal) anaesthesia**
    - ▸ Inject into subarachnoid space cerebrospinal fluid (CSF).
    - ▸ Use small volume of concentrated solution.
    - ▸ Sensory <u>and</u> motor functions are blocked.
    - ▸ Use for urologic, lower abdominal, pelvic, lower extremity, and some OB/GYN procedures.
  - **Complications**[4,14,17]
    - ▸ **Hypotension:** A complication that results from vasodilation, especially with hypovolemia.
    - ▸ **"Wet" epidural:** Puncturing the dura with a 17-gauge needle results in a 75% chance that a
      young patient develops a postdural puncture headache.

▶ **"High spinal":** A spinal anaesthetic that migrates toward the head (cephalad). If it reaches T1-4, this can block sympathetic innervation to the heart, which results in bradycardia and a decrease in cardiac output. If the anaesthetic travels above C4 (the level of the phrenic nerve), apnea may result.

▶ **Spinal headache:** A consequence of a continued CSF leak through the dura. The low CSF pressure results in traction on pain-sensitive structures, especially in the upright position, and results in headache. Treat with fluids, caffeine, and blood patch.

▶ **Urinary retention:** A very common complication (4.1% of all spinals).

▶ **Spinal cord damage:** A very rare complication, but the primary concern among patients. It is extremely important to document any preexisting neurologic or neuromuscular disorders or chronic back pain **before** the anaesthetic is given.

TOPICAL ANAESTHETICS

TIP: Consider using topical anaesthetic products for children (before administering a subcutaneous injection of anaesthetics) for cleaning and suturing close superficial wounds for superficial wound work in adults (Table 8-4).

Table 8-4   *Topical Anaesthetics*[5]

Betacaine Enhanced Gel, Betacaine Plus
• Topical 4% or 5% lidocaine gel
• Clean skin with alcohol before applying
• No occlusive dressing (like an OpSite) is necessary
• Anaesthetic effect seen 20-30 minutes after application
LMX4, LMX5
• Topical 4% or 5% lidocaine gel
• Clean skin with mild soap and water *(no alcohol)* before applying
• No occlusive dressing (like an OpSite) is necessary
• Anaesthetic effect seen 20-30 minutes after application
• Previously called ELA-Max
EMLA
• A 2.5% lidocaine and 2.5% prilocaine cream
• Occlusion required (like an OpSite)
• Anaesthetic effect seen 60 minutes after application
Viscous Lidocaine
• Comes in 2% or 5% concentrations
• Best on mucosal surfaces (especially useful before injecting local anaesthetic for a block, such as in the mouth)
Cryoanaesthetics
• Using ice to numb the skin just before using an injectable anaesthetic

GENERAL ANAESTHETICS[18]

GOALS
- Analgesia
- Amnesia
- Preservation of vital functions
- Quiet, relaxed field for surgeon

TYPES (USED IN BALANCED ANAESTHESIA)
- **Nitrous oxide** (Table 8-5)
  - Moves rapidly in and out of the body, increasing the volume or pressure within closed body compartments (e.g., pneumothorax, bowel lumen, pressure in sinuses)
- **Halogenated agents** (Table 8-5)
  - Halothane
  - Enflurane
  - Isoflurane
  - Methoxyflurane

Table 8-5   *Characteristics of Inhaled Agents*

Characteristics	Halothane	Enflurane	Isoflurane	Nitrous Oxide
Arrhythmias	Increased	—	—	—
Sensitivity to catecholamines	Increased	Slightly increased	—	—
Cardiac output	Decreased	Decreased then recovers	Decreased	—
Blood pressure	Decreased	Decreased then recovers	Decreased	—
Respiratory reflexes	Inhibited	Inhibited	Initial stimulation	—
Hepatic toxicity	High risk	Some risk	—	—
Anaesthetic	Very Potent	Potent	Potent	Weak
Analgesic	Weak	Some	Some	Potent

BALANCED ANAESTHESIA
- General anaesthesia is essential to surgical practice, because it renders patients analgesic, amnesic, and unconscious while causing muscle relaxation and suppression of undesirable reflexes.
- No single drug is capable of achieving all these effects rapidly and safely. Rather, several different categories of drugs are used to produce *balanced anaesthesia.*
- With a balanced approach, less of each drug is used, and the desired anaesthetic plane is achieved with less toxicity.

STAGES OR PLANES OF ANAESTHESIA

Stage I
Amnesia (begins with induction of anaesthesia and continues to loss of consciousness)
Threshold of pain perception not lowered

Stage II
Delirium (characterized by uninhibited excitation and potentially injurious responses to noxious stimuli, including vomiting, laryngospasm, hypertension, tachycardia, and uncontrolled movement)
Most dangerous stage

Stage III
Surgical anaesthesia (the target "depth" for anaesthesia)
Painful stimulation does not elicit somatic reflexes or deleterious autonomic response (HTN or tachycardia)

Stage IV
Overdose (commonly called "too deep")
Characterized by shallow or absent respirations, dilated and nonreactive pupils, and hypotension that may progress to circulatory failure

PATIENT CLASSIFICATION FOR ANAESTHESIA

AMERICAN SOCIETY OF ANESTHESIOLOGISTS (ASA) SCALE

ASA I: Healthy individual with no systemic disease
ASA II: Individual with one-system, well-controlled disease
ASA III: Individual with multisystem or well-controlled major system disease
ASA IV: Individual with severe, incapacitating, poorly controlled, or end-stage disease
ASA V: Patient in imminent danger of death with or without operation
"E":   Emergency operation qualifier

ADJUNCTS TO ANAESTHETICS
- **Preanaesthetic medications**
  - Anticholinergics
  - Antiemetics
  - Antihistamines
  - Barbiturates
  - Benzodiazepines
  - Opioids

MUSCLE RELAXANTS
- Succinylcholine
- Vecuronium
- Rocuronium

INTRAVENOUS ANAESTHESIA[19,20]

- **Barbiturates:** Short-acting hypnotics that are used for induction (includes thiopental [Pentothal]).
- **Ketamine:** A phencyclidine (PCP) derivative that produces a dissociative state characterized by mental disconnection and profound analgesia. It is commonly used during conscious sedation for dressing changes and in children and emergency room procedures (see later). Adverse effects are nightmares, hallucinations, and emergence delirium in up to 30% of adults.
- **Benzodiazepines:** Used as a sedative-hypnotic adjuvant for induction or premedication (diazepam [Valium] and midazolam [Versed]).
- **Opioids/narcotics:** Interfere with the processing of pain information and produce analgesia and sedation (morphine, meperidine, fentanyl, and sufentanil).

MUSCLE RELAXANTS

- Allows use of less inhaled agents to achieve a patient relaxation
- **Depolarizing muscle relaxant:** Succinylcholine
- **Nondepolarizing agents:** Vecuronium, atracurium

CONSCIOUS SEDATION[16,21,22] (Table 8-6)

- The administration of pharmacologic agents to produce a medically controlled state of depressed consciousness that:
  - Allows protective reflexes to be maintained
  - Retains the patient's ability to maintain a patent airway independently and continuously
  - Permits appropriate responses by the patient
- **Goals** of conscious sedation are to:
  - Facilitate the performance of a procedure
  - Control behavior, including anxiety
  - Return the patient to a state in which safe discharge is possible
- **Candidates**
  - Patients who are ASA I or II are good candidates for conscious sedation in an office or emergency room setting.
  - Infants and elderly patients are good candidates.
  - ASA III and IV patients may have conscious sedation, but it should be performed in a well-controlled environment (e.g., operating room) with constant monitoring by anaesthesia personnel.
- **Documentation** of conscious sedation should include:
  - Patient consent to procedure (consent required from parent or legal guardian with minors)
  - Compliance with dietary precautions that are consistent with accepted norms for general anaesthesia when applicable (e.g., no solids during the preceding 6 hours and nothing but clear fluids up to 4 hours before the procedure)
  - Medical history
  - General health of the patient as noted from a previous physical examination
  - Vital signs during the procedure (heart rate, respiratory rate, and oxygen saturation)
  - Medication used and route administered during the procedure
- **Personnel**
  - A physician responsible for administering the drugs (and possibly treating the patient) and a physician, registered nurse, or nurse anaesthesiologist not involved in the administration of drugs must be present to monitor the patient throughout the procedure.
  - When conscious sedation is performed for an emergency room procedure, the emergency room physician is responsible for the conscious sedation orders, because he or she must be immediately available until the patient is alert.

Table 8-6 *Commonly Used Drugs for Conscious Sedation*[19,22-24]

Medication	Dose	Comments
Sedatives		
Chloral hydrate	50-100 mg/kg po or pr	Up to 1 g/single dose Maximum dose: 2 g
Diazepam	0.1 mg/kg IV (slowly over 3 min) 0.15-0.3 mg/kg po	
Droperidol	0.02-0.05 mg/kg IV (slowly over 3 min)	Onset: 3-10 min Peak: 30 min Duration: 2-4 hr
Ketamine	3-4 mg/kg IM, 1-2 mg/kg IV (slowly over 1 min), or 10 mg/kg pr	Patients should also receive atropine (0.02 mg/kg IV) to decrease secretions
Midazolam	0.05 mg/kg IV (slowly over 3 min); 0.1-0.3 mg/kg IM; 0.5-0.7 mg/kg pr	Frequently given with ketamine to minimize the emergence phenomenon
Narcotics*		
Meperidine	1 mg/kg IM, SQ, or IV (slowly)	
Morphine	0.1 mg/kg IM, SQ, or IV (slowly)	
Butorphanol	0.01-0.02 mg/kg IV (slowly)	
Fentanyl	1-3 μg/kg (0.001-0.003 mg/kg)	Diminished sensitivity to CO_2 stimulation may persist longer than depression of respiratory rate
Antagonists		
Naloxone (for narcotics)	0.01-0.10 mg/kg IV to desired effect	Brief duration of action (30-45 min)
Physostigmine (for anticholinergic syndrome)	0.015-0.025 mg/kg to desired effect	Watch for cholinergic side effects (bradycardia, emesis, cramping, salivation)
Flumazenil (for benzodiazepines)	0.1-0.2 mg (partial antagonism) 0.4-1.0 mg (complete antagonism) Note: Pediatric dose not yet established	Benzodiazepine withdrawal-induced seizures; residual sedation/ hypoventilation

*Not to be used with infants less than 3 months old.
IM, Intramuscularly; *IV,* intravenously; *po,* per os (by mouth); *pr,* per rectum; *SQ,* subcutaneously.

■ **Intraoperative assessment**
- Continuous monitoring of appropriate parameters such as oxygen saturation, pulse rate, and blood pressure (discretion used for monitoring respiratory rate and cardiac rhythm)
- Documenting the vital signs by appropriate frequency during the procedure (frequency generally determined by type and amount of medication administered, length of the procedure, and general condition of the patient)
- Complete documentation of the procedure, medications, their effect, and any untoward incidents required

KEY POINTS

✔ The maximum safe dose of lidocaine without epinephrine is 4 mg/kg and with epinephrine is 7 mg/kg.

✔ The safe dose of epinephrine to be used in a delayed skin flap is 1:200,000.

✔ Loss of temperature sensation accompanies safe and adequate analgesia from local anaesthetic.

✔ Only the amino-ester class of local anaesthetics are associated with a true allergic reaction from the by-product of metabolism (PABA)

✔ Halothane is a general anaesthetic most associated with cardiac arrhythmias.

✔ Conscious sedation requires meticulous documentation in the clinic procedure room or in the emergency room.

REFERENCES

1. Covino BG. Local anesthesia. N Engl J Med 286:975-983, 1972.
2. Butterworth JF IV, Strichartz GR. Molecular mechanisms of local anesthesia: A review. Anesthesiology 72:711-734, 1990.
3. Troullos ES. Local anesthetics: A review of their pharmacology and clinical use. Compendium 8:774, 776, 1987.
4. Vaughan TA, Burt J. Local anesthetics. SRPS 9:1-11, 1999.
5. Broughton G. Clinical Survival Guide for Nurse Practitioner Students. San Antonio: Compass Publishing, LP, 2004, p 476.
6. Capogna G, Celleno D, Laudano D, et al. Alkalinization of local anesthetics. Which block, which local anesthetic? Reg Anesth 20:369-377, 1995.
7. Candido KD, Winnie AP, Covino BG, et al. Addition of bicarbonate to plain bupivacaine does not significantly alter the onset or duration of plexus anesthesia. Reg Anesth 20:133-138, 1995.
8. de Jong RH, Bonin JD. Mixtures of local anesthetics are no more toxic than the parent drugs. Anesthesiology 54:177-181, 1981.
9. Reinisch J, Myers B. The effect of local anesthesia with epinephrine on skin flap survival. Plast Reconstr Surg 54:324-327, 1974.
10. Wilhelmi BJ, Blackwell SJ, Miller JH, et al. Do not use epinephrine in digital blocks: Myth or truth? Plast Reconstr Surg 107:393-397, 2001.
11. Wu G, Calamel PM, Shedd DP. The hazards of injecting local anesthetic solutions with epinephrine into flaps: Experimental study. Plast Reconstr Surg 62:396-403, 1978.
12. Denkler K. A comprehensive review of epinephrine in the finger: To do or not to do. Plast Reconstr Surg 108:114-124, 2001.
13. Chen AH. Toxicity and allergy to local anesthesia. J Calif Dent Assoc 26:683-692, 1998.
14. Knudsen K, Beckman Suurkula M, Blomberg S, et al. Central nervous and cardiovascular effects of i.v. infusions of ropivacaine, bupivacaine and placebo in volunteers. Br J Anaesth 78:507-514, 1997.
15. Salinas FV, Liu SS. Spinal anaesthesia: Local anaesthetics and adjuncts in the ambulatory setting. Best Pract Res Clin Anaesthesiol 16:195-210, 2002.
16. Bitar G, Mullis W, Jacobs W, et al. Safety and efficacy of office-based surgery with monitored anesthesia care/sedation in 4778 consecutive plastic surgery procedures. Plast Reconstr Surg 111:150-156; discussion 157-158, 2003.
17. Lau H, Lam B. Management of postoperative urinary retention: A randomized trial of in-out versus overnight catheterization. ANZ J Surg 74:658-661, 2004.
18. Campagna JA, Miller KW, Forman SA. Mechanisms of actions of inhaled anesthetics. N Engl J Med 348:2110-2124, 2003.

19. McCarty EC, Mencio GA, Walker LA, et al. Ketamine sedation for the reduction of children's fractures in the emergency department. J Bone Joint Surg Am 82:912-918, 2000.
20. Choyce A, Peng P. A systematic review of adjuncts for intravenous regional anesthesia for surgical procedures. Can J Anaesth 49:32-45, 2002.
21. Lazzaroni M, Bianchi Porro G. Preparation, premedication and surveillance. Endoscopy 35:103-111, 2003.
22. Scheer B. Conscious sedation. Br Dent J 197:593; discussion 593, 2004.
23. Heinrich M, Wetzstein V, Muensterer OJ, et al. Conscious sedation: Off-label use of rectal S(+)-ketamine and midazolam for wound dressing changes in paediatric heat injuries. Eur J Pediatr Surg 14:235-239, 2004.
24. Holas A. Sedation for locoregional anaesthesia. Adv Exp Med Biol 523:149-159, 2003.

9. Photography for the Plastic Surgeon

Holly P. Smith

BASICS OF STANDARDIZED PHOTOGRAPHY

Photographic documentation serves medicolegal functions and has many educational, research, clinical, and marketing applications. It provides a means to assess surgical success or failure and leads to better communication between the patient and physician. It is one of the most useful tools to the plastic surgeon, but it can also be one of the most fallible. If quality and proper standardizations are not maintained, medical photographs can become misleading and unable to provide accurate photographic documentation.

ELEMENTS OF STANDARDIZED PATIENT PHOTOGRAPHY

A routine standardized procedure saves time, because decisions are determined by existing rules.[1] Standardization requires planning, a systematic approach, adherence to protocols, and attention to detail.[2,3]

- **Use a standardized series** (a predetermined set of photographs per procedure) to ensure that the same views are photographed each time.
- **Use Cardiff scales of reproduction with 35 mm film.**[4]
  - Advocates using a lens with focal length equal to at least twice the diagonal of the image plane to avoid unwanted image distortion
  - Controls magnification and perspective and ensures standardization among photographs taken by different photographers
- Use a flash for **consistent lighting.**
- **Color management**
  - Use an 18% gray card to balance color.
  - White balance the camera.
- **Attention to detail**
  - Remove jewelry, glasses, and heavy makeup.
  - Keep area clean.
  - Use a background.

VARIABLES WITH DIGITAL CAMERAS

- **Camera type**
  - Digital single lens reflex (SLR) with interchangeable lenses
  - Digital compact with zoom lens
- **Method of focusing and positioning**
  - Automatic focus using anatomic regions for positioning
  - Manual focus using set distances and focal lengths

NOTE: For clinical settings, a digital SLR camera with interchangeable, fixed focal length lenses is highly recommended. This allows for setting the distance on the lens and ensures an accurate and reproductive focal length. Choose a set meter on the lens and achieve focus by moving the camera closer to or farther from the subject. This will ensure consistent comparative views when photographing a patient over periods of time.

NOTE: In an operative setting where comparative views are not a priority, a compact camera with a swivel body or a twist LCD enables better flexibility. Cameras with bodies that swivel are especially useful for taking pictures directly over a supine or prone patient.

TERMINOLOGY

APERTURE
Aperture *refers to the size of the adjustable opening (iris) of a lens that determines the amount of light falling onto the film or sensor.*
- The size of the opening is measured using an *f-number* or *f-stop* (f 8, f 11, etc.).
- Because f-numbers are fractions of the focal length, larger f-numbers represent smaller apertures.
- The smaller the aperture, the greater the depth of field.

SHUTTER SPEED
Shutter speed *determines how long the iris of the camera is open to expose the film or sensor to light (e.g., a shutter speed of 1/125s will expose the sensor for 1/125th of a second).*
- Electronic shutters act by switching on the light-sensitive photodiodes of the sensor for as long as requested by the shutter speed.

DEPTH OF FIELD
Objects within a certain range behind or in front of the main focus point appear sharp. Depth of field *refers to the distance between the closest and farthest in-focus area of a photograph (also called the* focal range*).*
- Depth of field is affected by the aperture, subject distance, focal length, and film or sensor format.
- The smaller the aperture, the greater the depth of field.

FOCAL LENGTH
Focal length *is the distance in millimeters from the optical center of the lens to the focal point, which is located on the sensor or film.*
- The longer the focal length, the narrower the field of view.
- The shorter the focal length, the larger the field of view.

LENSES
Camera lenses are categorized **normal, telephoto,** *and* **wide angle,** *according to focal length and film size.*
- **Normal:** When the focal length of a lens is close to the diagonal measurement of the film/sensor's format, the lens is said to be *normal.* For example, 43.27 mm is the length of the diagonal in a 35 mm (35 mm $\times$ 24 mm) film plane. The closest equivalent lens is 50 mm. A 50 mm lens has a field of view of 46 degrees.
- **Wide angle:** When the focal length is shorter than the film/sensor's diagonal, the lens is *short* or *wide angle.* For example, using a 20 mm lens with a 35 mm film plane is wide angle. A 20 mm lens has a field of view of 94 degrees.

- **Telephoto:** When the focal length of a lens is longer than the film/sensor's diagonal, the lens is *long* or *telephoto*. For example, using a 105 mm lens with a 35 mm film plane is telephoto. A 105 mm lens has a field of view of 23 degrees.

NOTE: On some digital cameras, an equivalent lens will have a much smaller focal length, because the image sensors are much smaller than 35 mm.

SINGLE LENS REFLEX
A single lens reflex camera of 35 mm or medium format has a system of mirrors that shows the user the image precisely as the lens renders it.

THROUGH THE LENS (TTL)
A through-the-lens metering system has a light-sensitive mechanism in the camera body that measures exposure from the image light passing through the lens.

DIGITAL TERMINOLOGY

RESOLUTION
A measurement of the pixel count of an image, given either as pixels per inch (ppi), or as total pixels.
- Digital cameras capture images using a sensor. The resolution is calculated by multiplying the pixels captured along the width and length of the sensor.
- The amount of resolution one needs can be determined by output needs. Images for use on the Internet or for PowerPoint presentations do not need as much resolution as images intended for output to a printer.

TIP: Increased resolution is not always better. Match your resolution to your output needs. The higher the resolution, the larger the file size, and the more storage is needed. This can become costly and slow down software applications and file transfer time.

RECOMMENDED RESOLUTION ACCORDING TO OUTPUT
- 72 ppi for Internet and e-mail
- 72-150 ppi for PowerPoint presentations
- 300 ppi for print publications

TIP: One way to estimate how much resolution is necessary for printing is to multiply the size of the image you want by 300 ppi (the standard for photographic quality) (Table 9-1).

Table 9-1 *How to Estimate Resolution Needed for Printing*

Print Size (Inches)	Multiply by 300	Resolution Needed (Pixels)
3 × 4	3(300) × 4(300)	900 × 1200
5 × 7	5(300) × 7(300)	1500 × 2100
8 × 10	8(300) × 10(300)	2400 × 3000

CAMERA SENSOR

A camera sensor is similar to a computer chip that senses light focused on its surface. It consists of an array of pixels that collect photons.

- The two most popular sensors in digital cameras are the charged couple device **(CCD)** and the complementary metal oxide semiconductor **(CMOS)**.

STORAGE CARDS

- Storage cards perform the function that film does in conventional cameras. They are removable drives that store captured data.
- The most commonly used storage drive at this time is the Compact Flash.
  - Compact Flash II / Micro drive
  - Compact Flash I
  - Memory Stick
  - Secure Digital
  - SmartMedia
  - MultiMedia Card
  - Memory Stick Duo
  - xD-Picture Card
  - Reduced Size MultiMedia Card

IMAGE COMPRESSION

- Compressing image files is sometimes necessary to reduce file size.
- The larger the resolution of a digital image the larger the file size, which can make demands on storage.
- Compressing the data is important if a lot of images need to be stored, or if they are to be published on the Internet.
- There are two compression types
  - **Lossless** doesn't lose any image data
  - **Lossy** reduces the image data each time it is saved

FILE TYPES

- Digital images may be saved as different file types.
  - **JPEG (Joint Photographic Expert Group)**
    - ▸ One of the most universally used formats—compatible with browsers, viewers, and image editing software
    - ▸ Lossy compression
    - ▸ *Considered the best compression file type for photographs*
  - **Raw**
    - ▸ The unprocessed original image as it comes off the sensor before in-camera processing
    - ▸ Similar to a negative in film photography
  - **TIFF (Tagged Image File Format)**
    - ▸ Universal image format compatible with most image editing viewing programs
    - ▸ Lossless uncompressed format that produces no artifacts commonly seen with other image formats such as JPEG

NOTE: Although the TIFF and RAW formats preserve image quality better, they are not practical for storing many files. Resaving often in a JPEG format degrades an image, which becomes noticeable over time. For images that are resaved often, work from a copy of the image rather than the original.

WHAT TO LOOK FOR IN A DIGITAL CAMERA

DIGITAL VERSUS OPTICAL ZOOM

- **Digital zoom** takes a part of the scene and interpolates data to fit on the CCD sensor plane.
  - It mimics a greater zoom without gaining any image detail.
  - It often results in a blurry and pixilated image.
- **Optical zoom** changes the amount of the scene falling on the CCD sensor.
  - Information is not interpolated and can be enlarged and cropped with good results.
  - A 3× optical zoom gives a focal length of 35-105 mm, which is the minimum necessary for photographing the face and body.

VIEWFINDERS

The viewfinder is the window you look through to compose a scene.[5]

- **Viewfinders**
  - **Optical viewfinder on a digital compact camera**
    - ▸ The optical viewfinder is positioned above the camera lens so what you see through the optical viewfinder is different from what the lens projects onto the sensor.
    - ▸ This type of sensor has parallax error which can make framing inaccurate when photographing close-ups.
  - **Optical viewfinder on a digital SLR camera (TTL)**
    - ▸ These viewfinders use a mirror and a prism to show what the lens will project on the sensor.
    - ▸ This type of viewfinder does not have parallax errors.
  - **LCD on a digital compact camera (TTL)**
    - ▸ An LCD shows in real time what is projected onto the sensor by the lens.
    - ▸ An LCD does not have parallax errors but does shorten battery life, and it can be difficult to see LCD screens in bright sunlight conditions.
  - **Electronic viewfinder (EVF) on a digital compact camera (TTL)**
    - ▸ An electronic viewfinder shows in real time what is projected onto the sensor by the lens.
    - ▸ It simulates in an electronic way the effect of the (superior) optical TTL viewfinders found on digital SLRs and doesn't suffer from parallax errors.
    - ▸ EVF allows accurate framing but can shorten battery life.

VIDEO

- Many consumer cameras come with digital video capability.
- Although video resolutions are small and the recording time depends on the size of storage, video can nevertheless be useful for relaying information between physicians and for media presentations.

FLASHES

- On-camera flash
- Hot shoe connection: User has more flash and remote synchronization options
- Flash synchronization port on camera: Multiple flash devices may be added

MAGNIFICATION

- The Westminster scales of reproduction established the principle of standardizing clinical photograph magnification.[6] The Cardiff scales of reproduction revised this scale because of the change in size of the average person.[4]
- Focal lengths provided throughout the series are intended for photographing in a clinical setting. They are also intended for 35 mm film and higher-end digital SLR cameras with interchangeable fixed lenses whose CCD sensor is equal in size to 35 mm film.
- If using a camera with a CCD sensor smaller than 35 mm film, the focal length modifier can be determined by dividing the 35 mm plane (43.3 mm) by the digital camera's sensor diagonal. The size of the sensor usually can be found in the camera's literature supplied by the manufacturer. The sensors on most consumer digital cameras are 1.5 times smaller than 35 mm film.
  - For instance, a 50 mm lens used on a digital camera with a focal length modification of 1.5 is equivalent to a 75 mm lens.
- It is important to correct for disparities in focal lengths, because they can make dramatic differences, especially in comparative views[4] (Fig. 9-1).

HEAD POSITIONING

The **Frankfort plane** is used as a reference line for correct head positioning for x-ray films and has been used by physicians as a standard for head alignment when photographing the face. Some physicians choose to use the natural horizontal facial plane for alignment[1] (Fig. 9-2).

- **Frankfort plane**

Horizontal plane that transverses the top of the tragus (external auditory canal) across the infraorbital rim[7]
  - Can cause noticeable changes in jaw definition and submental soft tissue[8]
- **Natural horizontal facial line**

Achieved when the patient looks straight ahead as if looking into a mirror at eye level.[9]
  - Preferred for rhinoplasty surgery
  - Used in patients who have low-set ears[9]
- **Positioning**
  - Anatomically correct (top of head should be nearest the top of photograph)
  - Arms and hands: Exception to anatomic rule
  - Photographs of the location should be taken in addition to close-ups for accurate perspective and proportion
- **Oblique variables**
  - Some physicians prefer the tip of the nose to touch the side of the far cheek for a rhinoplasty series, whereas others want the dorsum of the nose to visually touch the medial eye (Fig. 9-3).
- **The true lateral**
  - Photographing the head overrotated or underrotated in lateral views is a common mistake (Fig. 9-4) but one that can be corrected easily by viewing straight across the two oral commissures[10] (Fig. 9-5).

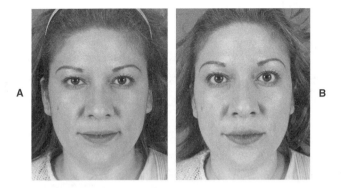

Fig. 9-1 Image **A** was created using a 105 mm lens 1:10. Image **B** was created with a 50 mm lens 1:10, which shows the lens distortion called a *barrel distortion*.

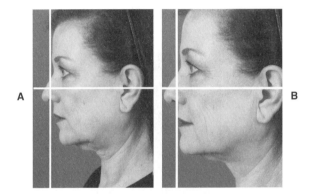

Fig. 9-2 Image **A** demonstrates the downfall to using the Frankfort plane in which neck retraction overemphasizes the degree of submental soft tissue. Image **B** shows the patient in the natural horizontal facial plane.

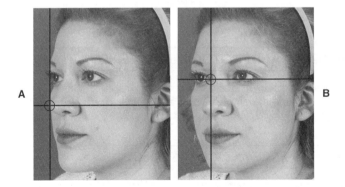

Fig. 9-3 For oblique views some physicians prefer the tip of the nose to touch the side of the far cheek for a rhinoplasty series **(A)**, whereas others want the dorsum to visually touch the medial eye **(B).**

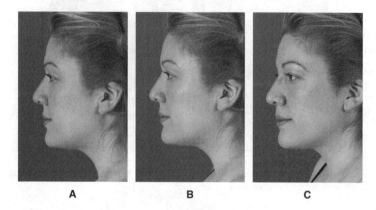

Fig. 9-4   Underrotation of the lateral view **(A)**, true lateral **(B)**, and overrotation of the lateral view **(C)**.

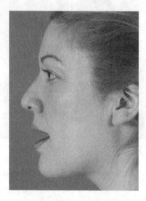

Fig. 9-5   A true lateral image may be obtained by viewing straight across the two oral commissures to verify correct rotation.

STANDARDIZED FACE PHOTOGRAPHIC SERIES (Fig. 9-6)

- Careful attention should be given to any tilting of the head that can distort the view.
- It is helpful to check earlobe symmetry from the anterior view to determine straightness of the head before photographing.[9]

STANDARDIZED FACE/NECK LIFT SERIES

- The contour of the neck can vary greatly depending on head and shoulder positions.
- Make sure that the head is in the standard anatomic position and that the patient is sitting straight.

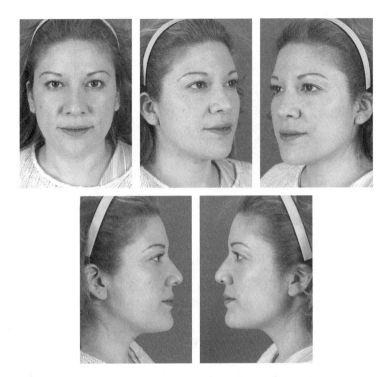

Fig. 9-6   Overview of standardized face series and set distances. Some of the photographs can be eliminated depending on the particular procedure performed.

- Any degree of neck flexion or head retraction can greatly enhance the submental fat at the jowl line. Conversely, neck extension can improve the jowl line.[8]
- A full-face series is photographed at 1 m with a 105 mm lens.

KEY POINTS FOR PHOTOGRAPHING FACE AND NECK SERIES (see Fig. 9-6)

- Photograph vertically.
- Photograph from top of hairline to sternal notch.
- Camera should be parallel with subject and positioned at midpoint of face (usually the nose).
- Ask patient to relax face and to not smile.
- Remove any distracting jewelry or heavily applied makeup.
- Fold down turtlenecks and turn collars away from neck.
- Pull hair back with neutral-colored headband.
- For oblique views, line the radix of the nose to touch the medial part of the opposite eye (see Fig. 9-3).

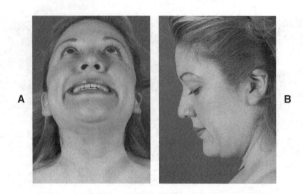

Fig. 9-7   View to show platysmal banding (teeth gritting) **(A)**. A reading view accentuates submental fat **(B)**.

SUPPLEMENTAL FACE/NECK VIEWS

■ When photographing for a neck or face lift series, views are typically added to show platysmal banding (teeth gritting), and a reading view accentuates submental fat as shown in Fig. 9-7.[11]

STANDARDIZED UPPER BROW/EYE SERIES

■ When photographing the eyes and brow, pay close attention to lower and upper lid excess, scleral show, ectropion, and upper lid hooding.

KEY POINTS FOR PHOTOGRAPHING BROW AND EYE SERIES

- Photograph horizontally.
- The close-up of the brow should extend below the lower crease of the lower eyelids to slightly above the hairline (Fig. 9-8, *A*).
- Ask patient to relax the brow while gazing upward (Fig. 9-8, *C*).
- Eyes should gaze downward to reveal any excess lower lid fat (Fig. 9-8, *D*).
- Make sure interpupillary line is horizontal in all views.

STANDARDIZED LASER/CHEMICAL PEEL SERIES (Fig. 9-9)

KEY POINTS FOR PHOTOGRAPHING LASER/CHEMICAL PEEL SERIES

- Remove heavy makeup.
- Close-up, oblique cheek views are photographed vertically at jaw line to slightly above eyebrow at 0.6 m.
- Lateral photographs taken further back (0.8 m) show tonal changes in the skin, if any, from cheek to jaw to neck.
- For a chemical peel of the chest area, an additional view is taken at 1 m as shown in the bottom of Fig. 9-9.

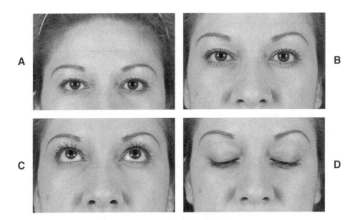

Fig. 9-8 When photographing the eyes and brow, these photographs are taken in addition to the standard face/neck lift series. Image **A** was photographed at 0.8 m. Images **B, C,** and **D** were photographed horizontally at 0.6 m with a 105 mm lens.

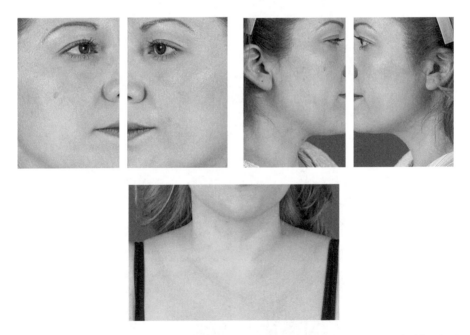

Fig. 9-9 Laser/chemical peel series. These photographs are taken in addition to the standard face/neck lift series. Close-ups are photographed at 0.6 m and 0.8 m with a 105 mm lens.

STANDARDIZED LIP SERIES (Fig. 9-10)

KEY POINTS FOR PHOTOGRAPHING THE STANDARDIZED LIP SERIES

- Remove lipstick and liners.
- Inferior philtral column should intersect cheek on opposite side in oblique view.
- Lips should be slightly parted and relaxed.

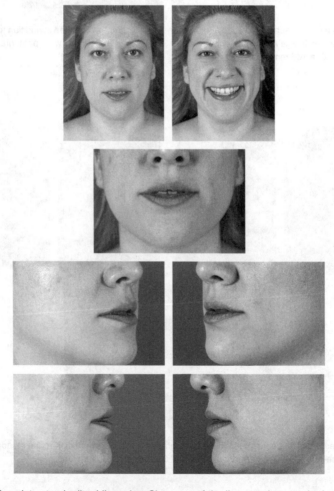

Fig. 9-10   Complete standardized lip series. Close-ups of the lips are photographed at 0.6 m with a 105 mm lens, whereas the full face is photographed at 1 m.

STANDARDIZED RHINOPLASTY/FACIAL FRACTURE SERIES (Fig. 9-11)

- The nose is often one of the most difficult series to photograph.
- It is often necessary to make small adjustments to the series.
- The oblique preference must be decided before photographing.
- The series can be used for facial fractures and for Mohs' reconstruction using forehead flaps or nasolabial flaps.

KEY POINTS FOR PHOTOGRAPHING THE STANDARDIZED RHINOPLASTY SERIES

- Photograph close-up views horizontally.
- Make sure camera is parallel to subject, focused on the midpoint (nose), and that a horizontal line can be drawn through the lower lateral eyes perpendicular to the dorsum.
- Line the tip of the nose between the eyebrows in the full basal view (Fig. 9-11, *A*). You may need to make adjustments for this view if the patient has low tip projection or a large upper lip that blocks the alar area.
- In the half basal view, set the tip of the nose just below the eyes (Fig. 9-11, *B*).
- Ask patient to relax face and to not smile.
- Remove any distracting jewelry.
- Pull hair back with neutral-colored headband.

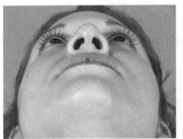
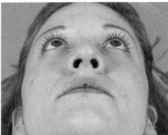
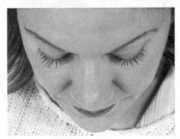

Fig. 9-11 Standardized rhinoplasty series. These photographs are taken in addition to the standard face/neck lift series. Close-up views are photographed with a 105 mm lens at 0.8 and 0.6 m.

SUPPLEMENTAL RHINOPLASTY VIEWS

- If the patient is having a depressor septi release, additional lateral and anterior views of the patient smiling are photographed (Fig. 9-12).
- A cephalic view is helpful to show nasal deviations[12] (Fig. 9-13).

STANDARDIZED BODY SERIES

- Contour and muscle structure can vary greatly depending on the positioning of the feet. Feet should always be parallel with weight distributed evenly[13] (Fig. 9-14).
- The body is photographed with a 50 mm lens at 1 m.

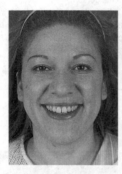 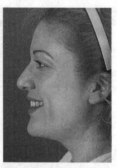

Fig. 9-12   Additional lateral and anterior views needed if the patient is having a depressor septi release.

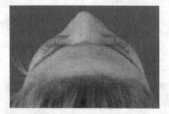

Fig. 9-13   A cephalic view is helpful to show nasal deviations.

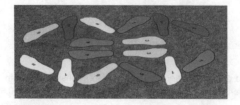

Fig. 9-14   For ease of positioning, place cut-out feet on the floor for the patient as a standing reference.

KEY POINTS FOR PHOTOGRAPHING THE BODY SERIES (Fig. 9-15)

- Photograph body vertically.
- Ask patient to distribute weight evenly between legs.
- Camera should be parallel with subject and positioned at midpoint of body (usually the abdomen).
- Legs should be set at hip width.
- Set knees straight, feet parallel with each other.
- Hands may be folded across breast area but no higher.
- Have patient relax abdomen.
- Use generic underwear.
- Photograph arms horizontally with elbows bent at 90 degrees and hands forward.
- Remove watches and jewelry.

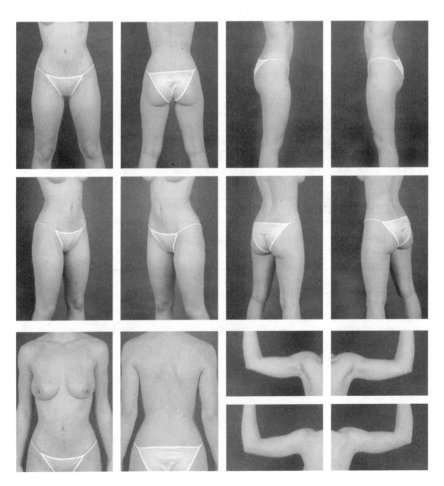

Fig. 9-15 Standardized body series.

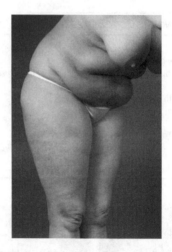

Fig. 9-16   The diver's view is an oblique view with the patient folded over while relaxing the abdomen.

SUPPLEMENTAL BODY CONTOURING SERIES

■ The diver's view is sometimes photographed to evaluate skin laxity[11] (Fig. 9-16).

STANDARDIZED BREAST SERIES (Fig. 9-17)

■ The breast series is photographed with a 50 mm lens at 1 m.

KEY POINTS FOR PHOTOGRAPHING THE BREAST SERIES

- Photograph horizontally.
- Photograph above shoulders and below navel for reference and proportion.
- Camera should be parallel with subject and positioned at midpoint of body (usually the areolas).
- Ask patient to relax shoulders.
- Reductions, mastopexies, and reconstructions should be photographed with arms positioned behind the body.
- The bottom set of photographs in Fig. 9-17 are specifically for latissimus flap breast reconstruction.
- Have patient remove necklaces, watches, and jewelry.

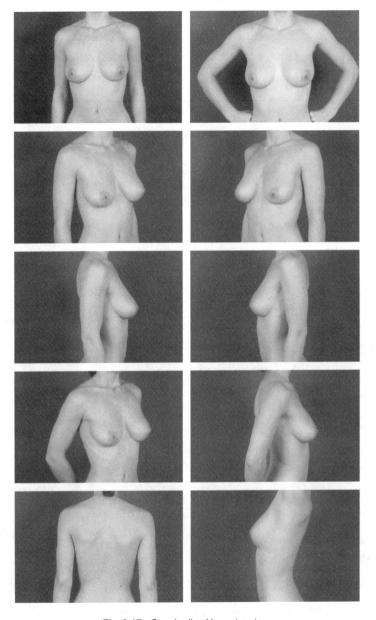

Fig. 9-17 Standardized breast series.

STANDARDIZED TRAM BREAST RECONSTRUCTION AND MALE BODY SERIES

■ The male body series and the TRAM breast reconstruction series are photographed at 1 m with a 50 mm lens.

KEY POINTS FOR PHOTOGRAPHING THE TRAM BREAST RECONSTRUCTION OR MALE BODY SERIES (Fig. 9-18)

- Photograph vertically.
- Photograph above shoulders and below navel.
- Camera should be parallel with subject and positioned at midpoint of body (usually the ribcage).
- Ask patient to relax shoulders.
- Position arms behind body in all views except the anterior and posterior.
- Remove any jewelry.
- Use generic undergarments.

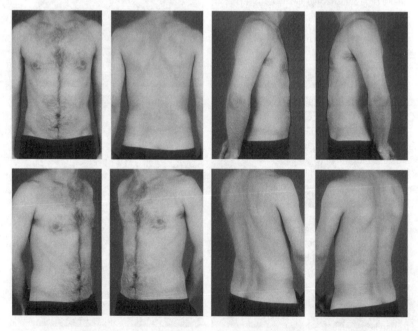

Fig. 9-18   The male body series and the TRAM breast reconstruction series.

PHOTOGRAPHING IN THE OPERATIVE SETTING

There is a lot more control of the lighting and background when photographing in a clinical setting versus an operative setting.

KEY POINTS FOR KEEPING PHOTOGRAPHS CLEAN

- Clear any unnecessary information and elements from photographs that may distract or misrepresent what the photograph intends to show.
- Cover unwanted areas with surgical towels.
- Clean blood off patient and clear surgical tools from frame before photographing.
- Have patient remove makeup if photographing the face.

KEY POINTS FOR KEEPING PHOTOGRAPHS GENERIC

- Use generic undergarments when photographing the body.
- Cover areas of clothing with towels or remove clothing.
- Remove large or distracting jewelry, hats, and sunglasses.
- Cover tattoos if possible.
- Keep a backdrop with you at all times to block out unnecessary people or furniture.
- If it is necessary to have a hand in the photograph, make sure examination gloves are used.
- Remove brand names from rules and equipment if possible.

PHOTOGRAPHIC CONSENT[12,14]

Along with keeping your patients generic, it is also important to maintain anonymity. The following are the standards used for the Health Insurance Portability and Accountability Act (HIPAA). Private or smaller entities may have different requirements.

- **Photographing for treatment**
  - Health care providers may photograph or create audio or video recordings of patients for treatment purposes without obtaining those patients' written authorization.
- **Photographing for nontreatment purposes**
  - If a patient agrees to be photographed or recorded for nontreatment purposes, the patient's written authorization must be obtained.
  - Nontreatment purposes that require patient authorization are:
    - Educational lectures and presentations for health care professionals (e.g., CME)
    - Scientific publications for which another authorization is not already on file
    - Patient education materials
    - Use in broadcast, print, or Internet media for educational or public interest purposes
- According to HIPAA, authorizations are not required if all identifiable patient information is removed from the photograph or recording.

NOTE: Although HIPAA does not require authorization for the use of photographs that have had all identifiable patient information removed, the healthcare provider may be liable for invasion of privacy. Courts have imposed liability primarily when the provider has exploited the patient for commercial benefit.[15]

- Identifiable patient information *cannot* be removed from any full-face or comparable images, which *always* require authorization.
- A photograph or electronic reproduction is considered to identify a patient if it shows the full face of the patient, or if any of the 19 elements of protected health information are present. These elements are:
  - Name
  - Date of birth
  - Address
  - Telephone number
  - Fax number
  - E-mail address
  - Social Security number
  - Medical record number
  - Account number
  - Driver's license number
  - Credit card number
  - Names of relatives
  - Name of employer
  - Health plan beneficiary number
  - Vehicle or other device serial number
  - Internet Universal Resource Locator (URL)
  - Internet Protocol (IP) address
  - Finger or voice prints
  - Date and time of treatment
- It is *not* satisfactory to "black out the eyes." Recognition of a patient applies to all distinguishing features of the face.[1] HIPAA does not specifically address masking the eyes, but it is strongly recommended to obtain a consent form when using any part of the face for purposes other than treatment.
- As standard practice, even if a patient has a photographic consent for nontreatment purpose on file, always contact the patient before potential nontreatment use.

KEY POINTS

✔ Uniformity and standardization are key to producing accurate photographic documentation.
✔ Lack of quality can distort clinical findings and lead to misrepresentation of images.
✔ Successful patient photography begins with a basic familiarity of both digital and conventional 35 mm photography.
✔ Special attention should be given to legal and ethical issues before undertaking any clinical photography.

REFERENCES

1. Grom RM. Clinical and operating room photography. Biomed Photogr 20:251-301, 1992.
2. Roos O, Cederblom S. A standardized system for patient documentation. J Audiov Media Med 14:135-138, 1991.
3. DiBernadino BE, Adams RL, Krause J, et al. Photographic standards in plastic surgery. Plast Reconstr Surg 102:559-568, 1998.
4. Young S. Maintaining standard scales of reproduction in patient photography using digital cameras. J Audiov Media Med 24:162-165, 2001.
5. Bockaert V. Viewfinder, 2005. Available at *www.dpreview.com/learn/?/Glossary/Camera_System/Viewfinder_01.htm*.
6. Williams AR. Clinical and operating room photography. In Vetter JP, ed. Biomedical Photography. Boston: Focal Press, 1992, pp 258-259.
7. Thomas JR, Tardy ME Jr, Przakop H. Uniform photographic documentation in facial plastic surgery. Otolaryngol Clin North Am 13:367-381, 1980.
8. Sommer DD, Mendelsohn M. Pitfalls of nonstandardized photography in facial plastic surgery patients. Plast Reconstr Surg 114:10-14, 2004.
9. Galdino GM, DaSilva D, Gunter JP. Digital photography for rhinoplasty. Plast Reconstr Surg 109:1421-1434, 2002.
10. Davidson TM. Photography in facial plastic and reconstructive surgery. J Biol Photogr Assoc 47:59-67, 1979.
11. Gherardini G. Standardization in photography for body contour surgery and suction-assisted lipectomy. Plast Reconstr Surg 100:227-237, 1997.
12. LaNasa JJ Jr, Smith O, Johnson CM Jr. The cephalic view in nasal photography. J Otolaryngol 20:443-544, 1991.
13. Williams AR. Positioning and lighting for patient photography. J Biol Photogr Assoc 53:131-143, 1985.
14. US Department of Health and Human Services. Standards for privacy of individually identifiable health information (45 CFR parts 160 and 164). Federal Register 65; Dec 28, 2000.
15. Roach WH Jr, ed. Medical Records and the Law. Gaithersburg, MD: Aspen Publishers,1994, pp 207-208.

PART II

Skin and Soft Tissue

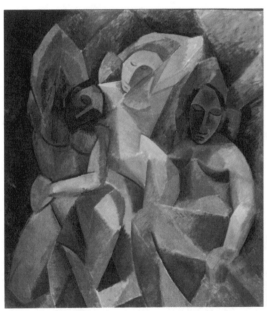

10. Structure and Function of Skin

John L. Burns

SKIN FUNCTIONS

- Largest body organ: 16% total body weight
- Protection: UV, mechanical, chemical, thermal, barrier to microorganisms
- Metabolic: Vitamin D synthesis
- Thermoregulation

ANATOMY OF SKIN (Fig. 10-1 and Table 10-1)

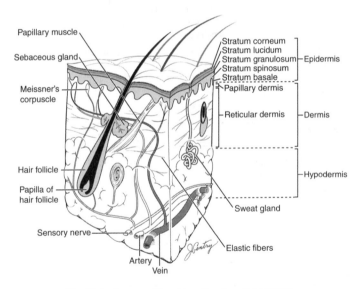

Fig. 10-1   Layers of the skin with adnexal structures.

Table 10-1   *Contents of Skin Layers*

	Cells	Appendages	Functions/Responses
Epidermis	Keratinocyte Melanocyte Langerhans Cell Merkel Cell		Protective barrier Pigmentation Immunity Touch reception
Dermis	Fibroblast		Collagen/elastic fiber, ground substance
	Macrophage Mast cell		Scavenger Allergic response
		Hair follicle Sebaceous gland Eccrine sweat gland Apocrine sweat gland Naked nerve fiber Meissner's, Pacini's, and Krause's corpuscles Blood vessel Lymph vessel	 Sebum Thermoregulation Sweat Pain Pressure, temperature
Hypodermis	Adipocyte		Insulation, energy
Muscle	Striated muscle cell		Movement

EMBRYOLOGY

- **Epidermis:** Derived from **ectoderm**
- **Dermis:** Derived from **mesoderm**
- **Immigrant cells**
  - Melanocytes: Neural crest origin
  - Merkel cells: Neural crest origin
  - Langerhans cells: Mesenchymal origin (from precursor cells of bone marrow)

HISTOLOGY[1,2]

EPIDERMIS (Table 10-2)

- Thickness varies by location, with average thickness being 100 μm (compared to 1500-4000 μm for full-thickness skin).
- **Keratinocyte** is the major cell. Keratinocyte differentiation occurs in 28-45 days, progressing from basal proliferative germinal layer to dead cornified layer.
- **Immigrant cells**
  - Melanocytes: Produce melanin to protect against UV radiation
  - Merkel cells: Slow adapting touch mechanoreceptors in glabrous areas
  - Langerhans cells: Antigen-presenting cells in spinous layer

Table 10-2   *Five Layers of Epidermis*

Layer	Cell Types	Characteristics
Stratum corneum	Nonviable keratinocytes	External barrier: 20-25 layers of stratified squamous keratinocytes that are constantly shed
Stratum lucidum	Nonviable keratinocytes	Translucent transitional layer present only in thick skin, offers additional protection
Stratum granulosum	Marginally viable keratinocytes	Transition zone, 3-4 layers thick, where keratinocytes flatten in their migration to the surface
Stratum spinosum	Viable keratinocytes	Part of malpighian (living) layer, which replaces nonviable cells
Stratum basale	Mitotically active keratinocytes, melanocytes, tactile cells, nonpigmented granular dendrocytes	Single layer in contact with the basement membrane where keratinocytes are regenerated

DERMIS

- The two layers, **papillary** and **reticular,** make up an integrated system of cells, fibrous amorphous connective tissue, neurovascular networks, and dermal appendages.
- **Papillary dermis**
  - Begins at basement membrane
  - Thickness similar to epidermis (100 μm)
  - High content of type III collagen, lesser type I
  - Collagenase activity
  - Mature elastic fibers absent
- **Reticular dermis**
  - Papillary dermis to hypodermis
  - Bulk of dermis (2000-2500 μm)
  - Primarily type I collagen organized into large fibers and bundles
  - Large, mature, bandlike, elastic fibers extend between collagen bundles
  - Elastic and collagen bundles progressively larger toward hypodermis
- **Structural components**[3]
  - **Collagen** (Table 10-3)
    - ▶ Principle building block of connective tissue
    - ▶ One third of total body protein content
    - ▶ Provides tensile strength
    - ▶ Adult skin: 4:1 ratio (type I/III)
    - ▶ Immature scar: 2:1 ratio (type I/III)
    - ▶ Collagen synthesis (Fig. 10-2)
      - ✦ Amino acid (AA) chains produced in fibroblast cytoplasm
      - ✦ Secreted into extracellular matrix in form of *tropocollagen*
      - ✦ 3 polypeptide alpha chains bind to form triple helix configuration
      - ✦ Disarrayed during relaxation and straight with parallel alignment during stretch
  - **Elastin**
    - ▶ Sheets of rubberlike material synthesized from fibroblasts
    - ▶ Precursor from *tropoelastin*

(Text continues on p. 113)

Table 10-3   *Five Types of Collagen*

Type	Structure	Distribution
Type I	Hybrid of two chains. Low in hydroxylysine and glycosylated hydroxylysine	Bone Tendon Skin Dentin Ligament Fascia Arteries Uterus
Type II	Relatively high in hydroxylysine and glycosylated hydroxylysine	Hyaline cartilage Eye tissues
Type III	High in hydroxyproline, contains interchain disulfide bonds	Skin Arteries Uterus Bowel wall
Type IV	High in hydroxylysine and glycosylated hydroxylysine; may contain large globular regions	Basement membrane
Type V	Similar to type IV	Basement membranes Perhaps other tissues

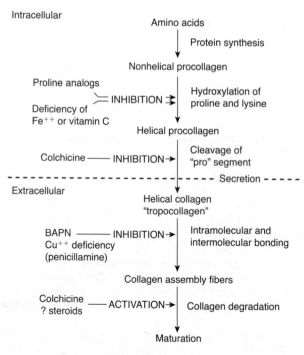

Fig. 10-2   Collagen synthesis.

- ▸ Polymerizes and interweaves with collagen
- ▸ *Fibrillin* needed for elastin deposition and fiber formation
- ▸ Confers stretch and elastic recoil
- ▸ Disruption leads to loss of recoil
- ▸ Fibers decrease with aging
- • **Ground substance**
  - ▸ Amorphous transparent material like semifluid gel
  - ▸ Permits metabolite diffusion
  - ▸ Composed of glycosaminoglycans in the form of hyaluronic acid and proteoglycans

AGING SKIN[4,5,6]

HISTOLOGIC EFFECTS OF AGING (Fig. 10-3 and Table 10-4)

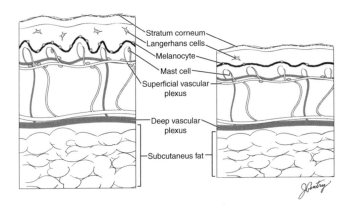

Fig. 10-3 Histology of aging skin. (Aging skin is shown on the right.)

Table 10-4 *Histologic Findings in Aging Skin*

Epidermis	Dermis
Compact laminated stratum corneum	Dermal atrophy
Flattened dermal-epidermal junction	Fibroblasts enlarge and decrease mitotic activity
Fewer layers of keratinocytes	30% reduction in vein cross section
Melanocyte density decreases	Pacini's and Meissner's corpuscles decrease in density by one third
Langerhans cells decrease	

PHOTOAGING (ACTINIC CHANGES) (Table 10-5)
- **Clinically evidenced by:**
  - Rhytids
  - Laxity
  - Pigmentary mottling

Table 10-5 *Histologic Findings in Photoaging*

Epidermis	Dermis
Atrophic and flat	Dermoelastosis
Loss of vertical polarity	*Grenz zone* is characteristic
Thick, ragged basement membrane	Increased ground substance
Pigmentary mottling	

PHYSIOLOGIC EFFECTS OF AGING
- Cell replacement decreases.
- Injury response decreases.
- Barrier function lessens.
- Chemical clearance worsens.
- Sensory perception decreases.
- Immune responsiveness decreases.
- Thermoregulation worsens.
- Vascular responsiveness decreases.
- Sweat production decreases.
- Vitamin D production decreases.

GENETIC DISORDERS OF THE SKIN[7-10]

EHLERS-DANLOS SYNDROME *(CUTIS HYPERELASTICA)*
- Incidence: 1:400,000
- Connective tissue disorder
- Hypermobile joints
- Thin, friable, hyperextensive skin
- Subcutaneous hemorrhages

CUTIS LAXA *(ELASTOLYSIS)*
- Incidence: Only several hundred cases known worldwide
- Degeneration of elastic fibers in the dermis
- Loose, inelastic skin

PSEUDOXANTHOMA ELASTICUM
- Incidence: 1:160,000
- Loose skin
- Degenerated elastic fibers

PROGERIA (HUTCHINSON-GILFORD SYNDROME)

- Incidence: 1:1,000,000
- Growth retardation
- Craniosynostosis, micrognathia
- Baldness
- Prominent ears
- Loss of subcutaneous fat

TIP: Avoid rejuvenation surgery for patients with Ehlers-Danlos syndrome and progeria because of wound healing issues.

Rejuvenating surgery is possible for patients with cutis laxa and pseudoxanthoma elasticum.

KEY POINTS

- ✔ The epidermis is composed of 5 layers, of which the most superficial 2 layers (stratum corneum and stratum lucidum) are composed of nonviable keratinocytes.
- ✔ Collagen provides the tensile strength of the skin.
- ✔ Adult skin contains a 4:1 ratio of type I/type III collagen.
- ✔ There are predictable physiologic and histologic skin changes that occur with age.
- ✔ Cutis laxa and pseudoxanthoma elasticum are the only congenital skin disorders that are responsive to surgical rejuvenation.

REFERENCES

1. Burkitt HG, Young B, Heath JW. Wheater's Functional Histology: A Text and Color Atlas, 3rd ed. New York: Churchill Livingstone, 1993.
2. Fawcett DW, Jensh RP. Bloom & Fawcett: Concise Histology. London: Hodder Arnold, 1997.
3. Gibson T. Physical properties of the skin. In McCarthy JG, ed. Plastic Surgery, vol 1. Philadelphia: WB Saunders, 1990.
4. Gilchrest BA. Age-associated changes in the skin. J Am Geriatr Soc 30:139-143, 1982.
5. Gilchrest BA. Aging of the skin. In Soter NA, Baden HP, eds. Pathophysiology of Dermatologic Diseases. New York: McGraw Hill, 1984.
6. Savin JA. Old skin. Br Med J 283:1422-1423, 1981.
7. Glat PM, Langaker MT. Wound healing. In Aston AJ, Beasley RW, Thorne CMH, eds. Grabb and Smith's Plastic Surgery, 5th ed. Philadelphia: Lippincott-Raven, 1997.
8. Kenedi RM, Gibson T, Daly CH. Bioengineering studies of the human skin. In Jackson SF, Harkness R, Partridge S, et al, eds. Structure and Function of Connective and Skeletal Tissues. London: Butterworths, 1965.
9. Robinson JB, Friedman RM. Wound healing and closure. Sel Read Plast Surg 8(1), 1997.
10. Ross R. Problems in Aesthetic Surgery: Biological Causes and Clinical Solutions. St Louis: Mosby, 1986, pp 49-64.

11. Basal Cell Carcinoma, Squamous Cell Carcinoma, and Melanoma

Danielle M. LeBlanc
Dawn D. Wells

BASAL CELL CARCINOMA (BCC)

DEMOGRAPHICS[1,2]
- BCC is the most common form of skin cancer.
- 95% of cases occur between 40 and 79 years of age.
- In lightly pigmented skin, male/female ratio is 1.5:1.
- In darkly pigmented skin, male/female ratio is 1.3:1.
- Head and neck sites account for 93% of all BCC; 26% of all BCC occur on the nose alone.[2]

RISK FACTORS
- Fitzpatrick skin type (Table 11-1)[3]
- Sun exposure
- Advancing age
- Immunosuppression: AIDS, organ transplant medications
- Carcinogen exposure: UV and ionizing radiation, arsenic, hydrocarbons[4-6]
- Premalignant lesions
  - Nevus sebaceus of Jadassohn
    - ▶ Present at birth on scalp and for face
    - ▶ Well-circumscribed, hairless, yellowish plaque that becomes verrucous and nodular at puberty
    - ▶ 10%-15% malignant degeneration to BCC
- Predisposing conditions
  - Nevoid basal cell syndrome (Gorlin's syndrome)[1,7]
    - ▶ Autosomal dominant inheritance pattern on chromosome 9q22.3–q31

Table 11-1 *Fitzpatrick's Classification of Sun-Reactive Skin Types*

Skin Type	Color	Reaction to First Summer Exposure
I	White	Always burn, never tan
II	White	Usually burn, tan with difficulty
III	White	Sometimes mild burn, tan average
IV	Moderate brown	Rarely burn, tan with ease
V	Dark brown*	Very rarely burn, tan very easily
VI	Black	Do not burn, tan very easily

*Asian Indian, Oriental, Hispanic, or light African descent.
From Fitzpatrick TB. The validity and practicality of sun-reactive skin types I through VI. Arch Dermatol 124:869, 1988.

- ▸ Multiple basal cells, odontogenic keratocysts, palmar and plantar pits, calcification of falx cerebri, bifid ribs, hypertelorism, broad nasal root
- **Xeroderma pigmentosum (XP)**
  - ▸ Autosomal recessive inheritance pattern
  - ▸ Impaired DNA repair mechanism
  - ▸ Intolerance to UV radiation
  - ▸ Multiple epithelial malignancies

RECURRENCE AND METASTASIS
- Risk of new primary 35% at 3 years and 50% at 5 years
- New lesions tend to be same histopathologic type as previous
- Metastasis rare, less than 0.1% incidence overall to lymph nodes, lungs, and bones

BIOLOGY
- Tumors originate from the pluripotential epithelial cells of epidermis and hair follicles (basal keratinocytes) at the dermoepidermal junction.

TYPES OF BASAL CELL CARCINOMAS[1,8-11]
There are **26** identified subtypes that follow certain histologic patterns (Fig. 11-1). Mixed patterns are found in 38.5% of cases.
- **Nodular**
  - Most common histologic type: 50%-60%
  - Flesh-colored, pearly nodule with overlying telangiectasias
  - May be ulcerated: Central ulcer surrounded by rolled border; historically called *rodent ulcer*
- **Superficial spreading**
  - 9%-15% of basal cell carcinomas
  - Lie in epidermis without dermal invasion
  - Usually multiple, occur on the trunk
  - Often mistaken for fungal infection or eczema
- **Micronodular**
  - 15% of basal cell carcinomas
  - Small rounded nodules of tumor the size of hair bulbs

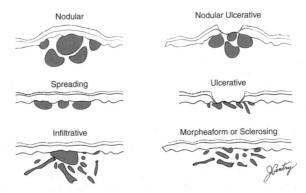

Fig. 11-1   Histologic types of basal cell carcinoma. (Modified from Jacobs GH, Rippey JJ, Altini M. Predication of aggressive behavior in basal cell carcinoma. Cancer 49:533, 1982.)

- **Infiltrative**
  - 7% of basal cell carcinomas
  - Tumor islands of variable size with jagged configuration
- **Pigmented**
  - 6% of basal cell carcinomas
  - Pigmentation from melanin
  - Often confused with melanoma
- **Morpheaform or sclerosing**
  - 2%-3% of basal cell carcinomas
  - Typically described by patients as an "enlarging scar" without any history of trauma
  - Usually an indurated, flat, or slightly elevated papule or plaque with white to yellow scarlike appearance
  - Rarely ulcerates
  - *High incidence of positive margins after excision*

TREATMENT

- Each case should be treated differently according to size, anatomic location, histologic type, and whether primary or recurrent.
- Patients treated for BCC should be observed periodically for 5 years or longer because of high rate of new primary cancers.
- Treatment modalities include *medical, destructive,* and *surgical excision.*
- **Medical**
  - **Imiquimod 5% (Aldara)**
    - ▸ Topical cream used daily for 6 weeks
    - ▸ Effective versus superficial lesions only

TIP: 5-fluorouracil (5-FU) should not be used for BCC because it may destroy surface cells without affecting deeper cells.

- **Radiotherapy**
  - ▸ Overall cure rate of primary lesions 92%[12]
  - ▸ Requires multiple treatments
  - ▸ Associated risks of osteitis and skin necrosis
  - ▸ Reserved for elderly patients who are not surgical candidates
- **Destructive**
  - **Electrodesiccation and curettage (ED&C)**
    - ▸ *Most common treatment modality*
    - ▸ Curette removes visible tumor, electrodesiccation removes residual tumor cells
    - ▸ Allows healing by secondary intention
    - ▸ Cure rates of 96%-100% for tumors less than 2 mm[13]
    - ▸ Overall cure rate 74%[12]
    - ▸ Not recommended in dense hair-bearing areas or if tumor extends into subcutaneous layer
  - **Cryosurgery[14]**
    - ▸ Cooling tumor cells to −40° C during repetitive freeze-thaw cycles destroys malignant tissue.
    - ▸ Appropriate for small-to-large BCCs of the nodular and superficial types with clearly definable margins (laterally and in depth).

  - ▸ Not indicated for tumors deeper than 3 mm unless thermocouples are used to measure depth of freeze.
  - ▸ Contraindications include cold intolerance, morpheaform or recurrent BCC, and cosmetically sensitive areas.
  - ▸ Treatment causes prolonged edema (4-6 weeks) and permanent pigment loss.
- **Laser phototherapy** (CO_2 laser)
  - ▸ Ablation of BCC confined to epidermis and papillary dermis
  - ▸ Disadvantage: Inability to evaluate surgical margins
- **Photodynamic therapy**
  - ▸ Light-activated photosensitizing drug (5-aminolevulinic acid) to create oxygen free radicals that selectively destroy target cells
  - ▸ Not currently approved by FDA for BCC (only for actinic keratosis)
- ■ **Surgical**
- **Primary surgical excision**
  - ▸ Current literature recommends 4 mm margin for small primary BCC on the face.[15]
  - ▸ Recommended margins are **3-5 mm** for well-demarcated lesions and **7 mm** for aggressive forms.
  - ▸ Lesions with high-recurrence risk are micronodular, infiltrative, and morpheaform.
- **Mohs' micrographic surgery**
Sequential horizontal excision using topographic map of lesion and repeat excision until all positive margins are tumor free
  - ▸ Performed under local anaesthesia in office
  - ▸ Cure rates 99% for primary tumors with significant tissue conservation[16]
  - ▸ **Indications**
    - ✦ Recurrent tumors
    - ✦ Cosmetically sensitive areas (periorbital, periauricular, paranasal)
    - ✦ Morpheaform/sclerosing types or aggressive malignant features
    - ✦ Poorly delineated margins in scar tissue
    - ✦ Other tumor types: Squamous cell with perineural invasion, dermatofibrosarcoma protuberans, microcystic adnexal carcinoma

CUTANEOUS SQUAMOUS CELL CARCINOMA (SCC)

DEMOGRAPHICS[17,18]
- ■ **SCC is second most common skin cancer after BCC**
- ■ North American incidence is 41:100,000.
- ■ Australian incidence is 201:100,000 (higher individual sun exposure).
- ■ Predilection in sun-exposed regions
- ■ In lightly pigmented skin, male/female ratio is 2.5:1
- ■ In darkly pigmented skin, male/female ratio is 1.3:1

RISK FACTORS
- ■ Fitzpatrick skin type
- ■ Sun exposure
- ■ Carcinogen exposure: Pesticides, arsenic, organic hydrocarbons
- ■ Viral infection: HPV and herpes simplex
- ■ Radiation: Long-term latency between exposure and disease

- Immunosuppression: 253-fold increased risk for SCC in renal transplant patients
- Chronic wound caused by thermal burn, discoid lupus, fistula tract, osteomyelitis
- PUVA (psoriasis treatment)
- **Premalignant lesions**
  - **Actinic keratosis/solar keratosis**
    - ▸ Occur in regions of sun exposure
    - ▸ Macular/papular lesions with scaly irregular surface
    - ▸ Malignant transformation is common
  - **Bowen's disease**
    - ▸ In situ demonstrates full thickness cytologic atypia of keratinocytes with normal basal cells
    - ▸ Erythematous plaque with sharp borders and slight scaling
    - ▸ <u>Erythroplasia of Queyrat:</u> Bowen's disease of the glans penis, vulva, or oral mucosa
  - **Leukoplakia**
    - ▸ *Most common premalignant lesion of oral mucosa*
    - ▸ Mucosal changes with white patch
    - ▸ Malignant transformation 15%
  - **Keratoacanthoma**
    - ▸ Smooth dome-shaped mass of squamous cells and keratin grow rapidly over 1-6 weeks and ulcerate with central crusting.
    - ▸ Once stabilized, tumors spontaneously regress over 2-12 months and heal with scarring.
    - ▸ Keratoacanthoma resembles SCC histologically.
    - ▸ Larger or atypical lesions should be treated as SCC.

RECURRENCE AND METASTASIS[1,19]

- **Lymph node examinations are mandatory.**
- Clinical lymphadenopathy with biopsy-proven metastatic disease warrants lymphadenectomy.
- Metastasis from primary occurs 2%-5% on trunk, 10%-20% on face/extremity.
- Local metastasis to regional nodal basin, but distant metastasis occurs by hematogenous dissemination most commonly to the lungs, liver, brain, skin, or bone.
- 3-year cumulative risk of a subsequent SCC after an index SCC is 18%.
- Presence of positive nodes from lesion on extremity carry a dismal 35% 5-year survival despite nodal dissection.

NOTE: Most SCC-related deaths are related to ear lesions.

- **Predictors of tumor recurrence for SCC**
  - **Degree of cellular differentiation**
    - ▸ Well-differentiated: 7% recurrence
    - ▸ Moderately differentiated: 23% recurrence
    - ▸ Poorly differentiated: 28% recurrence
  - **Depth of tumor invasion**
  - **Perineural invasion**

TIP: All recurrent SCC should be considered to have perineural invasion until proven otherwise.
Tumors that penetrate dermis or are thicker than 8 mm are associated with high risk for death.

BIOLOGY
- SCC arise from the malpighian or basal layer of epidermis.

TYPES OF SQUAMOUS CELL CARCINOMAS
- All types are histologically similar with irregular masses of squamous epithelium proliferating downward toward dermis.
- Tumor grade is the degree of cellular differentiation and measures the ratio of atypical pleomorphic and anaplastic cell to the normal epithelium.
- **Verrucous**
  - Exophytic and slow growing
  - Common on palms and soles
  - Less likely to metastasize
- **Ulcerative**
  - Aggressive with raised borders and central ulceration
  - Commonly metastasizes to regional lymph nodes
- **Marjolin's ulcer[20]**
  - Arise in chronic wounds (burn scars, fistulas, osteomyelitis tracks)
  - Burn scars have 2% lifetime malignant degeneration potential
  - Latency period proportional to age of injury, but average interim is **32.5 years**
  - Commonly metastasize to lymph nodes
- **Subungual**
  - Squamous changes involving the nail bed
  - Presents as erythema swelling and localized pain followed by nodularity and ulceration

TREATMENT
Treatment modalities include **medical, destructive,** and **surgical excision.** Annual full skin evaluation follow up is recommended.
- **Medical**
  - **Radiation[21]**
    - ▶ Cure rate for primary radiotherapy is 90%.
    - ▶ Reserved for:
      - ✦ Debilitated patients who are poor surgical candidates
      - ✦ Adjuvant therapy in management of high-stage large tumors
      - ✦ Recurrent tumors that require multimodal therapy
  - **Topical**
    - ▶ 5-FU excellent for treating premalignant lesions (e.g., actinic keratosis)
    - ▶ Not recommended for treatment of SCC
  - **Photodynamic therapy**
    - ▶ Better against premalignant lesions
  - **Chemotherapy**
    - ▶ Usually reserved for adjuvant therapy with large tumors or recurrent disease
- **Destructive**
  - **Electrodesiccation and curettage and cryosurgery**
    - ▶ Reserved for small superficial lesions
    - ▶ Does not produce a surgical specimen for histology and margin analysis

- **Surgical**
  - **Excision**
    - ▸ Wide local excision is a good treatment option with 95% cure rate.
    - ▸ Most recent recommendations are based on size, grade, location of tumor, and depth of invasion.[1,22]
      - ✦ Smaller than 2 cm, grade 1, low-risk region, depth to dermis—**4 mm** margins
      - ✦ Larger than 2 cm, grade 2, 3, or 4, high-risk region, depth to subcutaneous fat—**6 mm** margins
    - ▸ Frozen sections often give false negatives.
  - **Mohs' micrographic surgery**
    - ▸ 95% cure rate for primary SCC
    - ▸ Lower recurrence rates with tissue preservation
    - ▸ 5-year recurrence rates for primary cutaneous SCC 3.1% (versus 8.1% for surgical excision, and 10% for radiotherapy)[21]
    - ▸ Same indications as BCC
  - **Lymphadenectomy**
    - ▸ Lymphadenectomy indicated for clinically palpable nodes.
    - ▸ Fine-needle aspiration (FNA) may be used to confirm metastatic disease first.
    - ▸ Sentinel lymph node dissection (SLND) maps the first node in basin by injection of radiolabeled technetium colloid and local lymphoscintigraphy with blue lymphangiography dye.
      - ✦ Determine nodal status of basin with less morbidity than total basin lymphadenectomy
      - ✦ Indicated for high-risk SCC without palpable nodes
    - ▸ Elective lymph node dissection (ELND) involves removal of clinically negative nodes from a nodal basin.
      - ✦ Indicated for tumor extending to parotid capsule or contiguous nodal drainage basin

MELANOMA

DEMOGRAPHICS[1,23]

- Caucasian North American lifetime risk is 1.4%.
- General population risk is 0.5%.
- 40,000 new cases are diagnosed per year in United States.

RISK FACTORS[1,24,25]

- **UV exposure**
  - High altitude
  - Extreme southern latitudes (Australia, New Zealand)
- **Age**
  - 50% occur in patients more than 50 years of age.
- **Family history**
  - History is positive in 10% of patients.
  - Risk may be up to 8 times higher depending on number of relatives.
  - Familial melanomas occur at a younger ages.
- **Phenotype**
  - Fitzpatrick type I, II
  - Light hair color

- ▶ **When compared with black hair:**
  - ✦ Redhead: 3.6 times higher
  - ✦ Brunette: 2.8 times higher
  - ✦ Blonde: 2.4 times higher
- ■ **Sex[26]**
  - Males: 1:49 lifetime risk; more common on trunk and head
  - Females: 1:72 lifetime risk; more common in lower extremity
- ■ **Race**
  - Risk is 10 to 20 times higher for Caucasians than blacks.
  - Prognosis in blacks is worse because of delayed diagnosis.
- ■ **Other**
  - Higher socioeconomic status yields higher risk
  - Immunosuppression
- ■ **Predisposing conditions**
  - **Atypical mole syndrome: B-K mole syndrome, familial atypical multiple mole melanoma (FAMMM)**
    - ▶ More than 100 melanocytic nevi measuring 6-15 mm
    - ▶ 1 or more measuring larger than 8 mm
    - ▶ 1 or more with clinically atypical features
    - ▶ 10% risk of melanoma
    - ▶ Nevi present at birth and increase in number around puberty
  - **Dysplastic nevus**
    - ▶ Atypical melanocytes with potential for transformation
    - ▶ **6%-10%** lifetime risk of malignant degeneration
    - ▶ Histopathologic diagnosis
    - ▶ Clinically indistinguishable from melanoma in situ
  - **Congenital nevus:** 6% lifetime risk depending on size
  - **Typical moles:** Increased risk if more than 50
  - **Melanoma in situ:** Lesions have intraepidermal proliferation with fully developed cellular atypia
  - **Xeroderma pigmentosum** (See description in BCC section)
  - **Lentigo maligna**
    - ▶ Also known as *Hutchinson freckle, senile freckle,* or *circumscribed precancerous melanosis*
    - ▶ Nonnested proliferation of variably atypical melanocytes and atrophic dermis

BENIGN PIGMENTED LESIONS MISTAKEN FOR MELANOMA[27]

TIP: Melanomas are characterized by ABCDs: Asymmetry, Border irregularity, Color variegation, and Diameter more than 6 mm. Any pigmented lesion greater than 5-10 mm in diameter is more likely to be malignant than benign.[28]

- ■ **Junctional nevi**
  - Flat, uniform color on palms, soles, genitalia, and mucosa
  - Pale to dark brown
  - Smooth macular and sharply defined
  - Appear usually around ages 4-12 and change little during childhood
- ■ **Compound nevi**
  - Darker and palpable raised border
  - Smooth or rough and can have hair

- Appear during puberty and fade
- *Halo nevus* is compound nevus surrounded by depigmented ring of skin
■ **Intradermal nevi**
  - Raised pale papules with pigment in flecks
  - Coarse dark terminal hairs may grow in lesions
  - Occur in second or third decade of life
  - Most commonly found on face and neck
■ **Blue nevi**
  - Blue-black lesion less than 5 mm in size that remains stable with time
  - Usually found on dorsa of hands or feet, head, neck, or buttocks
  - Very rare degeneration potential
■ **Spitz nevus**
  - Juvenile melanoma of children and young adults
  - Smooth surface, dome shaped, red or pink
  - Telangiectasias typically are present
  - Most common on head and neck
  - Typically less than 6 mm in diameter
  - Often noticed after rapid change in size or color
  - Proliferation of enlarged spindled/epithelioid melanocytes
■ **Lentigo**
  - Pigmented macular lesions with reticulated pattern
  - Most common in middle age from sun exposure
  - <u>Simple lentigo:</u> Common brown/black mole
  - <u>Solar lentigo:</u> Liver spot or age spot
■ **Seborrheic keratosis**
  - Multiple variously colored raised verrucous papules
  - Most commonly found on trunk

TIP: Seborrheic keratosis can mimic melanoma.

■ **Pyogenic granulomas**
  - Short development course of days to weeks
  - Commonly occurs at site after minor trauma
  - Raised with surrounding inflammation
  - Painless
  - Most common on hands and around mouth
■ **Pigmented BCC**

MELANOMA GROWTH PATTERNS[29,30]
■ **Superficial spreading melanoma**
  - **Most common:** 70%
  - Usually arises from preexisting nevus
  - Average size 2 cm
  - Typical appearance: Flat junctional nevus, asymmetric borders, and color variegation
■ **Nodular melanoma**
  - 15%-30% of all cases
  - Aggressive

- Typically arises denovo in normal skin
- More common in men (2:1)
- 1-2 cm dome shaped
- Resembles a blood blister
- Keeps sharp demarcation because of lack of horizontal growth pattern
- 5% amelanotic
- **Lentigo maligna**
  - 4%-10% of all cases
  - *Least aggressive subtype*
  - Clearly related to sun exposure
  - Appearance of skin stain in multiple shades of brown
  - More common in women
  - Radial growth phase of precursor lesion *(Hutchison freckle)*
  - Transition to vertical growth marks transition to melanoma
- **Acral-lentiginous melanoma**
  - 2%-8% of cases in whites, but 35%-60% of cases in nonwhites
  - *Usually on palms, soles of feet, subungual*
  - Melanonychia: Linear pigmented streak in the nail
  - 3 cm, usually flat with irregular border and multiple color shades
  - Long radial growth phase, transition to vertical growth increases metastatic risk
- **Desmoplastic melanoma**
  - 1% of all cases
  - *Propensity for perineural invasion*
  - Immunohistochemical stain reactive to S-100 protein
  - High rate of regional lymph node spread
- **Amelanotic melanoma**
  - No pigment by light microscopy
  - Diagnosis by immunohistochemical staining
  - Usually diagnosed in vertical growth phase
- **Noncutaneous melanoma**
  - 2% of all cases
  - Mucosal melanoma
  - Arises on mucosal surfaces
  - Usually large at diagnosis
  - Poor prognosis
- **Ocular melanoma**
  - 2%-5% of all cases
  - Vision interference leads to earlier diagnosis
  - Liver metastases are common

MELANOMA STAGING[31,32]

- Histologic analysis of full thickness biopsy specimen is categorized by microstaging.
  - **Breslow thickness:** Measurement of tumor thickness in millimeters
  - **Clark's level:** Level determined by histologic invasion through skin layers[31] (Fig. 11-2)

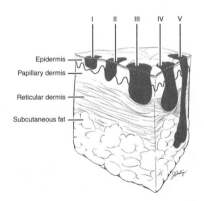

Fig. 11-2 Levels of tumor invasion by the Clark microstaging criteria. (Modified from McGovern VJ, Mihm MC Jr, Bailly C, et al. The classification of malignant melanoma and its histologic reporting. Cancer 32:1446, 1973.)

- A new tumor node metastasis (TNM) melanoma staging system was introduced by the American Joint Committee on Cancer (AJCC) in 2002 based on data from 17,000 patients and 13 international centers[32] (Tables 11-2 and 11-3).
  - **Tumor thickness (Breslow thickness) replaces level of invasion (Clark's level) as the most important prognostic variable of primary tumor invasion that best predicts survival.**
  - Ulceration of the primary tumor (microscopic histopathologic ulceration) upstages the disease to the next highest T substage.
  - The number of metastatic lymph nodes replaces the size of lymph nodes in the N stage.
  - Lymphatic mapping data (lymphoscintigraphy) and micrometastatic local regional disease within lymph nodes is incorporated in clinical and pathologic staging.
  - Subcategorization of stage IV metastatic disease is based on anatomic site of the metastasis and elevated serum LDH.

Table 11-2   *AJCC Melanoma Staging System 2002: Tumor/Node/Metastasis Classification for Melanoma*

Tumor Classification		Clinical
T1	<1.0 mm (depth of invasion)	a: Without ulceration
T1		b: With ulceration or Clark's level IV or V
T2	1.01-2.0 mm (depth of invasion)	a: Without ulceration
T2		b: With ulceration
T3	2.01-4.0 mm (depth of invasion)	a: Without ulceration
T3		b: With ulceration
T4	>4.0 mm (depth of invasion)	a: Without ulceration
		b: With ulceration
Node Classification		
N1	One lymph node	a: Micrometastasis
		b: Macrometastasis
N2	2-3 lymph nodes	a: Micrometastasis
		b: Macrometastasis
		c: In-transit metastases/satellites without metastatic lymph nodes
N3	4 or more metastatic lymph nodes, matted lymph nodes, or combinations of in-transit metastases/satellites, or ulcerated melanoma and metastatic nodes	
Metastasis Classification		
M1a	Distant skin, subcutaneous, or lymph node metastases	Normal LDH
M1b	Lung metastases	Normal LDH
M1c	All other visceral metastases Any distant metastases	Normal LDH Elevated LDH with any M

Modified from Balch CM, Buzaid AC, Soong SJ, et al. Final version of the American Joint Committee on Cancer staging system for cutaneous melanoma. J Clin Oncol 19:3635, 2001.

Table 11-3 *Pathologic Stage Grouping*

Stage	Tumor	Node	Metastasis	Overall Survival		
				1-Year	5-Year	10-Year
0	Tis	N0	M0		100%	100%
IA	T1a	N0	M0		95%	88%
IB	T1b	N0	M0		91%	83%
	T2a	N0	M0		89%	79%
IIA	T2b	N0	M0		77%	64%
	T3a	N0	M0		79%	64%
IIB	T3b	N0	M0		63%	51%
	T4a	N0	M0		67%	54%
IIC	T4b	N0	M0		45%	32%
IIIA	T1-4a	N1a	M0		69%	63%
	T1-4a	N2a	M0		63%	57%
IIIB	T1-4b	N1a	M0		53%	38%
	T1-4b	N2a	M0		50%	36%
	T1-4a	N1b	M0		59%	48%
	T1-4a	N2b	M0		46%	39%
	T1-4a/b	N2c	M0		30%-50%	34%
IIIC	T1-4b	N1b	M0		29%	24%
	T1-4b	N2b	M0		24%	15%
	Any T	N3	M0		27%	18%
IV	Any T	Any N	Any M	59%	19%	16%
	Any T	Any N	Any M	57%	7%	3%
	Any T	Any N	Any M	41%	9%	6%

Modified from Balch CM, Buzaid AC, Soong SJ, et al. Final version of the American Joint Committee on Cancer staging system for cutaneous melanoma. J Clin Oncol 19:3635, 2001.

TREATMENT OF MELANOMA[33-38]

■ **Biopsy technique**
- 5-7 mm punch biopsy adequate but may miss thickest portion of tumor
- Incisional biopsy for low suspicion lesion or in cosmetically sensitive region
- Excisional biopsy recommended for lesions less than 1.5 cm in diameter
- Shave biopsy forfeits ability to stage on thickness
- Full-thickness biopsy not required in subungual melanoma because it offers no prognostic information

---

TIP: Avoid cauterizing because margins may be distorted.

■ **Surgical excision**
- **Wide local excision** (WLE) with surgical margins based on tumor thickness
  - ▶ **In situ:** 0.5 cm margin
  - ▶ **Less than 1 mm:** 1 cm margin
  - ▶ **1-4 mm:** 2 cm margin
  - ▶ **Greater than 4 mm:** 2-3 cm margin

- Depth of resection should **not** include fascial layer, because this increases risk of metastatic disease without improving long-term survival.
- For subungual melanoma, amputation is recommended proximal to distal interphalangeal joint (or IP joint of thumb).

- **Lymph nodes**
  - **Sentinel lymph node biopsy (SLNB)**
    - Staging procedure, **not** a therapeutic treatment
    - Performed in conjunction with WLE of primary tumor
    - Skip metastasis reported 0%-2%
    - **Indications**
      - Male truncal melanoma less than 0.76 mm
      - All patients with 0.76-1.0 mm
      - All melanomas less than 1.0 mm thick
  - **ELND**
    - No survival benefit except with 1-2 mm intermediate thickness melanomas
  - **Therapeutic lymph node dissection**
    - Performed for positive SLNB patients or clinically palpable disease
    - Only potential cure for metastatic nodal disease
    - Patients with clinically palpable nodes have poor prognosis

- **Adjuvant therapy**
  - More effective against subclinical micrometastases than primary tumors, and against residual disease after removal of gross disease
  - No adjuvant therapy is so effective that it is routinely recommended
  - May benefit patients by palliation of symptoms, prolongation of life
    - **Interferon**
      - **Interferon α-2b:** Recombinant version of naturally occurring leukocyte α interferon
      - Several studies from the Eastern Cooperative Oncology Group (ECOG) document disease-free survival benefit of treatment with interferon α-2b.
      - Appropriate in patients with regional nodal/in-transit metastasis or node-negative patients with primary melanomas deeper than 4 mm.
      - Inappropriate for node-negative patients with nonulcerated lesions smaller than 4 mm.
      - *Uncertain in patients with ulcerated lesions of intermediate depth (2-4 mm).*
    - **Chemotherapy**
      - Agents such as dacarbazine (DTIC), carmustine, cisplatin, and tamoxifen
      - Generally palliative only, with some success for regression of tumor burden
    - **Radiotherapy**
      - Rarely indicated as primary treatment of cutaneous melanoma, except lentigo maligna or desmoplastic melanomas
      - Can be used as preoperative or postoperative treatment of primary site, in unresectable lymph node basins, or in palliation of metastatic disease
    - **Immunotherapy**
      - Melanoma vaccines are currently awaiting approval by the FDA.
      - Interleukin 2 has been approved for stage IV disease.

SURVEILLANCE AND RECURRENCE[37,39]

- Local recurrence usually occurs within 5 cm of original lesion within 3-5 years, usually resulting from incomplete resection of primary tumor.
- Reports of second primary melanomas is 2%-3.4%.
- Guidelines of any follow-up program include early detection and treatment of recurrent disease.
  - Indiana University Interdisciplinary Melanoma Program (Table 11-4)
    - Asymptomatic patients
      - LDH and alkaline phosphatase
      - CXR
      - Other common sites of recurrence: Skin, subcutaneous tissues, lymph nodes, and distant sites
    - Reexcision primary treatment of small recurrences
- Regional recurrence can also be treated with radiation or chemotherapy.
- Outcomes show stable mortality at 2.2 per 100,000 annually (Fig. 11-3).

Table 11-4   *Current Clinical Follow-up Guidelines at the Indiana University Interdisciplinary Melanoma Program**

| | Follow-Up† | | |
AJCC Stage	Physical Examinations	Laboratory	CXR
Stage 0 (in situ)	Initial and yearly up to 10 years	None	None
Stage Ia (<0.75 mm)	Every 6 months for 2 years, yearly up to 10 years	Initial	Yearly
Stage Ib (0.76-1.5 mm)	Every 6 months for 4 years, yearly to 10 years	Yearly	Yearly
Stage II (1.5-4.0 mm)	Every 3-4 months for 4 years, every 6 months for 1 year, yearly to 10 years	Yearly	Yearly
Stage III (>4.0 mm, node-negative)	Every 3 months for 4 years, every 6 months for 1 year, yearly to 10 years	Yearly	Every 6 months for 2 years, yearly to 10 years
Stage III (node-positive or recurrent)	Every 3 months for 4 years, every 6 months for 1 year, yearly to 10 years	Yearly	Every 6 months for 3 years, yearly to 10 years
Stage IV	Every 1-3 months, depending on disease status, symptoms, etc.	Every 6 months if NED, otherwise as clinically indicated	

From Wagner JD, Gordon MS, Chuang TY, et al. Current therapy of cutaneous melanoma. Plast Reconstr Surg 105:1774, 2000.
CXR, posteroanterior and lateral chest radiographs; *NED*, no evidence of disease after therapy.
*Patients at high risk for second primary melanomas may require more frequent visits. Symptoms, physical examinations, abnormal surveillance laboratory results, or abnormal skull x-ray direct additional laboratory or radiographic tests.
†Laboratory serum alkaline phosphatase and lactate dehydrogenase.

Fig. 11-3 Fifteen-year survival results for more than 4000 melanoma patients treated at University of Alabama at Birmingham and the Sydney Melanoma Unit by AJCC stage. Distribution of patients shown in parentheses. (Modified from Stadelmann WK, Rapaport DP, Seng-jaw S, et al. Prognostic clinical and pathologic features. In Balch CM, Houghton AN, Sober AJ, et al, eds. Cutaneous Melanoma, 3rd ed. St Louis: Quality Medical Publishing, 1998.)

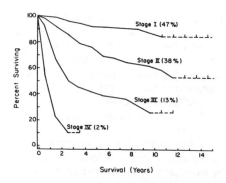

Survival (Years)

KEY POINTS

✔ BCC is the most common type of skin cancer.
✔ Nevus sebaceus of Jadassohn has a 10%-15% incidence of malignant degeneration to BCC.
✔ Nodular BCC is the most common histologic subtype.
✔ Recommended surgical margins for BCC are usually 3-5 mm.
✔ Mohs' surgery has specific indications.
✔ Erythroplasia of Queyrat is Bowen's disease of the glans penis, vulva, or oral mucosa.
✔ Leukoplakia is the most common premalignant lesion of oral mucosa.
✔ Most SCC-related deaths are associated with ear lesions.
✔ Marjolin's ulcers are SCC that arise in chronic wounds.
✔ Surgical margins for SCC are usually 4-6 mm, sometimes more.
✔ Superficial spreading is the most common growth pattern of melanoma.
✔ Acral-lentiginous melanoma usually occurs on the palms and soles and is more common in blacks.
✔ Breslow thickness is the most important prognostic variable that predicts survival (melanoma).
✔ WLE margins in melanoma are based on tumor thickness.

REFERENCES

1. Habif TP. Clinical Dermatology: A Color Guide to Diagnosis and Therapy, 4th ed. St Louis: Mosby, 2004.
2. Shanoff LB, Spira M, Hardy SB. Basal cell carcinoma: A statistical approach to rational management. Plast Reconstr Surg 39:619, 1967.
3. Fitzpatrick TB. The validity and practicality of sun-reactive skin types I through VI. Arch Dermatol 124:869, 1988.
4. Kubasiewicz M, Starzynski Z. Case-referent study on skin cancer and its relation to occupational exposure to polycyclic aromatic hydrocarbons. Pol J Occup Med 2:221, 1989.
5. Hutchinson J. Arsenic cancer. Br Med J 2:1280, 1888.
6. Lever LR, Farr PM. Skin cancers or premalignant lesions occur in half of high-dose PUVA patients. Br J Dermatol 131:215, 1994.
7. Gorlin RJ, Goltz RW. Multiple nevoid basal epithelioma, jaw cysts and bifid ribs: A syndrome. N Engl J Med 262:908, 1960.
8. Jacobs GH, Rippey JJ, Altini M. Prediction of aggressive behavior in basal cell carcinoma. Cancer 49:533, 1982.
9. Bolognia JL, Jorizzo J, Rapini R. Dermatology, vol 2. St Louis: Mosby, 2003.
10. SEER cancer statistics review, 1973-1995. Bethesda, MD: National Cancer Institute, 1998. National Institute of Health Publication No. 98-2789.

11. Pollack SV, Goslen JB, Sheretz EF, et al. The biology of basal cell carcinoma: A review. J Am Acad Dermatol 7:569, 1982.
12. Dubin N, Kopf AW. Multivariate risk score for recurrence of cutaneous basal cell carcinomas. Arch Dermatol 119:373, 1983.
13. Salasche SJ. Curettage and electrodesiccation in the treatment of midfacial basal cell epithelioma. J Am Acad Dermatol 8:496, 1983.
14. Zacarian SA. Cryosurgery of cutaneous carcinomas: An 18 year study of 3022 patients with 4228 carcinomas. J Am Acad Dermatol 9:947, 1983.
15. Kimyai-Asadi A, Alam A, Goldberg LH, et al. Efficacy of narrow-margin excision of well-demarcated primary facial basal cell carcinomas. J Am Acad Dermatol 53:464, 2005.
16. Cottel WI, Proper S. Mohs' surgery, fresh tissue technique: Our technique with a review. J Dermatol Surg Oncol 8:576, 1982.
17. Vitaliano PP, Urbach F. The relative importance of risk factors in nonmelanoma carcinoma. Arch Dermatol 116:454, 1980.
18. Gallagher RP, Hill GB, Coldman AJ, et al. Sunlight exposure, pigmentation factors, and risk of nonmelanotic skin cancer. II. Squamous cell carcinoma. Arch Dermatol 131:164, 1995.
19. Immerman SC, Scanlon EF, Christ M, et al. Recurrent squamous cell carcinoma of the skin. Cancer 51:1537, 1983.
20. Lawrence EA. Carcinoma arising in the scars of thermal burns. Surg Gyecol Obstet 95:579, 1952.
21. Rowe DE, Carroll RJ, Day CL Jr. Prognostic factors for local recurrence, metastasis, and survival rates in squamous cell carcinoma of the skin, ear, and lip. J Am Acad Dermatol 26:976, 1992.
22. Broadland DG, Zitelli JA. Surgical margins for excision of primary cutaneous squamous cell carcinoma. J Am Acad Dermatol 27:108, 1992.
23. National Cancer Institute. What you need to know about melanoma: Information about detection, symptoms, diagnosis and treatment of melanoma. NIH Pub No 02-1563, 2003.
24. Crombie IK. Racial differences in melanoma incidence. Br J Cancer 40:185, 1979.
25. Devesa SS, Silverman DT, Young JL Jr, et al. Cancer incidence and mortality trends among whites in the United States, 1947-1984. J Natl Cancer Inst 79:701, 1987.
26. Surveillance, Epidemiology, and End Results (SEER) Program. SEER 17 incidence and mortality, 2000-2003. National Cancer Institute, 2006. Available at http://seer.cancer.gov/faststats.
27. Rhodes AR. Potential precursors of cutaneous melanoma. In Lejeune FJ, Chaudhuri PK, Das Gupta TK, eds. Malignant Melanoma: Medical and Surgical Management. New York: McGraw-Hill, 1994, p 97.
28. Elwood JM, Gallagher RP, Hill GB, et al. Pigmentation and skin reaction to sun as risk factors for cutaneous melanoma: Western Canada Melanoma Study. Br Med J 288:99, 1984.
29. Mihm MC Jr, Fitzpatrick TB, Brown MM, et al. Early detection of primary cutaneous malignant melanoma: A color atlas. N Engl J Med 289:989, 1973.
30. Milton GW. Clinical diagnosis of malignant melanoma. Br J Surg 55:755, 1968.
31. McGovern VJ, Mihm MC Jr, Bailly C, et al. The classification of malignant melanoma and its histologic reporting. Cancer 32:1446, 1973.
32. Balch CM, Buzaid AC, Soong SJ, et al. Final version of the American Joint Committee on Cancer staging system for cutaneous melanoma. J Clin Oncol 19:3635, 2001.
33. Balch CM, Buzaid AC. Finally, a successful adjuvant therapy for high risk melanoma. J Clin Oncol 4:1, 1996.
34. Kim CJ, Dessureault S, Gabrilovich D, et al. Immunotherapy for melanoma. Cancer Control 9:22, 2002.
35. Morton DL, Wen DR, Wong JH, et al. Technical details of intraoperative lymphatic mapping for early stage melanoma. Arch Surg 127:392, 1992.
36. Gershenwald JE, Fischer D, Buzaid AC. Cutaneous melanoma: Clinical classification and staging. Clin Plast Surg 27:361, 2000.
37. Wagner JD, Gordon MS, Chuang TY, et al. Current therapy of cutaneous melanoma. Plast Reconstr Surg 105:1774, 2000.
38. Reintgen DS, Rapaport DP, Tanabe KK, et al. Lymphatic mapping and sentinel lymphadenectomy. In Balch CM, Houghton AN, Sober AJ, et al, eds. Cutaneous Melanoma, 3rd ed. St Louis: Quality Medical Publishing, 1998.
39. Brobeil A, Rappaport D, Wells K, et al. Multiple primary melanomas: Implications for screening and follow up programs for melanoma. Ann Surg Oncol 4:19, 1997.

12. Burns

John L. Burns

DEMOGRAPHICS

INCIDENCE[1]
- 1.2 million cases in the United States each year
  - 60,000 require hospitalization
  - 5000 deaths
- **High-risk groups:** Children, the elderly, the disabled

OVERALL INCIDENCE
- Since 1971, deaths attributed to burns have decreased more than 40%
  - Dramatic improvement is because of preventive measures and advanced critical care. However, with improved survival come many more patients with more reconstructive and functional needs.

PATHOPHYSIOLOGY

BURN WOUNDS CLASSIFIED BASED ON DEPTH OF PENETRATION
- **First degree**
  - *Epidermis only*
    - ▸ Skin erythema
    - ▸ No blistering
    - ▸ Sensate
    - ▸ Blanches with pressure
- **Second degree**
  - **Superficial:** *Papillary dermis sparing skin appendages*
    - ▸ Sensate
    - ▸ Blanches with pressure
    - ▸ Blistering
  - **Deep:** *Reticular dermis with skin appendages*
    - ▸ Decreased sensation
    - ▸ No capillary refill
    - ▸ White
    - ▸ Blistering
- **Third degree**
  - *Entire dermis and adnexal structures*
    - ▸ Blistering absent
    - ▸ Insensate
    - ▸ Charred with gradation in color

Table 12-1   *Burn Tissue Histology*

Zone	Clinical Finding	Treatment
Zone of coagulation (necrosis)	Nonviable necrotic tissue in center of burn wound	Excision and grafting
Zone of stasis (edema)	Surrounds zone of coagulation, initially viable	Aggressive resuscitation can improve perfusion and prevent transformation to necrosis
Zone of hyperemia (inflammation)	Outermost zone, viable	Aggressive resuscitation

INDICATIONS/PATIENT SELECTION[2]

CRITERIA FOR TRANSFER TO A BURN CENTER

- Second-degree burns over more than 10% of total body surface area (TBSA)
- Third-degree burns
- Burns involving face, hands, feet, genitalia, perineum
- Chemical burns
- Electrical burns, including lightning strikes
- Any burn with concomitant trauma where burn poses greatest risk to patient
- Inhalation injury
- Preexisting medical disorders that could affect mortality
- Hospitals without qualified personnel or equipment for care of burned children

TIP: The criteria for transfer to a burn center are frequently asked on exams and Boards.

PREOPERATIVE TREATMENT

FACIAL BURNS[3]

- Fluorescent staining
- Ophthalmology consult

INHALATION INJURY

- Arterial blood gas analysis
- Chest x-ray examination
- Carboxyhemoglobin
- Bronchoscopy

COMPARTMENT SYNDROME

- Pain on passive stretch
- Paresthesias
- Pallor
- Tense compartments to palpation
- Poikilothermia

- Loss of pulse (late sign)
- Doppler flowmeter
- Compartment testing with pressure more than 30 mm Hg (indication for escharotomy/fasciotomy)

ELECTRICAL INJURIES
- ECG
- Cardiac monitoring
- Renal function testing with urine myoglobin
- Maintain urine output at 30-50 ml/hr

CHEMICAL BURNS
- **Hydrofluoric acid:** Treat topically with calcium gel or intradermal calcium gluconate
- **Alkalines:** Copious irrigation, avoid neutralization with weak acids
- **Acids:** Copious irrigation
- **Phenol:** Irrigate and treat with polyethylene glycol
- **Phosphorus:** Stain particles with 0.5% copper sulfate and surgically remove

TIP: These chemical injuries and their treatments are frequently on tests.

RESUSCITATION: PARKLAND FORMULA[4]

- **4 ml × Weight (kg) × %TBSA burned** (Fig. 12-1)
- Half of the total amount in Ringer's lactate given over the first 8 hours from the time of injury and the second half over the next 16 hours

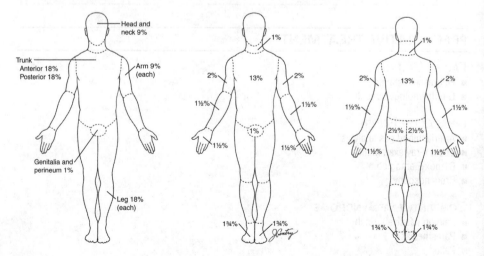

Fig. 12-1   Calculation of total body surface area.

TIP: Adequate volume resuscitation is paramount because this can preserve the zone of stasis
(edema) and prevent further tissue loss.

OPERATIVE TREATMENT[5,6]

- **Excision**
  - Fascial excision results is less blood loss than tangential excision but creates a more severe deformity.
  - The decision on how much to excise during a single setting is determined by the patient's comorbid conditions, blood availability, and the ability to close the wound.
- **Grafting** (Table 12-2)
  - **Autografting:** Meshed autograft allows coverage of a larger area
  - **Homograft** (cadaveric skin) or **xenograft** (different species) when donor sites are not available in large burns

TIP: Plan for surgical blood loss of 0.5 ml/cm^2 (area of burn excision).

Table 12-2   *Mechanism of Skin Graft Take*

Stage	Timing	Histology
Plasmatic imbibition	First 48 hours	Wound exudate diffuses into graft preventing desiccation of graft and graft loss
Inosculation	48-72 hours	Vascular channels either reconnect or are newly established
Capillary ingrowth	4-5 days	Full circulation is restored

POSTOPERATIVE TREATMENT

- **Systemic antibiotics**
  - Culture guided: Sputum, blood, tissue, urine
- Topical antimicrobials (Table 12-3)
- **Nutrition**
  - Metabolic demands can be increased 200%.
  - Malnutrition results in delayed wound healing, organ failure, compromised immune system
  - Enteral feeding is preferred to TPN.
  - **Curreri formula** is used to calculate caloric needs:
    - **25 kcal/kg/day + 40 kcal/%TBSA/day**
  - Dedicate 1-2 gm/kg/day of protein, providing a calorie to nitrogen ratio of 100:1.

Table 12-3   *Commonly Prescribed Topical Antimicrobials for Burn Wounds*

Drug	Target Organism	Properties and Side Effects
Silver sulfadiazine (Silvadene)	Broad spectrum with gram-positive and gram-negative coverage	Transient leukopenia Penetrates eschar poorly
Mafenide acetate (Sulfamylon)	Gram-positive	Potent carbonic anhydrase inhibitor Hyperchloremic metabolic acidosis Compensatory hyperventilation Penetrates deeply
0.5% silver nitrate solution	Staphylococcus species and gram-negative aerobes (Pseudomonas)	Hyponatremia Hypokalemia
Sodium hypochlorite	Broad spectrum	At 0.025% is bactericidal without inhibiting fibroblasts or keratinocytes
Nystatin	Fungus	Powder easily mixed with other antimicrobials

COMPLICATIONS

- **Care related[5]**
  - **Pneumonia:** *Most common cause of death in burn patients*
  - Sepsis
  - Gastrointestinal complications: Ileus and ulceration are common
  - Renal failure: ATN from underperfusion
  - Shock: Inadequate end-organ perfusion

TIP: 5 cardinal signs of sepsis:

1. Hyperventilation
2. Thrombocytopenia
3. Hyperglycemia
4. Obtundation
5. Hypothermia

- **Surgical**
  - Graft loss
  - Burn scar contracture
  - Wound breakdown

TIP: 3 most common causes of skin graft loss:

1. Hematoma
2. Infection
3. Shear

KEY POINTS

✔ Decreased sensation occurs with second-degree and deeper burns.
✔ Know the criteria for admission for burn injuries—they are frequently tested.
✔ The Parkland formula is used to calculate initial resuscitation for the first 24 hours after burn injury. The time of injury, **not** the time of presentation, is used to figure the rate.
✔ Silver sulfadiazine can cause leukopenia.
✔ Mafenide acetate can cause metabolic acidosis secondary to its inhibition of carbonic anhydrase.

REFERENCES

1. Ryan CM, Schoenfeld DA, Thorpe WP, et al. Objective estimates of the probability of death from burn injuries. N Engl J Med 338:362-366, 1998.
2. Boswick JA, ed. The Art and Science of Burn Care. Rockville, MD: Aspen Publishers, 1987.
3. Feldman J. Facial burns. In McCarthy JG, ed. Plastic Surgery, vol 3. Philadelphia: Saunders, 1990, pp 2153-2236.
4. Herndon DN, ed. Total Burn Care, 2nd ed. London: WB Saunders, 2002.
5. Tobin MJ. Advances in mechanical ventilation. N Engl J Med 344:1986-1996, 2001.
6. Hendon DN, Barrow RE, Rutan RL, et al. A comparison of conservative versus early excision therapies in severely burned patients. Ann Surg 209:547-552, 1989.

13. Vascular Anomalies

John L. Burns

CLASSIFICATION (Table 13-1)

Table 13-1 *Classification Schemes for Vascular Anomalies*

Classification	Definition	Example
Descriptive	Colloquial terms	Strawberry angioma or cherry angioma
Anatomic/Physiologic	Histologic findings	Capillary versus cavernous hemangiomas
Embryologic	Vascular anomalies result from errors in embryogenesis	Capillary versus cavernous hemangiomas reflect errors occurring during different periods of embryogenesis
Biologic	Vascular lesions are classified as hemangiomas or malformations on the basis of cellular features	Hemangiomas versus venous, lymphatic, or arteriovenous malformations

TIP: Accurate terminology is critical for both diagnosis and treatment.

Hemangiomas will involute and often do not require surgery.

Port wine stain is a widely accepted term for capillary malformation.

Lymphatic malformation should be used instead of *cystic hygroma* or *lymphangioma*.

HEMANGIOMAS[1,2]

EPIDEMIOLOGY
- **Most common tumors of infancy**
- Incidence: 1:10 by age of 1 year
- Female/male ratio: 3:1
- 60% occur on head and neck

PATHOGENESIS
- **True neoplasms** that grow by endothelial proliferation
- Mast cells are abundant
- Growth inhibited by steroids

CLINICAL COURSE (7 STAGES)
- **Origin (first weeks of life):** Herald spot, small telangiectasia

- **Initial growth (2-5 weeks):** Gradual appearance of closely packed pinhead lesions
- **Intermediate growth (2-10 months):** Enlargement of bright red, tense lesion
- **Completed growth (6-20 months):** Stationary period, becomes quiescent
- **Initial involution (6-24 months):** Lesion becomes softer, flatter, and color fades
- **Intermediate involution (1.5-5 years):** Decreased size with blanching and fibrosis
- **Completed involution (>5 years):** Variable degrees of atrophy and contour deformity

---

TIP: Prognostic signs in hemangiomas:

- Neither the size of the hemangioma nor the sex of the patient influences the speed or completeness of resolution.
- The site of the hemangioma has minimal effect on the final result.
- Multiple hemangiomas do not necessarily resolve at the same time or speed.
- The presence of subcutaneous elements of the tumor has no effect on the final outcome.
- Early dramatic growth is not a prognostic sign of resolution.
- The time of involution is indicative of outcome.
- The presence of ulceration has no prognostic significance except for scar consequences.

TREATMENT

- **Conservative management:** Total involution occurs in 50%-65% of hemangiomas by 5 years, in 70% by 7 years, and in more than 90% by 9 years.
- **Steroids:** In the growth phase oral or intralesional steroids can arrest the growth of the hemangioma but will not cause regression.
- **Laser:** Pulsed dye and Nd:YAG lasers can cause involution of hemangiomas.
- **Surgery:** Depending on the circumstances, surgery is usually delayed until the child is of school age and beginning to experience psychological consequences.

COMPLICATIONS

- **Bleeding:** Usually responds to pressure and rarely requires surgical ligation.
- **Ulceration:** Most common complication occurs in less than 5% of patients.
- **Infection:** Infections are rare, but are more common with intraoral or perianal hemangiomas.
- **Visual obstruction:** Visual obstruction during the first year of life for a period of 1 week can result in deprivation amblyopia or anisometropia.
- **Nasolaryngeal obstruction:** Hemangiomas proliferating in the subglottic airway are potentially life-threatening and should be treated aggressively with steroids, surgery, or laser treatment.
- **Auditory canal obstruction:** Obstruction can result in mild to moderate conductive hearing loss.
- **Kasabach-Merritt syndrome:** Profound thrombocytopenia can occur in conjunction with a hemangioma or hemangiomatosis.
- **Congestive heart failure:** Sometimes congestive heart failure is seen in association with neonatal hemangiomatosis or large visceral hemangiomas.
- **Multiple neonatal hemangiomatosis:** Mortality in infants with multiple neonatal hemangiomatosis is 54%.
- **Skeletal distortion:** Bones are typically deformed by pressure from the hemangioma, bony hypertrophy is rarely seen.
- **Emotional/psychological distress:** Children become aware of their deformity around age 5 and treatment should be more aggressive at this time.

ASSOCIATED DISORDERS (Table 13-2)

Table 13-2   *Associated Disorders*

Disorder	Comments
Maffucci's syndrome	Enchondromatosis associated with multiple cutaneous hemangiomas
Von Hippel-Lindau disease	Hemangiomas of the retina, hemangioblastomas of the cerebellum, commonly associated with cysts of the pancreas, liver, adrenal glands, and kidneys Seizures and mental retardation may be present
PHACE syndrome	Large facial hemangiomas associated with **p**osterior fossa malformations, **h**emangiomas, **a**rterial anomalies, **c**oarctation of the aorta and other cardiac defects, and **e**ye abnormalities
Epithelioid hemangioma	Rare tumor of adulthood with borderline malignant potential

VASCULAR MALFORMATIONS[3] (Table 13-3)

- Structural and morphologic anomalies resulting from faulty embryonic morphogenesis
- **Present at birth,** grow proportionately with the child, and do not regress, unlike hemangiomas

Table 13-3   *Vascular Malformations*

Malformation	Comments
Port wine stains	Capillary malformation most commonly seen on the face in trigeminal nerve distribution
Venous malformation	Venous anomaly swells in the dependent position
Lymphatic malformation	Lymphatic anomaly, frequently infected
Arteriovenous malformation (AVM)	High-flow lesion causes local destruction and can result in heart failure and profound consumptive coagulopathy

From Mulliken JB. Classification of vascular birthmarks. In Mulliken JB, Young AE. Vascular Birthmarks: Hemangiomas and Malformations. Philadelphia: WB Saunders, 1988, pp 24-37.

PATHOGENESIS

- **3 stages**
  1. Capillary network of interconnected blood lakes form with no identifiable arterial or venous channels.
  2. Venous and arterial channels appear on either side of the capillary network on day 48 of gestation. Errors in this stage could result in vascular malformations.
  3. Vascular channels mature and further differentiate.
     - *The autonomic nervous system also influences the development of the vascular system.* Port wine stains often occur along the trigeminal nerve distribution.

PORT WINE STAINS (Table 13-4)

EPIDEMIOLOGY
- 0.3% of newborns affected
- Most frequent in the face: 80%
- Correspond to the distribution of the **trigeminal nerve**
- Sometimes accompanied by ocular and central nervous system disorders
- Female/male ratio: 3:1

TREATMENT
- Left untreated, 70% progress to cobblestoning ectasia
- Photocoagulation with the pulsed dye laser (585 nm) or Nd:YAG laser
  - Multiple treatments necessary
- Ophthalmologic evaluation for glaucoma if V1 lesions

Table 13-4 *Syndromes With Port Wine Stains*

Syndrome	Comments
Sturge-Weber syndrome	Large facial port wine stain with V1 and commonly V2 trigeminal nerve distribution. Associated with leptomeningeal venous malformations and frequent mental retardation.
Klippel-Trénaunay syndrome	Patchy port wine stain on an extremity overlying a deeper venous and lymphatic malformation with associated skeletal hypertrophy.
Parkes-Weber syndrome	Similar to Klippel-Trénaunay but distinguished by the presence of an arteriovenous fistula.

VENOUS MALFORMATIONS

EPIDEMIOLOGY
- Incidence: 1%-4%
- Most common presentation in adults: Varicosity of the superficial veins of the leg

DIAGNOSIS
- Blue or purple lesions with spongy texture
- Swell in the dependent position
- **Decrease in size when elevated**
- Aching in extremity lesions
- Can be hormone sensitive and enlarge during puberty and with pregnancy

TREATMENT
- Many lesions amenable to sclerotherapy
- Extremity aching managed with compression garments and analgesics
- Laser treatment: Nd:YAG or argon laser
- Surgical resection

LYMPHATIC MALFORMATIONS

DIAGNOSIS
- Clear cutaneous vesicles signify a dermal lymphatic component in a vascular malformation
- Soft and compressible
- **Often cause bony overgrowth**

PATHOGENESIS
- Combined venous and lymphatic vascular anomalies are frequent.

TREATMENT
- Injection with sclerosing agent
- Laser ablation for cutaneous blebs
- Surgery

COMPLICATIONS
- Frequent infection: Aggressive antibiotic therapy is crucial.
- Surgical morbidity is high with lymphatic formation of blebs through the surgical area, prolonged draining, slow wound healing, and potential infection.

ARTERIOVENOUS MALFORMATIONS[4] (Table 13-5)

DIAGNOSIS
- **Pulsatile high-flow lesion**
- Angiography defines anatomy and hemodynamics
- MRI also useful in determining extent of the lesion

TREATMENT
- Preoperative medical management of any underlying coagulation defect secondary to thrombotic consumption
- Preoperative embolization followed by surgical resection within 72 hours
- Wide local excision because recurrence rates are very high
- Use of ischemic suture techniques, hypotensive anaesthesia, and even cardiopulmonary bypass to control bleeding
- Postexcisional reconstruction with flaps often necessary

Table 13-5   *Syndromes With Vascular Anomalies*

Syndrome	Comments
Bannayan-Zonana syndrome	Microcephaly, multiple lipomas, and multiple vascular malformations
Riley-Smith syndrome	Pseudopapilledema, microcephaly, and vascular malformations
Blue rubber bleb nevus syndrome	Similar to Klippel-Trénaunay syndrome but distinguished by the presence of an arteriovenous fistula
Osler-Weber-Rendu disease (hereditary hemorrhagic telangiectasia)	Multiple malformed ectatic vessels in the skin, mucous membranes, and viscera

COMPLICATIONS

- Consumptive coagulopathy
- Congestive heart failure
- Local destruction of normal anatomy
- Surgical bleeding

KEY POINTS

✔ Arteriovenous malformations frequently require preoperative embolization immediately before surgical resection.

✔ Hemangiomas are the most common tumor of infancy and frequently involute spontaneously (general rule: 70% involute by 7 years).

✔ Treat hemangiomas nonsurgically unless they involve bleeding, ulceration, or obstruction of an orifice.

✔ Vascular malformations are present at birth (in contrast to hemangiomas) and do not regress.

✔ Port wine stains typically affect the area along the distribution of the trigeminal nerve.

✔ Venous malformations swell in the dependent position and can be hormone sensitive.

✔ Lymphatic malformations often cause bony overgrowth.

REFERENCES

1. Drolet BA, Esterly NB, Frieden IJ. Hemangiomas in children. N Engl J Med 341:173, 1999.
2. Folkman J. Successful treatment of an angiogenic disease. N Engl J Med 320:1211, 1989.
3. Young AE. Pathogenesis of vascular malformations. In Mulliken JB, Young AE. Vascular Birthmarks: Hemangiomas and Malformations. Philadelphia: WB Saunders, 1988, pp 107-113.
4. Kohout MP, Hansen M, Pribaz JJ, et al. Arterio-venous malformations of the head and neck: Natural history and management. Plast Reconstr Surg 102:643, 1998.

14. Congenital Nevi

Dawn D. Wells
John L. Burns

DEMOGRAPHICS

INCIDENCE[1]
Lesion must be present at birth to be classified as congenital.
- Equal prevalence in males and females
- Occurrence in all races
- One percent incidence in newborns, with greater incidence in blacks (1.8%)
- Giant congenital nevocytic nevi (CNN) (>20 cm): 1:20,000

CLASSIFICATION

- Classification based on size and clinical appearance (Table 14-1)

Table 14-1 *Classification of Congenital Nevi*

Size	Comments
Small (<1.5 cm²)	Tan to brown irregularly shaped maculae or papules with mottled freckling Darken with puberty May become elevated and develop hair
Medium (1.5 cm²-20 cm²)	Same properties as small congenital nevi
Giant (>20 cm²)	Dark, hairy, with verrucous texture Satellite lesions often present Also called *bathing suit nevi, stocking,* or *coat-sleeve* May extend into the leptomeninges and have associated neurologic manifestations such as epilepsy Those that overlie the vertebral column may be associated with spina bifida or meningomyelocele May be associated with neurofibromatosis

TIP: After birth, CNN grow in proportion to overall increase in body size.

HISTOLOGY

DISTINGUISHING FEATURES
- CNN are usually characterized as nevus cells between collagen bundles located in the deeper dermis, but they may also invade appendages, vessels, and nerves.
- Acquired nevi are usually composed of nevus cells limited to papillary and upper reticular dermis and do not involve skin appendages.
- Giant CNN have similar histopathology as small and medium nevi, except they may extend into muscle, bone, dura mater, and cranium.

RISK OF MALIGNANT TRANSFORMATION

The risk of malignant transformation is a controversial topic for which there are many opinions.[2-5]
- Small CNN lifetime risk of melanoma development is 1%-5%.
- Medium CNN lifetime risk of melanoma development is uncertain.
- Small- and medium-sized nevi rarely change into melanoma before puberty.
- Of giant nevi, 5%-10% result in melanoma, and 50% usually arise between 3 and 5 years.
- Melanoma development with giant CNN has a poor prognosis.

CLINICAL FINDINGS
- Rapid increase in size
- Irregularity of border
- Development of asymmetry
- Variation of color within the nevus
- Development of satellite lesions
- Changes in texture

MANAGEMENT

Management is controversial and is based on risk of malignant transformation, cosmetic appearance, risk of scarring, and psychological issues
- CNN occurring within the first 2 years of life are called *congenital nevus tardive* and should be managed according to appearance and growth pattern.
- Nongiant nevi should be observed annually for changes. If suspicious, a biopsy should be performed, or the nevi should be removed by prophylactic excision, especially if they are anatomically difficult to monitor (e.g., on the back or scalp).
- Nevi smaller than 1.5 cm not known to be present at birth should be treated like acquired nevi and managed according to their color, growth, and pattern.
- Atypical-appearing CNN should be removed regardless of size.
- Giant CNN should be completely excised as soon as possible.
- Surgical techniques include skin grafts, flaps, tissue expanders, or tissue culture using the patient's own healthy skin.
- Patients with giant nevi should have imaging studies performed to rule out CNS involvement.
- Other modalities (e.g., laser or curettage) to remove congenital nevi have high recurrence rates.

DIFFERENTIAL DIAGNOSIS

The following lesions can sometimes be confused with CNN:

- **Café au lait spot:** May be present at birth but usually develops in childhood; well-circumscribed, homogenous color of coffee with milk, oval, completely macular
- **Nevus spilus:** Usually acquired, but some are congenital; tan macula commonly 1-4 cm in diameter and speckled with dark brown papules or maculae 1-6 mm in diameter
- **Epidermal nevus:** Present at birth or develop in early childhood; tan or brown warty papules, linear array without plaques or hair; most commonly located on extremities
- **Common acquired nevus:** Few nevi present in early childhood; may be brown, tan, or skin-colored; round or ovoid lesions
- **Atypical (dysplastic) nevus:** Occurs during puberty or later; usually more than one color of brown, irregular lesion; usually larger than 6 mm; most commonly found on trunk
- **Blue nevus:** Usually appears in late adolescence; generally smaller than 1 cm; firm, dark-blue to gray-black, sharply defined round papule; most commonly found on dorsa of hands or feet, head, and neck
- **Becker's nevus:** Onset at adolescence; lesions commonly found on the shoulders of males in unilateral distribution; color varies from uniformly tan to dark brown; margins usually irregular; hair usually develops after pigmentation; mean size 125 cm²
- **Halo nevus:** Generally seen in individuals younger than 20 years; appears as white halo around nevus; most commonly found on upper backs of teenagers
- **Mongolian spot:** Steel-blue macula present at birth or first few weeks of life in lumbosacral area; size ranges from a few centimeters to 20 cm or more; more common in darkly pigmented races; usually disappears in early childhood
- **Nevus of Ota:** Onset at birth or less than 1 year and around puberty; especially found in Asians and blacks; blue-brown unilateral periocular macula; size varies from a few centimeters in diameter to lesions covering half the face; areas follow the distribution of the first two branches of the trigeminal nerve
- **Nevus of Ito:** Usually appears at birth; typically found in Asians and blacks; large, blue-brown macula located on posterior shoulder, areas innervated by posterior supraclavicular and lateral cutaneous brachial nerves
- **Spitz nevus:** Usually appears at birth; red or pigmented smooth dome-shaped papule; telangiectasia is a frequent finding; average diameter 8 mm; most commonly found on head and neck
- **Nevus sebaceus:** Onset at birth; solitary yellowish-orange, waxy plaque; usually found on scalp

KEY POINTS

✔ Congenital nevi *must* be present at birth.
✔ Congenital nevus *tardive* are nevi that occur within the first 2 years of life.
✔ Giant congenital nevi are usually classified as those nevi larger than 20 cm², covering more than 1% of total body surface area (TBSA), or bigger than the size of a palm.
✔ CNN cells invade skin appendages, whereas acquired nevi cells do not.
✔ Giant nevi have a malignant transformation rate of 5%-10% (melanoma).
✔ Imaging studies are necessary for patients with giant nevi to rule out CNS involvement.
✔ Blue nevi commonly occur on the dorsa of hands or feet, head, and neck.
✔ A nevus of Ota follows the distribution of V_1 and V_2.
✔ A nevus of Ito is located on the posterior shoulder along the distribution of the posterior supraclavicular and lateral cutaneous brachial nerves.

REFERENCES

1. Bett BJ. Large or multiple congenital melanocytic nevi: Occurrence of cutaneous melanoma in 1008 persons. J Am Acad Dermatol 52:793-797, 2005.
2. Marghoob AA. Congenital melanocytic nevi. Evaluation and management. Dermatol Clin 20:607-616, 2002.
3. Patterson WM, Lefkowitz A, Schwartz RA, et al. Melanoma in children. Cutis 65:269-272, 2000.
4. Rhodes AR, Silverman RA, Harrist TJ, et al. A histologic comparison of congenital and acquired nevomelanocytic nevi. Arch Dermatol 121:1266-1273, 1985.
5. Rhodes AR, Wood WC, Sober AJ, et al. Nonepidermal origin of malignant melanoma associated with a giant congenital nevocellular nevus. Plast Reconstr Surg 67:782-790, 1981.

PART III

Head and Neck

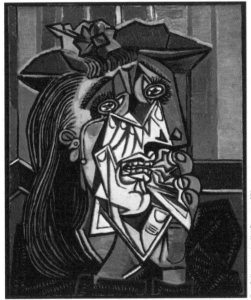

15. Head and Neck Embryology

Thornwell Hay Parker III

THE BUILDING BLOCKS[1]

TRILAMINAR DISC
- **Ectoderm:** Nervous system, skin (epidermis and appendages), and neural crest cells and derivatives
- **Mesoderm:** Bone, cartilage, muscles, connective tissue (dermis), dura mater, heart, vessels, blood, reproductive organs, and genitourinary system
- **Endoderm:** Gastrointestinal and respiratory lining and digestive organ parenchyma

BRANCHIAL STRUCTURES

- Neural crest migration is critical to branchial arch and facial development, influencing development of nerves, arteries, muscles, and skeletal structure.
- The **branchial arches** develop as mesenchymal swellings around the primitive pharynx and form a three-layer cylinders of ectoderm, mesoderm, and endoderm.
  - Different from the **somites,** which are mesodermal swellings around the neural tube
- **Branchial clefts** develop on the *external* surface, and **branchial pouches** develop on the *internal* surface as grooves between each arch.

BRANCHIAL ARCHES

Typically **six** arches are described; however, the first four are the most prominent.
  Arch I: Produces **maxillary (Ia)** and **mandibular (Ib)** arches with significant contributions to middle and lower facial development, contains **muscles of mastication,** and carries trigeminal nerve distribution **(V$_2$/V$_3$)**
  Arch II: **Hyoid arch** (provides soft tissue coverage of face and neck including frontalis; **muscles of facial expression;** and platysma, ossicles, and hyoid bone), carries facial nerve distribution **(VII)**
  Arch III: Contribution to hyoid bone, **stylopharyngeus muscle,** and glossopharyngeal nerve distribution **(IX)**
  Arches IV-VI: Laryngeal and thyroid cartilages, **pharyngeal and laryngeal musculature,** levator veli palatini muscle, and vagus nerve distribution **(X)**

TIP: The boldface structures above are usually tested on written examinations.

BRANCHIAL CLEFTS

- **Cleft I:** Significant, it becomes the **external auditory canal.**
- **Clefts II-IV:** *Operculum flap* grows downward from arch II and fuses below cleft IV to create the *cervical sinus.*
  - The cervical sinus disappears by week 6, and failure to do so results in **branchial cleft cysts, sinus tracts,** or **fistulas.**
  - These anomalies are often detected in the second decade of life and are palpable at the **anterior border of the sternocleidomastoid (SCM).**
  - Anomalies from **cleft II** are the most common, running under the middle/lower SCM, over the glossopharyngeal nerve, and between the external carotid artery and internal carotid artery (over the internal artery) toward the tonsillar fossa.
  - Anomalies from cleft III are similar but run under the internal carotid artery.

BRANCHIAL POUCHES

All pouches become important structures.
- **Pouch I:** Internal auditory canal
- **Pouch II:** Palatine tonsil
- **Pouch III:** Inferior parathyroid and thymus
- **Pouch IV:** Superior parathyroid **(pouch IV migrates above pouch III)**
- **Pouch V:** Ultimobranchial body (thyroid C-cells)

BONES

- **Intramembranous ossification**
  - Any cartilaginous precursors resorb
  - De novo bone formation from neural crest derivatives
  - Forms flat, squamous bones of cranium, orbit, nose, zygoma, maxilla, palate, and mandible
- **Endochondral ossification**
  - Cartilaginous precursors vascularized and ossified
  - Forms cranial base (occipital, squamous temporal, and sphenoid bone), ossicles, and hyoid bone

SCALP AND SKULL

- **Components**
  - Ectoderm forms skin (epidermis) and appendages.
  - Neural crest derivatives form skin (dermis), fat, squamous bone, and dura mater.
  - Neural tube derivatives form arachnoid, pia mater, and brain.
- **Growth**
  - Cranial vault grows in response to brain growth.
  - Bone growth proceeds **perpendicular** to orientation of sutures.
  - **Craniosynostosis:** Sutures fuse prematurely (see Chapter 21).
    - ▶ **Virchow's law:** Following suture fusion, growth proceeds **parallel** to suture instead of perpendicular.

MOUTH

- **Stomodeum:** Primitive mouth forms 3-4 weeks from invagination of ectoderm around buccopharyngeal membrane.
- Ectodermal derivatives form mouth anterior to the tonsils.

FACE[2-4] (Fig. 15-1)

THEORIES OF GROWTH

- **Fusion of processes:** Distinct facial processes grow toward one another, contact, and fuse by mechanisms similar to wound healing; *failure of contact and fusion results in clefts* (Meckel[2]).
- **Mesodermal penetration:** There are no distinct processes; instead elevations and depressions form with mesodermal penetration between the ectoderm and endoderm to maintain the confluence of elevations; *failure of mesodermal penetration results in clefts* (A. Fleischmean[2]).

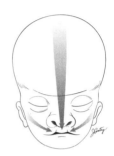

Fig. 15-1 Migratory pattern of ectomesenchyme to form the facial processes.

TERMINOLOGY (PROCESSES VERSUS PROMINENCES)

- Because many feel the mesodermal penetration theory is more accurate, the term *prominence* has been favored over *process*.

PROCESSES/PROMINENCES (Fig. 15-2)

- **Frontonasal prominence**
  - Pulled down ventrally during craniocaudal flexion, positioned just cranial to stomodeum
- **Nasal placodes:** Ectodermal densities develop at inferior end of frontonasal prominence
- **Nasal pit:** Develops as placodes deepen, eventually rupturing into mouth because the palate has not closed
- **Medial and lateral nasal swellings:** Develop along the rim of the deepening nasal pits and become the **medial and lateral nasal prominences**
  - Develops into three components during weeks 4-5
    1. **Frontal prominence**
    2. **Medial nasal prominence**
    3. **Lateral nasal prominence**
- **Maxillary prominences**
  - Medial growth during weeks 5-6 compresses the medial nasal prominences toward each other.
  - Lateral nasal prominences are compressed superiorly, separated from the maxillary prominences by the nasolacrimal groove, which closes to form the nasolacrimal duct system.

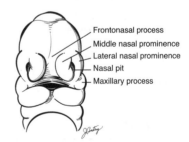

Frontonasal process
Middle nasal prominence
Lateral nasal prominence
Nasal pit
Maxillary process

Fig. 15-2 Some features of the human embryo at 5-6 weeks gestation.

Summary of Prominence Derivatives (Fig. 15-3)

- **Frontal prominence:** Forehead and apex of nose
- **Medial nasal prominence:** Primary palate, midmaxilla, midlip, philtrum, central nose, and septum
- **Lateral nasal prominences:** Nasal ala
- **Maxillary prominences:** Secondary palate, lateral maxilla, lateral lip
- **Mandibular prominences:** Mandible, lower lip, and lower face

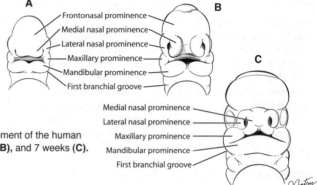

Fig. 15-3   Embryonic development of the human face at 5 weeks **(A)**, 6 weeks **(B)**, and 7 weeks **(C)**.

PALATE

- **Primary palate:** 5-6 weeks, medial nasal prominences come together to form the primary palate, midmaxilla, and septum
- **Secondary palate:** 9-12 weeks, lateral palatine shelves initially hang vertically but assume a horizontal position as tongue drops with mandibular growth; the right palate drops first, which may explain the higher incidence of clefts on the left side
- **Incisive foramen:** Lies between the primary and secondary palate

TONGUE

- **Arch I:** Forms **anterior** two-thirds (from three ventral wall swellings), two lateral lingual, and the tuberculum impar (the lower midline swelling)
- **Arch II:** No contribution
- **Arch III:** Forms **posterior** one-third from ventral wall midline swelling
- **Occipital myotomes:** Migrate to provide lingual musculature, bringing lingual nerve motor distribution (XII)

EXTERNAL EAR

CLEFT AND ARCH CONTRIBUTION

- **Branchial arch I:** Three anterior hillocks form **tragus, root of helix,** and **superior helix**
- **Branchial cleft I:** Forms **external auditory canal**
- **Branchial arch II:** Three posterior hillocks form **antihelix, antitragus,** and **lobule**

TIP: These are frequent test questions.

- The ear develops in neck region—arrested growth (microtia) usually results in inferiorly displaced auricle

---

KEY POINTS

✔ **Arch I**
- Produces maxillary and mandibular arches
- Forms muscles of mastication and carries CN V
- Three anterior hillocks: Form tragus, root of helix, and superior helix

✔ **Cleft I**
- Becomes external auditory canal

✔ **Arch II**
- Forms muscles of facial expression, carries CN VII
- Three posterior hillocks: Form antihelix, antitragus, and lobule

✔ **Frontal prominence:** Forehead and apex of nose.

✔ **Medial nasal prominence:** Primary palate, midmaxilla, midlip, philtrum, central nose, and septum.

✔ **Lateral nasal prominences:** Nasal ala.

✔ **Maxillary prominences:** Secondary palate, lateral maxilla, and lateral lip.

✔ **Mandibular prominences:** Mandible, lower lip, and lower face.

✔ Anomalies of **branchial cleft II** are the most common and typically are present over the SCM.

✔ **Branchial pouch III** becomes the **inferior** parathyroid glands, and **branchial pouch IV** becomes the **superior** parathyroid glands.

REFERENCES

1. Gosain AK, Moore FO. Embryology of the head and neck. In Aston SJ, Beasley RW, Thorne CHM, eds. Grabb and Smith's Plastic Surgery, 5th ed. Philadelphia: Lippincott-Raven, 1997.
2. Millard DR Jr. Cleft Craft I: The Evolution of Its Surgery, vol 1. Boston: Little Brown, 1976.
3. Cochard LR. Netter's Atlas of Human Embryology. Teterboro, NJ: Icon Learning Systems, 2002.
4. Persaud M. The Developing Human: Clinically Oriented Embryology, 7th ed. Philadelphia: WB Saunders, 2003.

16. Craniosynostosis

Thornwell Hay Parker III

DEFINITION

Premature fusion of cranial suture

INCIDENCE[1]
1:1000-2000 in general population

NORMAL PHYSIOLOGY[2]

- **Normal cranial growth**
  - Growth responds to increasing brain volume: Brain size triples by 1 year, quadruples by 2 years, and approximates 85% adult growth by 3 years of age.
  - Normal growth occurs perpendicular and parallel to sutures.
- **Normal suture anatomy**
  - Sutures are joints (syndesmoses) between the cranial bones. They have miniature ball and socket configurations along their lengths, which allow for stability and continued growth (Fig. 16-1).
- **Normal suture fusion**
  - **Metopic:** 2 years
  - **Sagittal:** 22 years
  - **Coronal:** 24 years
  - **Lambdoidal:** 26 years
- **Normal fontanelle closure**
  - **Posterior fontanelle:** 3-6 months
  - **Anterior fontanelle:** 9-12 months

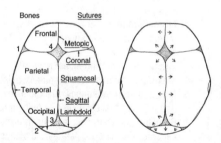

Fig. 16-1 Cranial sutures in the human fetus. Premature closure produces growth restriction perpendicular to the line of the suture and compensatory overgrowth parallel to it. (From Carson BS, Dufresne CR. Craniosynostosis and neurocranial asymmetry. In Dufresne CR, Carson BS, Zinreich SJ, eds. Complex Craniofacial Problems. New York: Churchill Livingstone, 1992, p 169.)

ETIOLOGIC FACTORS AND PATHOPHYSIOLOGY

VIRCHOW'S LAW
Premature suture fusion results in cranial growth predominately parallel to sutures (rather than perpendicular).

THEORIES OF SUTURE CLOSURE

- **Cranial base**
  - Synostoses result from abnormal tension exerted by cranial base through the dura.
  - Theory does *not* account for isolated synostoses.
- **Intrinsic suture biology**
  - Synostoses result from the osteoinductive properties of dura mater, which contains osteoblastlike cells.
- **Extrinsic factors**
  - Synostoses result from extrinsic forces or systemic disease.
    - In utero compression
    - Hydrocephalus decompression
    - Abnormal brain growth (e.g., microcephaly)
    - Systemic pathology (e.g., hypothyroidism or rickets)

GENETICS

- 50% of syndromic synostoses are hereditary.
- 2% of isolated synostoses are hereditary.
- Links have been found to mutations of FGFR2, FGFR3 (isolated unicoronal), MSX2 (Boston type), TWIST (S-C), and long arm of 10 (Crouzon's disease).

INDICATIONS FOR TREATMENT

- Early suture closure may **decrease intracranial volume, restrict brain growth,** and cause **intracranial hypertension** (<15 mm Hg).
  - Mental impairment/neuropsychiatric disorders
  - Growth impairment
  - Optic atrophy and vision loss
- More involved sutures correlates with increased intracranial pressures (ICP).[3]
  - 13% incidence of increased ICP with **isolated** synostosis
  - 42% incidence of increased ICP with **multiple** suture synostoses
- More involved sutures correlates with increased mental impairment.
- Mental insults are gradual, irreversible, and difficult to detect.
- Cosmetic deformity and difficult social interactions.

DIAGNOSIS AND EVALUATION

- **History**
  - Headache
  - Irritability
  - Difficulty sleeping
- **Physical examination**
  - No movement at sutures
  - Palpable ridges (especially metopic)
  - Bulging or closed fontanelles
  - Abnormal cranial morphology, orbital rim relationship to cornea, abnormal/asymmetric facial features

- **Imaging studies**
  - **Radiographic film**
    - ▶ Anteroposterior, lateral, and Townes; C-spine (for associated C-spine anomalies)
    - ▶ Plain films often adequate for diagnosis and operative planning
    - ▶ Suture fusion revealed by **absence of suture line**
    - ▶ Elevated ICP revealed by late findings of cortical thickening, fingerprinting, beaten copper (Luckenschadel), loss of cisternae
  - **CT scan**
    - ▶ Not required for isolated craniosynostosis
    - ▶ Used routinely in syndromic synostoses
    - ▶ Three-dimensional imaging to better define suture fusion, abnormal morphology, and intracranial volume
    - ▶ Detect hydrocephalus, signs of elevated ICP, and other bone/brain abnormalities seen in some syndromes
  - **MRI**
    - ▶ Usually unnecessary
    - ▶ Used for select syndromes (Apert's or Pfeiffer syndrome) with suspicion of brain abnormalities

CLASSIFICATION (Fig. 16-2)

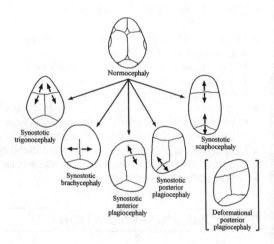

Fig. 16-2 Skull shapes and affected sutures in craniosynostosis. (From Cohen MM Jr, MacLean RE. Anatomic, genetic, nosologic, diagnostic, and psychosocial considerations. In Cohen MM Jr, MacLean RE, eds. Craniosynostosis: Diagnosis, Evaluation, and Management, 2nd ed. New York: Oxford University Press, 2000, pp 119-143.)

SAGITTAL SYNOSTOSIS
- Incidence: 50% of craniosynostosis
- Morphology: **Scaphocephaly;** also called *dolichocephaly*
  - Increased AP diameter and decreased biparietal width
  - Frontal bossing and occipital bulge
- Male/female ratio: 4:1

UNILATERAL CORONAL SYNOSTOSIS
- Incidence: 20% of craniosynostosis
- Morphology: **Anterior plagiocephaly**
  - Ipsilateral frontal flattening and contralateral bossing
  - Ipsilateral occipitoparietal flattening, ipsilateral occipitomastoid bossing, and contralateral parietal bossing
  - Ipsilateral ear posteriorly displaced
  - Recessed supraorbital and lateral rim; shallow orbit
  - **Harlequin deformity:** Lack of descent of greater wing of the sphenoid (also ipsilateral)
  - Recessed zygoma and inferior rim
  - Root of nose constricted and deviated to ipsilateral side
  - Cranial base short in AP direction

BILATERAL CORONAL SYNOSTOSIS
- Incidence: 20% of craniosynostosis
- Morphology: **Brachycephaly**
  - Most common deformity in Apert's syndrome and Crouzon's syndrome
  - Recession of supraorbital ridges with bulging forehead
  - Shallow orbits and hypertelorism
  - Anterior cranial base wide, but short in AP direction

METOPIC SYNOSTOSIS
- Incidence: 10% of craniosynostosis
- Morphology: **Trigonocephaly**
  - Most obvious with midline vertical forehead ridge and keel shaped forehead
  - Bitemporal narrowing, hypotelorism, upward slant of bilateral canthi
  - Anterior cranial base increased in the AP dimension
- ICP elevation: 4%-10%

LAMBDOID SYNOSTOSIS
- Incidence: Less than 3% of craniosynostosis
- Morphology: **Posterior plagiocephaly** or **occipital plagiocephaly**

DEFORMATIONAL PLAGIOCEPHALY (Table 16-1)
- Incidence: 1:300 in the general population

TIP   Often mistaken for lambdoidal or coronal plagiocephaly

- Head assumes *parallelogram* configuration
- Ipsilateral occipital flattening and frontal bossing
- Ear displaced anteriorly

- Not true craniosynostosis, but deformation secondary to external forces
  - **Supine positioning: American Academy of Pediatrics** recommends infants sleep supine to lessen risk of sudden infant death syndrome (SIDS); this has led to an increasing incidence of deformities.
  - **Rotational forces:** Torticollis, vertebral abnormalities, and visual field deficits may all cause preferential rotation and unequal pressure on the occiput.

Table 16-1   *Anatomic Features That Differentiate Synostotic and Deformational Frontal Plagiocephaly*

Anatomic Feature	Synostotic	Deformational
Ipsilateral superior orbital rim	Up	Down
Ipsilateral ear	Anterior and high	Posterior and low
Nasal root	Ipsilateral	Midline
Ipsilateral cheek	Forward	Backward
Chin deviation	Contralateral	Ipsilateral
Ipsilateral palpebral fissure	Wide	Narrow
Anterior fontanel deviation	Low contralateral	High none

From Hansen M, Mulliken JB. Frontal plagiocephaly: Diagnosis and treatment. Clin Plast Surg 21:543-553, 1994.

OTHER MORPHOLOGIC VARIANTS

- **Turricephaly:** Excessive skull height and vertical forehead from **untreated brachycephaly**
- **Oxycephaly:** Pointed head; forehead retroverted and tilted back; from **fusion of multiple sutures**
- **Kleeblattschaedel (cloverleaf deformity):** Secondary to **pansutural** synostosis

SYNDROMIC CRANIOSYNOSTOSIS[4]

- **Crouzon's syndrome**
  - Autosomal dominant
  - Incidence: 1:25,000
  - Intracranial: Hydrocephalus, ICP elevation in 43%, usually mild mental impairment
  - Cranial/upper face: **Turribrachycephaly,** coronal and lambdoidal synostoses
  - Orbits: Exorbitism/proptosis leads to conjunctivitis/keratitis
  - Midface: Hypoplasia
  - **Extremities: Normal**
- **Apert's syndrome**
  - Autosomal dominant
  - Incidence: 1:100,000-160,000
  - Intracranial: ICP elevation in 66%, ventriculoperitoneal (VP) shunts often needed, **mental impairment common,** cerebral palsy
  - Cranial/upper face: Only bicoronal synostoses, but significant **turribrachycephaly**
  - Orbits: Proptosis, downslanting palpebral fissures, and hypertelorism
  - Midface: Hypoplasia, nose turned down with depressed dorsum and septal deviation
  - Extremities: **Severe syndactyly of hands and feet** (usually two to four fingers or toes)
  - **Other: Acne**
- **Pfeiffer syndrome**
  - Autosomal dominant
  - Intracranial: **Usually normal mental status**
  - Cranial/upper face: **Turribrachycephaly;** coronal, sometimes sagittal synostoses
  - Orbits: Shallow, exorbitism, hypertelorism, downslanting palpebral fissures
  - Midface: Hypoplasia, nose turned down with low nasal bridge

- Extremities: **Broad thumbs and halluces,** mild cutaneous syndactyly (second and third fingers, second through fourth toes)
- Other: Also called *lower Apert's syndrome*
- Cohen[5] divided into three types
  - ▸ Type I: Classical (most common)
  - ▸ Type II: Severe cloverleaf
  - ▸ Type III: Intermediate

■ **Saethre-Chotzen syndrome**
- Autosomal dominant, TWIST gene mutation
- Incidence: 1:25,000-50,000
- Intracranial: **Mental status usually normal**
- Cranial/upper face: **Asymmetric brachycephaly**
- Orbits: **Ptosis of eyelids**
- Midface: Hypoplasia, facial asymmetry, hypoplastic nasal septum, narrow palate
- Extremities: Partial syndactyly
- Other: **Low hairline,** also called *upper Apert's syndrome*

■ **Carpenter's syndrome**
- **Autosomal recessive**
- Intracranial: **Mental impairment associated**
- Cranial/upper face: **Brachycephaly,** asymmetric, variable suture involvement
- Orbit: Displaced medial canthi
- Extremities: Preaxial syndactyly of feet, soft tissue syndactyly of third or fourth fingers
- Other: **ventricular septal/atrial septal defects in 33%, possible venous and bony abnormalities, low-set ears**

TREATMENT

■ Multidisciplinary team approach
- Plastic surgeon, neurosurgeon, oral surgeon/dentist/orthodontist, ear/nose/throat surgeon, ophthalmologist, speech therapist, pediatrician, geneticist, child psychologist, nurses

SURGERY

TIMING

■ Usually treat craniosynostosis between **3 months and 1 year of age,** but earlier if pansutural involvement
■ **Earlier:** More malleable, may lessen concomitant facial deformities, heal and regenerate bone faster
■ **Later:** Potentially less need for revision
■ **General timeline**
- Cranial vault reshaping/frontoorbital advancement: 3-12 months
  - ▸ When staged, usually perform posterior craniotomy first, then anterior craniotomy 3 weeks later
- Midface (Le Fort III ± I): 6-12 years
- Mandible: 14-18 years

GOALS
- Allow normal brain growth
- Achieve normal craniofacial contour (social)

TYPICAL SEQUENCE
- Use transcoronal incision.
- Dissect subperiosteally.
  - If dissecting to supraorbital rims, release supraorbital nerve with osteotome.
- Craniotomy: Drill burr holes and connect them with craniotome.
- Carefully elevate bone flaps off dura.
- Elevate temporalis, then cut and advance frontal bar.
- Cut barrel staves, and outfracture as needed.
- Split bone graft as needed with osteotome.
- Mold bone flaps as needed with burr, scoring, and radial osteotomies.
- Replace bone flaps.
- Fixate with absorbable hardware.
- Apply additional bone grafts, bone dust, and exogenous grafts (hydroxyapatite) as needed to close.
- Place drain and close scalp.

TECHNIQUES
- **Plagiocephaly and brachycephaly:** Bifrontal craniotomy, frontoorbital advancement repositioning frontal bar, recontouring frontal bone with radial osteotomies and repositioning with 180-degree turn, barrel staves
- **Scaphocephaly:** Possible bifrontal and biparietooccipital craniotomies, radial osteotomies, central bar widened with graft, barrel staves, outfracturing of temporal and parietal bone, frontoorbital advancement (may stage operation as anterior and posterior stages)
- **Trigonocephaly:** Bifrontal craniotomy, frontal reshaping with burr and radial osteotomies, fronto-orbital advancement, possible bone grafting
- **Posterior plagiocephaly:** Biparietooccipital craniotomies and contouring
- **Deformational plagiocephaly:** Mostly nonoperative management; address preventable causes; helmet molding: Helmet worn up to 23 hours a day, in three different stages

ALTERNATIVE APPROACHES
- **Strip craniectomy**
  - Still under study
  - Primarily for isolated sagittal synostoses when less than 4 months of age
  - High recurrence rate
  - Open versus endoscopic approaches
  - Helmet molding applied postoperatively

FIXATION
- **Hardware**
  - Wires
  - Titanium screws and plates
  - Absorbable hardware
  - **LactoSorb**[6] (Lorenz Surgical, Jacksonville, FL)
    - Absorbable hardware
    - Made of polylactic and polyglycolic acid

▸ Resorbs in 9-15 months by hydrolysis
▸ May avoid growth restriction

GRAFTS

- **Autologous bone grafts**
  - **Split calvarial:** Usually parietal bone split ex vivo
  - **Split rib:** Leave periosteum intact for rib regeneration, harder to mold and increased resorption
  - **Iliac wing, split tibia**
- **Methylmethacrylate:** Resin
- **Hydroxyapatite:** Calcium phosphate, which is 70% human bone
  - Preformed ceramics or moldable nonceramic (but small pores for vascular ingrowth)
  - Replamineform: Heat coral with aqueous phosphate
- **Others:** Porous polyethylene (Medpor; Porex, Newnan, GA), bioactive glass (bonds with tissues), demineralized bone
- **Bone tissue engineering**

POSTOPERATIVE CARE

- Observation in ICU for 24-48 hours
- Close monitoring: Neurologic examination every 2 hours; hematocrit and sodium every 6 hours for 24 hours
- Transfusions commonly given if hematocrit falls below 30
  - 10 ml/kg over 4 hours
- Head dressing and drain removed 1 day postoperatively
- Parents instructed to guard against head trauma, but otherwise may hold and lay child down as usual
- Return to clinic every 4-6 months until 3 years, then once a year until 5 years, then every other year

COMPLICATIONS

- 1%-2% mortality with surgery
- Plate migration
- Bleeding: Most require transfusions; large surface area of raw bone bleeds most over the first 24 hours
- Venous air embolism
- Infection: Although postoperative fever is very common, it does not warrant extensive workup unless other clinical signs of infection[7]
- Cerebrospinal fluid leak: Check intraoperatively with Valsalva maneuver
- Visual changes or compromise
- Reoperation rates higher for syndromic craniosynostosis: 27% versus 5.9% for isolated; highest with bilateral coronal synostosis

KEY POINTS

- ✔ Cranial growth is normally perpendicular but predominantly parallel after fusion.
- ✔ Brain size triples by 1 year and quadruples by 2 years.
- ✔ If suture is fused, then no suture is seen on plain radiographic films.
- ✔ Involved sutures
  - Sagittal (50%): Leads to scaphocephaly
  - Unicoronal (20%): Leads to anterior plagiocephaly
  - Bicoronal (20%): Leads to brachycephaly/turribrachycephaly
  - Metopic (10%): Leads to trigonocephaly
  - Lambdoid (<3%): Leads to posterior plagiocephaly
- ✔ Lambdoidal plagiocephaly
  - Trapezoid configuration
  - Posterior displacement of ear
- ✔ Deformational plagiocephaly
  - Parallelogram configuration
  - Anterior displacement of ear
- ✔ Syndromes
  - Crouzon's disease: Normal extremities
  - Apert's syndrome: Acne, common mental impairment, severe syndactyly
  - Pfeiffer syndrome: Broad thumbs/halluces, usually no mental impairment
  - Saethre-Chotzen syndrome: Low hairline and eyelid ptosis
  - Carpenter's syndrome: Autosomal recessive, VSD/ASD in 33% of cases

REFERENCES

1. Pyo DJ, Persin JA. Craniosynostosis. In Aston SJ, Beasley RW, Thorne CHM, eds. Grabb and Smith's Plastic Surgery, 5th ed. Philadelphia: Lippincott-Raven, 1997.
2. Hunt JH, Flood J. Craniofacial anomalies II: Syndromes and surgery. Sel Read Plast Surg 9(25), 2002.
3. Renier D, Sainte-Rose C, Marchac D, et al. Intracranial pressure in craniostenosis. J Neurosurg 57:370-377, 1982.
4. Katzen JT, McCarthy JG. Syndromes involving craniosynostosis and midface hypoplasia. Otolaryngol Clin North Am 33:1257-1284, 2000.
5. Cohen MM Jr. Pfeiffer syndrome update: Clinical subtypes and guidelines for differential diagnosis. Am J Med Genet 45:300-307, 1993.
6. Tharanon W, Sinn DP, Hobar PC, et al. Surgical outcomes using bioabsorbable plating systems in pediatric craniofacial surgery. J Craniofac Surg 9:441-444, 1998.
7. Hobar PC, Masson JA, Herrera R, et al. Fever after craniofacial surgery in the infant under 24 months of age. Plast Reconstr Surg 102:32-36, 1998.

17. Craniofacial Clefts

Melissa A. Crosby

EMBRYOLOGY[1]

- **3-8 weeks:** Facial development occurs (Fig. 17-1).[2]
  - **3-4 weeks:**
    - ▶ Frontonasal prominence of forebrain results in nasal and olfactory placodes that become medial and lateral processes.
      - ✦ **Medial nasal process:** Nasal tip, columella, philtrum, and premaxilla
      - ✦ **Lateral nasal process:** Nasal ala
    - ▶ Mandibular arch bifurcates to form mandibular processes that move toward midline to form lower mouth.
  - **5-6 weeks:**
    - ▶ Nasal processes enlarge, migrate, and coalesce in midline to unite with maxillary process to form upper lip; completes growth of midface when coalesced.

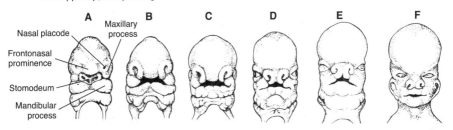

Fig. 17-1 Embryonic development of the human face. **A,** 4-week embryo. **B,** 5-week embryo. **C,** 6-week embryo. **D,** 6½-week embryo. **E,** 7-week embryo. **F,** 8-week embryo. (From Kawamoto H Jr. Rare craniofacial clefts. In McCarthy J, ed. Plastic Surgery: Cleft Lip and Palate and Craniofacial Anomalies, vol 4. Philadelphia: WB Saunders, 1990, pp 2945-2951.)

PATHOGENESIS

THEORIES

- **Classic**[3,4]
  - Failure of facial processes to fuse.
  - Face forms as maxillary processes meet and coalesce with paired globular processes beneath the nasal pits.
  - Epithelial contact is established, and mesodermal penetration completes fusion forming lip and hard palate.
  - Cleft forms when process disrupted.
- **Mesodermal penetration**[5-8]
  - Face consists of a bilaminar ectodermal membrane with epithelial seams demarcating major processes.

165

- Mesenchyme migrates into double wall of ectoderm penetrating and smoothing out seams.
- Dehisces and cleft produced if penetration fails and epithelial walls unsupported.

CLASSIFICATION[1,9,10]

■ **Anatomic:** A number is assigned to each malformation according to its position relative to midline (Fig. 17-2).[11]

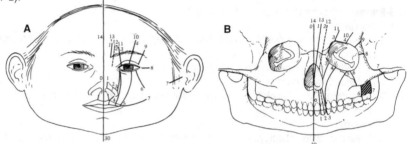

Fig. 17-2 Tessier classification of clefts. **A,** Paths of various clefts on the face. **B,** Location of the clefts on the facial skeleton. (From Tessier P. Anatomical classification of facial, cranio-facial, and latero-facial clefts. J Maxillofac Surg 4:69-92, 1976.)

■ **Embryologic:** Craniofacial skeleton develops along a helical course symbolized by the letter S (not commonly used as a classification system).[12]

ORAL-NASAL CLEFTS
Oral-nasal clefts occur between the midline and Cupid's bow, disrupting both the lip and nose.
■ **Cleft no. 0**
  - Directly in midline of lip and nose
  - Can continue as cleft no. 14
■ **Cleft no. 1**
  - Cleft through lateral margin of Cupid's bow progressing into nose through the parasagittal dorsum on one side
  - Classified as *nasoschizis* (subtype of nasal dysplasia)
  - Can continue as cleft no. 13
■ **Cleft no. 2**
  - Extremely rare
  - Originates at lateral margin of Cupid's bow and extends into the middle third of the nostril as deficiency and flattening of soft tissue of nose
  - Can extend as cleft no. 12
■ **Cleft no. 3**
  - Common
  - Unilateral or bilateral
  - Can continue as cleft no. 10 or cleft no. 11
  - Originates from lateral margin of Cupid's bow and extends across the base of the nasal ala into normal union between the medial nasal process and the maxillary process; extends through the nasolacrimal duct and into lacrimal groove

ORAL-OCULAR CLEFTS

*Clefts that connect the oral and orbital cavities without disrupting the integrity of the nose; occur lateral to Cupid's bow, extending through the soft tissue of the cheek and maxillary process; called **meloschisis** (includes Tessier clefts nos. 4-6)*

- **Cleft no. 4**
  - One of most disruptive and complicated clefts
  - Unilateral, bilateral, or combined with other clefts
  - Begins lateral to Cupid's bow between commissure of mouth and philtral crest, passes onto cheek lateral to nasal ala, and curves into lower eyelid terminating medial to punctum
  - Lower canniculus usually disrupted along with most of the inferior supporting structures to the eye
  - Medial canthal ligament and lacrimal apparatus usually intact
  - **Osseous:** Begins between lateral incisor and canine teeth onto anterior surface maxilla lateral to piriform aperture, medial to infraorbital nerve; medial and inferior portions of orbital wall disrupted
- **Cleft no. 5**
  - **Rarest** of oral-ocular clefts
  - Lip is cleft medial to but near the commissure extending laterally on cheek into lateral third of lower eyelid
  - **Osseous:** Lateral to canine extending lateral to the infraorbital foramen entering lateral half of orbit
- **Cleft no. 6**
  - Includes incomplete forms of Treacher Collins syndrome
  - Transition between oral-ocular and lateral facial clefts
  - Extends lateral to oral commissure and across lateral portion of maxilla and zygoma to terminate in a **coloboma** (soft tissue deformity of the lower lid in the lateral third)
  - Ear normal
  - **Osseous:** Molar area on the involved side hypoplastic, and extends into the zygomatic maxillary suture with malar hypoplasia extending into lateral third of orbit

LATERAL FACIAL CLEFTS

Include Tessier clefts nos. 7-9, Treacher Collins syndrome, Goldenhar's syndrome, hemifacial microsomia, and necrotic facial dysplasia

- **Cleft no. 7**
  - ***Most common of all craniofacial clefts***
  - Males affected more frequently than females
  - 10% bilateral
  - Occurs in 1-6 of 8000 births in sporadic fashion
  - Has been postulated that cleft is a result of disruption of **stapedial artery** in embryogenesis
  - Originates in the lip at the oral commissure and extends laterally toward the ear, ceasing at the anterior border of the masseter muscle
  - Variable degrees of soft tissue deformity
  - Worst form may see maldevelopment of external ear
  - Middle ear, zygoma, maxilla, and mandible affected
  - Mandible deficiency in condyle, ascending ramus, and temporomandibular joint
  - Open bite or crossbite seen
  - Paresis of CN V and CN VII common
- **Cleft no. 8**
  - Rare—almost always exists in combination with another rare cleft
  - Isolated largely to orbital area
  - Lateral canthal irregularity accompanied by dermoid

- Involves the frontozygomatic suture
- Associated with Goldenhar's syndrome
■ **Cleft no. 9**
  - Extremely rare
  - Involves the superolateral orbit dividing lateral third of eyelid and brow
  - Superior orbital rim and temporal bone involved
  - May be accompanied by encephaloceles

TREACHER COLLINS SYNDROME (Fig. 17-3)
■ Bilateral combination of Tessier cleft nos. 6-8
■ Described by Treacher Collins in 1900
■ **Autosomal dominant** with incidence of 1:10,000 live births
■ Change in gene on chromosome 5
■ Includes coloboma and retraction of lower lid (antimongoloid slant), with hypoplasia of lower lid lashes
■ Upper lid redundant in lateral half and gives false impression of ptosis
■ Lateral canthus displaced inferiorly
■ Absence of zygomatic arch
■ Hypoplasia of temporalis muscle
■ Ear malformations
■ Abnormalities of hairline including tongue-shaped processes extending toward cheeks
■ Absence of lateral inferior orbital rim
■ Hypoplasia of malar bones and mandible
■ **Airway management priority** in newborn because of narrow pharyngeal diameter and mandibular shortening

GOLDENHAR'S SYNDROME
■ Sporadic occurrence
■ Prominent frontal bossing
■ Low hairline
■ Mandibular hypoplasia
■ Low-set ears
■ Colobomas of upper eyelid
■ Epibulbar dermoids
■ Bilateral anterior accessory auricular appendages (Fig. 17-4)
■ Vertebral abnormalities

CRANIAL CLEFTS
Clefts extend superiorly from the lateral orbit to the midline and proceed through the frontal bone and often into the base of the cranial vault.
■ **Cleft no. 10**
  - Corresponds to the cranial branch of cleft no. 4
  - Positioned in the center of the upper lid, brow, and orbit
  - Coloboma in mid-upper lid and irregular retracted central brow
  - **Osseous:** Divides central superior orbital rim, underlying cranial bone, and frontal bone
  - May include encephaloceles and hypertelorism from inferolateral rotation of orbit
■ **Cleft no. 11**
  - Found in combination with cleft no. 3
  - Cleft in medial eyebrow and lid with some soft tissue irregularity over forehead

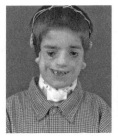
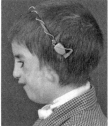

Fig. 17-3   Patient with Treacher Collins syndrome and tracheostomy for airway management. (Courtesy Craniofacial Clinic UT Southwestern.)

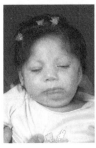
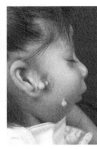
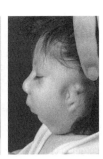

Fig. 17-4   Patient with Goldenhar's syndrome demonstrating anterior accessory auricular appendages. (Courtesy Craniofacial Clinic UT Southwestern.)

- **Osseous:** Extends through cranial base and into ethmoid sinuses
- Encephaloceles and hypertelorism may be present
- **Cleft no. 12**
  - Extension of cleft no. 2
  - Encephalocele and disruption of medial eyebrow margin seen
  - Orbital hypertelorism
  - **Osseous:** Involves frontal bone extending inferiorly to the frontal process of maxilla into ethmoid labyrinth
  - Cribriform plate normal
- **Cleft no. 13**
  - Extension of cleft no. 1
  - Extends through olfactory groove with widening of cribriform plate
  - Massive encephaloceles visible when bilateral
  - Irregularity of medial eyebrow with displacement into orbit
- **Cleft no. 14**
  - Midline facial clefts accompanying central nervous system abnormalities
  - Extension of cleft no. 0
  - If true cleft, see herniation of intracranial contents resulting in arrest of normal migration of orbit
  - Hypertelorism and cranium bifida may be present
  - Cribriform plate displaced inferiorly
  - Olfactory grooves widely separated
  - Frontal nasal encephalocele is present
  - If dysgenesis or agenesis occurs, may see cyclopia

- Holoprosencephaly: Hypotelorism, microcephaly, and severe CNS abnormalities
- Life expectancy severely limited

RECONSTRUCTION

MULTIDISCIPLINARY APPROACH
- Initially focuses on soft tissue closure, with excision of all scar within clefts until normal tissue is reached, followed by meticulous layered closure of soft tissue
- Skeletal reconstruction often necessary but delayed until child is older

GOALS
- Functional correction of macrostomia
- Soft tissue reconstruction of eyelid to prevent globe exposure
- Separation of the confluent oral, nasal, and orbital spaces
- Aesthetic correction of deformity

KEY POINTS
- ✔ The most common craniofacial cleft is no. 7.
- ✔ Treacher Collins syndrome involves Tessier clefts nos. 6-8.
- ✔ Goldenhar's syndrome is associated with Tessier cleft no. 8.
- ✔ Know the Tessier diagram and location of each cleft based on midline.

REFERENCES

1. Hunt JA, Hobar PC. Common craniofacial anomalies: Facial clefts and encephaloceles. Plast Reconstr Surg 112:606-616, 2003.
2. Kawamoto HK Jr. Rare craniofacial clefts. In McCarthy JG, ed. Plastic Surgery: Cleft Lip and Palate and Craniofacial Anomalies, vol 4. Philadelphia: WB Saunders, 1990, pp 2945-2951.
3. Dursy E. Zur Entwicklungsgeschichte des Kopfes des Menschen und der hoeheren Wirbelthiere. Tubingen, Verlag der H Lauppschen-Buchhandlung, 1869, p 99.
4. His W. Die Entwickelung der menschlichen und tierischer Physiognomen. Z Arch Anat Entwicklungsgesch, 1892, p 384.
5. Pohlmann EH. Die embryonale Metamorphose der Physiognomie und der Mundhoehle des Katzenkopfes. Morphol Jahrb Leipzig 41:617, 1910.
6. Veau V. Hasencharten menschlicher Keimlinge auf der Stufe 21-23 mm SSL. Z Anat Entwiklunsgesch 108:459, 1938.
7. Stark RB. The pathogenesis of harelip and cleft palate. Plast Reconstr Surg 13:20, 1954.
8. Stark RB, Saunders DE. The first brachial syndrome: The oral-mandibular-auricular syndrome. Plast Reconstr Surg 29:299, 1962.
9. Argenta LC, David LR. Craniofacial clefts and other related deformities. In Achauer BM, Eriksson E, Kolk CV. Plastic Surgery: Indications, Operations, and Outcomes. St Louis: Mosby, 2000, pp 741-754.
10. Hunt J, Flood J. Craniofacial anomalies II: Syndromes and surgery. Sel Read Plast Surg 3(25), 2002.
11. Tessier P. Anatomical classification of facial, cranio-facial, and latero-facial clefts. J Maxillofac Surg 4:69-92, 1976.
12. Van der Meulen JC, Mazzola R, Vermey-Keers C, et al. A morphogenetic classification of craniofacial malformations. Plast Reconstr Surg 71:560, 1983.

18. Distraction Osteogenesis

Jeffrey E. Janis
Jason E. Leedy

DEFINITION

Distraction osteogenesis (DO) is a surgical technique by which new bone is generated in the gap between two bone segments in response to tensile stress across the gap after osteotomies are performed. The overlying soft tissue elongates and undergoes hypertrophy as well.

PHYSIOLOGY[1]

Tension-stress effect occurs when normal human tissue that is placed under a consistent, moderate tension responds by regenerating (i.e., forming new tissue of identical type).

BONE
- DO allows generation of **bone** and **soft tissue.**
- Bone gap is created, and, through the continued application of tension across the gap, soft callus does not progress to hard callus and fracture union.
- Bone gap has four zones.
  1. **Fibrous central zone:** New collagen fibers form parallel to the axis of distraction
  2. **Transition zone:** Early formation of bone
  3. **Bone remodeling zone:** Primary mineralization found with bone spicule formation
  4. **Mature bone zone:** Progressive calcification of the primary mineralization front with formation of lamellar bone and marrow elements
- At the cessation of distraction the mineralizing fronts fuse, giving fracture union.
- *The bone formed through the process of DO is indistinguishable from natural mature bone.*

SOFT TISSUE
- Muscles elongate and undergo hypertrophy *(distraction histogenesis).*
- "Soft tissue memory" may result in relapse after removal or cessation of distraction.

DISTRACTION PROCESS[1]

- **Corticotomy or osteotomy**
  - Fracture created through cortical bone preserving periosteal attachments and medullary continuity
- **Application of distraction device**
- **Latency**
  - Period between corticotomy or osteotomy and commencement of distraction
  - Usually 5-7 days
  - Allows formation of a bridge of fibrovascular tissue

171

- *Rate*
  - ▸ Number of millimeters the gap is widened daily
    - ✦ Usually 1 mm/day
  - ▸ Less can lead to premature ossification, local ischemia, or both
- *Rhythm*
  - ▸ Number of times per day the distractor is activated
  - ▸ Usually 0.5 mm twice a day or 0.25 mm four times a day
- **Activation phase**
  - Period between corticotomy and conclusion of distraction
- **Consolidation phase**
  - Period between the conclusion of distraction to evidence of bony remineralization
  - Usually 8 weeks
  - Distractor left in place, although no active distraction occurring
  - Check quality of new bone with radiographs (Fig. 18-1)
- **Removal of distraction device**
  - Performed when cortical outline is seen on postoperative radiograph

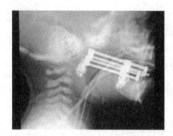

Fig. 18-1 Radiographs can be used to check new bone quality during consolidation phase of mandibular distraction.

INDICATIONS FOR DISTRACTION

- **Mandibular lengthening**
  - Hemifacial microsomia
  - Micrognathia
  - Airway compromise in the newborn secondary to micrognathia
- **Le Fort I advancement**
  - Cleft lip patients with premaxillary retrusion
- **Le Fort III/monobloc advancement**
  - Syndromic patients with midface retrusion

DISTRACTION DEVICES

EXTERNAL
- Uses percutaneous pins and external distractor device
- Can have multiple vectors
- Device removal does not require operation
- Percutaneous scars may require revision

INTERNAL
- Use internal distraction devices placed directly on bone
- Single vector
- Device removal requires operation
- Avoids cutaneous scarring

RESORBABLE
- Available, but not commonly used because of postoperative complications

MANDIBULAR DISTRACTION

GOALS
- Achieve proper occlusion
- Lengthen the ramus/body
- Reconstruct a mandibular defect
- Reconstruct the temporomandibular joint

OPERATIVE TECHNIQUE
1. Gain adequate exposure of mandible through an intraoral incision.
2. Identify proposed site of osteotomy or osteotomies based on preoperative imaging.

> TIP: Avoid disruption of tooth buds through preoperative dental examinations, radiographs, and CT scans.

3. Place the distraction device.
4. Perform the osteotomies.
- Vertical osteotomy on ramus to give horizontal advancement
  ‣ Make C-shaped osteotomy to exclude coronoid process (and pull from temporalis) from anterior segment (Fig. 18-2)
- Oblique osteotomy on lower ramus to give both horizontal and vertical advancement
- Horizontal osteotomy on ramus to give vertical lengthening
5. Perform closure

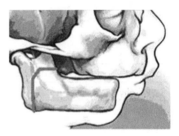

Fig. 18-2   C-shaped mandibular osteotomy.

MIDFACE/MAXILLARY DISTRACTION OSTEOGENESIS

GOALS
- **Achieve proper occlusion**
- **Correct midface retrusion**
  - Useful if more than 1 cm of advancement desired because gradual process with distraction allows soft tissues to accommodate better than if advancement performed immediately
- **Improve aesthetic appearance**

> TIP: Improves hypernasality.

OPERATIVE TECHNIQUE

1. Gain adequate exposure of midface/maxilla through a gingivobuccal incision and/or a coronal incision if necessary.
2. Identify proposed site of osteotomy or osteotomies based on preoperative imaging (Le Fort I, II, or III).

TIP: Again, *always* avoid tooth bud disruption!

3. Mobilize soft tissues.
4. Place the distraction device.
5. Perform closure.

COMPLICATIONS (Table 18-1)

- Scarring (distractor pin site)
- Infection
- Fibrous nonunion
- Premature ossification
- Tooth bud disruption
- Inappropriate vector

Table 18-1 *Incidence of Complications in Craniofacial Distraction Osteogenesis*

Complication	Frequency (%)
Compliance problems	4.7
Hardware failure	4.5
Device dislodgement	3.0
Premature consolidation	1.9
Pain preventing distraction	1.0
Fibrous nonunion	0.5
Inappropriate vector (single vector device)	8.8
Inappropriate vector (multivector device)	7.2
Pin tract infection	5.2

From Mofid MM, Manson PN, Robertson BC, et al. Craniofacial distraction osteogenesis: A review of 3278 cases. Plast Reconstr Surg 108:1103, 2001.

TIP: Bone grafting may be required if distraction failure occurs.

KEY POINTS

✔ Distraction osteogenesis involves corticotomy, latency, activation phase, and consolidation phase.
✔ Soft tissue accommodation may prevent relapse as seen in single-stage advancements.

REFERENCE

1. Hunt J, Flood J. Craniofacial anomalies II: Syndromes and surgery. Sel Read Plast Surg 9(25), 2002.

19. Cleft Lip

Amanda A. Gosman

EMBRYOLOGY

- The **primary palate** includes lip, nostril sill, alveolus, and hard palate **anterior** to incisive foramen.
  - The medial and lateral nasal prominences of the frontonasal process fuse with the maxillary prominence to form the primary palate during weeks 4 to 7 of gestation.
- Cleft lip results from failure of the medial nasal prominence and the maxillary prominence to fuse.
- Cleft lip with or without cleft palate (CL/P) is an embryologically, anatomically, and genetically distinct entity from isolated cleft palate (CP).

ANATOMY

NORMAL UPPER LIP ANATOMY
- **Surface landmarks**
  - **Philtral columns:** Bilateral vertical bulge created by dermal insertion of orbicularis oris fibers
  - **Philtral dimple:** Concavity between columns created by relative paucity of muscle fibers
  - **White roll:** Prominent ridge just above cutaneous-vermilion border
  - **Vermilion:** Red mucosal portion of the lip divided into *dry* (keratinized) and *wet* (nonkeratinized)
  - **Red line:** Junction between the dry and wet vermilion mucosa
  - **Cupid's bow:** Curvature of central white roll; two lateral peaks are the inferior extension of the philtral columns
  - **Tubercle:** Vermilion fullness at central inferior apex of Cupid's bow
- **Muscles**
  - **Orbicularis oris[1]:** Fibers decussate in midline and insert into dermis of opposite philtral columns
    - **Deep portion:** Functions as a sphincter; continuous fibers pass from commissure to commissure across midline and extend deep to vermilion
    - **Superficial portion:** Functions in speech and facial expression; originates from muscles of facial expression
  - **Levator labii superioris:** Inserts inferiorly on white roll, contributes to peaks of Cupid's bow, and functions to elevate lip
- **Blood supply and innervation**
  - **Arterial supply:** Bilateral superior labial arteries
  - **Sensory:** Trigeminal nerve (V_2)
  - **Motor:** Facial nerve (VII)

CLEFT LIP ANATOMY
- A cleft lip is the projection and outward rotation of the premaxilla with retropositioning of the lateral maxillary segment.
- The vertical height of the lip is decreased.
- Two thirds of Cupid's bow, one philtral column, and philtral dimple are preserved on the noncleft side.

- The superficial portion of the orbicularis oris parallels the cleft margin and abnormally inserts into the cleft side alar base and the base of the columella on the noncleft side.
- The deep portion of the orbicularis oris is interrupted but does not abnormally insert.
- The musculature between the philtral midline and cleft margin on the noncleft side is hypoplastic.
- In bilateral clefts the prolabial segment between the clefts does not contain muscle.
- If an incomplete cleft is less than two thirds of the lip height, some muscle fibers may cross the cleft.
- Muscle continuity is disrupted in a **microform** cleft.
- **Simonart's band** is a skin bridge without muscle that crosses the nasal sill.

ANATOMY OF THE CLEFT NASAL DEFORMITY (Fig. 19-1)
- Caudal septum deviated to the noncleft side
- Posterior septum convex on cleft side, impinging on airway
- Columella shortened, and base deviated to the noncleft side
- Nasal tip deviated to noncleft side, and dome depressed on cleft side

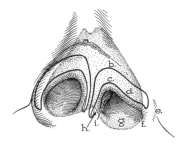

Fig. 19-1   The unilateral cleft nasal deformity. *a,* Nasal tip deviated. *b,* Alar cartilage displaced caudally. *c,* Angle between medial and lateral crura more obtuse. *d,* Buckling in the lateral crura. *e,* Flattened alar facial angle. *f,* Deficiency in bony development. *g,* Widened nostril floor. *h,* Columella and anterior caudal septal border deviated. *i,* Posterior septum convex on cleft side causing varying degrees of obstruction. (From Spira M, Hardy SB, Gerow FJ. Correction of nasal deformities accompanying unilateral cleft lip. Cleft Palate J 7:112, 1970.)

- Lower lateral cartilage attenuated and caudally displaced
  - Medial crura separated at the dome from the noncleft side
  - Lateral crura flattened and spans cleft in an obtuse angle
- Loss of overlap of upper and lower lateral cartilages with inferior displacement and hooding of alar rim
- Alar base outwardly rotated, flared, posteriorly displaced, and farther from midline than noncleft side
- Absent alar-facial groove on cleft side
- Hypoplastic maxilla and posterior displaced piriform margin on cleft side
- Widened nostril floor on cleft side
- Vestibular lining deficient on the cleft side

CLASSIFICATION

CLEFT LIP
- Unilateral versus bilateral
- Complete versus incomplete
  - **Complete clefts:** Extend through lip into nasal floor
  - **Incomplete clefts:** Varies in the extent of deformity
    - **Microform** *(forme fruste):* A mild incomplete cleft characterized by:
      - Vertical scar or furrow extending from vermilion to nasal floor
      - Notch in vermilion border
      - Varying degrees of vertical lip shortness
      - Alar deformity

ALVEOLAR CLEFT
- Unilateral versus bilateral
- Complete versus incomplete
- Wide versus narrow
- Collapse versus no collapse of alveolar arch segments

DIAGRAMMATIC SCHEMES
- Smith's modification of Kernohan's "striped Y" classification accurately describes cleft varieties using an alphanumeric system[2] (see Chapter 20).

INCIDENCE AND ETIOLOGIC FACTORS

- **CL/P incidence**
  - Racial distribution[3]
    - Asians: 2.1:1000
    - Whites: 1:1000
    - African Americans: 0.4:1000
  - Gender distribution: CL/P more frequent in males (male/female: 2:1)
- **Lateral positions**
  - *Left unilateral CL/P most common*
  - Left/right/bilateral: 6:3:1
- **Associated anomalies**
  - Incidence of isolated associated anomalies with CL/P is 7%-14%[4]
    - More common with bilateral clefts
    - Congenital heart anomalies most common
  - Incidence of CL/P associated with a syndrome (more than one malformation involving more than one developmental field) is 13.8%[5]
- **Genetics**
  - Combination of multiple interacting major genes and multifactorial inheritance[6,7]
  - Familial risk of CL/P (see Chapter 20)
- **Environmental and other associated risk factors** (see Chapter 20)

MANAGEMENT PRINCIPLES

MULTIDISCIPLINARY TEAM APPROACH
Initial evaluation by the CP team should be performed shortly after birth to assess feeding and associated anomalies, to provide genetic counseling, to outline the treatment plan, and to start presurgical orthopedics.
- **Feeding**
  - Special bottle-feeding techniques may be required (squeezable bottles and cross-cut nipples).
  - Monitor closely for appropriate weight gain.
- **Presurgical orthopedics:** Methods to narrow and align cleft segments
  - **Passive:** Nasoalveolar molding[8]
    - Reduces severity of cleft lip and nasal deformity and optimize results of initial surgical repair
    - Reduces alveolar gap and promotes arch alignment
  - **Active:** Pin retained appliance (Latham)
    - Screw activation expands palate and retracts premaxilla

- ▸ May adversely affect maxillary growth
- ▸ Reserved for severe deformities
- **Lip adhesion:** Preliminary closure of cleft to decrease tension of definitive repair
  - ▸ May be indicated for wide clefts if presurgical orthopedics is not available
  - ▸ Significant risk of dehiscence, and scar interferes with definitive repair

TIMING AND SEQUENCE OF TREATMENT

- **Primary cleft lip repair**
  - **3 months of age is standard**
  - **Goals**
    - ▸ Reconstruction of philtrum, Cupid's bow, and tubercle
    - ▸ Functional muscle reconstruction
    - ▸ Symmetry
    - ▸ Minimal scarring
- **Primary cleft nasal repair**
  - Performed at time of primary lip repair (3 months)
  - Release and repositioning of cleft nasal components and alar cartilages successfully integrated into primary lip repair without significant growth impairment
- **Columellar lengthening** (bilateral cleft lip)
  - 12-24 months of age
  - May be performed at time of palate repair
- **Alveolar cleft repair**
  - **Gingivoperiosteoplasty**
    - ▸ Gingivoperiosteoplasty is the primary closure of alveolar cleft by advancing bilateral mucoperiosteal flaps; it is performed at the time of primary cleft lip repair.
    - ▸ Presurgical orthopedics are usually needed to narrow cleft and align segments so that primary repair is technically feasible.
    - ▸ Of patients who underwent nasoalveolar molding and gingivoperiosteoplasty, 60% did not require secondary bone grafting.[9]
  - **Primary alveolar bone grafting** (before 2 years of age)
    - ▸ Rib graft is placed under mucosal flaps in upper buccal sulcus.
    - ▸ Multiple studies report associated growth impairment.[10]
    - ▸ Modified techniques that limit dissection and avoid the use of vomerine flaps reportedly have improved dental outcomes without growth impairment.[11]
  - **Secondary bone grafting**
    - ▸ Early secondary: 2-5 years old
    - ▸ Secondary: 5-16 years old
    - ▸ Late secondary: >16 years old

TIP: Secondary bone grafting is most successful when performed during transitional dentition when the canine root is incompletely formed (usually between 8 and 12 years of age).

- ▸ Iliac crest cancellous bone graft preferred
- ▸ Cancellous graft packed into cleft after closure of nasal and oral mucosal flaps
- ▸ Maxillary arch alignment optimized orthodontically before graft placement

- **Repair of secondary cleft lip deformities**
  - **Optimal timing** depends on the severity of the deformity and its effect on the psychosocial development of the patient. Most commonly performed during:
    - ▶ Preschool: When developing peer interaction
    - ▶ Adolescence: Optimal results after cessation of facial growth
  - **Common deformities that require correction:**
    - ▶ White roll deformities
    - ▶ Deficient vermilion *(Whistle deformity)*
    - ▶ Buccal sulcus deformity
    - ▶ Short lip
    - ▶ Long lip (bilateral cleft)
    - ▶ Tight lip
- **Repair of secondary cleft lip nasal deformity**
  - Preschool age
    - ▶ Risk of growth disturbance with septoplasty
    - ▶ May result in bulbous tip in adolescence because of accumulation of fibrofatty tissue and scar
  - Adolescence
    - ▶ Definitive osteoplastic rhinoplasty and septoplasty after cessation of facial growth
- **Orthognathic surgery**
  - Treatment of maxillary hypoplasia with Le Fort I advancement during adolescence

---

TECHNIQUES OF PRIMARY CLEFT LIP REPAIR

UNILATERAL CLEFT LIP

- **Straight-line repair (Rose-Thompson)** (Fig. 19-2, *A*)
  - Original cleft lip repairs involved excision of cleft margin and primary straight-line closure; have been replaced by repairs that incorporate Z-plasty to establish normal vertical height of lip
  - Limited application for correction of minimal incomplete clefts and vermilion notching (microform cleft)
- **Triangular flap repair (Randall-Tennison)** (Fig. 19-2, *B*)
  - Incorporates Z-plasty at vermilion border
  - May result in excessive vertical height of lip
  - Unfavorable oblique scar crosses the projected line for the philtrum and violates Cupid's bow
  - May be used for wide clefts

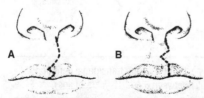

Fig. 19-2 A, Straight-line repair (Rose-Thompson) for unilateral cleft lip. **B,** Triangular flap repair (Randall-Tennison) for unilateral cleft lip. (From Byrd HS. Unilateral cleft lip. In Aston SJ, Beasley RW, Thorne CHM, eds. Grabb and Smith's Plastic Surgery, 5th ed. Philadelphia: Lippincott-Raven, 1997, p 246.)

- **Rotation-advancement repair (Millard)** (Fig. 19-3)
  - **Most commonly used repair**
  - Incorporates Z-plasty superiorly
  - Upper triangular flap from lateral segment advanced into the back cut of the medial rotation flap
  - Resultant scar follows projected line of philtral column and preserves Cupid's bow

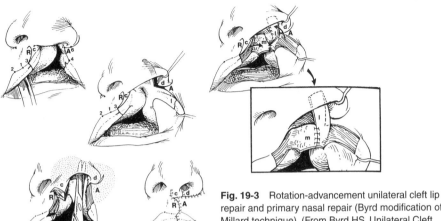

Fig. 19-3 Rotation-advancement unilateral cleft lip repair and primary nasal repair (Byrd modification of Millard technique). (From Byrd HS. Unilateral Cleft Lip. In Aston SJ, Beasley RW, Thorne CHM, eds. Grabb and Smith's Plastic Surgery, 5th ed. Philadelphia: Lippincott-Raven, 1997, p 250.)

- Medial C-flap used for columellar lengthening
- Nasal lining augmented with L-flap from mucosal portion of lateral segment
- Gingivolabial sulcus augmented with M-flap from mucosal portion of medial segment
- Triangular lateral vermilion flap used to augment deficient vermilion under Cupid's bow on medial segment and establish normal continuity of red line
- Accurate repair and alignment of the superficial and deep (under vermilion) components of the orbicularis oris critical for restoration of dynamic lip function
- May be difficult in wide clefts

BILATERAL CLEFT LIP

- **Millard repair** (Fig. 19-4, *A*)
  - Philtral flap is created from central skin of prolabium.
  - Prolabial parings are banked for future columellar lengthening.
  - Prolabial white roll and vermilion is discarded; remaining mucosa from prolabium is used to reconstruct central gingivolabial sulcus.
  - Lateral lip segments are advanced medially beneath elevated philtral flap.
  - Cupid's bow and the central tubercle are reconstructed from the white roll and vermilion of lateral lip segments.
  - Orbicularis oris muscle is reconstructed beneath the elevated philtral flap.
  - Significant widening of the prolabium may occur.
  - White roll (from lateral lip segments) may look unnatural.
  - Incidence of whistle deformity is low.
- **Modified Manchester repair** (Fig. 19-4, *B*)
  - Preserves white roll and vermilion from the prolabium for reconstruction of Cupid's bow and tubercle.
  - Philtral flap is cut to desired width, and prolabial parings are mostly discarded.
  - Small flaps from prolabial paring can be used to surface nasal floor.
  - Lateral muscle elements are sutured to prolabial subcutaneous tissue.

• If the prolabial white roll and vermilion are of poor quality, the reconstruction of Cupid's bow is compromised, and the central vermilion may have an abnormal patchy appearance. A Millard-type repair may be preferred.

Fig. 19-4   A, Millard repair for bilateral cleft lip. **B,** Modified Manchester repair for bilateral cleft lip. (From Pantaloni M, Byrd HS. Cleft lip I: Primary deformities. Sel Read Plast Surg 9[21], 2001.)

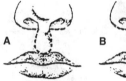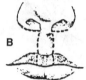

KEY POINTS

✔ CL/P is an embryologically, anatomically, and genetically distinct entity from isolated CP.
✔ The incidence of CL/P varies according to race, whereas the incidence of CP does not.
✔ The orbicularis oris has a superficial and a deep component. Accurate reconstruction of these components during cleft lip repair is critical to restoring the dynamic function of the lip.
✔ Presurgical nasoalveolar molding can optimize primary repair of the cleft lip, nose, and gingiva.
✔ Primary cleft nasal repair can be integrated successfully into primary lip repair.
✔ Accurate primary cleft lip repair is the best treatment for secondary deformities.
✔ Correction of secondary deformities is optimized when performed after the cessation of facial growth.
✔ Many successful modifications of the standard repair techniques have been described.

REFERENCES

1. Nicolau PJ. The orbicularis oris muscle: A functional approach to its repair in the cleft lip. Br J Plast Surg 36:141, 1983.
2. Smith A, Khoo AK, Jackson IT. A modification of the Kernahan "Y" classification in cleft lip and palate deformities. Plast Reconstr Surg 6:1842, 1998.
3. Sullivan W. Cleft lip with or without cleft palate in blacks: An analysis of 81 patients. Plast Reconstr Surg 84:406, 1989.
4. Witkop C. Cleft lip with or without cleft palate. In Bergsma D, ed. Birth Defects Compendium. New York: Wiley & Sons, 1979, p 223.
5. Jones M. Facial clefting: Etiology and developmental pathogenesis. Clin Plast Surg 20:599, 1993.
6. Carreno H, Paredes M, Tellez G, et al. Association of nonsyndromic cleft lip and cleft palate with microsatellite markers located in 6p. Rev Med Chil 127:1189, 1999.
7. Chung CS, Bixler D, Watanabe T, et al. Segregation analysis of cleft lip with or without cleft palate: A comparison of Danish and Japanese data. Am J Hum Genet 39:603, 1986.
8. Grayson BH, Maull D. Nasoalveolar molding for the infant born with clefts of the lip, alveolus, and palate. Clin Plast Surg 31:149, 2004.
9. Santiago P, Grayson B, Cutting CB, et al. Reduced need for alveolar bone grafting by presurgical orthopedics and primary gingivoperiosteoplasty. Cleft Palate Craniofac J 35:77, 1998.
10. Burt JD, Byrd HS. Cleft lip: Unilateral primary deformities. Plast Reconstr Surg 105:1043, 2000.
11. Rosenstein SW, Grasseschi M, Dado DV. A long-term retrospective outcome assessment of facial growth, secondary surgical need, and maxillary lateral incisor status in a surgical-orthodontic protocol for complete clefts. Plast Reconstr Surg 111:1, 2003.

20. Cleft Palate

Amanda A. Gosman

EMBRYOLOGY

PRIMARY PALATE

- The lip, nostril sill, alveolus, and hard palate **anterior** to the incisive foramen.
- The medial and lateral nasal prominences of the frontonasal process migrate and fuse with the maxillary prominence to form the primary palate during weeks 4-7 of gestation.
- The median palatine process forms by the fusion of the bilateral median nasal prominences and gives rise to the premaxilla.
- Interruption of the migration or fusion of these processes may result in a cleft of the primary palate.

SECONDARY PALATE

- The hard palate **posterior** to the incisive foramen and the soft palate.
- Migration and fusion of the lateral palatal processes of the maxillary prominence form the secondary palate between 5 and 12 weeks of gestation.
- At 8 weeks of gestation the lateral palatal processes are vertical.
- As the tongue drops, the palatal processes rotate into a horizontal position and fuse from anterior to posterior.
- Fusion takes 1 week longer in females and may contribute to increased incidence of isolated cleft palate in females.
- The right lateral palatal process becomes horizontal before the left process. The greater incidence of left-sided clefts may be related to the longer period of rotation.

NORMAL ANATOMY (Fig. 20-1)

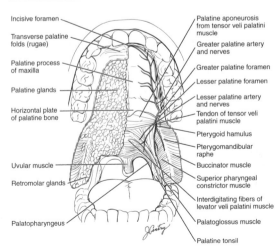

Incisive foramen

Transverse palatine folds (rugae)

Palatine process of maxilla

Palatine glands

Horizontal plate of palatine bone

Uvular muscle

Retromolar glands

Palatopharyngeus

Palatine aponeurosis from tensor veli palatini muscle

Greater palatine artery and nerves

Greater palatine foramen

Lesser palatine foramen

Lesser palatine artery and nerves

Tendon of tensor veli palatini muscle

Pterygoid hamulus

Pterygomandibular raphe

Buccinator muscle

Superior pharyngeal constrictor muscle

Interdigitating fibers of levator veli palatini muscle

Palatoglossus muscle

Palatine tonsil

Fig. 20-1 Anatomy of the normal palate.

183

HARD PALATE BONY ANATOMY

- **Primary palate**
  - Premaxillary portion of maxilla: **Anterior to the incisive foramen**
- **Secondary palate**
  - Palatine processes of maxilla
  - Palatine processes of the palatine bone

SOFT PALATE (VELUM)

Six paired muscles of velopharyngeal closure separate the oropharynx and nasopharynx; velopharyngeal closure is necessary for proper phonation, swallowing, and breathing.

- **Levator veli palatini (LVP)**
  - Originates from temporal bone and eustachian tube; bilateral muscles interdigitate at midline behind palatal aponeurosis to form a sling
  - **Function:** Elevates velum and pulls it posteriorly
- **Superior pharyngeal constrictor**
  - Broad muscle courses anteriorly within the pharyngeal wall to attach to the velum
  - **Function:** Medial movement of the lateral pharyngeal wall
- **Palatopharyngeus**
  - Arises from posterior pharynx, passes through posterior tonsillar pillar, and inserts on velum
  - **Function:** Depresses palate
- **Tensor veli palatini (TVP)**
  - Arises from membranous wall of eustachian tube; tendon passes around the pterygoid hamulus and gives rise to the palatal aponeurosis, which fuses to the posterior hard palate
  - **Function:** Opens eustachian tube
- **Uvula**
  - Extends behind the levator to the tip of the uvula
  - **Function:** Upward movement and shortening of the uvula
- **Palatoglossus**
  - Originates from tongue, passes through anterior tonsillar pillar, and inserts on anterior velum
  - **Function:** Depresses palate

BLOOD SUPPLY AND INNERVATION

- **Hard palate**
  - *Greater palatine artery* (from the maxillary artery) and *greater palatine nerve* (CN V) pass through the greater palatine foramen.
  - *Nasopalatine nerve* (CN V) communicates with the greater palatine nerve at the incisive foramen to supply the premaxilla.
- **Soft palate**
  - *Lesser palatine artery* (maxillary artery) and *lesser palatine nerve* (CN V) pass through the lesser palatine foramen.
  - *Ascending pharyngeal artery* (external carotid) and *ascending palatine branch of the facial artery* contribute to blood supply of lateral structures.
  - All muscles of velum are innervated by the *pharyngeal plexus* (CN IX, CN X, and with contributions from CN XI), **except for the TVP, which is supplied by CN V.**

TIP: The following question is typically asked on written examinations: Which muscle of the velum is not innervated by the pharyngeal plexus, and what is its innervation?

CLEFT CLASSIFICATION AND ANATOMY

PRIMARY PALATE CLEFTS
Primary palate clefts can involve the lip, nostril sill, alveolus, and/or hard palate **anterior** to the incisive foramen
- **Complete versus incomplete**
  - Complete clefts penetrate the entire structure.
- **Bilateral versus unilateral**

SECONDARY PALATE CLEFTS
Secondary palate clefts can involve the hard palate **posterior** to the incisive foramen, the velum, or both
- **Complete versus incomplete**
- **Bilateral versus unilateral**
  - In unilateral clefts, the noncleft side of the palate is fused with the nasal septum, whereas in bilateral clefts there is no fusion between the palate and the nasal septum.
- **Midline isolated cleft palate**
  - Isolated cleft palates associated with a high and hypoplastic vomer may represent a distinct midline defect. Significant hypoplasia of related midline structures distinguishes this entity from the bilateral cleft palate.
- **Bifid uvula (most common palatal cleft)**
- **Submucous cleft**
  - Bifid uvula
  - Notching of posterior hard palate
  - Zona pellucida: Thin central area created by diastasis of soft palate musculature with intact mucosa
  - *Velopharyngeal incompetence (VPI) only indication for surgical intervention*
- **Cleft velum**
  - The levator muscle abnormally inserts into the posterior margin of the hard palate; all muscles that normally join at the midline are parallel to the cleft margin (Fig. 20-2).
  - Velopharyngeal closure is insufficient, resulting in reflux of oral contents into nasopharynx, speech disturbances, and possible eustachian tube dysfunction that results in hearing loss.

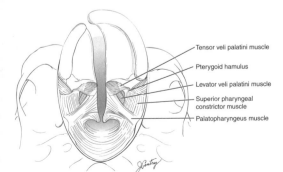

Tensor veli palatini muscle
Pterygoid hamulus
Levator veli palatini muscle
Superior pharyngeal constrictor muscle
Palatopharyngeus muscle

Fig. 20-2   Anatomy of the cleft palate. (Modified from Ross RB, Johnston MC. Cleft Lip and Palate. Baltimore: Williams & Wilkins, 1972, pp 68-91.)

KERNAHAN'S STRIPED Y CLASSIFICATION

- Smith's modification of Kernahan's striped Y classification accurately describes cleft varieties using an alphanumeric system[1] (Fig. 20-3).

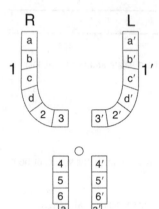

Fig. 20-3 Smith modification of the Kernahan striped Y classification. Boxes are shaded to indicate extent of cleft. The circle represents the incisive foramen. All right-sided clefts are designated by numerals without prime, and left-sided clefts are designated by numerals with prime. Incomplete cleft lips vary from microform to one third to two thirds, and these are classified as *a-c* or *a'-c'* for right and left, respectively. Lips with Simonart's band are classified as *d*. The alveolus is documented as *2* or *2'*. The palate anterior to the incisive foramen and posterior to the alveolus is documented as *3* or *3'*. The secondary palate, lying posterior to the incisive foramen, is subdivided into three segments based on the anatomic segments involved in the cleft. *4* denotes a cleft up to the palatine process of the maxillary bone, *5* is a cleft up to the palatine process of the palatine bone, *6* is a cleft including the soft palate only, and *a* denotes a submucous cleft. (From Smith AW, Khoo AK, Jackson IT. A modification of the Kernahan "Y" classification in cleft lip and palate deformities. Plast Reconstr Surg 6:1842-1847, 1998.)

EPIDEMIOLOGY

OVERALL INCIDENCE OF ORAL CLEFTS

Cleft lip, with or without cleft palate (CL/P), is genetically, embryologically, and anatomically distinct from isolated cleft palate (CP).

- **1:750 live births**[2]
- 46% CL/P
- 33% CP
- 21% CL
- Bifid uvula in 2% of the population[3]

RACIAL DISTRIBUTION

- **CL/P**[4]
  - Asians: 2.1:1000
  - Whites: 1:1000
  - Blacks: 0.4:1000
- **Isolated CP**
  - 0.5:1000 births
  - No racial variation

GENDER DISTRIBUTION

- Male/female CL/P: 2:1
- Male/female isolated CP: 1:2

LATERAL POSITIONS
- **Left unilateral CL/P most common**
- Left/right/bilateral CL/P: 6:3:1

FAMILIAL
CL/P and isolated CP are genetically distinct entities. Patients with one do not have relatives with increased frequency of the other entity.
- **CL/P**[5]
  - Normal parents (with or without a family history of CL/P), one child with CL/P: Frequency of CL/P in next child is 4%
  - ✱ Normal parents, two children with CL/P: Risk for next child is 9%
  - Parent with CL/P, no affected children: Risk for next child is 4%
  - Parent with CL/P, one child with CL/P: Risk for next child is 17%
  - Risk of CL/P in siblings increases with severity of deformity (bilateral greater than unilateral)[6]
    - ▶ Child with unilateral CL: Risk of CL/P for next child is 2.5%
    - ▶ Child with bilateral CL and CP: Risk of CL/P for next child is 5.7%
- **Isolated CP**[5]
  - Normal parents, one child with CP: Frequency of CP in next child is 2%
  - Normal parents, family history of CP, one child with CP: Risk for next child is 7%
  - Normal parents, two children with CP: Risk for next child is 1%
  - Parent with CP, no affected children: Risk for next child is 6%
  - Parent with CP, one child with CP: Risk for next child is 15%

ASSOCIATED ANOMALIES

- **Anomalies are more common with isolated CP.**
- All infants with clefts must be evaluated carefully for the presence of other anomalies.

NONSYNDROMIC CLEFT
Nonsyndromic cleft is characterized by one defect or multiple anomalies that are the result of a single initiating event or primary malformation.
- **Incidence of isolated associated anomalies**
  - More common with **bilateral clefts**
  - CL/P: 7%-14%[7]
    - ▶ Congenital heart anomalies most common
  - CP: 71%[8]
    - ▶ If Pierre Robin sequence excluded, then incidence closer to 17%[9]
- **Pierre Robin sequence** most common associated anomaly
  - Clinical features are micrognathia, glossoptosis, and CP.
  - Palatal clefts are wide, U-shaped midline defects as opposed to V-shaped clefts found in patients without associated anomalies.
  - Patients may have difficulty maintaining an adequate airway.

SYNDROMIC CLEFT

Syndromic cleft is characterized by more than one malformation involving more than one developmental field.

- More than 300 syndromes include some form of CP.
- **Incidence**[6]
  - CL/P: 13.8%
  - CP: 41.8%
- **Common syndromes**
  - **Stickler syndrome:** 25% of syndromic CP[10]
    - ► Autosomal dominant
    - ► Mutation in gene for type 2 collagen
    - ► Pierre Robin sequence, ocular malformations, hearing loss, and arthropathies
  - **Velocardiofacial (Shprintzen's) syndrome:** 15% of syndromic CP[10]
    - ► Autosomal dominant with variable expression
    - ► 22q11 "Catch 22" chromosomal deletion (diagnose with fluorescence in situ hybridization [FISH])
    - ► Cardiovascular abnormalities, abnormal facies, developmental delay
  - **Van der Woude's syndrome:** 19% of syndromic CL/P and CP[6]
    - ► Autosomal dominant with 70%-100% penetrance
    - ► CL/P or CP and bilateral lower lip pits

ETIOLOGIC FACTORS

GENETIC FACTORS

The genetic contribution to nonsyndromic oral clefts is estimated to be 20%-50%. Remaining percentages are attributed to environmental or gene-environment interactions.[11]

- **Nonsyndromic CP**
  - Mode of inheritance likely a recessive single gene model, several interacting loci, or both[12,13]
- **Nonsyndromic CL/P**
  - Combination of multiple interacting major genes and multifactorial inheritance[14,15]

ENVIRONMENTAL AND OTHER ASSOCIATED FACTORS

- **Maternal smoking:** Inconsistent data associated with increased risk of clefts
- **Maternal alcohol and caffeine ingestion:** Not associated with increased risk of isolated oral clefts[16]
- **Maternal corticosteroid use:** Associated with increased risk of CL/P and CP[17]
- **Teratogens** (e.g., alcohol, anticonvulsants, retinoids): Associated with multiple malformations, which may include oral clefts but not associated with isolated oral clefts
- **Folic acid and multivitamin supplements:** Lower incidence of CL/P births[18] when taken by pregnant women with family history of CL/P
- **High altitude:** Increased relative risk of CL/P[19]
- **Parental age:** Increased incidence of CL/P if both parents more than 30 years, *paternal age more significant than maternal age*

MANAGEMENT PRINCIPLES

MULTIDISCIPLINARY TEAM APPROACH
- Optimal management is provided by a coordinated team of professionals with a specific interest in clefts. Team members include:
  - Pediatrician
  - Plastic surgeon
  - Pediatric otolaryngologist
  - Speech pathologist
  - Pediatric dentist
  - Orthodontist
  - Oral surgeon
  - Audiologist
  - Psychologist
  - Social worker
  - Geneticist
- Initial team evaluation should be performed shortly after birth to assess airway, feeding, middle ear disease, and associated anomalies; to provide genetic counseling; and to explain the treatment plan.

AIRWAY MAINTENANCE
- Airway problems are rarely seen in the absence of other associated anomalies.
- **Pierre Robin syndrome is the most common cause of airway problems associated with cleft palate.**
- Treatment options for airway obstruction include the following:
  - Prone positioning until neuromuscular control improves
  - Nasal CPAP
  - Mandibular distraction
  - Tracheostomy as a last resort

FEEDING
- Inability to generate adequate suction and nasal spillage interfere with normal feeding.
- Children with CP are significantly more underweight than noncleft children.[20]
- Strategies for and adjustments to bottle-feeding techniques to overcome the lack of negative pressure during sucking usually facilitate successful feeding. Examples include the following:
  - Nipples with large cross-cut fissures
  - Squeezable bottles
  - Palatal obturator
- Steady weight gain is the most important indicator of adequate intake and should be closely monitored.

MIDDLE EAR DISEASE
- Abnormal eustachian tube function and inadequate ventilation may result from abnormal insertion of velopharyngeal musculature.
- **The incidence of otitis media in patients with cleft palate is 97%.**[21]
- Early myringotomy and grommet tube placement is recommended for all children with CP and has been associated with better hearing and speech outcomes.[22]

GOALS AND TIMING OF CLEFT PALATE REPAIR

GOALS
- **Normal speech**
  - Speech pathology is intrinsic to the anatomic derangement of cleft.
  - Normal speech development requires a competent velopharyngeal mechanism.
  - Prelinguistic babbling in infants is important for normal speech development.
  - Normal children speak their first words by 13 months and integrated speech develops by 2 years.
- **Normal maxillofacial growth**
  - Surgical repair and scar formation are considered the most important cause of maxillary growth restriction for patients with CL/P.
  - CP patients have some intrinsic growth deficiency of the maxilla that varies with the severity of clefting.
  - Lip repair, alveolar repair, and dissection of the vomer have a significant effect on facial growth.
  - Soft palate repair **is not** associated with growth restriction.
  - The timing of CP repair before 8 years of age has not conclusively demonstrated differences in the degree of facial growth restriction.
    - ▶ Repair between 8 and 12 years of age (phase of rapid maxillary growth) is associated with the most severe growth restriction.
    - ▶ Repair after adolescence is associated with normal facial growth.[23]
- **Normal hearing**
  - Abnormal hearing capacity interferes with normal speech development.
  - The average incidence of hearing loss in CP patients is **50%**.[24]
  - Hearing loss is primarily attributed to **eustachian tube dysfunction** and **recurrent otitis media**.
  - *The incidence of hearing loss is reduced with early palate closure.*[25]

TIMING
- **Early repair** (before 12 months of age) is associated with better speech and hearing but may impair facial growth.
- **Delayed repair** is associated with better facial growth but also with poor speech and hearing outcomes.
- *The optimal timing of repair is controversial.* Most surgeons favor early repair, because facial growth imbalance can be surgically corrected later.
- Two-stage palate repair with early closure of the soft palate (3-6 months) and delayed repair of the hard palate (15-18 months) avoids periosteal undermining of palatal and vomerine tissue and has the advantage of early velar function necessary for normal speech development.[26]

SURGICAL REPAIR

SOFT PALATE REPAIR
- **Intravelar veloplasty**[27]
  - LVP muscle is dissected from abnormal insertion on posterior hard palate, reoriented transversely, and sutured in midline to reconstitute the levator sling.
  - Oral and nasal mucosa are closed in separate layers.
  - Speech outcome may be equivalent to veloplasty with side-to-side muscle repair. Anatomic repositioning of LVP may be unnecessary.[28]
- **Double opposing Z-plasty**[29] (Fig. 20-4)

- Two Z-plasties based on cleft midline are designed from oral and nasal surface of soft palate.
  - ▶ Anteriorly based flaps contain only mucosa, and posteriorly based flaps contain mucosa and levator muscle complex.
  - ▶ Nasal mucosal flaps are transposed and closed, the levator sling is reoriented transversely, and the oral mucosal flaps are transposed and closed.
- Soft palate is lengthened, but transverse dimension is shortened, making the closure of wide clefts difficult.
- Speech outcomes are superior to Von Langenbeck repair, but incidence of fistula is greater in wide clefts.[30]
- Relaxing incisions in the hard palate mucosa, the use of a vomer flap, or both may be required to achieve tension-free closure and reduce risk of fistula.[31]

Fig. 20-4   Furlow's double opposing Z-plasty palatoplasty technique. (From Furlow L. Cleft palate repair by double opposing Z-plasty. Plast Reconstr Surg 78:724-738, 1986.)

HARD PALATE REPAIR
- **Von Langenbeck palatoplasty** (Fig. 20-5)
- Bilateral, bipedicled, mucoperiosteal flaps
  - ▶ Parallel incisions along cleft margin and lingual side of alveolus
  - ▶ Nasal and oral mucosal flaps mobilized and approximated in the midline
- Poor speech outcomes attributed to the creation of a short immobile palate[32]
- Good speech outcomes when combined with intravelar veloplasty[33,34]

Fig. 20-5   Von Langenbeck palatoplasty. (From Randall P, LaRossa D. Cleft Palate. In McCarthy JG, ed. Plastic Surgery. Philadelphia: WB Saunders, 1990, p 2743.)

- **V-Y pushback palatoplasty** (Veau-Wardill-Kilner) (Fig. 20-6)
- Bilateral mucoperiosteal flaps based on greater palatine arteries
  - ▶ V-Y closure anteriorly to lengthen palate
  - ▶ Fracture of the hamulus
  - ▶ Levator muscle repair
  - ▶ Nasal and oral mucosa closed in separate layers
- Denuded anterior palatal bone may adversely affect facial growth
- Superior speech outcomes with V-Y lengthening of palate unsubstantiated and do not justify associated increased morbidity, risk of growth disturbance, and higher incidence of fistula[33,35,36]

Fig. 20-6 V-Y pushback palatoplasty (Veau-Wardill-Kilner). (From Randall P, LaRossa D. Cleft palate. In McCarthy JG, ed. Plastic Surgery. Philadelphia: WB Saunders, 1990, p 2744.)

- **Two-flap palatoplasty** (Bardach) (Fig. 20-7)
  - Bilateral mucoperiosteal flaps based on greater palatine arteries
    - ▶ Lateral incisions along lingual side of alveolus extend anteriorly to cleft margin
    - ▶ Wide mobilization of palatal tissue permits tension-free closure
    - ▶ Levator sling reconstruction
    - ▶ Nasal and oral mucosa closed in separate layers
  - Speech results comparable to other techniques

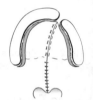

Fig. 20-7 Two-flap palatoplasty. (Modified from Afifi GY, Kaidi AA, Hardesty RA. Cleft palate repair. In Evans GRD, ed. Operative Plastic Surgery. New York: McGraw Hill, 2000, pp 487-498.)

- **Vomer flaps** (Fig. 20-8)
  - Can be used to close hard palate defect
  - Can be inferiorly or superiorly based and bilateral or unilateral
  - Useful in the closure of wide or bilateral clefts
  - Scarring thought to interfere with maxillary growth along the vomeropalatine suture[37]
  - Use in *early* palatoplasty is controversial because of the risk of facial growth disturbance

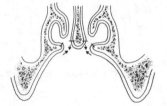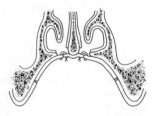

Fig. 20-8 Bilateral, inferiorly based vomer flaps. (From Nguyen PN, Sullivan PK. Issues and controversies in the management of cleft palate. Clin Plast Surg 20:671-682, 1993.)

POSTOPERATIVE CARE

- **Monitor for airway obstruction.**
  - Continuous pulse oximetry
  - Tongue suture
  - May need nasopharyngeal airway
- **Monitor for postoperative bleeding.**
  - Confirm adequate hemostasis at end of operation.
    - ▸ Repeat infiltration with 0.5% lidocaine with 1/100,000 epinephrine.
    - ▸ Pack raw areas with fibrillar collagen or other hemostatic agent.
  - Manage postoperative bleeding with intranasal oxymetolazone (Afrin) or with pressure applied to palate.
  - Bleeding may lead to airway obstruction.
- **Elevate head to 30 degrees.**
- **Apply elbow extension splints.**
- Arrange **feeding.**
  - Liquid diet via cup or **syringe** for 24 hours after surgery, then advance to soft diet
  - Soft diet until postoperative day 10 with avoidance of any hard objects in mouth
- Apply **medications.**
- Use antibiotics (cephalexin) for 5 days.
- Use Tylenol with codeine (or equivalent) as needed for pain.
- **Discharge when tolerating adequate diet,** usually postoperative day 1.

COMPLICATIONS

ACUTE

- Operative mortality from cleft palate surgery is 0.5%.[38]
- Life-threatening complications include the following:
  - Bleeding
  - Airway compromise

FISTULA

- Incidence ranges 5%-60%
  - Risk factors
    - ▸ Severity of cleft (incidence highest in bilateral clefts)
    - ▸ V-Y pushback repairs associated with highest incidence
    - ▸ Wound tension
    - ▸ Single-layer repair
    - ▸ Dead space under mucoperiosteal flaps
    - ▸ Maxillary expansion
- **Type**
  - *Most common location is the postalveolar portion of the hard palate.*
  - Primary fistulas occur after cleft palate surgery.
  - Secondary fistulas occur after maxillary expansion for orthodontic alignment.

- **Clinical significance**
  - Depends on size and location of fistula
  - Problems
    - ▸ Speech impairment because of nasal escape
    - ▸ Oronasal reflux
    - ▸ Poor hygiene from food trapping
- **Treatment**
  - **Surgical options**
    - ▸ Mobilization of surrounding palatal tissue and primary closure with or without bone graft
    - ▸ Tongue flaps
    - ▸ Facial artery myomucosal (FAMM) flap
    - ▸ Pharyngeal flap
    - ▸ Free radial forearm flap
  - **Nonsurgical**
    - ▸ Obturator

POOR MAXILLOFACIAL GROWTH
- Coordinated monitoring of growth with team orthodontist and oral surgeon during development
- Evaluate and prepare for indicated orthognathic procedures when growth complete

VELOPHARYNGEAL INCOMPETENCE (see Chapter 21)
- Incomplete closure of velum against posterior pharynx during speech characterized by:
  - Hypernasal resonance
  - Nasal air escape
  - Compensatory articulation patterns

KEY POINTS

- ✔ Cleft lip with or without cleft palate (CL/P) is genetically, embryologically, and anatomically distinct from isolated cleft palate (CP).
- ✔ If the greater palatine artery pedicle is accidentally divided when performing a unipedicled palatal flap repair, then the flap usually survives off of the posterolateral supply from the lesser palatine, ascending pharyngeal, and ascending palatine arteries.
- ✔ The tensor veli palatini is the only muscle in the velum not supplied by the pharyngeal plexus. It is supplied by the trigeminal nerve (CN V).
- ✔ Associated anomalies and syndromes are more common with isolated CP than with CL/P.
- ✔ Pierre Robin sequence is the most common anomaly associated with CP.
- ✔ Optimal management of patients with cleft palate requires a multidisciplinary team.
- ✔ Speech and hearing outcomes are best with early palate repair.
- ✔ The degree of facial growth restriction with early palate repair is unclear.
- ✔ The palate should be repaired and functioning before the development of integrated speech at age 2 years.
- ✔ Levator muscle repair greatly improves speech outcomes and should be combined with hard palate repair.

REFERENCES

1. Smith AW, Khoo AK, Jackson IT. A modification of the Kernahan "Y" classification in cleft lip and palate deformities. Plast Reconstr Surg 6:1842-1847, 1998.
2. Sadove AM, van Aalst AJ, Culp JA. Cleft palate repair: Art and issues. Clin Plast Surg 31:231-241, 2004.
3. Lindemann G, Riss B, Severin I. Prevalence of cleft uvula among 2732 Danes. Cleft Palate J 14:226-229, 1977.
4. Sullivan W. Cleft lip with or without cleft palate in blacks: An analysis of 81 patients. Plast Reconstr Surg 84:406-408, 1989.
5. Fraser F. Etiology of cleft lip and palate. In Grabb WC, Rosenstein SW, Bzoch KR, eds. Cleft Lip and Palate. Surgical, Dental, and Speech Aspects. Boston: Little Brown, 1971.
6. Jones MC. Facial clefting: Etiology and developmental pathogenesis. Clin Plast Surg 20:599-606, 1993.
7. Witkop C. Cleft lip with or without cleft palate. In Bergsma D, ed. Birth Defects Compendium. New York: Wiley & Sons, 1979, p 222.
8. Morris HL, Bardach J, Ardinger H, et al. Multidisciplinary treatment results for patients with isolated cleft palate. Plast Reconstr Surg 92:842-851, 1993.
9. Hagberg C, Larson O, Milerad J. Incidence of cleft lip and palate and risks of additional malformations. Cleft Palate Craniofacial J 35:40-45, 1998.
10. Coleman JR, Sykes JM. The embryology, classification, epidemiology, and genetics of facial clefting. Fac Plast Surg Clin North Am 9:1-13, 2001.
11. Marazita ML, Mooney MP. Current concepts in the embryology and genetics of cleft lip and palate. Clin Plast Surg 31:124-140, 2004.
12. Christensen K, Mitchell LE. Familial recurrence-pattern analysis of nonsyndromic isolated cleft palate: A Danish Registry study. Am J Hum Genet 58:182-190, 1996.
13. Carinci F, Pezzetti F, Scapoli L, et al. Genetics of nonsyndromic cleft lip and palate: A review of international studies and data regarding the Italian population. Cleft Palate Craniofacial J 37:33-40, 2000.
14. Carreno H, Paredes M, Tellez G, et al. Association of nonsyndromic cleft lip and palate with microsatellite markers located in 6p. Rev Med Chil 127:1189-1198, 1999.
15. Chung CS, Bixler D, Watanabe T, et al. Segregation analysis of cleft lip with or without cleft palate: A comparison of Danish and Japanese data. Am J Hum Genet 39:603-611, 1986.
16. Natsume N, Kawai T, Ogi N, et al. Maternal risk factors in cleft lip and palate: A case control study. Br J Oral Maxillofac Surg 38:23-25, 2000.
17. Carmichael SL, Shaw GM. Maternal corticosteroid use and risk of selected congenital anomalies. Am J Med Genet 86:242-244, 1999.
18. Tolarova M, Harris J. Reduced recurrence of orofacial clefts after periconceptional supplementation with high dose folic acid and multivitamins. Teratology 51:71-78, 1995.
19. Castilla EE, Lopez-Camelo JS, Campana H. Altitude as a risk factor for congenital anomalies. Am J Med Genet 86:9-14, 1999.
20. Lazarus DDA, Hudson DA, Fleming AN, et al. Are children with clefts underweight for age at time of primary surgery? Plast Reconstr Surg 103:1624-1629, 1999.
21. Dhillon R. The middle ear in cleft palate children pre and post palatal closure. J Roy Soc Med 81:710-713, 1988.
22. Hubbard TW, Paradise JL, McWilliams BJ, et al. Consequences of unremitting middle-ear disease in early life. Otologic, audiologic, and developmental findings in children with and without cleft palate. N Eng J Med 312:1529-1534, 1985.
23. Koberg W, Koblin I, Speech development and maxillary growth in relationship to technique and timing of palatoplasty. J Maxillofac Surg 1:44-50, 1973.
24. Yules RB. Current concepts of treatment of ear disease in cleft palate children and adults. Cleft Palate J 12:315-322, 1975.
25. Watson DJ, Rohrich RJ, Poole ME, et al. The effect on the ear of late closure of the cleft hard palate. Br J Plast Surg 39:190-192, 1986.
26. Rohrich RJ, Love EJ, Byrd HS, et al. Optimal timing of cleft palate closure. Plast Reconstr Surg 106:413-421, 2000.

27. Kriens OB. An anatomical approach to veloplasty. Plast Reconstr Surg 43:29-41, 1969.
28. Marsh JL, Grames LM, Holtman B. Intravelar veloplasty. Cleft Palate J 26:46-50, 1989.
29. Furlow L. Cleft palate repair by double opposing Z-plasty. Plast Reconstr Surg 78:724-738, 1986.
30. Spauwen PH, Goorhuis-Brouwer SM, Schutte HK. Cleft palate repair: Furlow versus von Langenbeck. J Craniomaxillofac Surg 20:18-20, 1992.
31. LaRossa D, Jackson OH, Kirschner RE, et al. The Children's Hospital of Philadelphia modification of the Furlow double-opposing Z-palatoplasty: Long-term speech and growth results. Clin Plast Surg 31:243-249, 2004.
32. Veau V. Discussion on the treatment of cleft palate by operation. Proc R Soc Med 20(Part III):156, 1926.
33. Dreyer TM, Trier WC. A comparison of palatoplasty techniques. Cleft Palate J 21:251-253, 1984.
34. Trier WC, Dreyer TM. Primary Von Langenbeck palatoplasty with levator reconstruction: Rationale and technique. Cleft Palate J 21:254-262, 1984.
35. Holtmann B, Wray RC, Weeks PM. A comparison of three techniques of palatorrhaphy: Early speech results. Ann Plast Surg 12:514-518, 1984.
36. Wray C, Dann J, Holtmann B. A comparison of three techniques of palatorrhaphy: In hospital morbidity. Cleft Palate J 16:42-45, 1979.
37. Delaire J, Precious D. Avoidance of the use of vomerine mucosa in primary surgical management of velopalatine clefts. Oral Surg 60:589-597, 1985.
38. Grabb W. General aspects of cleft palate surgery. In Grabb WC, Rosenstein SW, Bzoch KR, eds. Cleft Lip and Palate. Surgical, Dental, and Speech Aspects. Boston: Little Brown, 1971.

21. Velopharyngeal Incompetence

Thornwell Hay Parker III

INCIDENCE

- Following primary cleft palate repair
  - 70%-80% achieve acceptable speech
  - 10%-15% achieve acceptable speech after additional speech therapy
  - 10%-30% have persistent velopharyngeal incompetence (VPI) requiring secondary operative intervention

NORMAL PHYSIOLOGY OF VELOPHARYNGEAL CLOSURE

- The velum and lateral and posterior pharyngeal walls act together as a sphincter or valve to separate the oral and nasal cavities during swallowing and speech, channeling airflow and acoustic energy.

PRINCIPAL MUSCLES (Fig. 21-1)
The first three muscles listed here are the most important
- **Levator veli palatini**
  - **Origin:** Cranial base (petrous temporal bone)
  - **Insertion:** Normally traverses the middle third of soft palate, fusing to the contralateral muscle, forming the levator sling
  - **Innervation:** CN IX-CN X
  - **Function:** Posterior and superior movement of velum
- **Superior pharyngeal constrictor**
  - **Origin:** Median raphe (posterior pharyngeal midline)
  - **Insertion:** Medial pterygoid and the pterygomandibular raphe
  - **Innervation:** CN X
  - **Function:** Mostly lateral wall motion
- **Palatopharyngeus**
  - **Origin:** Posterior and lateral pharyngeal walls

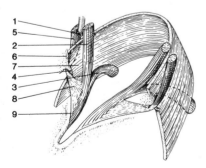

1, 5, 2, 6, 7, 4, 3, 8, 9

Fig. 21-1 Anatomy of the soft palate in congenital clefts. *1,* Eustachian tube orifice; *2,* levator veli palatini; *3,* palatopharyngeus; *4,* hamulus; *5,* tensor veli palatini; *6,* medial pterygoid; *7,* superior constrictor; *8,* palatal aponeurosis; *9,* posterior margin of the hard palate. (From Furlow LT Jr. Cleft palate repair by double opposing Z-plasty. In Vistnes LM, ed. How They Do It: Procedures in Plastic and Reconstructive Surgery. Boston: Little Brown, 1992.)

- **Insertion:** Velum via posterior tonsillar pillar
- **Innervation:** CN X
- **Function:** Mostly lateral wall motion
■ **Tensor veli palatini**
  - **Origin:** Membranous wall of eustachian tube
  - **Insertion:** Pterygoid hamulus
  - **Innervation:** CN V
  - **Function:** Opens eustachian tube
■ **Muscle of uvula**
  - **Origin:** Posterior velum
  - **Insertion:** Mucous membrane of the uvula
  - **Innervation:** CN X
  - **Function:** Upward movement and shortening of the uvula
■ **Palatoglossus muscle**
  - **Origin:** Tongue
  - **Insertion:** Anterior velum
  - **Innervation:** CN X
  - **Function:** Depresses palate

> TIP: All of the aforementioned muscles are innervated by CN X, **except** for the tensor veli palatini. (This is a frequently asked question in exams.)

PATHOLOGY[1]

VPI results from incomplete closure of the velum against the pharyngeal walls. Most typically seen after cleft palate repair, the deficiency being secondary to **poor posterior excursion of the velum.**

ETIOLOGIC FACTORS
■ **Unrepaired cleft palate or submucosal cleft**
■ **Other structural anomalies**
  - Short palate
  - Large nasopharynx
  - Tonsillar atrophy
  - Tonsillectomy 1:1500-10,000
  - Le Fort I and Le Fort II advancement
■ **Immobility**
  - Scar
  - Neurogenic dysfunction of velum or lateral pharyngeal wall

DIAGNOSIS AND EVALUATION[2]

SCREENING
■ Usually begins at 4 years of age, when able to assess speech

CLINICAL EVALUATION

- **Intraoral examination**
  - Anatomy: Tonsils, velum, lateral pharyngeal wall
  - Unrepaired cleft palate
  - Submucosal clefts: *Calnan's triad*
    - ▶ Bifid uvula: 20% have VPI
    - ▶ Zona pellucida: Pale line running longitudinally in soft palate midline secondary to muscular diastasis with intact mucosa; nearly 100% have VPI
    - ▶ Palpable notch at posterior edge of hard palate
  - Palatal fistulas
- **Tongue test**
  - Pull out the patient's tongue, then have the patient seal his or her lips around it and inflate his or her cheeks. With VPI, the patient is unable to maintain oropharyngeal pressure to inflate the cheeks.
- **Intranasal examination**
  - Septal deviation
  - Septal fistulas
  - Hypertrophied turbinates
- **Reflex and voluntary behavior**
  - Nasal regurgitation when swallowing liquids
  - Fatigue or abnormal movements with repetitive gag stimulation
  - Velar motion with sustained phonation of "a"
- **Speech evaluation:** Abnormal valving mechanism leads to four particular speech problems
  1. **Hypernasality (resonance)**
     - ▶ Manifests as nasal vibrations produced during vowel production of "e," "i," and "u"
  2. **Nasal emissions (airflow)**
     - ▶ Audible or inaudible
     - ▶ Inaudible nasal emissions detected by placing mirror under nares to check for fogging with vowel production
  3. **Imprecise consonants (air pressure)**
     - ▶ Inability to build pressure in oral cavity to produce consonants, particularly plosives (e.g., "p") and fricatives (e.g., "f")

TIP: Test for imprecise consonants with the phrase "I pet puppies."

---

  4. **Compensatory articulations**
     - ▶ Using other anatomic areas to produce deficient articulations: **Glottal stops, pharyngeal fricatives,** pharyngeal stops, velar fricatives, posterior nasal fricatives, and middorsal fricatives
     - ▶ May persist despite good technical correction of VPI; the older the age at time of repair, the more difficult to correct these articulations with speech therapy

DIRECT AND INDIRECT METHODS OF OBJECTIVE ASSESSMENT

- **Objectives**
  - Determine velar length
  - Palatal elevation and level of attempted closure
  - Velopharyngeal gap size
  - Excursion

- Pattern of closure
- Nasopharyngeal depth
■ **Modalities**
  - **Lateral cephalogram**
    ▸ Static image at rest and during sustained production for "-ee"
    ▸ Demonstrates soft palate elevation and contact with posterior wall
  - **Multiview videofluoroscopy**
    ▸ *Modality of choice*
    ▸ Barium swallowed and dynamic views taken in sagittal, coronal, and transverse planes (lateral, frontal, submentovertex views)
    ▸ Lateral view
      ✦ Similar to lateral cephalogram
      ✦ Shows palatal and post pharyngeal movement
      ✦ Demonstrates the level of the palate
    ▸ Frontal view
      ✦ Shows medial motion of lateral wall
      ✦ Grade on scale as 0/5 to 5/5
      ✦ *Assists in determination of pharyngeal flap width*
  - **Nasopharyngoscopy**
    ▸ Achieves direct view, facilitates observing pattern of closure
    ▸ Standard views difficult; may miss small gaps, and patient cooperation may be problematic
  - **MRI**
    ▸ Not very useful in preoperative evaluation
    ▸ Used in velocardiofacial syndrome to evaluate for medially displaced internal carotid arteries
  - **Phototransduction:** Intranasal fiberoptic light is measured by intraoral detector, quantifies changes with velopharyngeal movement
  - **Aerodynamics:** Study of pressure and flow
  - **Acoustics:** Quantifies changes in nasal resonance, helpful for biofeedback speech training
■ **Other preoperative procedures**
  - **Tonsillectomy and adenoidectomy** (T&A)
    ▸ Always should be performed *before* pharyngoplasty if future T&A anticipated
    ▸ Avoids recurrence following spontaneous tonsillar involution and improves quality of suture repair by removing friable lymphoid tissue
    ▸ Performed at least 3 months before, with an otorhinolaryngologist familiar with pharyngoplasty techniques
    ▸ Reevaluate speech, videofluoroscopy, and nasal endoscopy 3 months after T&A

TREATMENT[3,4]

NONOPERATIVE
■ **Speech therapy**
  - Articulation therapy, sucking and blowing exercises, electrical and tactile stimulation, biofeedback
■ **Prosthetics**
  - **Two types**
    1. Obturator prosthesis: Fills residual gaps when tissue is deficient
    2. Palatal lift prosthesis: Used when there is adequate tissue but poor coordination and movement

- May improve the intrinsic capability for velopharyngeal closure and eventually allow weaning from prosthesis (controversial)

TIP: A prosthesis may also be used as a temporary, reversible trial to test the expected effectiveness of surgical interventions.

OPERATIVE

VPI repair typically corrects incompetence that persists despite cleft repair.

- **Intravelar veloplasty:** Component of cleft palate repair, reapproximating the velar musculature and mucosa at the midline, restoring velopharyngeal competence and closure
- **Timing:** When patient begins speaking
- **Surgical approaches**
  - Palatoplasty
    - ▶ Used for unrepaired cleft palates that are typically repaired at a younger age (see Chapter 20)
    - ▶ Examples: V-Y pushback and double opposing Z-plasty
  - Pharyngoplasty
    - ▶ **Pharyngeal flap** (Fig. 21-2)
      - ✦ *Technique of choice for almost all VPI*

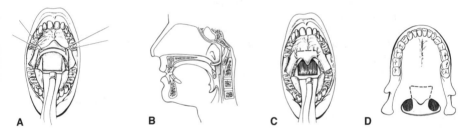

Fig. 21-2 Technique of nonobstructing pharyngeal flap. **A,** Incision; **B,** flap insertion to the dorsum of the soft palate; **C,** flap is hidden behind soft palate; **D,** healed flap represented as a narrow tube, note large lateral ports. (Modified from Argamaso RV. The pharyngeal flap. In Kernahan DA, Rosenstein SW, eds. Cleft Lip and Palate. A System of Management. Baltimore: Williams & Wilkins, 1993, pp 263-269.)

- ✦ Creates a static central obstruction to compensate for the anteroposterior deficiency seen with poor posterior velar excursion (the most common deficiency after cleft palate repair)
- ✦ **Flap width:** Critical to achieving good outcome; width determined by lateral wall excursion seen on multiplane videofluoroscopy and endoscopy, graded 0/5 to 5/5
  - - **Too wide:** Hyponasality, mouth breathing, obstructive sleep apnea
  - - **Too narrow:** Continued VPI symptoms
  - - Width determined historically by direct visualization intraoperatively
- ✦ **Superiorly versus inferiorly based pharyngeal flaps**
  - - **Superiorly based flap:** More length and lies closer to palatal plane but more difficult to raise
  - - *Technique:* Incise down to prevertebral fascia, elevate to level of palatal plane (usually 1-2 cm above tubercle of the atlas [C1 vertebra] but ultimately determined from lateral view of videofluoroscopy)

CAUTION: Be aware of potential medial ICA displacement.

* **Inferiorly based flap:** Easier to raise but shorter and tethers velum inferiorly; good for short gap and lower lying palatal plane
  - *Technique:* Incision just below adenoid pad
▶ **Sphincter pharyngoplasty**
  * Recent widespread use but less reliable outcome data available to compare with pharyngeal flap
  * **Possible indications: Mild hypernasality with absent or minimal medial excursion of lateral walls,** short AP deficiency, and circular velopharyngeal closure pattern
  * Provides static and possibly dynamic lateral and posterior obstruction, creating a smaller central orifice
  * **Hynes[5]:** Elevated lateral pharyngeal flaps 3-4 cm long with salpingopharyngeus muscle, sutured anterior to Passavant's ridge
  * **Orticochea modification[6]:** Incorporated posterior tonsillar pillar with palatopharyngeus muscle
  * **Jackson modification[7]:** Added small superior pharyngeal flap
▶ **Posterior pharyngeal wall augmentation**
  * Creates static posterior pharyngeal obstruction
  * Used with small coronal gaps
  * Placement of filler substance behind mucosa of posterior pharyngeal wall
    - Collagen, cartilage, petroleum jelly, paraffin, Silastic, Teflon, Proplast
  * **Advantages:** Quicker, simpler, reversible, less alteration of airway and musculature
  * **Disadvantages:** Much less effective, migration, extrusion, and resorption
▶ **Palatal lengthening**
  * Typically used in primary palate repair not secondary repair
  * Sparse data concerning secondary repair
  * Usually achieves much less gain in length than expected
  * Indications: Most useful for small gaps

POSTOPERATIVE CARE

■ Typically 1-night hospitalization to monitor airway
  * Syndromic conditions may need further observation
  * Liquid or soft diet until good wound healing (approximately 3 weeks)
■ Continue multidisciplinary team approach
  * Every 3 months for the first year, then once a year for their remaining developmental years
  * Follow closely with speech evaluation and taped recordings
  * Continue speech and behavioral therapy as needed
  * Videofluoroscopy, nasal endoscopy, or both as needed

COMPLICATIONS

■ **Airway obstruction**
  * 9% with significant airway obstruction, usually within 24 hours; only 1% require reintubation
  * **Risk factors:** Microretrognathia (Pierre Robin sequence syndrome), other congenital syndromes, perinatal respiratory dysfunction, early age, upper respiratory tract infection
  * Obstructive sleep apnea: Reports of up to 90% with initial sleep apnea for 1-2 days, resolving as edema resolves

- **Bleeding:** 8%
- **Dehiscence:** Usually when pharyngoplasty flaps have been sutured to friable tonsillar tissues or flaps are atrophic and scarred from previous tonsillectomy
- **Recurrence:** Results from narrow pharyngeal flaps, contracture or scarring, tonsillar atrophy, and Le Fort I, Le Fort II, or Le Fort III

KEY POINTS

- ✔ VPI results from incomplete closure of the velum against the pharyngeal walls.
- ✔ Following primary cleft palate repair, 10%-30% of patients have persistent VPI and unacceptable speech despite speech therapy, and secondary operative intervention is required.
- ✔ Multiview videofluoroscopy is the primary modality for preop planning. The lateral view shows the level of the palatal plane, and the frontal view shows lateral wall motion, determining the width of flap needed.
- ✔ Operative treatment typically creates a static obstruction to lessen the amount of dynamic obstruction required for pharyngeal closure.

REFERENCES

1. Panataloni M, Hollier L. Cleft palate and velopharyngeal incompetence. Sel Read Plast Surg 9(23), 2001.
2. Johns D, Rohrich R, Awada M. Velopharyngeal incompetence: A guide to clinical evaluation. Plast Reconstr Surg 112:1890-1897; quiz 1898, 1982, 2003.
3. Hobar PC, Johns DF, Flood J. Cleft palate repair and velopharyngeal insufficiency. In Aston SJ, Beasley RW, Thorne CHM, eds. Grabb and Smith's Plastic Surgery, 5th ed. Philadelphia: Lippincott-Raven, 1997.
4. Witt P. Velopharyngeal insufficiency. In Auchauer B, Eriksson E, Vander Kolk C, et al, eds. Plastic Surgery: Indications, Operations, and Outcomes. St Louis: Mosby, 2000.
5. Hynes W. Pharyngoplasty by muscle transplantation. Br J Plast Surg 3:128, 1950.
6. Orticochea M. Construction of a dynamic muscle sphincter in cleft palates. Plast Reconstr Surg 41:323, 1968.
7. Jackson IT, Silverton JS. The sphincter pharyngoplasty as a secondary procedure in cleft palates. Plast Reconstr Surg 59:518, 1977.

22. Microtia

Danielle M. LeBlanc

DEMOGRAPHICS

- Incidence ranges 0.76-2.35 per 10,000 births[1]
- Male predominance 2:1
- More common in Asians (Japanese) and Hispanics than Caucasians
- Relatively higher incidence rate (0.1%) among Navajo tribe Native Americans[2]
- Estimated ratio of right/left/bilateral: 5:3:1
- Maternal parity effect seen with increased risk noted at more than four pregnancies[3]

EMBRYOLOGY

- **First (mandibular)** and **second (hyoid)** branchial arches are responsible for auricular development (Fig. 22-1).
- Failure of development or adverse effects within 6-8 weeks of gestation lead to clinical variations of microtia. Popular theories include:
  - **Teratogens:** Accutane, retinoic acid, thalidomide
  - **Ischemia:** Decreased blood supply in utero
  - **Genetic:** Syndromic causes
- Later insults in gestational development cause less severe auricular deformities.

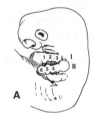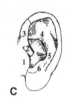

Fig. 22-1 Embryology of the external ear. **A,** Hillock formation in an 11 mm human embryo. **B,** Hillock configuration in a 15 mm embryo at 6 weeks of gestation. **C,** Adult auricle with hillock derivations. (From Beahm EK, Walton RL. Auricular reconstruction for microtia. Part I: Anatomy, embryology and clinical evaluation. Plast Reconstr Surg 109:2473, 2002.)

ASSOCIATED ABNORMALITIES

Middle ear and **external auditory canal defects** are commonly associated, although there is no correlation between severity of external defect and middle ear function. Defects in hearing are 80%-90% conductive and 10%-15% sensorineural.[4]

CAUSES OF HEARING DEFECTS
- Ossicular chain disruption (fusion/hypoplasia of malleus, incus)
- Absence of ossicles
- Atresia of tympanic cavity (lack of external auditory canal)

- Variable degrees of auricular malformation seen in syndromes
  - Branchial arch syndromes
  - Goldenhar's syndrome
  - Treacher Collins syndrome
  - Oculoauriculovertebral dysplasia
  - Facial nerve abnormalities
  - Cleft lip/palate
  - Mandibular hypoplasia
  - Hemifacial microsomia

TIP: Isolated microtia is the mildest form of hemifacial microsomia.[1,5,6]

OTHER MALFORMATIONS ASSOCIATED WITH MICROTIA AND ANOTIA[1]
- 30%: Facial clefts and cardiac defects
- 14%: Anophthalmia/microphthalmia
- 11%: Limb reduction defects or renal malformations
- 7%: Holoprosencephaly

INDICATIONS FOR AURICULAR REPAIR

- **Primary goal**
  - Improvement of acoustic function (sound localization, speech perception)
- **Secondary goals**
  - Speech
  - Social acceptance
  - Emotional development

TIMING OF AURICULAR RECONSTRUCTION

PRIMARY FACTORS INFLUENCING TIMING[1]
- **Age of external ear maturity**
  - 85% of ear development is attained by age 4.
  - Ear width continues to grow until age 10.
- **Availability of adequate donor rib cartilage**
  - Usually adequate by age 5-6
- **School age and psychological factors of peer ridicule**
- **Need for middle ear (acoustic) surgery**
  - Auricular reconstruction is commonly performed **before** middle ear surgery when possible.
  - If acoustic surgery is performed first, the otologist must coordinate with the plastic surgeon to establish:
    - ► Canal position
    - ► Vascular axis of flaps
    - ► Location of incisions used in auricular reconstruction

- Most hearing deficits (especially in bilateral microtia) are treated with conductive hearing aids. Osseointegrated or bone-anchored devices must be placed to achieve good coaptation and avoid surgical incision sites.
- **Different techniques** more appropriate for different ages to achieve optimal reconstruction
- **Brent technique:** Wait until **age 4-6,** allowing for ear maturity and appropriate school age.
- **Nagata technique:** Wait until **age 10,** or when **chest circumference at xyphoid is 60 cm,** to allow additional cartilage for use in integrated tragal reconstruction.

PREOPERATIVE WORKUP

The microtia patient is evaluated by both plastic surgeon and otologist within the first 12 months of life and then is seen annually until reaching optimal age for reconstruction.
- **Family history** of syndromes, genetic counseling
- **Complete physical examination**
  - Evaluation of ear structure
  - Evaluation of facial symmetry, animation, and dental occlusion
- **Diagnostic studies**
  - Complete audiometric testing to determine conductive versus sensorineural defect
    ▸ Presence of cholesteatoma (squamous epithelium trapped in middle ear)
  - Temporal bone imaging
    ▸ High-resolution CT scan for evaluating middle ear ossicles and cleft to help plan future otologic surgery
    ▸ MRI to determine course of facial nerve, which can be displaced—especially in absence of pneumatized mastoid[7]

CLASSIFICATION

Many attempts have been made to classify microtia based on embryologic development and severity of deformity[7]

CURRENT CLASSIFICATION SYSTEM
Current system (Nagata,[8] Tanzer[9]) divides categories **based on surgical correction** of the deformity.
- **Anotia:** Absence of auricular tissue
- **Lobular type:** Remnant ear with lobule and helix but without concha, acoustic meatus, or tragus
- **Conchal type:** Remnant ear and lobule with concha, acoustic meatus, and tragus
- **Small conchal type:** Remnant ear and lobule with small indentation of concha
- **Atypical microtia:** Cases that do not fall into the previous categories

TREATMENT OPTIONS

AUTOGENOUS COSTAL CARTILAGE GRAFT
- **Tanzer[9]**
- Remains best long-term reconstructive option
- Modified by Brent and Nagata (see later in this chapter)

- Shortcomings
  - Donor site morbidity and postoperative sequelae (pulmonary)
  - Chest wall deformity
  - Number of staged procedures

SILASTIC® FRAMEWORK (Dow Corning, Midland, MI)
- **Cronin**[10]
- Excellent aesthetic appearance
- No donor site morbidity
- Discontinued because of:
  - Spontaneous extrusion
  - Susceptibility to minor trauma
  - Unacceptable long-term failure rates

POROUS POLYETHYLENE IMPLANT
- **Reinisch**[11]
- Good short-term results with regard to aesthetics and extrusion rates
- No long-term data available

PROSTHETIC/OSSEOINTEGRATED RECONSTRUCTION
- Limited by available technology and skill of anaplastologist
- Variable cost depending on quality
- Lifespan/durability depends on age of patient
- Excellent alternative for patients with poor local tissue or high operative risk
  - Failed autologous reconstruction
  - Trauma
  - Radiation
  - Cancer
  - Elderly patient

TISSUE ENGINEERING
- Scaffolding remains a critical component of successful engineering.
- Nonhuman experimental chondrocyte studies have yielded de novo neocartilage that can be rendered into shapes.[12]

MOST COMMONLY USED TREATMENT TECHNIQUES

BRENT TECHNIQUE[13-15]
Four-stage reconstruction beginning at **4-6 years of age**

Stage I: A high-profile ear framework is fabricated from **contralateral** costochondral rib cartilage of synchondrosis of the **sixth to eighth ribs** and placed in a subcutaneous pocket at the posterior/inferior border of the ear vestige (Fig. 22-2).

Stage II: Lobule transposition occurs several months after framework.

Stage III: Projection of the construct is performed through an incision along the margin of the rim. The posterior capsule is elevated, and projection is stabilized by a wedge of banked costal cartilage placed subfascially. Polyethylene blocks may also be used as a wedge. The retroauricular skin is advanced to minimize visible scarring, and a split-thickness graft (harvested from hip) is used to cover the posterior defect and is secured with a tie-over bolster.

Stage IV: Tragus construction, conchal excavation, and symmetry adjustment. The tragus is fashioned from composite graft from contralateral conchal vault, or in bilateral cases using an anteriorly based conchal flap with cartilage support.

NOTE: Recently Brent[14] incorporated a tragal component in his initial framework to decrease the total number of stages.

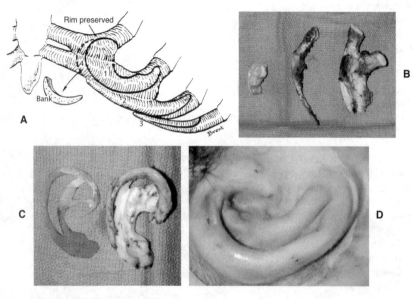

Fig. 22-2   **A,** Rib cartilages used for total ear construction. *1,* Synchondrotic block used for body of framework; *2,* floating rib used for helix; *3,* strut used for tragus; *4,* extra cartilage wedge to be banked for use during elevation procedure. **B,** Synchondrosis of ribs 7 and 8 and floating rib. **C,** Autogenous cartilage framework construct with contralateral acetate template. **D,** Subcutaneous placement of cartilaginous framework. (**A** from Brent B. Technical advances in ear reconstruction with autogenous rib cartilage grafts: Personal experience with 1200 cases. Plast Reconstr Surg 104:319, 1999.)

NAGATA TECHNIQUE[16,17]

Involves **two stages** starting about **age 10.** Several modifications are involved, depending on the type of microtia present.

Stage I: Ipsilateral rib cartilage high-definition framework from the **sixth through ninth ribs** leaving most of the perichondrium in situ to minimize chest wall deformity. Framework constructed **with a tragal component** and placed in a subcutaneous pocket through a W-shaped flap. The lobule is transposed in this stage.

Stage II: Framework elevation staged at 6 months. Additional cartilage harvested from the fifth rib through previous incision to use as wedge, and temporoparietal fascia flap is elevated and tunneled subcutaneously to cover posterior cartilage grafts. After advancement of retroauricular skin, the remaining defect is covered with skin graft (split thickness from occipital scalp) and secured with bolster.

POSTOPERATIVE CARE

- **Hemostasis and skin coaptation**
  - Closed suction drain: Brent advocates silicone catheter and red-top vacuum tube system to prevent skin necrosis from pressure dressing.
  - Tie-over bolster: Nagata advocates bolster secured for 2 weeks.
- **Monitoring**
  - Frequent postoperative monitoring is imperative for the detection of infection, hematoma, or exposure.
- **Limit activity**
  - To protect framework
  - 3-6 week restriction of sports because of chest wall donor site

COMPLICATIONS

SKIN LOSS

- Rates are variable, depending on technique.
- **Prevention strategy is best.**
  - Perform meticulous dissection to preserve subdermal plexus.
  - Avoid injury to superficial temporal vessels and protect temporoparietal fascia salvage resource.
  - Avoid pressure dressings.
  - Brent noted closed suction drains instead of compression bolster decreased skin-related complications from 33% to 1%.[15]
- **Early intervention can save the framework.**[13]
  - Small skin loss (<1 cm) may be managed conservatively with local wound care.
  - Larger areas must be debrided and exposed construct covered with local skin and fascia flaps to prevent loss of framework.

INFECTION

- Uncommon (<0.5%)[15]
- Arises from:
  - Construct exposure
  - External ear pathogens
- Typical presentation
  - Erythema
  - Edema
  - Subtle fluctuance or drainage
- Rarely presents as pain or fever
- Prevention
  - Meticulous preoperative cleaning of external ear
  - Understanding and recognizing middle ear pathology (otitis/cholesteatoma)
- Treatment: Immediate antibiotic irrigation of flap

HEMATOMA

- Condition is rare (0.3%) but devastating.
- **Early recognition is vital.**
- Treatment is immediate drainage.

CHEST WALL DONOR SITE COMPLICATIONS

- **Pneumothorax** (rate unknown)
  - May require intraoperative catheter to evacuate air
- **Atelectasis**
  - Improved with infusion pumps of local anaesthetics
- **Chest wall deformity rates vary by age**
  - Up to 64% at age 10 or younger
  - 20% in older children
  - Reduced by amount of perichondrium left intact at donor site
- **Hypertrophic scar**
  - Important to consider for placing donor site incision in inframammary fold with female patients

LONG-TERM COMPLICATIONS

- **Suture extrusion**
  - Minor
  - Treatment is excision
- **Cartilage resorption rates**
  - Rates variable
  - Require regrafting if framework shape altered
  - Avoid placing new cartilage in scarred bed; avoid tight sutures
- **Low hairline complications**
  - Can be prevented
    - ▸ Preoperative laser treatment
    - ▸ Intraoperative destruction of follicles
  - Native skin always preferable to skin graft
- **Relative size discrepancy**
  - Brent[15] noted trend in growth rates of reconstructed ears
    - ▸ 48%: Same
    - ▸ 41.6%: Larger
    - ▸ 10.3%: Smaller

KEY POINTS

- ✔ The first and second branchial arches are responsible for auricular development.
- ✔ Ear reconstruction is usually undertaken when the patient is at least 6 years old.
- ✔ Autogenous ear reconstruction (with costal cartilage) is the preferred method of reconstruction.
- ✔ A temporoparietal fascia flap can be used for soft tissue coverage over the underlying autogenous framework.

REFERENCES

1. Beahm EK, Walton RL. Auricular reconstruction for microtia. Part I: Anatomy, embryology and clinical evaluation. Plast Reconstr Surg 109:2473, 2002.
2. Aase JM, Tegtmeier RE. Microtia in New Mexico: Evidence of multifactorial causation. Birth Defects Orig Artic Ser 13:113, 1977.
3. Harris J, Kallen B, Robert E. The epidemiology of anotia and microtia. J Med Genet 33:809, 1996.
4. Llano-Rivas I, Gonxales-del Angel A, del Castillo V, et al. Microtia: A clinical and genetic study at the National Institute of Pediatrics in Mexico City. Arch Med Res 30:120, 1999.
5. Bennun RD, Mulliken JB, Kaban LB, et al. Microtia: A microform of hemifacial microsomia. Plast Reconstr Surg 76:859, 1985.
6. Figueroa AA, Friede H. Craniovertebral malformations in hemifacial microsomia. J Craniofac Genet Dev Biol Suppl 1:167, 1985.
7. Rogers BO. Microtic, lop, cup and protruding ears: Four directly inheritable deformities? Plast Reconstr Surg 41:208, 1968.
8. Nagata S. A new method for total reconstruction of the auricle for microtia. Plast Reconstr Surg 92:187, 1993.
9. Tanzer RC. Total reconstruction of the external ear. Plast Reconstr Surg 23:1, 1959.
10. Cronin TD. Use of a Silastic frame for total and subtotal reconstruction of the external ear: Preliminary report. Plast Reconstr Surg 37:399, 1966.
11. Reinisch J. Microtia reconstruction using a polyethylene implant: An eight year surgical experience. Presented at the Seventy-eighth Annual Meeting of the American Association of Plastic Surgeons, Colorado Springs, CO, May 1999.
12. Walton RL, Beahm EK. Auricular reconstruction for microtia. Part II: Surgical techniques. Plast Reconstr Surg 110:234, 2002.
13. Brent B. Technical advances in ear reconstruction with autogenous rib cartilage grafts: Personal experience with 1200 cases. Plast Reconstr Surg 104:319, 1999.
14. Brent B. Modification of the stages in total reconstruction of the auricle: Parts I to IV (discussion). Plast Reconstr Surg 93:267, 1994.
15. Brent B. Auricular repair with autogenous rib cartilage grafts: Two decades of experience with 600 cases. Plast Reconstr Surg 90:355, 1992.
16. Achauer BM, Eriksson E, Guyuron B, et al. Plastic Surgery: Indications, Operations, and Outcomes. St Louis: Mosby, 2000, p 1023.
17. Nagata S. A new method for total reconstruction of the auricle for microtia. Plast Reconstr Surg 92:187, 1993.

23. Prominent Ear

Jeffrey E. Janis

NORMAL EAR ANATOMY (Fig. 23-1)[1-5]

- Lateral skin is dense, adherent, and thin.
- Medial skin is loose, fibrofatty, and thick.
- By the third year of life, the ear has attained 85% of its adult size.
- Ear width reaches its mature size in boys at 7 years and in girls at 6 years.
- Ear length matures in boys at 13 years and in girls at 12 years.
- The older a person becomes, the stiffer and more calcified the cartilage.
- Cartilage is much floppier and more malleable as a neonate.

> TIP: Nonoperative correction of some congenital ear anomalies can be performed by molding if initiated within the first 72 hours of life to take advantage of cartilage malleability, which is secondary to circulating maternal hormones.

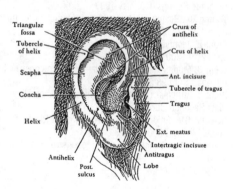

Fig. 23-1 Anatomy of the external ear. (From Janis JE, Rohrich RJ, Gutowski KA. Otoplasty. Plast Reconstr Surg 115:60e-72e, 2005.)

EMBRYOLOGIC ORIGINS

- **Mandibular branchial arch (first):** Anterior hillock—Contributes the tragus, root of helix, and superior helix only (upper one third of ear)
- **Hyoid branchial arch (second):** Posterior Hillock—Contributes the remainder (antihelix, antitragus, lobule) (lower two thirds of ear)
- Ear begins to protrude from developing face approximately 3-4 months of gestation

VASCULARITY (Fig. 23-2)

- Terminal branches of the external carotid artery
- Posterior auricular artery
- Superficial temporal artery

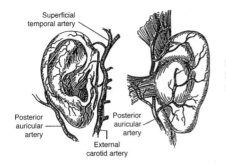

Fig. 23-2   Vascularity of the ear. (From Aston SJ, Beasley RW, Thorne CHM, et al. Grabb and Smith's Plastic Surgery, 5th ed. Philadelphia: Lippincott, 1997.)

INNERVATION (Fig. 23-3)

AURICULOTEMPORAL NERVE
- Branch of the trigeminal nerve
- Provides sensitivity to the tragus and crus helicis

GREAT AURICULAR NERVE
- Separates into anterior and posterior divisions
- Branch of the cervical plexus (C2-3)
- Supplies rest of ear

AURICULAR BRANCHES OF THE VAGUS (ARNOLD'S NERVE)
- Supplies the external acoustic meatus

LESSER OCCIPITAL NERVE

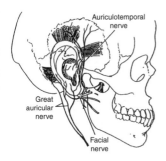

Fig. 23-3   Innervation of the ear. (From Aston SJ, Beasley RW, Thorne CHM, et al. Grabb and Smith's Plastic Surgery, 5th ed. Philadelphia: Lippincott, 1997.)

NORMAL EAR AESTHETIC PROPORTIONS[4,6]

SUMMARY OF NORMAL EAR AESTHETICS

- The long axis of the ear inclines posteriorly approximately 20 degrees from the vertical.
- The ear axis does not normally parallel the bridge of the nose (the angle differential is approximately 15 degrees).
- The ear is positioned approximately one ear length (5.5-7 cm) posterior to the lateral orbital rim between horizontal planes that intersect the eyebrow and columella.
- The width is approximately 50%-60% of the length (width 3-4.5 cm; length 5.5-7 cm).
- The anterolateral aspect of the helix protrudes 21-30 degrees from the scalp.
- The anterolateral aspect of the helix is approximately 1.5-2 cm from the scalp (although there is a large amount of racial and gender variation).
- The lobule and antihelical fold lie in a parallel plane at an acute angle to the mastoid process.
- The helix should project 2-5 mm more laterally than the antihelix in the frontal view.

From Janis JE, Rohrich RJ, Gutowski KA. Otoplasty. Plast Reconstr Surg 115:60e-72e, 2005.

EPIDEMIOLOGY[7]

- Relatively common, with an incidence in Caucasians of about **5%.**
- **Autosomal dominant** trait
- Despite benign physiologic consequences, numerous studies attest to the psychological distress, emotional trauma, and behavioral problems this deformity can inflict on children[5,8-10]
- **Commonly caused by a combination of two defects:**
  1. Underdevelopment of antihelical folding
  2. Overdevelopment of the conchal wall

PREOPERATIVE EVALUATION

The following should be assessed[11]:
- Degree of antihelical folding
- Depth of the conchal bowl
- Plane of the lobule and deformity, if present
- Angle between the helical rim and the mastoid plane
- Quality and spring of the auricular cartilage

MAJOR ANATOMIC CHARACTERISTICS

1. Poorly defined antihelical fold
2. Conchoscaphal angle more than 90 degrees
3. Conchal excess (can be determined by placing medial pressure along helical rim)

NONSURGICAL TREATMENT[2,3]

- **Molding techniques initiated within the first 72 hours of birth**
  - Takes advantage of circulating maternal hormones that result in more pliable and malleable cartilage
  - Perform continuously for 6-8 weeks
  - May avoid surgical treatment

GOALS OF SURGICAL TREATMENT[12]

- All traces of protrusion in the upper third of the ear must be corrected (some remaining protrusion in the middle or lower portions may be acceptable, provided that the top is thoroughly corrected; but the reverse does not hold true).
- From the front view, the helix of both ears should extend beyond the antihelix (at least down to the midear and preferably all the way down).
- The helix should have a smooth and regular line throughout.
- The postauricular sulcus should not be marked, decreased, or distorted.
- The ear should not be placed too close to the head, especially in boys (posterior measurement from the outer edge of the helix to the skin of the mastoidal region should be **10-12 mm** at the top, **16-18 mm** in the middle third, and **20-22 mm** in the lower third).
- The positions of the two ears (i.e., the distances from the lateral borders to the head) should match fairly closely—to within **3 mm** at any given point.

TIMING OF SURGERY

- Timing depends on a rational approach based on auricular growth and age of school matriculation.
- Because the ear is nearly fully developed by age 6-7 years, correction may be performed by this time.
  - In 76 patients who underwent cartilage excision otoplasty for prominent ears, Balogh and Millesi[13] demonstrated that auricular growth was not halted after a 7-year mean follow-up.

SURGICAL TECHNIQUES

MOST COMMON
- **Mustarde**[14]: Cartilage molding
- **Furnas**[15]: Cartilage molding
- **Converse–Wood-Smith**[16]: Cartilage breaking

OTHERS
- **Stenstrom**[17]: Cartilage scoring
- **Chongchet**[18]: Cartilage scoring

NOTE: Cartilage scoring techniques are based on the observation that cartilage curls away from a cut surface, which has been attributed to "interlocked stresses" that are released when the perichondrium is incised.[19,20]

MUSTARDE TECHNIQUE (Fig. 23-4)

- Used to correct **upper third** deformities, most often a poorly defined antihelical fold
- **Technique:**
  - Press medially on the ear and mark the concha and outer portion of the antihelical fold with a methylene-blue–dipped 25-gauge needle (full thickness to tattoo the postauricular skin).
  - Mark the postauricular skin excision between the marks.
  - Excise the skin and carry incision down to raw cartilage.
  - Place permanent mattress sutures (clear nylon or Mersilene [Ethicon, Cornelia, GA]) full thickness through the cartilage along the tattooed marks, making sure to capture the anterior perichondrium without piercing the anterior skin.
  - Tie sutures down to effect (may require "floating" sutures).
  - Close and dress with compression dressing of choice.
  - Patient should wear elastic ski band continuously for 3 weeks and avoid strenuous activity.

CAUTION: Watch for iatrogenic narrowing of the external auditory canal.

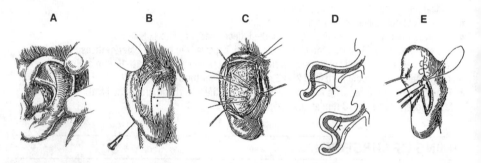

Fig. 23-4   The Mustarde technique. **A,** Several pairs of ink marks are made on the concha and outer aspect of the antihelix. **B,** Several 23-gauge needles dipped in ink are used to transfer the ink marks to the postauricular skin. **C,** The skin excision is carried down to cartilage. After hemostasis is obtained, several sutures are placed through the full thickness of cartilage. Usually two or three well-placed sutures are all that are required. **D,** The sutures are tied simultaneously. **E,** A subcuticular 4-0 nylon suture is used for closure. (From Aston SJ, Beasley RW, Thorne CHM, et al. Grabb and Smith's Plastic Surgery, 5th ed. Philadelphia: Lippincott, 1997.)

FURNAS TECHNIQUE (Fig. 23-5)

- Used to correct deformities of the **upper two thirds** of the ear, most often conchal excess
- Can be combined with other techniques (e.g., Mustarde technique for correcting an absent antihelical fold)
- **Technique:**
  - Perform a postauricular skin excision down through perichondrium to raw cartilage.
  - Dissect medially and laterally to expose the postauricular muscles and ligaments.

CAUTION: Avoid injuring branches of the great auricular nerve.

  - Resect a segment of mastoid fascia to expose underlying periosteum.
  - Place several permanent mattress sutures (clear nylon or Mersilene) full thickness through the conchal cartilage to the mastoid fascia/periosteum (capturing the anterior perichondrium).

- Tie sutures down to effect (may require "floating" sutures).
- Close and bolster
- Patient should wear elastic ski band continuously for 3 weeks and avoid strenuous activity.

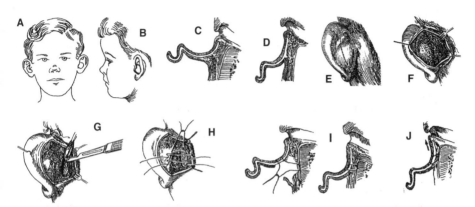

Fig. 23-5   The Furnas technique. **A** and **B**, The Furnas technique is best used for patients with prominence of the superior two thirds of the ear. **C** and **D**, The deeply cupped and enlarged conchal cartilage of the prominent ear *(C)* is contrasted with normal conchal cartilage *(D)* in cross-section. **E**, An ellipse of skin is excised in the postauricular sulcus. **F**, Exposure of the posterior auricular muscles and ligaments. **G**, Dividing and resecting the posterior auricular muscles and ligaments. **H**, Several mattress sutures are used to attach conchal cartilage to the mastoid fascia. **I**, The mattress sutures should be placed through the full thickness of conchal cartilage. **J**, The sutures are tied simultaneously. (From Aston SJ, Beasley RW, Thorne CHM, et al. Grabb and Smith's Plastic Surgery, 5th ed. Philadelphia: Lippincott, 1997.)

CONVERSE–WOOD-SMITH TECHNIQUE
- A **cartilage-breaking** technique, rather than cartilage-molding technique, as in the previous examples
- Useful when dealing with the stiffer cartilage of young adults and adults
- **Useful for correcting more severe prominent ear deformities (e.g., when entire ear is involved)**
  - Conchal excess
  - Loss of antihelical fold
  - Increased conchoscaphal angle
- **Drawbacks**
  - Secondary sharp ridging
  - Contour irregularities
- **Technique:**
  - Press helix medially against the scalp.
  - Mark the superior rim of the triangular fossa, the upper border of the superior crus, and the junction of the helix and scapha.
  - Mark the full length of the conchal rim.
  - Transpose these marks to the postauricular skin using full-thickness punctures with methylene-blue–dipped 25-gauge needles.
  - Demarcate the area of postauricular skin resection and excise. Dissect down to raw cartilage.

- Perform cartilage-breaking incisions sharply.
- Reform the antihelix by placing full-thickness mattress sutures with permanent suture material (clear nylon or Mersilene) and tie down to effect.
- Estimate amount of conchal excess by pressing inward on the newly created antihelix and excise.
- Approximate the newly cut edges of the concha and antihelix with permanent suture and tie down to effect.

> TIP: Do not evert edges, because doing so will cause permanent ridging.

- Close and bolster.
- Patient should wear elastic ski band continuously for 3 weeks and avoid strenuous activity.

CORRECTION OF LOBULE PROMINENCE (LOWER THIRD) (Fig. 23-6)
- Corrected using the **modified fishtail excision** (Wood-Smith)[21]
- **Technique:**
  - Mark a "V extension" from the inferior aspect of the postauricular incision used for correction of prominent ear deformity (e.g., Mustarde, Furnas, etc).
  - Transpose the marking to the mastoid skin while the ink is still fresh, forming a mirror image pattern in the shape of a fishtail.
  - Excise along the demarcated line.
  - Close and dress.

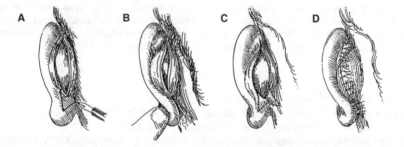

Fig. 23-6 Correction of prominent lobules. **A,** A V extension of the posterior auricular incision is drawn on the posterior surface of the lobule. **B,** While the ink is still wet, the lobule is pressed against the mastoid skin. **C,** The mirror impression of the V is transposed to the mastoid skin. Excision of all skin within the borders of the modified fishtail design is carried out. **D,** Closure is performed with a running 4-0 nylon suture.

COMPLICATIONS[22]

HEMATOMA
- **Most immediate and pressing postoperative problem**
- If sudden onset of persistent, unilateral pain, then suspect hematoma
- **Management**
  - Dressing removal, suture removal, and evacuation of clot
  - Reapplication of dressings with mild compression
  - To operating room for reexploration and hemostasis, if active

INFECTION
- Rare
- Usually from *Staphylococcus* or *Streptococcus,* occasionally *Pseudomonas*
- Sulfamylon useful in preventing spread of infection and chondritis
- Long-term problem is from infection

CHONDRITIS
- Surgical infection requiring prompt reexploration and excision of necrotic cartilage

LATE DEFORMITY
- Usually manifests within 6 months of surgery
- More often operator dependent than technique dependent
- Tan[23] found:
  - 24% of patients undergoing the Mustarde technique required "reoperation."
  - 10% of patients undergoing the Stenstrom technique required "reoperation."
    - Reason: Presence of sutures resulted in sinuses and wound infection in 15% of cases
  - Cartilage-breaking techniques (e.g., Luckett, Converse, and Wood-Smith) leave more "sharp edges" and "contour irregularities" than do non–cartilage-breaking techniques (e.g., Mustarde and Stenstrom).

TIP: Need to "break the ring of cartilage" to prevent telephone ear deformity.

KEY POINTS
- ✔ Ear cartilage is very malleable right after birth, and deformities can sometimes be corrected nonsurgically through molding techniques.
- ✔ Otoplasty for prominent ear deformities usually is done around age 6-7 years.
- ✔ The three typical deformities that make up the prominent ear deformity are: A poorly defined antihelical fold, a conchoscaphal angle greater than 90 degrees, and/or conchal excess.
- ✔ There are three approaches to treating prominent ear: Cartilage scoring, cartilage molding, and cartilage breaking.
- ✔ Hematoma and infection are rare, but need to be treated immediately and aggressively.
- ✔ The most common long-term complication is recurrence of the deformity, which is technique and surgeon dependent.

REFERENCES
1. Allison GR. Anatomy of the external ear. Clin Plast Surg 5:419, 1978.
2. Tan ST, Abramson DL, MacDonald DM, et al. Molding therapy for infants with deformational auricular anomalies. Ann Plast Surg 38:263, 1997.
3. Tan ST, Shibu M, Gault DT. A splint for correction of congenital ear deformities. Br J Plast Surg 47:575, 1994.

4. Farkas LG, Posnick JC, Hreczko TM. Anthropometric growth study of the ear. Cleft Palate Craniofac J 29:324, 1992.
5. Adamson JE, Horton CE, Crawford HH. The growth pattern of the external ear. Plast Reconstr Surg 36:466, 1965.
6. Farkas LG. Anthropometry of normal and anomalous ears. Clin Plast Surg 5:401, 1978.
7. Adamson PA, Strecker HD. Otoplasty techniques. Facial Plast Surg 11:284, 1995.
8. Campobasso P, Belloli G. [Protruding ears: The indications for surgical treatment.] Pediatr Med Chir 15:151, 1993.
9. Bradbury ET, Hewison J, Timmons MJ. Psychological and social outcome of prominent ear correction in children. Br J Plast Surg 45:97, 1992.
10. Macgregor FC. Ear deformities: Social and psychological implications. Clin Plast Surg 5:347, 1978.
11. Ellis DA, Keohane JD. A simplified approach to otoplasty. J Otolaryngol 21:66, 1992.
12. McDowell AJ. Goals in otoplasty for protruding ears. Plast Reconstr Surg 41:17, 1968.
13. Balogh B, Millesi H. Are growth alterations a consequence of surgery for prominent ears? Plast Reconstr Surg 89:623, 1992.
14. Mustarde JC. The correction of prominent ears using mattress sutures. Br J Plast Surg 16:170, 1963.
15. Furnas DW. Correction of prominent ears by conchamastoid sutures. Plast Reconstr Surg 42:189, 1968.
16. Converse JM, Wood-Smith D. Technical details in the surgical correction of the lop ear deformity. Plast Reconstr Surg 31:118, 1963.
17. Stenstrom SJ. A natural technique for correction of congenitally prominent ears. Plast Reconstr Surg 32:509, 1963.
18. Chongchet V. A method of antihelix reconstruction. Br J Plast Surg 16:268, 1963.
19. Gibson T, Davis W. The distortion of autogenous cartilage grafts: Its cause and prevention. Br J Plast Surg 10:257, 1958.
20. Fry HJH. Interlocked stresses in human nasal septal cartilage. Br J Plast Surg 19:276, 1966.
21. Wood-Smith D. Otoplasty. In Rees T, ed. Aesthetic Plastic Surgery. Philadelphia: Saunders, 1980, p 833.
22. Furnas DW. Complications of surgery of the external ear. Clin Plast Surg 17:305, 1990.
23. Tan KH. Long-term survey of prominent ear surgery: A comparison of two methods. Br J Plast Surg 39:270, 1986.

24. Facial Skeletal Trauma

Jason K. Potter

GENERAL

- **Trauma** is the number one cause of death in individuals less than 40 years of age.
- Death secondary to injury accounts for 80% of all deaths among teens and young adults.
- Traumatic injury is the number one cause of lost productivity.
- There are approximately 1.6 million head injuries annually in the United States.
- Alcohol is a contributing factor in almost 50% of head injuries.
- A review of the Maryland Shock Trauma Registry (1986-1994) reported that 11% of trauma patients (2964 of 25,758) sustained maxillofacial fractures requiring subspecialty intervention.[1]

EPIDEMIOLOGY

- Applied force and facial injury
  - Severity of injury is a function of energy delivered. Kinetic energy: $K = mv^2$
  - Moving object strikes head or moving head strikes static object.
- Variables affecting type and severity of injury
  - **Area of strike:** Specific anatomic location that receives energy
  - **Resistant force:** Resultant movement of head
  - **Angulation of strike:** More severe injury with perpendicular delivery of energy than with tangential delivery

CLASSIFICATION

ASSAULT
- Males, 18-25 years old, are typically attacked by unknown assailants.
- Females are typically attacked by known assailants.
- 40% of ER visits result from assault.
  - 30% present with fracture, 80% of these involve facial bone.
- Elevated blood alcohol reported in 50% of incidents.
- Incidence ranking: Nasal > mandible > zygoma > midface

MOTOR VEHICLE COLLISION
- Males 18-25 years old
- Associated with more severe trauma
- Frequently involves midface structures (nose, zygoma, maxilla)
- Overall reduction in number of injuries by more than 30% as a result of modernized auto safety systems
  - 1948-1955, 54% reduction of Le Fort II/III injuries
  - 1988-1993, 9.6% reduction of Le Fort II/III injuries
  - Seat belt laws: Incidence of facial injury reduced from 21% to 6% in 2 years

FALLS

- Bimodal age group
  - Toddlers
  - Elderly
- Common cause of facial injury in developing countries because of lack of safety measures
- Hands-out fall: Fractures of zygoma and lateral face
- No-hands fall: Fractures of central face and dentoalveolar structures

WAR

- Head and neck involvement in 16% of injuries
- Modern high-velocity weapon injuries of head and neck frequently fatal

SPORTS

- Relatively low incidence, secondary to mouth guards and protective headgear

CLINICAL SIGNIFICANCE

- Face provides anterior protection for the cranium.
- Facial appearance is highly valued by most cultures.
- Maxillofacial region is associated with a number of important functions of daily life: Seeing, smelling, eating, breathing, and talking.
- Maxillofacial injuries may occur as isolated injuries or as part of polytrauma.
- In general, maxillofacial injuries are a low priority in the management of the polytrauma patient but are addressed in the Advance Trauma Life Support (ATLS) tertiary survey.
  - Exceptions that can lead to life-threatening or irreversible injury:
    - Life-threatening hemorrhage
    - Loss of airway
    - Cervical spine injury
    - Neurologic injury

LONG-TERM PHYSICAL IMPAIRMENT

- A direct relationship has been demonstrated between severity of injury and work disability in patients with complex facial fractures.[1]
  - These patients reported higher incidence of somatic complaints than general trauma patients.
  - Residual cranial nerve deficits, facial numbness, persistent facial pain, headaches, and sinus problems were unrelated to severity of injury.

PATIENT EVALUATION

DETAILED HISTORY

- **Method of injury:** Include mechanism and specifics for severity of injury, (e.g., assault with weapon delivers more force than fists alone)
- **Location of injury**
- **Time of injury:** Length of time from injury to presentation

- **Loss of consciousness**
- **Subjective complaints**
  - Double vision
  - Loss of vision
  - Hearing loss
  - Otorrhea or rhinorrhea
  - Malocclusion
- Inquire about any **environmental considerations** that may affect management: Chemical, agricultural, or farm injuries.
- **Preexisting conditions**
  - Many patients who present to the ER for facial trauma have been there before.

TIP: Preexisting enophthalmos or malocclusions can mislead and result in significant waste of resources if appropriate inquiries are not made.

- **Identify potentially devastating injuries**
  - **Life-threatening hemorrhage**
    - ▶ **Internal maxillary artery** most common source associated with facial fractures
    - ▶ **Management**
      - ◆ Posterior nasal packing
      - ◆ Immediate reduction of fractures
      - ◆ Consideration of angiography and selective embolization for a stable patient or ligation of external carotid for a hemodynamically unstable patient
  - **Loss of airway**
    - ▶ May result from massive edema or loss of anterior support of the tongue, resulting in obstruction at the level of the hypopharynx

TIP: Be wary of loss of airway in the patient with multiple fractures of the anterior mandible.

- ▶ **Four indications for tracheotomy**[2]
  1. Acute airway obstruction and failed endotracheal intubation
  2. Expected prolonged mechanical ventilation
  3. Multiple facial fractures associated with basilar skull injuries
  4. Destruction of nasal anatomy associated with facial fractures
- **Cervical spine injury**
  - ▶ Spinal injury accounts for 6%-8% of trauma admissions: 30% involve the cervical spine, and 50% have concomitant injury of the cord.
  - ▶ 15%-20% of all cervical spine injuries are associated with facial bone fractures. Conversely, 1%-4% of all facial injuries are associated with cervical spine injury.[3]
  - ▶ Most importantly, there is a delay in diagnosis of cervical spine injury in 10%-25% of patients, when associated with facial injury.

CAUTION: Spinal precautions should be used with every patient.

- **Neurologic injury**
  - ▶ Estimated 1.6 million brain injuries annually in the United States
  - ▶ 60,000 deaths, 70,000-90,000 cases of permanent neurologic disability

▸ 13-75 times greater risk of death from neurologic injury with any middle or upper facial fracture compared with isolated mandibular fracture[4]
▸ **Risk for intracranial injury**
  ✦ Presence of skull fracture implies transmission of a large force.
  ✦ Incidence of intracranial injury, with loss of consciousness, is 1.3%-17.2%.[5]
  ✦ Incidence increases with a Glasgow Coma Score (GCS) less than 15 and longer unconsciousness.
  ✦ Closed head injury (CHI) occurs in 17.5% of patients with facial fractures.[6]
  ✦ Midfacial fractures have more frequent association with closed head injury than do mandible fractures.[6]
  ✦ Patterns of facial fractures tend to be more severe in patients with CHI.[6]
▸ **Classification of neurologic injury**
  ✦ **Primary injury** is the initial injury and the cause of presentation.
  ✦ **Secondary injury** is a result of damage to neurons because of systemic physiologic responses to the initial injury.
    - **Hypotension** and **hypoxia** are the major causes of secondary injury.

PHYSICAL EXAMINATION

Examination of the maxillofacial complex is a detailed process and therefore requires an organized approach to prevent omitting key elements. Before beginning, the patient should be cleansed of all dried blood and dirt that may obscure underlying injury.

INSPECTION
■ Thoroughly inspect all areas of the head and neck to assess for contusions, lacerations, edema, hematomas, asymmetries, or obvious deformities.
■ Inspect pupils for symmetry and reaction to light; inspect the external auditory canal for lacerations and tympanic membrane for rupture, hemotympanum, or otorrhea. This information should help guide the physical examination.

PALPATION
■ Begin in the frontal region.
  • Palpate the frontal process, orbital rims, nasal bones, and zygomas.

> TIP: Bimanual or bilateral palpation helps identify side to side differences that may indicate fractures.

  • Note any step-offs, crepitus, or gross deformity.
■ Palpate in the region of any laceration or contusion for underlying fracture.
■ Proceed intraorally and run fingers along the zygomaticomaxillary buttresses, noting step-offs, ecchymosis, or lacerations.
  • Note any gingival lacerations and assess whether all teeth are present and nonmobile.
■ Place the nondominant hand on the nasal dorsum and, using the dominant hand, grasp the anterior maxilla (dentition) and assess for mobility.
■ Grasp the mandible bimanually and assess for mobility along its length.
■ Note any ecchymosis on the floor of mouth.

- Assess occlusion.
- Palpate cervical spine and note any tenderness or step-offs.

EVALUATE CRANIAL NERVES II-XII (see Chapter 27).

Note: Determine whether there are any paresthesias or functional deficits.

DIAGNOSTIC IMAGING

- **For diagnostic purposes, patients with abnormal findings during physical examination should have computed tomography (CT) of the maxillofacial complex in both axial and coronal planes.**
- CT scans are the gold standard for middle and upper facial fractures.
- Plain films are not necessary for evaluation of midfacial fractures (unlike mandibular fractures) when CT is available.
- Reconstructed coronal images are not of acceptable quality and should only be tolerated when patient positioning for coronal imaging is precluded by cervical spine precautions.

TIMING OF OPERATIVE INTERVENTION

- Prevention or minimization of secondary injury is of primary importance.[7]
- Initial management of the head-injured patient should be similar to that for the polytrauma patient without head injury, focusing on control of hemorrhage and restoration of perfusion.
- Maintenance of cerebral perfusion pressure (CPP) greater than 70 is mandatory during the preoperative, perioperative, and postoperative periods.
- Brain injury increases with inadequate resuscitation and with operative procedures that allow hypotension or low CPP.
- Treatment protocol is based on individual patient's clinical assessment and treatment needs.

FRONTAL SINUS FRACTURES

- **The frontal bone requires the greatest force of any facial bone to fracture;** it can withstand 800-1600 pounds of force (Fig. 24-1).[8]
- The sinus is contained within the frontal bone and drains beneath the **middle meatus** into the nasal cavity through the **nasofrontal ducts.**
- The sinus is not present at birth; development begins at about age 2 years and does not reach adult size until about age 12 years.

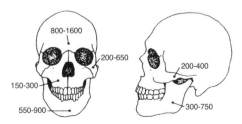

Fig. 24-1 The forces (measured in pounds) necessary to fracture the frontal sinus are 2 to 3 times greater than those needed to fracture the zygoma, maxilla, or mandible. (From Nahum AM. The biomechanics of maxillofacial trauma. Clin Plast Surg 2:59-64, 1975.)

- The sinus is not identifiable radiographically until about age 8 years.
- Two indications for treatment are cosmesis and obstruction of normal sinus drainage.

CLINICAL PRESENTATION
- Upper face edema and ecchymosis
- Palpable deformity of frontal bone
- Laceration of forehead
- Paresthesias of supraorbital or supratrochlear nerves
- Cerebrospinal fluid (CSF) rhinorrhea
  - Occurs with dural laceration in region of cribriform plate or adjacent to posterior table fractures
  - Diagnostic laboratory confirmation with a β-transferrin test
  - *Ring test* for bedside evaluation
- Globe displacement (forward and inferiorly)
  - May occur when orbital roof is involved

IMAGING
- **CT scans are required.**
- **Evaluate for:**
  - Involvement of anterior and or posterior tables
  - Degree of posterior table displacement or comminution
  - Pneumocephalus
  - Level of injury relative to superior orbital rim
  - Associated injuries
- Direct evidence of ductal injury cannot be obtained from CT.
- Only isolated anterior table fractures and transverse linear fractures through both tables, but above level of sinus floor, are assumed to have no associated duct injury.[9]

MANAGEMENT
- **Treatment is based on:**
  - Contour deformity secondary to displacement of anterior table
  - Presence of CSF leak
  - Likelihood of nasofrontal duct obstruction
  - Degree of displacement or comminution of posterior table
- Surgical access is provided through a coronal flap or existing lacerations.
- The coronal flap should be elevated in the **subgaleal plane** to allow easy and atraumatic elevation of a pericranial flap, when needed.
- **Open reduction with internal fixation (ORIF) of anterior table**
  - Reserved for isolated anterior table fractures without involvement of nasofrontal duct
  - Used when there is no associated CSF leak
  - Fixation provided with low-profile miniplates (1.3 mm system; Synthes, West Chester, PA)
- **Sinus obliteration**
  - Indicated for fractures of anterior table combined with involvement of nasofrontal ducts
  - Used when posterior table displacement minimal and no CSF leak
  - Sinus mucosa completely removed with rotary burs and ducts obstructed obliterated grafts
  - Obliteration performed with fat grafts, pericranial flap, spontaneous osteogenesis, or bone grafts

> TIP: It is not advisable to obliterate the sinus with bone cement because of complications from infection.

- **Cranialization**
  - Indicated for fractures of anterior table combined with involvement of **CSF leak, significant displacement, or comminution of posterior table**
  - Procedure performed in conjunction with neurosurgery
  - Posterior table removed, remaining mucosa removed, ducts obliterated, nasal cavity isolated from cranial cavity by interposition of pericranial flap along floor of anterior cranial fossa
  - Anterior table reconstructed as for posterior table
  - Algorithm for management presented in Figs. 24-2 and 24-3[10]

PEDIATRIC CONSIDERATIONS
- None; frontal sinus not developed in children

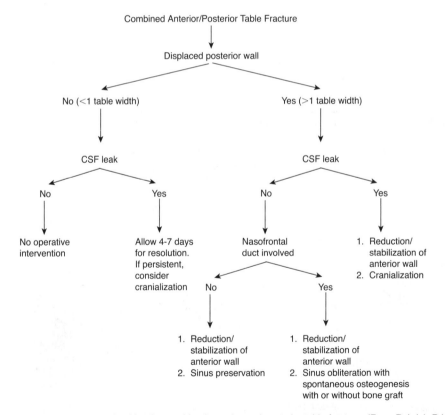

Fig. 24-2 Management algorithm for combined anterior and posterior table fracture. (From Rohrich RJ, Hollier LH. Management of frontal sinus fractures: Changing concepts. Clin Plast Surg 19:219, 1992.)

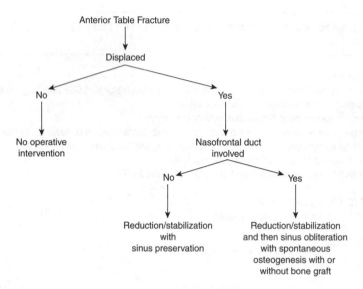

Fig. 24-3 Management algorithm for anterior table fracture. (From Rohrich RJ, Hollier LH. Management of frontal sinus fractures: Changing concepts. Clin Plast Surg 19:219, 1992.)

NASOORBITAL ETHMOID FRACTURES

- Fractures of the nasoorbital ethmoid complex (NOE) represent the most problematic fractures to repair and probably result in the most noticeable postinjury change in facial appearance.
- Fractures in this region alter the soft tissue–bony relationships of the nasal dorsum, nasoorbital valley, and medial canthus.
- By definition, these fractures involve the nasal and ethmoid bones of the medial orbit.
- **Markowitz classification** is based on the central fragment, which bears the medial canthal tendon (Fig. 24-4).
  - **Type I:** A single, noncomminuted, central fragment without medial canthal tendon disruption

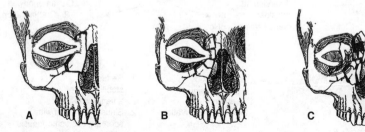

Fig. 24-4 Classification of NOE fractures. **A,** Type I; **B,** Type II; **C,** Type III. See text for description. (From Markowitz BL, Manson PN, Sargent L, et al. Management of the medial canthal tendon in nasoethmoid orbital fractures: The importance of the central fragment in classification and treatment. Plast Reconstr Surg 87:843-853, 1991.)

- **Type II:** Comminuted central fragment without medial canthal tendon disruption
- **Type III:** Severely comminuted central fragment with disruption of the medial canthal tendon
- Surgical access is provided through a coronal approach or existing lacerations.

CLINICAL PRESENTATION
- Telecanthus: Sometimes **not** present in monobloc type I fracture
- Loss of dorsal nasal projection
- Periorbital edema or ecchymosis
- Step-offs at orbital rims
- Subconjunctival hemorrhage

RADIOGRAPHIC EVALUATION
- CT scans are diagnostic.
- Axial and coronal images are required for complete evaluation.
- Assess for comminution in region of medial canthi, degree of orbital involvement, degree of posterior nasal displacement, and possible frontal sinus involvement.

TREATMENT
Treatment is directed at reconstituting intercanthal relationship, nasal projection, and internal orbital structures.[11,12]
- Wide exposure is provided through coronal flap.
- Bony structures are reduced and stabilized with low-profile miniplates.
- Cranial bone grafts are harvested to reconstruct nasal projection.
- Canthal tendons are reconstructed with transnasal wiring.
- Minimal hardware should be placed in nasoorbital valley to reduce bulk.
- Soft tissues of nasoorbital valley should be redraped with bolsters or thermoplastic nasal splints; if not done, this region thickens, creating an uncorrectable deformity.

PEDIATRIC CONSIDERATIONS
- Nasal reconstruction is aimed at reduction and stabilization.
- Dorsal nasal bone grafts should be reserved for severe injuries and older children.
- Resorbable fixation systems are used when feasible.
- The septum is a major growth center of the face, and parents should be counseled about potential growth disturbances.

NASAL FRACTURES

- **The most common fractures of facial bones.**
- Often occur in isolation or as part of a complex fracture pattern.

TIP: During examination, it is important to determine whether a NOE component is present.

- Posttraumatic deformity of the nose common following treatment and reported in up to 50% of patients.
  - Can be minimized by accurate diagnosis and reduction during a thorough external and internal nasal examination.
- Septal fractures frequently undiagnosed and untreated, resulting in late deformity.

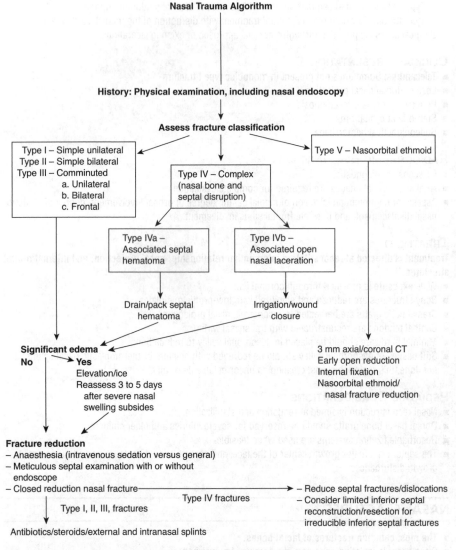

Nasal Trauma Algorithm

History: Physical examination, including nasal endoscopy

Assess fracture classification

Type I – Simple unilateral
Type II – Simple bilateral
Type III – Comminuted
    a. Unilateral
    b. Bilateral
    c. Frontal

Type IV – Complex
(nasal bone and
septal disruption)

Type V – Nasoorbital ethmoid

Type IVa –
Associated septal
hematoma

Type IVb –
Associated open
nasal laceration

Drain/pack septal
hematoma

Irrigation/wound
closure

Significant edema
No → **Yes**
Elevation/ice
Reassess 3 to 5 days
after severe nasal
swelling subsides

3 mm axial/coronal CT
Early open reduction
Internal fixation
Nasoorbital ethmoid/
    nasal fracture reduction

Fracture reduction
– Anaesthesia (intravenous sedation versus general)
– Meticulous septal examination with or without
   endoscope
– Closed reduction nasal fracture —————————————→ – Reduce septal fractures/dislocations
                            Type IV fractures   – Consider limited inferior septal
    Type I, II, III, fractures   reconstruction/resection for
                                          irreducible inferior septal fractures

Antibiotics/steroids/external and intranasal splints

Fig. 24-5 Nasal fracture algorithm delineating trauma classification and respective treatments. (From Rohrich RJ, Adams WP. Nasal fracture management: Minimizing secondary deformities. Plast Reconstr Surg 106:266, 2000.)

CAUTION: It is essential to identify septal hematomas and provide timely drainage to prevent late destruction of the septum.

CLINICAL PRESENTATION
- Nasal deformity
- Nasal edema
- Laceration
- Epistaxis
- Crepitus
- Tenderness
- Septal deviation
- Septal hematoma

IMAGING
- Nasal fractures usually can be diagnosed clinically at the initial setting or once edema resolves.
- CT for isolated injuries is unnecessary and is a poor use of resources.
- Standard radiographs are of limited value.

TREATMENT
- Anatomic reduction of nasal bones and septum is needed to prevent late deformity.
- Algorithm for management is presented in Fig. 24-5.[13]

ORBITAL FRACTURES (Fig. 24-6)

- Fractures of the bony orbit may occur alone or as part of complex facial fractures.
- The bony orbit consists of **seven** individual bones that vary significantly in thickness.
- The thinnest region is along the medial wall **(lamina papyracea).**
- Isolated fractures may occur (without associated fracture of orbital rim) of the floor and medial wall.
    - These fractures are postulated to occur either from increased pressure that develops within the orbit (from posterior displacement of orbital tissues) or when deformation of the orbital bones occurs from a blow, so that fractures of thin portions of the floor result without fracture of the orbital rim.[14]
- Without treatment, orbital fractures may result in **dystopia** (vertical globe malposition) or **enophthalmos** (posterior malposition).
    - **Dystopia** results from the loss of bony support maintaining globe position.
    - **Enophthalmos** results from **two factors.**
        1. Fractures of the orbit result in increased intraorbital volume and disrupt the fine ligamentous system within the periorbita.
        2. When healing occurs, the periorbita assumes a spherical shape that has a smaller volume than its previous conical shape.

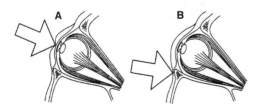

Fig. 24-6 Mechanism of injury from orbital blowout fractures. **A,** Hydraulic theory. **B,** Bone conduction theory. (From Waterhouse N, Lyne J, Urdang M, et al. An investigation into the mechanism of orbital blowout fractures. Br J Plast Surg 52:607-612, 1999.)

TIP: Simply put, a smaller volume in a larger orbit results in enophthalmos.

CLINICAL PRESENTATION
- Periorbital edema or ecchymosis
- Step-offs at orbital rims
- Subconjunctival hemorrhage: Disruption of periosteum that may occur with or without orbital fracture
- Limited eye excursions
  - True entrapment is rare in adults and usually is a result of edema.
  - In children entrapment of recti must be ruled out.
- Enophthalmos or exophthalmos
- Diplopia
- Infraorbital nerve paresthesia

IMAGING
- CT scans are diagnostic.
- Axial and coronal images are required for complete evaluation.
- Assess for location and size of defect.
- Soft tissue images identify herniation of orbital contents and possible entrapment.

TREATMENT
- Treatment aims to restore orbital contours and volume.
- A decision to operate should be based on size of defect and presence of enophthalmos or diplopia.
  - All patients should be observed during the 2 weeks after injury to assess development or resolution of symptoms (enophthalmos or diplopia) as edema resolves.
  - A decision to operate should be made during this interval because cicatricial healing will compromise the ability to restore premorbid orbital position later.

TIP: In general, defects smaller than 1 cm do not require operative treatment unless enophthalmos or diplopia persists at 2 weeks.

   Large defects should be treated regardless of symptoms because enophthalmos is likely to occur.

- Surgical access to the orbital floor is provided through subtarsal or transconjunctival (with or without canthotomy) incisions.
- Subciliary incisions should be avoided because of increased lower lid deformities associated with this approach.[15]
- Access to the medial wall, above the level of the canthus, requires either addition of a coronal approach or a transcaruncular extension of the transconjunctival approach.
- Many materials are available for reconstruction of the orbital walls.[16]
  - Titanium mesh
  - Autologous bone
  - Polyethylene (Mylar)
  - Porous polyethylene (Medpor®; Porex Surgical, Newnan, GA)
  - Nylon sheets (SupraFoil®; S. Jackson, Inc., Alexandria, VA)

PEDIATRIC CONSIDERATIONS
- Pediatric bone is more likely to deform and recoil after fracture and may result in muscle entrapment.
  - This represents a relatively emergent situation because true entrapment results in ischemia and necrosis of the muscle, further resulting in movement dysfunction.
  - 62% of patients with true entrapment present with pain from eye movement or nausea and vomiting.
- **Use resorbable fixation systems when feasible.**

ZYGOMATICOMAXILLARY COMPLEX (ZMC) FRACTURES

- **The zygoma has four articulations.**
  - Frontal
  - Maxillary
  - Sphenoid
  - Temporal
- ZMC fractures usually disrupt most of these relationships, allowing malposition of the zygoma in the anteroposterior, vertical, and horizontal dimensions.
- To accurately reduce these fractures, at least three of four articulations must be assessed intraoperatively.
- ZMC fractures should be classified as **low-energy** or **high-energy,** based on the comminution at each articulation.
  - **High-energy** fractures demonstrate comminution at each articulation and therefore require surgical exposure of each to assure accurate reduction.
  - **Low-energy** fractures are noncomminuted and generally do not require surgical exposure as aggressive as for high-energy fractures.
- ZMC fractures, when treated appropriately, do not leave deformities, and complications of lower lid incisions may be the only telltale sign of treatment.
  - Exposure of the orbital floor should be for planned reconstruction rather than exploration.[17]

CLINICAL PRESENTATION
- Malar flattening
- Step-offs at orbital rims, zygomatic arch, zygomaticomaxillary buttress
- Enophthalmos or dystopia
- Infraorbital paresthesia
- Trismus
- Downsloping palpebral fissure

IMAGING
- CT scans are diagnostic.
- Axial and coronal images are required for complete evaluation.
- **Assess for:**
  - Degree of comminution (high- or low-energy)
  - Medial or lateral rotation of zygoma
  - Anteroposterior projection of zygoma
  - Position of lateral orbital wall
  - Need for reconstruction of orbital floor

TREATMENT

Treatment usually requires open reduction and stabilization with internal fixation. Occasionally, minimally displaced injuries may be stable after initial reduction and do not need fixation.

- **Low-energy injuries**[18]
  - These injuries are usually exposed intraorally at the zygomaticomaxillary (ZM) buttress and using an upper blepharoplasty incision.
  - The upper lid incision allows visualization of the zygomaticofrontal (ZF) and zygomaticosphenoid (ZS) articulations.
  - **The ZS articulation is the most important to assess for reduction.**

> **TIP:** A Carroll-Girard screw can be used to provide three-dimensional control of the segment for reduction.

  - Initial stabilization of the ZF with a malleable miniplate (1.3 mm system; Synthes) sets the vertical height and allows continued manipulation of the segment in anteroposterior and horizontal dimensions.
  - Perform ZM articulation fixation.
  - Additional fixation may be placed along the ZS articulation.
  - Lower lid incisions and exposure of the floor are not needed to assess reduction with exposure of ZF, ZM, and ZS articulations and should be reserved for reconstruction of the floor, when indicated.
- **High-energy injuries**
  - Require wide exposure through coronal flap to include exposure of the temporal articulation
  - More frequently require reconstruction of the orbital floor
  - Following wide exposure, resuspension of malar soft tissues critical to prevent malar ptosis and soft tissue deformity
- Algorithm for management shown in Fig. 24-7

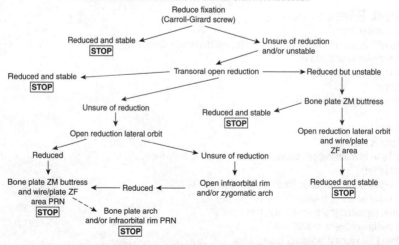

Fig. 24-7   Treatment algorithm for ZMC fractures. (From Ellis E III, Kittidumkerng W. Analysis of treatment for isolated zygomaticomaxillary complex fractures. J Oral Maxillofac Surg 54:386-400, 1996.)

PEDIATRIC CONSIDERATIONS

CAUTION: Permanent dentition development is at risk when placing fixation screws at the ZM buttress.

- **Resorbable fixation systems used when feasible**

ZYGOMATIC ARCH FRACTURES

Fractures of the zygomatic arch are almost a purely aesthetic concern, except in the rare instances when the fracture segment impedes mandibular excursion by interfering with the coronoid process.

CLINICAL PRESENTATION
- Palpable deformity
- Contour deformity
- Trismus

TREATMENT
- Uncomplicated fractures can be elevated using **Gillies approach.**
- Stabilization is generally unnecessary.

MAXILLARY FRACTURES

- The maxilla constitutes the majority of the midface skeleton.
- It contains the maxillary sinus and dentition.
- **Three major buttresses provide strength** (Fig. 24-8).
  1. Nasomaxillary
  2. Zygomatic
  3. Pterygomaxillary

TIP: These regions also present the best quality bone for using rigid fixation.

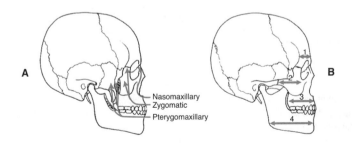

Fig. 24-8   A, Facial buttresses responsible for vertical support: Nasomaxillary, zygomatic, and pterygomaxillary. **B,** Anteroposterior buttresses: frontal *(1)*, zygomatic *(2)*, maxillary *(3)*, and mandibular *(4)*.

CLASSIFICATION

- **Dentoalveolar**
  - Involves teeth and supporting osseous structure
- **Le Fort I** (Fig. 24-9, *A*)
  - *Separates tooth-bearing maxilla from midface*
  - Extends from piriform aperture posteriorly through the nasal septum, lateral nasal walls, anterior maxillary wall, through the maxillary tuberosity or pterygoid plates
  - Upper jaw clinically mobile
- **Le Fort II** (Fig. 24-9, *B*)
  - *Pyramidal fracture*
  - Extends through frontonasal junction along medial orbital wall, usually passing through inferior orbital rim at the zygomaticomaxillary suture; continues posteriorly through tuberosity or pterygoid plates
  - Upper jaw and nasal bones clinically mobile as solitary unit
- **Le Fort III** (Fig. 24-9, *C*)
  - *Craniofacial disjunction*
  - Extends through frontonasal junction along medial orbital wall and inferior orbital fissure and out lateral orbital wall
  - Fractures through pterygoid plates at high level
  - Clinically, simultaneous mobility at maxilla and at nasofrontal and zygomaticofrontal regions

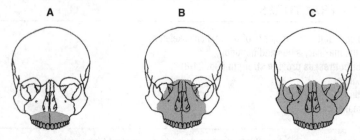

Fig. 24-9   Le Fort midfacial fractures. **A,** Le Fort I fracture separating inferior portion of maxilla in horizontal fashion, extending from piriform aperture of nose to pterygoid maxillary suture area. **B,** Le Fort II fracture involving separation of maxilla and nasal complex from cranial base, zygomatic orbital rim area, and pterygoid maxillary suture area. **C,** Le Fort III fracture (i.e., craniofacial separation) is complete separation of midface at level of nasoorbital ethmoid complex and zygomaticofrontal suture area. Fracture also extends through orbits bilaterally.

TIP: This system provides for a good description of injury; however, rarely do these injuries occur in isolation. There usually are multiple fracture patterns in a patient, making the system clinically less useful.

CLINICAL PRESENTATION

- Facial edema
- Periorbital ecchymosis
- Epistaxis

- Malocclusion: Anterior open bite secondary to posterior-inferior displacement of maxilla
- Tenderness during palpation at buttresses
- Crepitus
- Mobility of maxilla
- Palpable step-offs

IMAGING
- CT scans diagnostic
- Axial and coronal images required for complete evaluation
- **Assess:**
  - Degree of comminution
  - Presence of sagittal fracture component
  - Fracture through pterygoid plates
  - Level(s) of injury

TREATMENT
- Treatment for isolated maxillary fractures is directed at **restoring normal premorbid occlusion.**
- Patients with dentoalveolar fractures require stabilization of the dentoalveolar segment with an arch bar for 4-6 weeks.
- During the ensuing weeks, referral to a dentist is appropriate for endodontic evaluation of avulsed teeth in the segment.
- Patients with Le Fort–type fractures require open reduction and rigid fixation.
- Closed reduction and maxillomandibular fixation (MMF) are **not** appropriate because they lead to facial lengthening by downward forces transmitted by the mandible.
- Arch bars should be applied to both dental arches and the fractures exposed using a maxillary circumvestibular incision from first molar to first molar.
- The maxillary segment is mobilized with Rowe disimpaction forceps or similar instruments.
- Once adequate mobility is present to allow passive reduction of the fracture, the segment is manually reduced and the jaws are placed into MMF.

TIP: Placing the jaws into MMF without providing passive reduction of the maxillary segment causes unseating of the mandibular condyles from their fossa and results in malocclusion when MMF is released and the condyles return to their natural position.

- Occasionally there is a nonreducible maxillary fracture (i.e., unable to obtain premorbid occlusion).
  - This may require performing a Le Fort I level osteotomy to correct the deformity at the time of fracture repair.
  - Fixation of fractures is provided by 1.5-2.0 mm miniplates on stable bone, usually at the region of the piriform (nasomaxillary buttress) or ZM buttress.

PEDIATRIC CONSIDERATIONS
- Treatment considerations are the same as for adults but may be technically more difficult.
  - Arch bars are difficult to place in the pediatric patient because of mixed dentition, missing teeth, and unfavorable dental anatomy of the primary teeth.
  - Difficulty in placing fixation systems is encountered secondary to developing tooth buds.
- Panoramic radiographs should be obtained to locate developing permanent dentition.

PANFACIAL FRACTURES

Panfacial fractures are fractures of the upper and midfacial skeleton associated with fractures of the mandible (see Chapter 30).
This represents a particularly difficult clinical situation because there is no stable reference from which to begin reduction of fractures.

> TIP: In general, treatment should proceed top to bottom, bottom to top, and back to front.

- Anatomic reconstruction of the mandible should be performed initially to provide a stable base from which to reconstruct the midface.
  - If bilateral condyle fractures are present, at least one intact condyle should be reconstructed to provide appropriate vertical height relationships for the midface.
- Anteroposterior reconstruction of the zygomas should be reestablished to provide accurate facial projection.
- Reconstruction then proceeds inferiorly from the stable frontal process to the level of the maxilla.
- Fixation across the Le Fort I level is the last area to be stabilized.
- Because of the severity of these injuries, some degree of malreduction inevitably will occur.
- By reestablishing the major determinants of facial form early (mandibular base, vertical height, antero-posterior projection) any subtle malreductions may be tolerated at the Le Fort I level *above* the dentition.

ASSOCIATED CONDITIONS

TEMPORAL BONE TRAUMA
- **Signs**
  - Otorrhea
  - Facial palsy
  - Hemotympanum
  - **Battle's sign:** Bruising over mastoid process that appears 24-48 hours after injury
- **Fracture patterns**
  - **Longitudinal**
    - ▶ Accounts for 80%-90% of temporal bone fractures
    - ▶ Bilateral in 8%-29% of patients
    - ▶ Facial nerve injury in 20% of patients
    - ▶ Hearing loss in 67% of patients
  - **Transverse**
    - ▶ Facial nerve injury in 40% of patients
    - ▶ Hearing loss in 100% of patients
- **Complications**
  - **Facial nerve paresis**
    - ▶ Paresis occurs in 10%-50% of temporal bone fractures, most commonly with transverse type.
    - ▶ **Management**
      - ✦ Surgery is not indicated for incomplete palsy.
      - ✦ Immediate paresis does not usually resolve and is an indication for exploration.
      - ✦ Delayed paresis generally has a good prognosis, and exploration is indicated when electrical evidence indicates nerve degeneration.

- **Hearing loss**
  - Tos[15] studied 248 temporal bone fractures.
    - 26 (10%) were transverse with 100% having total hearing loss.
    - 222 (90%) were longitudinal with 67% having hearing loss.
    - Patients with sensorineural hearing loss did not improve.
    - Patients with conductive hearing loss (CHL) eventually improved, except when ossicular chain disruption was present.
  - **CHL present for longer than 2 months suggests ossicular chain disruption and need for exploration.**
- **Vestibular dysfunction**
  - Nystagmus suggests vestibular injury.
  - Peripheral vestibular nystagmus occurs with vertigo.
  - Spontaneous nystagmus in head-neutral position is pathologic.
  - **Fast component beats away from injured ear.**
  - Finding horizontal nystagmus that is greater with eyes closed suggests peripheral injury.
  - Management is supportive; prognosis is generally good, with most recovering in 6 months.
- **CSF leak**
  - CSF otorrhea occurs in 25% of temporal bone fractures.
  - Onset generally occurs within 24 hours.
  - Most close spontaneously in 24 hours.

OPHTHALMIC CONSEQUENCES

- Ocular injuries reported as high as **30%** following orbital trauma.
- **Only two ocular emergencies require treatment within minutes.**
  1. Chemical burns
  2. Central retinal artery occlusion
- **Anterior segment trauma**
  - **Corneal abrasion**
    - Cornea reepithelializes in 1 day under a patch.
    - Use of steroids or topical anaesthetic is contraindicated.
  - **Iridodialysis:** Avulsion from the iris root
  - **Traumatic mydriasis**
    - Pupillary sphincter rupture produces a widely, permanently dilated pupil.
    - The pupil does not react to direct or consensual stimuli.
  - **Hyphema**
    - Blood in the anterior chamber is most readily visible with a hand-held light.
    - Document visual acuity and height of the hyphema.
    - 3%-30% of patients will rebleed in 3-5 days.
    - Prognosis is worse with a rebleed.
    - Complications include corneal pigment staining, anterior synechia, and glaucoma.
    - Management focuses on preventing rebleed: Elevate head of bed, encourage bed rest, and give atropine drops to decrease iris movement.
- **Posterior segment trauma**
  - **Vitreous hemorrhage:** Vision returns with resolution
  - **Scleral rupture**
    - 18% associated with orbital fracture
    - Repair indicated to prevent hypotonia or fibrous ingrowth

- ▶ Retinal detachment
- ▶ Optic nerve avulsion
- **Sympathetic ophthalmia**
  - Bilateral granulomatous inflammation of uvea that usually occurs as complication of penetrating trauma or intraocular surgery
  - Pathogenesis unknown but thought that privileged intraocular antigens, exposed to regional lymph nodes following injury, stimulate cell-mediated response against eye
  - Exact incidence unknown, but estimated at 0.19% with trauma
  - Nontraumatized eye inflamed within 1 year of injury: 65% within 2 months; 80% within 3 months
  - Prevention: Enucleation of severely traumatized, sightless eye within 2 weeks of injury
  - Treatment difficult: If inflammation in sympathizing eye, outcome generally not improved by enucleation of traumatized eye
- **Traumatic optic neuropathy (TON)**
  TON is a traumatic loss of vision without external or initial ophthalmoscopic evidence of injury to the eye or its nerve.
  - **Etiologic factors**
    - ▶ Direct injury to globe
    - ▶ Retinal vascular occlusion
    - ▶ Orbital compartment syndrome
    - ▶ Injury to proximal neural structures
  - TON may occur without any fracture because of deceleration forces acting within the fixed intracanalicular portion of optic nerve.
  - **The only objective finding is the presence of a relative afferent pupillary defect.**
  - Optic atrophy will appear weeks later.
  - Improvement in visual acuity may occur in 30%-50% of patients.
  - **Treatment includes:**
    - ▶ Observation
    - ▶ High-dose steroids
      - ◆ Use of steroids has been extrapolated from the Second National Acute Spinal Cord Injury Study,[19] in which patients with spinal injury treated early with high-dose steroids demonstrated increased neurologic function at 6 weeks.
    - ▶ Surgical decompression
      - ◆ There is presently no data, similar to that for steroids, to support use of decompression in traumatic optic neuropathy.
    - ▶ *Two different studies have investigated treatment of TON.*
      - ◆ *In 1996, a meta-analysis demonstrated that steroids, extracranial decompression, or both are no better than no treatment.[20]*
      - ◆ *In 1999, the International Optic Nerve Trauma Study[21] found no clear benefit for either corticosteroid therapy or optic canal decompression. "These results and the existing literature provide sufficient evidence to conclude that neither corticosteroids nor optic canal decompression should be considered the standard of care for traumatic optic neuropathy."*
- **Superior orbital fissure syndrome (SOFS)**
  - Incidence is about 1 out of 130 patients with Le Fort II, III, or zygomatic-orbital fractures.
  - Diagnosis is by **clinical presentation.**
  - **Components**
    - ▶ Oculomotor nerve
      - ◆ Trochlear nerve
      - ◆ Abducens nerve

- Trigeminal nerve (lacrimal, frontal, nasociliary branches)
- Ophthalmic vein
▸ **Signs**
  - Ipsilateral ptosis of upper lid
  - Proptosis
  - Ophthalmoplegia
  - Anaesthesia in distribution of V_1
  - Dilation and fixation of ipsilateral pupil
▸ **Treatment**
  - Operative reduction of fractures results in improvement or resolution.
  - Recovery time is reported as 4.8-23 weeks.
  - Role of steroids is unclear.
- **Orbital apex syndrome**
  - Syndrome presents **similarly to SOFS,** but the patient also presents with **loss of vision** because of optic nerve involvement at the orbital apex.
- **Traumatic carotid-cavernous sinus fistula**
  - Fracture results in laceration or tear in arterial wall, allowing blood to shunt from the internal carotid artery to the cavernous sinus. Signs and symptoms may develop several days after the initial injury.
  - **Signs**
    ▸ Proptosis
    ▸ Ocular bruit
    ▸ Marked injection and chemosis of affected eye
    ▸ Ophthalmoplegia of CNs III, IV, or VI
    ▸ Dilated ophthalmic vein on CT of orbit
  - **Diagnosis is provided by angiography.**
  - **Prognosis is generally good** and not life threatening.
    ▸ Fistula may close spontaneously, commonly after angiography.
    ▸ Ischemic events may occur secondary to steal phenomena or embolism.
  - Treatment includes **surgical ligation of carotid artery** or **interventional placement of coils** to obliterate the fistula.

KEY POINTS

✔ Many patients presenting to the ER have been there before; remember to identify preexisting conditions.

✔ Before examination, patients should be cleaned of all dried blood and dirt that may obscure underlying injuries.

✔ Reconstructed coronal imaging should be accepted only when formal coronal CT scans are precluded by cerebrospinal injury.

REFERENCES

1. Girotto JA, MacKenzie E, Fowler C, et al. Long-term physical impairment and functional outcomes after complex facial fractures. Plast Reconstr Surg 108:312-327, 2001.
2. Hackl W, Fink C, Hausberger K, et al. The incidence of combined facial and cervical spine injuries. Trauma 50:41-45, 2001.
3. Marik PE, Varon J, Trask T. Management of head trauma. Chest 122:1-21, 2002.
4. Plaisier BR, Punjabi AP, Super DM, et al. The relationship between facial fractures and death from neurologic injury. J Oral Maxillofac Surg 58:708-712, 2000.
5. Cheung DS, Kharasch M. Evaluation of the patient with closed head trauma: An evidence based approach. Emerg Med Clin North Am 17:9-23, 1999.
6. Haug RH, Savage JD Likavek MJ, et al. A review of 100 closed head injuries associated with facial fractures. J Oral Maxillofac Surg 50:218-222, 1992.
7. Giannoudis PV, Veysi VT, Pape HC, et al. When should we operate on major fractures in patients with severe head injuries? Am J Surg 183:261-267, 2002.
8. Nahum AM. The biomechanics of maxillofacial trauma. Clin Plast Surg 2:59-64, 1975.
9. Stanley RB, Becker TS. Injuries of the nasofrontal orifices in frontal sinus fractures. Laryngoscope 97:728-731, 1987.
10. Rohrich RJ, Hollier LH. Management of frontal sinus fractures: Changing concepts. Clin Plast Surg 19:219-232, 1992.
11. Markowitz BL, Manson PN, Sargent L, et al. Management of the medial canthal tendon in nasoethmoid orbital fractures: The importance of the central fragment in classification and treatment. Plast Reconstr Surg 87:843-853, 1991
12. Ellis E III. Sequencing treatment for naso-orbito-ethmoid fractures. J Oral Maxillofac Surg 51:543-558, 1993.
13. Rohrich RJ, Adams WP. Nasal fracture management: Minimizing secondary nasal deformities. Plast Reconstr Surg 106:266-273, 2000.
14. Waterhouse N, Lyne J, Urdang M, et al. An investigation into the mechanism of orbital blowout fractures. Br J Plast Surg 52:607-612, 1999.
15. Tos M. Course of and sequelae to 248 petrosal fractures. Acta Otolaryngol 75:353-354, 1973.
16. Potter JK, Ellis E III. Biomaterials for reconstruction of the internal orbit. J Oral Maxillofac Surg 62:1280-1297, 2004.
17. Ellis E III, Reddy L. Status of internal orbit after reduction of zygomaticomaxillary fractures. J Oral Maxillofac Surg 62:275-283, 2004.
18. Ellis E III, Kittidumkerng W. Analysis of treatment for isolated zygomaticomaxillary complex fractures. J Oral Maxillofac Surg 54:386-400, 1996.
19. Bracken MB, Shepard MJ, Collins WF, et al. A randomized, controlled trial of methylprednisolone or naloxone in the treatment of acute spinal-cord injury: Results of the Second National Acute Spinal Cord Injury Study. N Engl J Med 322:1405-1411, 1990.
20. Cook MW, Levin LA, Joseph MP, et al. Traumatic optic neuropathy: A meta-analysis. Arch Otolaryngol Head Neck Surg 122:389-392, 1996.
21. Levin LA, Beck RW, Joseph MP, et al. The treatment of traumatic optic neuropathy. The International Optic Nerve Trauma Study. Ophthalmology 106:1268-1277, 1999.

25. Facial Soft Tissue Trauma

Jason K. Potter

GENERAL[1]

- Injuries range from superficial abrasions to lacerations of skin and nearby specialized structures.
- Thorough assessment is essential to fully diagnose the extent of injury and provide appropriate treatment.
- Particular attention should be given to the **mechanism of injury** and **quality of the wound.**
  - Crush injuries result in significantly greater tissue injury than injuries from sharp lacerations.
  - Wounds with gross contamination and foreign bodies must be debrided and receive appropriate prophylaxis.

EXAMINATION

- Examination follows the principles given in Chapter 24.
- Special attention is given to specialized structures near the soft tissue injury.
  - Lacrimal apparatus
  - External auditory meatus
  - Facial nerve
  - Parotid duct
- Wounds should be examined during the initial assessment and, following administration of local anaesthesia, should be reexamined to determine the depth and extent of the wound.

GENERAL CONSIDERATIONS FOR ALL WOUNDS

TIMING OF REPAIR
- Management of soft tissue injuries may be delayed until the patient is stabilized.
- The rich vascularity of the head and neck helps provide resistance to infection in the open wound.
- **Wounds should be kept moist** with saline-soaked gauze until closure is completed.

BLEEDING
- The vascularity of the region can lead to **significant blood loss** from laceration.
- Control of hemorrhage is usually amenable to local measures.
- Suction, packing, and irrigation should be used to identify the source.

CAUTION: Avoid blind clamping to prevent iatrogenic injury to specialized structures.

- Local anaesthetic with epinephrine may be used to provide vasoconstriction in the region.

TIP: Identify potential injury to the facial nerve before administration of local anaesthesia.

■ Although hemorrhage from facial injury may lead to hypovolemic shock, it is uncommon and usually represents significant delay in presentation, severe injuries, or hemorrhage from another associated injury. **It is imperative to thoroughly evaluate these patients to avoid missing critical injuries.**

DEBRIDEMENT

■ Debridement and irrigation of wounds is **mandatory** before closure to reduce the risk of infection.
■ Risk for infection increases the longer the wound remains open.
■ Debridement should remove all foreign bodies, dirt, and devitalized tissue.
■ Devitalized tissue is removed with sharp dissection.
  • Conservation of tissue is the goal.
  • This is especially important in areas of specialized tissue (e.g., nose, periorbital region, lips, ears, and hair-bearing skin).

TIP: The vascularity of the face allows surprisingly small portions of tissue to survive.

■ Wounds are irrigated with sterile saline solution until clear of debris.
  • Pulsed jet-irrigation devices are usually unnecessary.
■ Road rash must be thoroughly scrubbed to remove all imbedded debris. Any remaining debris creates unsightly tattooing.
■ **All patients should have their tetanus status updated.**

TIP: Drains may be fashioned from 21-gauge butterfly catheters and red-top tubes. Small perforations are made in the distal end of the tubing (<50% of the diameter of the tube to prevent the catheter breaking in vivo). The needle is inserted into the red-top tube using its negative pressure for suction. Tubes are changed every 2-3 hours or when half full.

MANAGEMENT

REPAIR
■ Tissues should be reapproximated anatomically.
■ Layered closure is ideal.
■ Local flaps should be avoided in the acute setting, especially in wounds with crush components, until the extent of devitalized tissue has declared itself.

TIP: It is always best to correct an unsightly scar caused by an injury than to correct an unsightly deformity caused by overly aggressive debridement and poor planning.

■ Large wounds may require small drains to evacuate dead space.

ABRASIONS
■ **The most important consideration for treating abrasions is complete removal of debris.**
  • Any residual debris within the dermis creates permanent tattooing.

- After adequate debridement, local wound care is instituted.
  - The wound should be kept moist.
  - Antibiotic ointment or Aquaphor® allows rapid reepithelialization.
- **Sun avoidance** is necessary for 6 months to 1 year because these wounds are susceptible to permanent hyperpigmentation from UV injury.

LACERATIONS
- Tissues should be handled gently.
- Hemostasis is mandatory, and dead space should be obliterated.
- Layered closure provides a tension free epidermal closure and reapproximates deeper tissues (muscle) to prevent contour deformity.
  - Deeper tissues should be approximated with 3-0 or 4-0 resorbable undyed suture.
  - Epidermal edges are reapproximated with interrupted or running 5-0 or 6-0 monofilament suture, ensuring wound eversion.
- Skin incisions, when necessary, should be planned within the relaxed skin tension lines.
- Sutures should be placed carefully in stellate lacerations to prevent strangling the blood supply to the tip of the flaps.

AVULSIVE WOUNDS
- Avulsive wounds should be repaired by local undermining, local flaps, or skin grafting.
- Delayed primary closure is effective when extensive soft tissue trauma is present to allow the wound to demarcate before definitive closure.

BITE WOUNDS
- **The face is the only region where consideration is given to primary closure of bite wounds.**
- These wounds *must* be aggressively irrigated.
- In addition to standard debridement, special attention is directed at antibiotic prophylaxis.
  - Antibiotic prophylaxis is best provided by amoxicillin/clavulanic acid (Augmentin®) or equivalent antibiotic.
- Infections secondary to bite wounds are usually polymicrobial, but certain species are characteristic of specific bite types.
  - *Eikenella* is a common pathogen from human bites.
  - *Pasteurella* and *Staphylococcus* are frequently acquired from **canine** and **feline bites.**
- **All animals must be investigated for current rabies vaccination.**

SPECIAL CONSIDERATIONS

TIP: In general it is not advisable to let facial wounds heal by secondary intention for aesthetic reasons.

SCALP
- Scalp wounds frequently present with profuse bleeding.
  - The use of local measures is effective.
    - ▸ Pressure
    - ▸ Injection of epinephrine containing local anaesthetics

- Larger vessels may be controlled with suture ligature.
- Cautery should be used cautiously to prevent alopecia.
■ The scalp is closed in layers.
- Galea is reapproximated with interrupted suture.
- The epidermal layer is reapproximated with either surgical staples or monofilament sutures.

EYEBROW

■ The eyebrow is one of the unique and irreplaceable structures of the face.
■ Only obviously necrotic tissue should be debrided to conserve the hair-bearing tissue.
■ After deep closure, hairlines are first approximated to prevent step-offs.

EYELID

■ Lacerations of the eyelid must be evaluated for injury to the septum and levator, because levator disruption may result in ptosis if not repaired.
■ Lacerations through the lid margin are closed in layers.
- Nonresorbable suture is placed in the tarsus to reconstruct continuity.
- Interrupted 6-0 silk sutures are then placed beginning at the gray line.
- **Eversion is necessary to prevent notching.**
- Sutures should be placed to prevent contact with the cornea.

LACRIMAL APPARATUS

■ Lacerations in the medial aspect of the lid must be assessed for injury to the lacrimal apparatus.
- This is facilitated by cannulation of the puncta with lacrimal probes.
- Laceration is identified by viewing the probe in the wound.
■ When lacrimal injury is present, the puncta are cannulated with Crawford tubes that are passed into the nose and maintained up to 4 weeks.
■ If cannulation of the lacrimal system is not possible, the lacerations are repaired, and the patient may be managed with dacryocystorhinostomy if epiphora is problematic.

EAR

■ Conservative debridement is important to maintain the size of the ear.
■ Soft tissue trauma to the ear frequently results in exposed cartilage.
- Cartilage that has been stripped of perichondrium should be debrided.
- Exposed cartilage that maintains viable perichondrium may be retained.
■ When portions of the ear are pedicled on narrow stalks, the ear should be repaired and leech therapy initiated for 3-5 days until venous connections begin to develop.
■ Circumferential lacerations of the external auditory meatus may heal with stenosis.
- Stenting of the canal should be performed with Merocel® wicks (Medtronic Ophthalmics, Jacksonville, FL) and mupirocin calcium (Bactroban®) ointment.
■ Hematomas **must** be evacuated and bolster dressing used when skin flaps are present.

CAUTION: Allowing hematomas to organize and fibrose causes a thickened ear.

NOSE

■ Small losses of nasal soft tissue can result in significant distortion of the nasal shape, and therefore conservative debridement is the rule.

- The nose consists of **three lamellae.**
  1. Skin and soft tissue
  2. Cartilaginous framework
  3. Mucosa (lining)
- **Lacerations of the nose require assessment of injury and repair to each lamella.**
- Full-thickness lacerations are best repaired from inside out.
  - The nasal mucosa is repaired with 4-0 chromic suture.
  - Transected cartilages should be reconstructed with 5-0 monofilament suture.
  - The skin is repaired with 6-0 vertical mattress sutures.
- Avulsive wounds must be repaired following the principles of nasal reconstruction (see Chapter 31).
- Avulsive wounds may be temporized with skin grafts or local wound care until definitive reconstruction is possible.

LIP

- Lip lacerations require careful reapproximation of the vermilion border and orbicularis oris muscle.
- The vermilion should be marked with methylene blue before infiltration of anaesthesia to prevent distortion of landmarks.
- Repairing the orbicularis oris is important to prevent retraction of the lacerated muscle, which creates unsightly depression and associated lateral bulging.
- Once the deep layers are closed the vermilion is approximated.
- Closure of the remaining epidermis and mucosa is then completed.
- For avulsive defects, lip repair follows the principles of lip reconstruction (see Chapter 34).

TONGUE

- Lacerations of the tongue notoriously break down because of the strength of the tongue musculature.
- Long-lasting resorbable suture is used to reapproximate the deep layer.
- 3-0 chromic suture is placed with knots buried to close the mucosal layer.

SALIVARY DUCTS

- Failure to identify lacerations of the salivary ducts results in sialocele or cutaneous fistula.
- Evaluation of parotid duct injury is as follows:
  - Cannulate Stenson's duct intraorally with a 24-gauge angiocatheter (at the level of the maxillary second molar).
  - Flush duct gently with saline and examine wound for extravasation of fluid.
  - Extravasation indicates duct injury that must be repaired.
- Parotid duct lacerations are best repaired with microsurgical techniques.
- Placement of Silastic® stents (Dow Corning, Midland, MI) is helpful, but they rarely maintain their positions long enough to provide benefit.
- Lacerations of the submandibular ducts may be marsupialized onto the floor of the mouth.

FACIAL NERVE

- Lacerations over the distribution of the facial nerve must be assessed for injury to the facial nerve.
  - **It is imperative to assess nerve function before administration of local anaesthesia.**
- Facial nerve lacerations medial to a line dropped from the lateral canthus to the corner of the mouth are too small to repair and may spontaneously recover.

- Lacerations lateral to this region should be repaired with microsurgical techniques.
  - Nerve injury is best repaired **within 72 hours,** because this allows using intraoperative nerve stimulation to identify the distal nerve end.
  - After 72 hours neurotransmitters are depleted in the distal nerve and stimulation is not possible.

KEY POINTS

- ✔ Watch for significant blood loss because of the vascularity of the face.
- ✔ Avoid blind clamping.
- ✔ Remove all embedded debris to avoid tattooing.
- ✔ Patient should avoid direct sunlight and use sunblock liberally to minimize scarring.
- ✔ It *may* be possible to primarily close bite wounds to the face after aggressive irrigation and debridement.
- ✔ *Meticulously* reapproximate vermilion border; use layers.
- ✔ *Always* evaluate ear hematomas.
- ✔ Close nasal lacerations in layers.
- ✔ It is important to identify lacerations of the parotid duct in susceptible wounds.
- ✔ Facial nerve injuries are best repaired within 72 hours of the transection.

REFERENCE

1. Fonseca RJ, Walker RV, Betts NJ, et al, eds. Oral and Maxillofacial Trauma, 2nd ed. Philadelphia: WB Saunders, 1997.

26. Mandibular Fractures

Jason K. Potter

EPIDEMIOLOGY

Two Most Common Causes
- Assault
- Motor vehicle collisions (MVCs)

Other Causes
- Gunshot wounds
- Falls
- Sports injuries

LOCATION OF FRACTURE

Fractures of the mandible usually are described by **location**, which affects the appropriate treatment.
- **Condyle:** Any fracture affecting condylar process of mandible; further classified as intracapsular, extracapsular, or neck
- **Coronoid:** Any fracture affecting coronoid process
- **Ramus:** Region superior to gonial angle up to sigmoid notch
- **Angle:** Including region of gonial angle to region of third molar
- **Body:** Including region anterior to third molar to approximately first premolar
- **Symphysis:** Region between mandibular canine teeth

INCIDENCE BY LOCATION (Fig. 26-1)

- **Ranking:** Angle > symphysis > body > condyle > coronoid > ramus
- **Assault** most commonly results in **angle** fractures.
- **MVCs** most commonly result in **body** fractures.

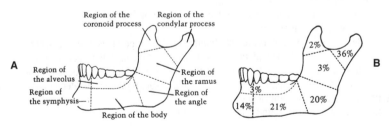

Fig. 26-1   A, Anatomic regions of the mandible. **B,** Frequency of fractures in those regions. (From Aston SJ, Beasley RW, Thorne CH, eds. Grabb and Smith's Plastic Surgery, 5th ed. Philadelphia: Lippincott, 1997.)

PATIENT EVALUATION

Any patient presenting with facial trauma requires a *complete* head and neck trauma exam (see Chapter 24).

PHYSICAL EXAMINATION
- Inspect occlusion.
  - Evaluate for presence of anterior or posterior open bite in centric occlusion
  - Evaluate for deviation of mandible during opening.
- Perform bimanual examination of the mandible to assess for mobility and tenderness.
- Palpate condyles, both preauricularly and with finger in external auditory canal, during excursion to elicit tenderness and assess translation.

TIP: Tongue blades should be used to retract the tongue and cheeks to allow for complete inspection.

- Evaluate the lingual and buccal aspects for evidence of trauma.
- All teeth should be accounted for and assessed for mobility.
- Document the presence of mental nerve paresthesias.

TIP: Ecchymosis in the floor of the mouth is pathognomonic for mandibular fractures.

Deviation of the chin may suggest condyle fracture.

Mental nerve paresthesia suggests fracture along the interosseous segment of infraalveolar nerve.

RADIOGRAPHIC EVALUATION
- Obtain two views of each region of the mandible.
- Inspect radiographs for the following:
  - Evidence of fractured mandible
  - Fractured teeth
  - Presence of teeth in the line of fracture
  - Degree of displacement
  - Direction of fracture (linear versus oblique)
  - Distance of alveolar nerve from teeth and inferior border of mandible
- Panoramic radiograph (Panorex):
  - Invaluable for assessment of mandibular trauma, because it provides views of all areas of mandibular corpus, teeth, and inferior alveolar nerve relationships in a single film.
  - It is the best single radiograph for screening the mandible, but it is not adequate alone.
- Mandible series includes posterior-anterior skull, lateral skull, right and left lateral oblique, Towne projection, and submental vertex images.
- CT images are not necessary with adequate quality radiographs.

TIP: Occasionally, because of the presence of cervical collars, adequate plain films are not possible and CT images are necessary.

GENERAL MANAGEMENT

ABCs

- Initial management always begins with Advance Training Life Support (ATLS) protocols.[1]
- Treatment of fractures of the mandible may be delayed up to 2 weeks, with appropriate oral and systemic antibiotic prophylaxis for critically injured patients.

ANTIBIOTICS

- All patients with mandible fractures should receive penicillin-based antibiotics (clindamycin [Cleocin®], if allergic to penicillin) prophylactically, beginning at presentation until reduction of fractures is performed.
  - This practice has been shown to reduce the incidence of postoperative infection to **6%**, compared with 50% in patients not receiving prophylactic antibiotics.[2]
- Use of postoperative antibiotics has not been shown to affect the incidence of postoperative infection.[3,4]

TIP: Oral chlorhexidine is useful for reducing bacterial counts in the oral cavity in the presence of open fractures.

TEETH IN THE LINE OF FRACTURE

- Fractures that contain teeth within the line of fracture are considered open fractures because of the communication of the fracture with the gingival sulcus and periodontal attachment.[5,6]
- Routine use of antibiotics and internal fixation allows preservation of most teeth within the line of fracture.
- **Six indications for teeth removal**
  1. Grossly mobile
  2. Periodontally compromised
  3. Nonrestorable
  4. Demonstrate periapical radiolucency
  5. Root fracture
  6. Exposed apices
- Nonrestorable teeth may be retained if removal would compromise accurate reduction of the fracture.
- Complete bony impactions typically require removal of large bony surfaces that otherwise would assist in reduction. These should be removed only when necessary.[5,6]

METHODS OF FIXATION

The mandible and muscles of mastication represent a complex biomechanical system that is beyond the scope of this text. Simply, two main trajectories of stress are present within the mandible: **Tensile and compression.** Neutralization of these stresses is necessary to achieve stability. Two fundamentally different systems have been advanced for the treatment of mandible fractures.

- **AO/Association for the Study of Internal Fixation (AO/ASIF)**
  - This system typically requires the use of large bulky plates.

■ **Champy system**
- Smaller, nonrigid plating system is used to neutralize unfavorable tensile forces, but it still allows transmission of more favorable compression forces.

AO/ASIF

■ The AO/ASIF was established in 1958 to define conditions for the highest quality bone surgery. It put forth **four conditions** that must be met to accomplish this goal.
1. Anatomic reduction of fragments
2. Functionally stable fixation of the fragments
3. Atraumatic operating technique
4. Early, active, pain-free mobility
■ **Methods of fixation**
- **Tension band and stabilization plate:** A small plate is placed at the alveolar border to neutralize tensile forces; a larger plate is placed at the inferior border to neutralize compression and torsion.
- **Reconstruction plate:** A large plate is placed at the inferior border when segmental loss or comminution preclude placement of tension band; a single plate neutralizes tensile, compression, and torsional stresses.

CHAMPY SYSTEM

This system advocates the use of monocortical miniplates. It originally was introduced by Michelet in 1967 and was later validated by Champy.[7]
■ The system is based on the concept that *only tensile stresses are harmful to fracture healing.*
■ In biomechanical studies to identify transmission of strains to the mandible, Champy defined the lines of ideal osteosynthesis.
- Proximal to the first premolar, a single plate is effective when placed in the midbody position.
- Anterior to the first premolar, 2 plates, 4-5 mm apart, are used.

TIP: This system requires bone to bone abutment of fracture segments and is not applicable to comminuted fractures or situations of segmental bone loss.

DEFINITIONS OF STABILITY

■ **Rigid (absolute) stability**
- No movement occurs across the fracture gap.
- Rigid stability is an ideal therapeutic principle, but no fixation provides absolute stability in all dimensions of a system as dynamic as the mandible.
■ **Functional stability**
- Movement is possible across the fracture gap but is balanced by external forces and remains within limits that allow the fracture to progress to union.
■ **Load-sharing stability**
- Functional stability is achieved by the fixation system in conjunction with stabilizing forces provided by anatomic abutment of noncomminuted fracture segments.
■ **Load-bearing stability**
- Functional stability, provided solely by the fixation system, is accomplished only by reconstruction plates.

IMPORTANCE OF STABILITY

- Primary bone healing is possible only in a stable system.
- Mobility leads to bone resorption and fibrous tissue ingrowth.
- When mobility is present, any internal device promotes resorption and infection.

MANAGEMENT OF SPECIFIC FRACTURE PATTERNS

- Operative treatment begins with extraction of indicated teeth followed by placement of arch bars (see Chapter 27).
- All fractures are exposed and reduced before placing maxillomandibular fixation (MMF).
- Once reduction is confirmed, MMF is placed, and fixation of fractures proceeds.

CONDYLE FRACTURES

Fractures of the mandibular condyle require early, active range-of-motion to rehabilitate the temporo-mandibular articulation.[8]

TIP: Regardless of whether closed or open techniques are used, beginning rehabilitation in the immediate postinjury period is probably the single most effective therapy.

- **Frequently treated by closed reduction techniques**
  - Difficulty with surgical access, risk to the facial nerve, and small fracture segments prevent widespread use of open reduction with internal fixation (ORIF) techniques.
- **Condyle fracture without malocclusion**
  - This fracture may be treated by soft diet and close observation.
  - If malocclusion develops (usually a deviation to the affected side with ipsilateral posterior open bite), arch bars should be placed, and occlusion should be controlled with elastics.
- **Condyle fracture with malocclusion**
  - **Closed reduction**
    - ▶ Arch bars are placed, and occlusion is controlled with elastics.
      - ✦ This is usually possible with a single class II elastic on the affected side.

TIP: Placement of MMF is *not* routinely necessary; it leads to stiffness and fibrosis within the masticatory apparatus, which inhibits rehabilitation.

  - **ORIF**
    - ▶ ORIF is necessary when:
      - ✦ Condylar segment is displaced and interferes with translation
      - ✦ Condyle is displaced into the middle cranial fossa
      - ✦ Combination of bilateral mandibular condyle fractures and midface fractures exist (must reestablish posterior vertical height)

ANGLE FRACTURES

Fractures of the mandibular angle are notorious for being associated with the highest complication rate of any single region of the mandible.

- ORIF techniques have complication rates equal to those of nonrigid techniques (requiring MMF).[8]

> TIP: Surgical access is provided through intraoral approaches, with the assistance of transfacial trocar when necessary.

BODY FRACTURES

Fractures of the mandibular body may be treated with either miniplate techniques or reconstruction plates.

- Miniplates are easier to adapt and place but are useful only in noncomminuted fractures, when accurate abutting of fracture segments provides *load-sharing.*
- Reconstruction plates are more difficult to adapt and place but may be used with comminuted fracture and when *load-bearing* fixation is necessary.

> TIP: Always give attention to the location of root apices and the inferior alveolar nerve in this region of the mandible. Use intraoral access.

SYMPHYSIS FRACTURES

Fractures of the symphysis may be treated with miniplates or reconstruction plates; these fractures frequently lend themselves to lag screws.

- Because of torsional forces generated at the symphysis, placement of two points of fixation are required, except when using reconstruction plates.
- Intraoral access is used.

SPECIAL CONSIDERATIONS

MULTIPLE FRACTURES

- With multiple fractures, the mandible has a tendency to splay, which, if not corrected and firmly stabilized, results in facial widening and significant deformity.[9]
- More rigid fixation systems should be used to prevent widening.

EDENTULOUS FRACTURES

Lack of dentition, small bone stock, and poor quality bone compromise the accuracy of reduction and the healing capacity.

- The Chalmers J Lyons Academy study of edentulous mandible fractures demonstrated the effectiveness of transfacial approaches to improve reduction and use of reconstruction plates to aid bony union in these situations.[10]
- Use of miniplates or closed reductions using patient's dentures are not recommended.
- In severely atrophic mandibles, bone grafting at the fracture may be necessary in the acute setting.

PEDIATRIC PATIENTS

- Stability of arch bars is compromised by unfavorable height of primary teeth contours or missing teeth (mixed dentition stage).
  - This can impact the quality of immobilization provided by MMF.

- The presence of developing tooth buds requires selective use of internal fixation to prevent injury.
  - Monocortical screw placement and miniplates can be used cautiously.
- Condyle fractures in the pediatric population must be followed very closely, because these fractures can lead to ankylosis and growth disturbances.
  - Start rehabilitation as early as possible.
- The favorable healing potential of children usually allows removal of MMF after 3-4 weeks, compared with 4-6 weeks in adults.
  - Prolonged MMF can significantly compromise rehabilitation.

KEY POINTS

✔ At least two radiographic views of each region of the mandible are required to evaluate injury effectively (mandible series or panoramic radiograph plus selected views).

✔ The proper treatment sequence is (1) exposure of all fractures, (2) reduction of all fractures, (3) placement of maxillomandibular fixation, and (4) fixation of fractures.

✔ Maxillomandibular fixation must be removed and occlusion reassessed after application of hardware. If the patient is to remain in MMF, it may be reapplied after confirming proper reduction.

✔ Restoration of premorbid occlusion must be precise in patients treated with internal fixation. Occlusal discrepancies that are present intraoperatively cannot be expected to resolve in the postoperative period.

✔ Most patients, especially those with fractures of the condylar process, require closely monitored physical therapy to rehabilitate the masticatory apparatus.

REFERENCES

1. American College of Surgeons. PHTLS: Basic and Advanced Prehospital Trauma Life Support, 5th ed. St Louis: Mosby, 2003.
2. Zallen RD, Curry JT. A study of antibiotic usage in compound mandibular fractures. J Oral Surg 33:431-434, 1975.
3. Miles BA, Potter JK, Ellis E III. The efficacy of postoperative antibiotic regimens in the open treatment of mandibular fractures: A prospective randomized trial. J Oral Maxillofac Surg 64:576-582, 2006.
4. Abubaker AO, Rollert MK. Postoperative antibiotic prophylaxis in mandibular fractures: A preliminary randomized, double-blind, and placebo-controlled clinical study. J Oral Maxillofac Surg 59:1415-1419, 2001.
5. Schnieder SS, Stern M. Teeth in the line of mandibular fractures. J Oral Maxillofac Surg 29:107-109, 1971.
6. Shetty V, Freymiller E. Teeth in the line of fracture: A review. J Oral Maxillofac Surg 47:1303-1306, 1989.
7. Throckmorton GS, Ellis E III. Recovery of mandibular motion after closed and open treatment of unilateral mandibular condylar process fractures. J Oral Maxillofac Surg 29:421-427, 2000.
8. Ellis E III. Treatment methods for fractures of the mandibular angle. J Craniomaxillofac Trauma 2:28-36, 1996.
9. Ellis E, Tharanon W. Facial width problems associated with rigid fixation of mandibular fractures. J Oral Maxillofac Surg 50:87-94, 1992.
10. Bruce RA, Ellis E III. The second Chalmers J Lyons Academy study of fractures of the edentulous mandible. J Oral Maxillofac Surg 51:904-911, 1993.

27. Basic Oral Surgery

Jason K. Potter

ANATOMY

DIVISIONS OF THE HEAD

- **Neurocranium:** Upper portion of head; responsible for housing and protecting the brain
- **Visceral cranium:** Lower portion of head; associated with visceral functions of breathing, smelling, eating, talking; may be subdivided into 5 regions
  1. Orbital region
  2. Infratemporal/temporal fossa
  3. Nasal region
  4. Maxilla (upper jaw)
  5. Mandible (lower jaw)

CRANIAL NERVES (Table 27-1)

Table 27-1 *Cranial Nerves*

Number	Name	Type	Foramen	Innervation	Function
I	Olfactory	Sensory	Cribriform plate	Nasal mucous membrane	Sense of smell
II	Optic	Sensory	Optic foramen	Retinas	Sense of sight
III	Oculomotor	Motor	Superior orbital fissure	Superior rectus, inferior rectus, medial rectus, inferior oblique, and the ciliary and sphincter pupillae muscles	
IV	Trochlear	Motor	Superior orbital fissure	Superior oblique muscle	
V	Trigeminal • Ophthalmic division (V_1) • Maxillary division (V_2) • Mandibular division (V_3)	Motor/sensory	• Superior orbital fissure • Foramen rotundum • Foramen ovale		• Sensation to upper one-third of face • Sensation to midportion of face • Sensation to lower face; motor supply to muscles of mastication
VI	Abducens	Motor	Superior orbital fissure	Lateral rectus	

Table 27-1   *Cranial Nerves—cont'd*

Number	Name	Type	Foramen	Innervation	Function
VII	Facial	Motor/ sensory	Styloid foramen		Taste to anterior two-thirds of tongue (through chorda tympani); motor supply to muscles of facial expression
VIII	Acoustic • Cochlear division • Vestibular division	Sensory	Internal acoustic meatus	• Organ of Corti • Semicircular canals	• Sense of hearing • Sense of equilibrium
IX	Glossopharyngeal	Motor/ sensory	Jugular foramen	Parotid gland	Sensation to oropharynx; motor supply to muscles of pharynx
X	Vagus	Motor/ sensory	Jugular foramen	Pharyngeal plexus	Sensation to larynx, trachea, and other aerodigestive mucous membranes; motor supply to muscles of larynx and levator veli palatini, palatoglossus, and palatopharyngeus
XI	Accessory	Motor	Jugular foramen	Sternocleidomastoid and trapezius muscles	
XII	Hypoglossal	Motor	Hypoglossal canal	Muscles of tongue	

BLOOD SUPPLY

- Arterial supply to the **neurocranium** is provided through the **internal carotid system** and the **vertebral system.**
- **Visceral cranium** is chiefly supplied by the **external carotid system.**
  - Midline structures of the forehead and midface receive dual vascularity from both the external and internal systems.
- Venous drainage is provided by the **internal jugular vein.**
  - Major drainage contributions from the face are provided by:
    - ▸ Facial vein
    - ▸ Retromandibular vein
    - ▸ External jugular vein

Muscle Groups

- **Six major muscle groups in the head assist with functions of the visceral cranium.**
  1. **Orbital muscles**
     - ▸ Include both *intrinsic* and *extrinsic* muscles
       - **Intrinsic muscles:** Associated with controlling light into the eye and lens control; the ciliary muscle, dilator, and constrictor pupillae
       - **Extrinsic muscles:** Responsible for eye movement; include the superior rectus, inferior rectus, medial rectus, lateral rectus, superior oblique, and inferior oblique muscles
  2. **Masticatory muscles**
     - ▸ Include the temporalis, medial and lateral pterygoids, and masseter muscles
     - ▸ Responsible for lower jaw movement
  3. **Muscles of facial expression**
     - ▸ Major muscles: The frontalis, orbicularis oculi and oris, zygomaticus major and minor, levator labii, depressor labii, and mentalis
  4. **Tongue muscles**
     - ▸ The **intrinsic muscles** responsible for changing the shape of the tongue include the superior and inferior longitudinal muscles, transverses, and verticalis.
     - ▸ **Extrinsic muscles** responsible for the gross tongue movements include the genioglossus, hyoglossus, styloglossus and palatoglossus muscles.
  5. **Pharynx muscles**
     - ▸ Include the superior, middle, and inferior pharyngeal constrictors
  6. **Larynx muscles**
     - ▸ Located within the larynx, these muscles are associated with producing voice.

Oral Cavity

- Extends from the oral aperture to the palatoglossal fold
- Important anatomic structures within the oral cavity:
  - **Wharton's ducts:** Salivary ducts for the submandibular and sublingual salivary glands on the floor of the mouth
  - **Stensen's ducts:** Salivary ducts for the parotid gland located on the buccal mucosa across from and at the level of the maxillary second permanent molar

Dentition

- **Pediatric (primary) dentition:** 20 teeth
  - 4 incisors, 2 canines, 4 molars per arch
  - No premolars in pediatric dentition.
  - Pediatric dentition referenced by letter beginning with the upper right second molar to upper left second molar (A-J) and continuing with the lower left second molar to lower right second molar (K-T)
- **Adult (secondary) dentition:** 32 teeth
  - 4 incisors, 2 canines, 4 premolars, 6 molars per arch
  - Adult dentition referenced by number beginning with the upper right third molar to upper left third molar (1-16) and continuing with the lower left third molar to lower right third molar (17-32)
- **Eruption sequence**
  - **Incisors:** 6-9 years
  - **Canines:** 9-10 years
  - **First premolars:** 10-12 years

- **Second premolars:** 11-12 years
- **First molars:** 6-7 years
- **Second molars:** 11-13 years
- **Third molars:** 17-20 years

DENTAL TERMINOLOGY

- **Occlusal:** Functional surface of the tooth
- **Apex:** Toward the root tip
- **Incisal:** Occlusal surface of anterior teeth
- **Mesial:** Toward the midline
- **Distal:** Away from the midline
- **Buccal:** Toward the cheek
- **Lingual:** Toward the tongue (mandibular)
- **Palatal:** Toward the palate (maxillary)
- **Overbite:** Amount of vertical overlap of incisal edges
- **Overjet:** Amount of horizontal overlap of incisal edges
- **Proclined:** Anterior tooth angulated toward the lip
- **Retroclined:** Anterior tooth angulated toward the tongue
- **Buccal version:** Posterior tooth angulated toward the cheek
- **Lingual version:** Posterior tooth angulated toward the tongue
- **Crossbite:** Horizontal malrelationship of teeth; may be classified as anterior or posterior
- **Open bite:** Occlusal surfaces not in contact when in centric occlusion; anterior open bite same as negative overjet
- **Centric occlusion:** Occlusion of teeth in maximal intercuspation
- **Centric relation:** Occlusion of teeth with condyle in its most anterior-superior position

MALOCCLUSION

Occlusion refers to the relationship of teeth to one another.

- Classes of malocclusion were first described by Edward H. Angle.
- Angle hypothesized that normal occlusion was based on the relationship of the first permanent molars so that the **mesiobuccal cusp of the maxillary first molar occludes in the buccal groove of the mandibular first molar.** When this relationship occurs, with the teeth located along a smoothly curving line of occlusion without individual teeth being malrotated or malposed, the patient has *normal occlusion.*
- Angle described **3 classes of malocclusion.**

   Class I: The mesiobuccal cusp of the maxillary first molar occludes in the buccal groove of the mandibular molar, but teeth are malposed or malrotated.

NOTE: Class I malocclusion is not normal occlusion.

   Class II: The mandibular molar is *distally* positioned relative to the maxillary molar.
   ▸ Two divisions describe the relationship of the incisor.
      Division I: Excessive overjet with normal angulation of incisor
      Division II: Incisor retroclined to some degree, resulting in less overbite and increased overjet
   Class III: The mandibular molar is *mesially* positioned relative to the maxillary molar.

LOCAL ANAESTHESIA

- Local anaesthesia of the intraoral structures and facial soft tissues may be provided by regional nerve blocks or infiltration in the area of interest.
- In general, for anaesthesia of the teeth, nerve blocks should be performed for the mandibular dentition because the mandibular bone thickness in most areas precludes diffusion of a local anaesthetic.
- Diffusion occurs easily across the thin maxillary bone to provide dental anaesthesia.

NERVE BLOCKS

INFRAORBITAL (Fig. 27-1)

- The infraorbital branch of V_2 can be palpated, exiting its foramen approximately 4-7 mm below the inferior orbital rim along a line dropped from the medial edge of the limbus.
- Several milliliters of local anaesthetic may be deposited at the foramen using either an intraoral or extraoral approach.
  - Intraorally, the lip is stretched to make the mucosa taut at the height of the anterior maxillary vestibule. The needle is inserted at the height of the vestibule to the level of the foramen. The plunger is pulled back slightly, and if clear the anaesthetic is deposited.
  - Extraorally, the foramen is palpated, the needle is inserted at the superior aspect of the nasolabial fold at an angle to the foramen. The plunger is pulled back slightly, and if clear the anaesthetic is deposited.
- An infraorbital nerve block provides anaesthesia of lip, medial cheek, lower lid, lateral nose, and buccal gingival to the mesial half of the first molar.
- Dental anaesthesia is provided to nearby teeth by diffusion.

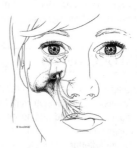

Fig. 27-1   The infraorbital nerve. (From Ellis E III, Kittidumkerng W. Analysis of treatment for isolated zygomaticomaxillary complex fractures. J Oral Maxillofac Surg 54:386-400, 1996.)

GREATER PALATINE (Fig. 27-2)

- Foramen is located halfway between the teeth and the palatal midline at about the second molar.
- Foramen is palpable as a soft depression in this location on the hard palate. Local anaesthetic (1-2 cc) is deposited after checking that the needle is not in a blood vessel.
- Provides anaesthesia of the palatal mucosa to the first premolar on its respective side.

NASOPALATINE (see Fig. 27-2)

- Foramen is located at the midline approximately 5-7 mm behind the maxillary incisors.
- Local anaesthetic (0.5-1 cc) is deposited after checking that the needle is not in a blood vessel.
- Provides anaesthesia of the palatal mucosa from canine to canine.

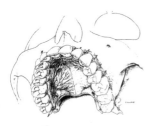

Fig. 27-2   The greater palatine nerve. (From Ellis E III, Kittidumkerng W. Analysis of treatment for isolated zygomaticomaxillary complex fractures. J Oral Maxillofac Surg 54:386-400, 1996.)

INFERIOR ALVEOLAR (Fig. 27-3)

- The inferior alveolar nerve enters the mandibular foramen on the medial ramus approximately 0.5-1 cm above the mandibular occlusal plane and 1.5-2 cm posterior to the anterior border of the ramus.
- With the patient's mouth open wide, the most medial aspect of the anterior surface of the ramus is palpated with the contralateral thumb.
- The needle is inserted at a 45-degree angle to the ramus entering at least 1 cm above the level of the occlusal plane (it is more effective to be higher than lower) and immediately adjacent to the antero-medial edge of the ramus.
- The needle is inserted until contact is made with bone. Check that the needle is not in a blood vessel, and inject several milliliters of solution.
- Provides anaesthesia of the entire mandibular hemidentition and buccal mucosa anterior to the second premolar.

LINGUAL (see Fig. 27-3)

- The lingual nerve is anaesthetized during the inferior alveolar block by withdrawing the needle approximately 0.5 cm and depositing 1-2 ml of solution.
- Provides anaesthesia of the entire lingual mucosa and respective half of the tongue.

BUCCAL (see Fig. 27-3)

- The buccal branch of V_3 is anaesthetized as it crosses the anterior border of the ramus.
- The needle is inserted into the retromolar mucosa over the anterior surface of the ramus, and several milliliters of solution are deposited after checking that the needle is not in a blood vessel.
- Provides anaesthesia of the buccal mucosa and gingiva anteriorly to the region of the first premolar.

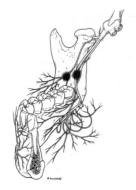

Fig. 27-3   The inferior alveolar nerve. (From Ellis E III, Kittidumkerng W. Analysis of treatment for isolated zygomaticomaxillary complex fractures. J Oral Maxillofac Surg 54:386-400, 1996.)

MENTAL

> TIP: The mental nerve is a distal branch of the inferior alveolar nerve. Therefore this block is not necessary when an inferior alveolar block has been performed.

- The mental nerve exits through its foramen below the second premolar. The lip is stretched, and the needle is inserted to the depth of the vestibule in this location.
- Several milliliters of solution are deposited after checking that the needle is not in a blood vessel.
- It provides anaesthesia of the buccal mucosa and gingiva anterior to the first premolar.

ODONTOGENIC INFECTIONS[2]

- Infections may range from localized infections without systemic manifestations to diffuse, systemic, life-threatening infections.
- Death from odontogenic infections still occurs and usually is a result of loss of airway or mediastinal extension of infection.
- Accurate evaluation of the patient and involved fascial spaces are requisite to proper management of these infections.

MICROBIOLOGY
- Almost all odontogenic infections are **polymicrobial.**
- Most common organisms include aerobic gram-positive cocci, anaerobic gram-positive cocci, and anaerobic gram-negative rods.
- **Approximately 60% of infections are mixed aerobic-anaerobic.** Important pathogens include *Streptococcus, Peptostreptococcus, Prevotella, Porphyromonas,* and *Fusobacterium.*

PATHOGENESIS
- Odontogenic infections arise from two major sources:
  1. **Periapical infection secondary to pulpal necrosis** leads to bacterial invasion in the periapical soft tissues.
  2. **Periodontal infection secondary to deep periodontal pocket** allows bacterial invasion in the surrounding tissue.
- **Periapical infection is the most common.**
  - From the periapical tissues the infection may erode through cortical bone into the facial soft tissues.
  - Location of infection is determined by the relationship of muscle attachments to the location of cortical perforation.
  - Example: A periapical infection of a mandibular premolar that erodes through the lingual bone will result in infection of the sublingual space because the mylohyoid attachment is inferior to the root apex, whereas the same process involving the second molar would present as a submandibular space infection, because the molar root apex lies below the mylohyoid attachment.

PRINCIPLES OF THERAPY

Standard history should be taken, and a physical should always be performed on all patients. Particular consideration should be given to the following:

DETERMINE SEVERITY OF INFECTION

- Signs of systemic involvement should be sought from the physical examination.
- Vital signs are reviewed for pyrexia, tachycardia, or hypotension.

CAUTION: Inability to control secretions or maintain a patent airway may indicate impending loss of airway and a need for emergent intervention.

- **Trismus** may be the only indication of a parapharyngeal space infection, and the clinician should take appropriate measures to thoroughly inspect the oropharynx.
- The source of infection should be identified (with assistance of panoramic radiography), with the adjacent fascial spaces examined directly for involvement.

ASSESS PATIENT'S HOST DEFENSE SYSTEM

- Patients with a medical history significant for conditions that produce immunodeficiency, such as diabetes, HIV, corticosteroid/chemotherapy usage, malnutrition, substance abuse, or other disease processes, require a more aggressive management approach.

PROVIDE SURGICAL DRAINAGE OF INFECTION

- Odontogenic infections should be treated by specialists trained in their management (when appropriate).
- The most important intervention after assessment and establishment of a secure airway is draining the infection and removing the source.

ADMINISTER APPROPRIATE ANTIBIOTIC COVERAGE

- *All odontogenic infections should be cultured.*
- Empiric therapy is begun with penicillin or clindamycin for allergic patients.
- Severe infections may require increased coverage for gram-negative and anaerobic bacteria.
- Antibiotic therapy should be guided by culture results.

ARCH BARS

- **Arch bars are used to:**
  - Stabilize dentoalveolar fractures
  - Provide stable base from which to institute maxillomandibular fixation
  - Control occlusion in the postinjury period
- The difficulty in placing arch bars depends on the age of the dentition (primary versus secondary or mixed) and the presence of partial edentulism.
- Arch bars are usually placed from first molar to first molar.
- In the setting of mandibular fractures, arch bars ideally extend **two teeth proximal to a fracture line** when possible.
- 24-gauge circumdental wires are used to secure the arch bar to each tooth.
- **Conventionally, wires are always:**
  - Twisted **clockwise** to tighten
  - Passed occlusal to the arch bar in the interproximal region of fractures to prevent the wire from interfering with reduction
  - Passed occlusal to the arch bar on the distal aspect of the last tooth and adjacent to edentulous spans
- Wires are typically applied from midline to posterior to prevent redundancy for arch bar.
- **Proper occlusion and fracture reduction must be established before completely tightening the cir-**

cumdental wires within the quadrant of the fracture to prevent maintenance of malreduction by the arch bar.
- This is facilitated by tightening the wires in the fracture segment after reducing the fracture and establishing maxillomandibular fixation.

DENTOFACIAL DEFORMITIES[3]

- Treatment of dentofacial deformities is an integrated orthodontic-surgical process.
- Dentofacial deformities are characterized by a skeletal discrepancy between mandible, maxilla, and skull base, or some combination thereof.
- Simple orthodontics do not correct the effects of malrelationship on facial balance but may camouflage malocclusion through creation of dental compensations.
- When skeletal elements are present the surgeon should be involved in early treatment planning to coordinate the orthodontic-surgical therapy.
- Orthodontic therapy proceeds to eliminate dental compensations and to level and align arch forms in anticipation of surgical correction of the skeletal component.

DENTAL EVALUATION

IDENTIFY
- Transverse and anterior-posterior discrepancies
- Open bites
- Tooth width discrepancies
- Excess arch curvatures (curve of Spee)
- Occlusal canting

CEPHALOMETRIC EVALUATION
- Cephalometric analysis allows standardized measurements from lateral cephalograms to determine the relationship between the skull base, maxilla, and mandible.
- These measurements evaluate dentofacial proportions and clarify the anatomic basis for the deformity.
- Cephalometric analysis should be used for diagnostic purposes but should not be the basis for planning surgery.
- Surgical decisions should be based on aesthetic evaluation of the face after considering the cephalometric diagnosis.
  - For example, patients with mild to moderate "cephalometrically" defined mandibular prognathism are usually best treated with maxillary advancement and not mandibular set-back (Fig. 27-4; Tables 27-1 and 27-2).

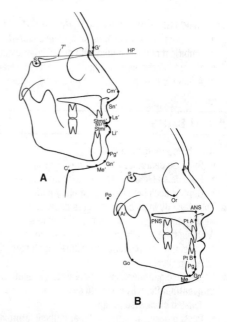

Fig. 27-4   A, Cephalometrics for soft tissue landmarks. **B,** Cephalometrics for hard tissue landmarks. (From Evans G. Operative Plastic Surgery. New York: McGraw-Hill, 2000.)

Aesthetic Evaluation

- Aesthetic evaluation includes frontal and profile evaluations.
- Frontal and profile evaluations are divided into evaluation of the upper, middle, and lower facial thirds in the vertical and horizontal dimensions.
- Balance of these regions is the goal.

Table 27-2 *Cephalometric Landmarks (Soft Tissue)*

G'	Soft tissue glabella: Most prominent point in the midsagittal plane of the forehead
Cm'	Columella point: Most anterior point on the columella of the nose
Sn'	Subnasale: Point at which the nasal septum merges with the upper cutaneous lip and the midsagittal plane
Ls'	Labrale superius: Mucocutaneous border of the upper lip in the midsagittal plane
Li'	Labrale inferius: Mucocutaneous border of the lower lip in the midsagittal plane
Pg'	Soft tissue pogonion: Most anterior point of the soft tissue chin
HP'	Horizontal plane: A plane drawn 7 degrees above the sella-nasion (S-N) plane, from which perpendicular lines are drawn to measure vertical soft tissue distances
Stms'	Stomion superius: Lowermost point of the vermilion of the lower lip
C'	Cervical point: Innermost point between the submental area and where the neck begins its vertical position
Me'	Soft tissue menton: Lowest point on the contour of the soft tissue chin
Gn'	Soft tissue gnathion: Constructed midpoint between soft tissue pogonion and soft tissue menton; located at the intersection of subnasale to soft tissue pogonion line and the line from C' to Me'.

Modified from Ferraro JW, ed. Fundamentals of Maxillofacial Surgery. New York: Springer-Verlag, 1997, p 241.

Table 27-3 *Cephalometric Landmarks (Hard Tissue/Bony Tissue)*

S	Sella: Center of the pituitary fossa—Sella turcica
N or Na	Nasion: Most anterior point at the junction of the nasal and frontal bones in the midsagittal plane
Po	Porion: Most superior point of the external auditory meatus
O or Or	Orbitale: Lowest point on the inferior bony border of the left orbital cavity as viewed from the lateral aspect
ANS	Anterior nasal spine: Most anterior tip of the maxillary nasal spine
PNS	Posterior nasal spine: Midline tip of posterior spine of hard palate in the midsagittal plane
P or Pg	Pogonion: Most anterior point on the contour of the mandibular symphysis
Pt A	Point A: Deepest midpoint on the maxillary alveolar process between anterior nasal spine and the crest of alveolar ridge
Pt B	Point B: Deepest midpoint on the alveolar process between the crest of the ridge and pogonion
Me	Menton: Lowest point on the contour of the mandibular symphysis
Gn	Gnathion: Most anterior-inferior point on the chin contour constructed point, determined by bisecting the angle formed by the facial and mandibular planes
Ar	Articulare: Junction of the basisphenoid and the posterior of the condyle of the mandible
Go	Gonion: Point at the angle of the mandible that is directed most inferiorly and posteriorly

Modified from Ferraro JW, ed. Fundamentals of Maxillofacial Surgery. New York: Springer-Verlag, 1997, p 241.

GENERAL DIAGNOSES

MAXILLARY EXCESS

- May occur in the anteroposterior, vertical, or transverse dimensions.
- **Vertical excess facial features include:**
  - Elongation of lower third
  - Narrow nasal base
  - Excessive incisal and gingival show
  - Lip incompetence
- May be associated with anterior open bite (apertognathia).
- Anteroposterior excess characteristically has a class II malocclusion with protrusion of maxillary incisors and convex facial profile.
- **Primary surgical correction involves Le Fort I osteotomy.**
- Segmental maxillary surgery can be performed for more complex deformities.

MAXILLARY DEFICIENCY

- May occur in the anteroposterior, vertical, or transverse dimensions.
- **Facial features include:**
  - Deficiency of infraorbital/paranasal regions
  - Inadequate upper tooth show
  - Short lower third
  - Deficient upper lip
- **Primary surgical correction involves Le Fort I osteotomy.**
- Segmental maxillary surgery can be performed for more complex deformities.
- Bone grafting may be required depending on the magnitude and vector of movement.

MANDIBULAR EXCESS (PROGNATHISM)

- Typically demonstrates class III molar and cuspid relationship and reverse overjet of the incisors.
- **Facial features include** prominent lower third.
- **Primary correction may involve maxillary advancement or mandibular setback depending on the facial analysis.**
- Mandibular setback is provided through bilateral sagittal split osteotomies (BSSRO) or intraoral vertical ramus osteotomies (IVRO).
- IVRO has the disadvantage of requiring maxillomandibular fixation.

MANDIBULAR DEFICIENCY (RETROGNATHISM)

- Typically demonstrates class II molar and cuspid relationship.
- May demonstrate excess overjet or deep bite.
- **Facial features include:**
  - Retruded position of chin
  - Acute labiomental fold
  - Abnormal lip posturing
  - Short thyromental distance
- **Primary surgical treatment involves mandibular advancement using BSSRO.**

STABILITY OF CORRECTION

- Relapse may occur following correction of dentofacial deformities.
- The factors that have the most influence on stability appear to be which jaw is being moved, the direction of movement, and the distance of movement.[4]
- **Orthodontic factors**
  - Inadequate removal of dental compensations
  - Inadequate leveling of dental arches
  - Presurgical orthodontic correction of skeletal transverse discrepancies
- **Surgical factors**
  - Inaccurate positioning of proximal mandibular segment and condyles
  - Inadequate fixation
  - Idiopathic condylar resorption

KEY POINTS

✔ Muscles of mastication include the temporalis, medial pterygoids, lateral pterygoids, and masseter.

✔ Stensen's duct is located adjacent to the second maxillary permanent molar.

✔ Children have 20 teeth (primary dentition).

✔ Adults have 32 teeth (secondary dentition).

✔ The adult dentition is numbered 1-32, starting with the upper right third molar and ending with the lower right third molar.

✔ Angle class I malocclusion is *not* necessarily normal occlusion.

REFERENCES

1. Hollinshead WH, ed. Anatomy for Surgeons: The Head and Neck, 3rd ed. Philadelphia: Lippincott, 1982.
2. Topazian RG, Goldberg MH, Hupp JR, eds. Oral and Maxillofacial Infections, 4th ed. Philadelphia: WB Saunders, 2002.
3. Epker BN, Stella JP, Fish LC. Dentofacial Deformities: Integrated Orthodontic and Surgical Approach, vol 1, 2nd ed. St Louis: Mosby, 1995.
4. Van Sickels JE, Richardson DA. Stability of orthognathic surgery: A review of rigid fixation. Br J Oral Maxillofac Surg 34:279, 1996.

28. Principles of Head and Neck Cancer: Staging and Management

Michael E. Decherd
Jeffrey E. Janis

CLASSIFICATION

The **American Joint Committee on Cancer** (AJCC) sets the standards for cancer staging. For every tumor there is a staging sheet that should be used to standardize cancer data collection.
- **The AJCC divides cancers of the head and neck into seven categories.**
   1. Lip and oral cavity
   2. Pharynx
   3. Larynx
   4. Paranasal sinuses
   5. Salivary glands
   6. Thyroid
   7. Esophagus
- The staging system uses the **TNM** method (tumor, nodes, metastasis) (Table 28-1).
   - **T:** 1-4
   - **N:** 0-3
   - **M:** 0-1 (may vary by tumor)

TIP: TNM is clinically more useful than stage. Even though a T3N0 and a T1N1 tumor are both stage III, they behave differently and may be treated differently.

Table 28-1   *General Staging Scheme for Head and Neck Cancer (May Vary by Tumor)*

	T1	T2	T3	T4
N0	Stage I	Stage II	Stage III	Stage IV
N1	Stage III	Stage III	Stage III	Stage IV
N2	Stage IV	Stage IV	Stage IV	Stage IV
N3	Stage IV	Stage IV	Stage IV	Stage IV

- The prefix **p** or **c** is used to designate how the stage is assigned (**p**athologic or **c**linical).
   - *Pathologic staging, if available, supersedes clinical staging.*
- The designators *m, y, r,* and *a* indicate *multiple tumors, following multimodal therapy, recurrent tumors,* and *at autopsy,* respectively.

- **Biologic factors:**
  - Perineural or perivascular invasion
  - Extracapsular spread (ECS)
    - ▸ Indicates a more aggressive tumor
    - ▸ Should be considered for radiation even if other criteria not met
- **Tumor grade** is not usually used clinically.
- Tumors should **not** be restaged.
  - Example: A patient that initially is M0 but turns up with pulmonary metastasis 6 months later is not changed to M1.

TUMOR STAGING

- Staging varies by **site.**
- **Oropharynx** and **oral cavity** approximately use the following (other subsites have their own systems):
  - **Tx:** No available information on primary tumor
  - **T0:** No evidence of primary tumor
  - **Tis:** Carcinoma in situ
  - **T1:** Greatest diameter of primary tumor 2 cm or less
  - **T2:** Greatest diameter of primary tumor more than 2 cm but not more than 4 cm
  - **T3:** Greatest diameter of primary tumor more than 4 cm
  - **T4:** Massive tumor more than 4 cm in diameter with deep invasion

NODAL METASTASIS[1]

- *Single greatest influence on survival is presence of nodal metastasis.*
- Nodal staging system is generally the same for upper aerodigestive tumors (except nasopharynx) (Fig. 28-1):
  - **Nx:** Nodes cannot be assessed
  - **N0:** No nodes containing metastasis
  - **N1:** A single ipsilateral node metastasis, 3 cm or less in diameter
  - **N2a:** A single ipsilateral positive node more than 3 cm but not more than 6 cm in diameter
  - **N2b:** Multiple positive ipsilateral nodes, none more than 6 cm in diameter
  - **N2c:** Bilateral or contralateral positive nodes, none more than 6 cm in diameter
  - **N3:** Adenopathy greater than 6 cm in diameter

NOTE: Older designations such as *fixed nodes* and *matted nodes* are no longer used.

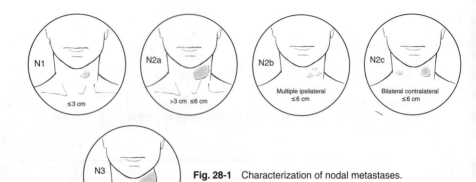

Fig. 28-1 Characterization of nodal metastases.

INCIDENCE

- Head and neck malignancy: 78,000 cases annually (7% of all cancers)
- Cancer deaths: 17,500 annually (4% of all cancers)
- 33% of patients with head and neck malignancy ultimately die of disease
- Alcohol and tobacco: 15-fold increased incidence over nonusers (squamous cell cancer)
- Male predominance

LEVELS OF THE NECK[2-6] (Fig. 28-2)

> TIP: The *levels* of the neck are different from the trauma *zones* of the neck.

Fig. 28-2 Levels of the neck.

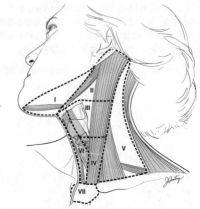

LEVEL I
- **Lymph node groups:** Submental and submandibular
- **Level Ia:** Submental triangle
  - **Boundaries:** Anterior bellies of the digastric muscle and the hyoid bone
- **Level Ib:** Submandibular triangle
  - **Boundaries:** Body of the mandible, anterior and posterior belly of the digastric muscle (includes the submandibular gland, pre- and postglandular lymph nodes, and pre- and postvascular lymph nodes [relative to facial vein and artery]).

LEVEL II
- **Lymph node groups:** Upper jugular
- **Boundaries**
  - **Anterior:** Lateral border of the sternohyoid muscle
  - **Posterior:** Posterior border of the sternocleidomastoid muscle
  - **Superior:** Skull base
  - **Inferior:** Level of the hyoid bone (clinical landmark); carotid bifurcation (surgical landmark)
- **Level IIa** and **IIb** arbitrarily designated anatomically by splitting level II with the *spinal accessory nerve*

LEVEL III
- **Lymph node groups:** Middle jugular
- **Boundaries**
  - **Anterior:** Lateral border of the sternohyoid muscle
  - **Posterior:** Posterior border of the sternocleidomastoid muscle
  - **Superior:** Hyoid bone (clinical landmark); carotid bifurcation (surgical landmark)
  - **Inferior:** Cricothyroid notch (clinical landmark); omohyoid muscle (surgical landmark)

LEVEL IV
- **Lymph node group:** Lower jugular
- **Boundaries**
  - **Anterior:** Lateral border of the sternohyoid muscle
  - **Posterior:** Posterior border of the sternocleidomastoid muscle
  - **Superior:** Cricothyroid notch (clinical landmark), omohyoid muscle (surgical landmark)
  - **Inferior:** Clavicle
- **Level IVa:** Lymph nodes that lie along the internal jugular vein but immediately deep to the **sternal head** of the sternocleidomastoid muscle
- **Level IVb:** Lymph nodes that lie deep to the **clavicular head** of the sternocleidomastoid muscle

LEVEL V
- **Lymph node groups:** Posterior triangle
- **Boundaries**
  - **Anterior:** Posterior border of the sternocleidomastoid muscle
  - **Posterior:** Anterior border of the trapezius muscle
  - **Inferior:** Clavicle
- **Level Va:** Lymphatic structures in the upper part of level V that follow the spinal accessory nerve
- **Level Vb:** Nodes that lie along the transverse cervical artery
  - Anatomically, the division between the two level 5 subzones is the *inferior belly of the omohyoid muscle.*

LEVEL VI
- **Lymph node groups:** Anterior compartment
- **Boundaries**
  - **Lateral:** Carotid sheath
  - **Superior:** Hyoid bone
  - **Inferior:** Suprasternal notch

LEVEL VII
- **Lymph node groups:** Upper mediastinal
- **Boundaries**
  - **Lateral:** Carotid arteries
  - **Superior:** Suprasternal notch
  - **Inferior:** Aortic arch

TREATMENT OF THE NECK[7-9]

GENERAL PRINCIPLES
- **Clinical N0 neck options (depends on primary tumor)**
  - Observation and serial exam
  - Staging neck dissections
  - Radiation
- With **clinical N+ neck,** comprehensive treatment of neck nodes usually required

NECK DISSECTIONS[10-19]

- **Radical neck dissection** (RND) removes[14,25]:
  - Lymph nodes in levels I through V
  - Sternocleidomastoid muscle
  - Internal jugular (IJ) vein
  - Spinal accessory nerve (CN XI)
- **Modified radical neck dissection** (mRND)
  - Preserves some or all nonlymphatic structures
  - Example: Modified radical neck dissection with preservation of the spinal accessory nerve and the internal jugular vein
- **Functional neck dissection**
  - Preserves all nonlymphatic structures (e.g., a modified radical neck dissection with preservation of CN XI, the IJ, and the sternocleidomastoid muscle)
  - Sometimes called a *Bocca* neck dissection[11]
  - Sometimes called a *mRND* type III
- **Comprehensive neck dissection**
  - Removes all standard lymphatic tissue
  - Includes radical and modified radical neck dissections
  - Typically required for N+ necks

- **Selective neck dissection**
  - Anything less than a comprehensive neck dissection
  - Removes only selected levels (e.g., levels II through IV)
  - Usually performed on N0 necks
- **Extended neck dissection**
  - Removes more than a standard neck dissection (e.g., the carotid artery)
  - Can still be a modified radical or radical

WORKUP

- **Complete head and neck exam**
  - Synchronous primaries in as many as **20%** of patients
  - Includes viewing the larynx and surrounding structures, as well as the nasopharynx (fiberoptic endoscopy may be needed)
- **Panendoscopy**
  - Direct laryngoscopy
  - Rigid bronchoscopy
  - Rigid esophagoscopy
- **Metastatic workup**
  - Somewhat controversial
  - Consider performing:
    - Chest x-ray examination (some prefer CT)
    - Basic chemistries, including calcium and liver function tests
    - Other workup basics according to symptoms (e.g., bone scan for bone pain)
- **Unknown primary**
  Malignant neck node with no obvious source
  - Management is controversial
  - Consider performing:
    - Ipsilateral tonsillectomy
    - Biopsies of nasopharynx (Rosenmüller's fossae in particular)
    - Biopsies of base of tongue
- **Neck mass**
  - Consider tissue diagnosis in any neck mass present for more than 2 weeks, especially in smokers over 40.
  - Initial test is **fine-needle aspiration** (FNA).
    - Excisional biopsy may increase metastasis if squamous cell carcinoma (SCC).
    - Excisional biopsy needed if FNA suggests lymphoma.
      - Send **fresh** for flow cytometry.

TREATMENT[20-23]

SALIVARY TUMORS
- **General**
  - Salivary gland tumors usually require operative intervention.
  - Most salivary gland tumors are in the parotid (80%), submandibular (10%-15%), and sublingual or minor salivary glands (5%-10%).

- ▸ **Parotid:** 80% benign; 20% malignant
- ▸ **Submandibular:** 50% benign; 50% malignant
- ▸ **Sublingual:** 40% benign; 60% malignant
- ▸ **Minor salivary:** 25% benign; 75% malignant

TIP: The smaller the gland, the higher the incidence of malignancy.

- All preauricular masses considered to be of parotid origin unless proven otherwise
- Children less frequent than adults
  - In **children,** most are **benign** (vasoformative lesions most frequent).
    - ▸ **Hemangioma is the most common tumor of the parotid in children.**
- **Most common benign neoplasms**
  - Pleomorphic (70%)
  - Warthin's tumor
- **Most common malignant neoplasms**
  - Mucoepidermoid
  - Adenoid cystic carcinoma
  - **Low-grade malignancies**
    - ▸ Low-grade mucoepidermoid
    - ▸ Acinic cell carcinoma
  - **High-grade malignancies**
    - ▸ High-grade mucoepidermoid
    - ▸ Adenoid cystic carcinoma
    - ▸ Squamous cell carcinoma
    - ▸ Adenocarcinoma
    - ▸ Undifferentiated

SIGNS AND SYMPTOMS
- Most patients present with **painless, asymptomatic mass.**
- **Physical signs suggestive of malignancy:**
  - Facial nerve weakness/paralysis
  - Lymphadenopathy
  - Skin changes
  - Pain (associated but *not* diagnostic)
- Patients with chronic inflammatory conditions (salivary stones or recurrent infections) or autoimmune diseases (Sjögren's syndrome) can have masses within the salivary glands.
- Malignant tumors of the head and neck, as well as of the kidney, prostate, and lymphoreticular system, can metastasize to the parotid.
  - **Exam**
    - ▸ Full head and neck exam, including external auditory canal, scalp, and intraoral with indirect laryngoscopy

TIP: Tumors occupying the deep lobe of the parotid can be clinically appreciated during intraoral exam as peritonsillar swellings.

- ► **Labs:** Complete blood cell count, liver function test
- ► **Imaging:** Chest radiography
- • **Diagnostics**
  - ► Fine-needle aspiration
  - ► Parotidectomy: May be necessary if nondiagnostic FNA
  - ► CT scan
  - ► MRI
    - ◆ Check for extension into deep lobe, parapharyngeal extension, nodal involvement, extension into skull, or carotid encasement.

CAUTION: Open incisional biopsies are usually contraindicated.

STAGING

- ■ **T1:** Less than 2 cm and without extraparenchymal extension
- ■ **T2:** 2-4 cm and without extraparenchymal extension
- ■ **T3:** Greater than 4 cm and/or tumor having extraparenchymal extension
- ■ **T4:** Greater than 6 cm or extension into, or involvement of, extraglandular tissues
- ■ **T4a:** Tumor invades skin, mandible, ear canal, and/or facial nerve
- ■ **T4b:** Tumor invades skull base and/or pterygoid plates and/or encases carotid artery
- ■ **N:** Regional lymph nodes (see Fig. 28-1)
- ■ **M:** Presence/absence of distant metastasis

TUMOR TYPES

BENIGN

- ■ **Mixed tumor (pleomorphic adenoma)**
  - • **Most common** (70%)
  - • Most frequently present as **asymptomatic mass**
  - • **Rare** facial nerve involvement
  - • Recur if they are shelled out of parotid gland or are incompletely excised
    - ► If recur then usually will reappear as multicentric nodular tumor implants in extraglandular tissue (with increased risk to the facial nerve)
  - • **Treatment**
    - ► **Superficial (also known as lateral) parotidectomy** for **superficial** lobe tumors
    - ► **Total parotidectomy** for those involving **deep** lobe
- ■ **Warthin's tumor (papillary cystadenoma lymphomatosum)**
  - • Second most common benign salivary tumor of the parotid
  - • Usually found in males over age 50
  - • **15% bilateral**

MALIGNANT

- ■ **Mucoepidermoid carcinoma**
  - • **Most common malignant tumor of the parotid**
  - • **Low grade:** Often indolent presentation
    - ► Treat with **superficial parotidectomy**
  - • **High grade:** Can be very aggressive

- **Adenoid cystic carcinoma**
  - **Most common malignant tumor in the minor salivary glands**
  - Usually firm, asymptomatic mass
  - Can spread perineurally and metastasize systemically
  - Does not tend to metastasize to cervical lymph nodes
  - Frequently invades extraglandular tissues by direct extension
  - Can recur after many years of disease-free survival
  - Must be followed at regular intervals for life; obtain chest radiographs every year
  - Has characteristic "swiss-cheese" appearance on pathology
- **Mixed tumor**
  - Can arise spontaneously, but many are thought to arise in *long-standing benign mixed tumors*
  - Aggressive
  - Tend to metastasize early

OTHER TUMOR TYPES
- Acinic cell carcinoma
- Squamous cell carcinoma
- Adenocarcinoma
- Lymphoma

INDICATIONS FOR RADICAL NECK DISSECTION

- Enlarged, palpable lymph nodes
- Large or rapidly growing tumors
- **Small tumors**
  - Squamous cell carcinoma
  - Adenoid cystic
  - Malignant mixed
  - High-grade mucoepidermoid

FIVE INDICATIONS FOR ADJUVANT RADIATION THERAPY

1. High-grade malignancies
2. Residual disease
3. Recurrent disease
4. Invasion of adjacent structures
5. T3 or T4 parotid malignancies

GENERAL TIPS

- Supraglottic cancers have high rates of occult metastasis and need some form of treatment for the neck.
- Neck specimens that show greater than N1 disease, or N1 disease that has biologic factors (such as perineural invasion) should be considered for postoperative radiation therapy.
- Bilateral sacrifice of internal jugular veins is survivable but has substantially increased morbidity.[24]
- Postradiation surgery has many more complications.
- Have a low threshold for performing a perioperative tracheotomy.
- Communication is crucial! Talk about a plan in detail ahead of time, because the surgeon doing the resection may be able to take measures to preserve vessels for free flaps.
- Laryngectomy patients will swallow better if you do either a pharyngeal plexus neurectomy or cricopharyngeal myotomy at time of surgery. They will also speak better if using esophageal or tracheoesophageal speech.
- Consider G-tube early for nutritional support.
- Be very aggressive with delirium tremens prevention postoperatively if there is any suspicion.
- Use high-output drains (especially with the left neck [but possible in the right]) in the early postoperative period or with feeding—be aware of potential chylous fistula.
- Be aware of early spiking fevers as an indicator of pharyngeal fistula.
- First feeding should be with dye before drains are out to check for fistula (and may help determine aspiration).

KEY POINTS

- ✔ The single greatest effect on survival is the presence of nodal metastasis.
- ✔ Alcohol and tobacco are predisposing factors for head and neck malignancy.
- ✔ The levels of neck dissection are **not** the same as the trauma zones of the neck.
- ✔ Mucoepidermoid carcinoma is the most common malignant salivary tumor.
- ✔ Pleomorphic adenoma is the most common benign salivary tumor.
- ✔ Warthin's tumors can be bilateral.

REFERENCES

1. Candela FC, Shah J, Jacques DP, et al. Patterns of cervical node metastases from squamous carcinoma of the larynx. Arch Otolaryngol Head Neck Surg 116:432-435, 1990.
2. Lindberg R. Distribution of cervical lymph node metastases from squamous cell carcinoma of the upper respiratory and digestive tracts. Cancer 29:1446-1449, 1972.
3. Martin H, DelValle B, Ehrlich H, et al. Neck dissection. Cancer 4:441-499, 1951.
4. Medina JE. A rationale classification of neck dissections. Otolaryngol Head Neck Surg 100:169-176, 1989.
5. Medina JE, Weisman RA. Management of the neck in head and neck cancer, part I. Otolaryngol Clin North Am 31(4), 1998.
6. Medina JE, Weisman RA. Management of the neck in head and neck cancer, part II. Otolaryngol Clin North Am 31(5), 1998.
7. Johnson JT, Myers EN. Cervical lymph node disease in laryngeal cancer. In Silver CE, ed. Laryngeal Cancer. New York: Thieme Medical, 1991, pp 22-26.

8. Kraus DH, Rosenberg DB, Davidson BJ, et al. Supraspinal accessory lymph node metastases in supraomohyoid neck dissection. Am J Surg 172:646-649, 1996.
9. Million RR. Elective neck irradiation of TxN0 squamous carcinoma of the oral tongue and floor of mouth. Cancer 34:149-155, 1974.
10. Anderson PE. The role of comprehensive neck dissection with preservation of the spinal accessory nerve in the clinically positive neck. Amer J Surg 168:499-502, 1994.
11. Bocca E, Pignataro O. A conservation technique in radical neck dissection. Ann Otol Rhinol Laryngol 76:975-987, 1967.
12. Pignataro O, Sasaki CT. Functional neck dissection: A description of operative technique. Arch Otolaryngol 106:524-527, 1980.
13. Byers RM, Wolf PF, Ballantyne AJ. Rationale for elective modified neck dissection. Head Neck 10:160-167, 1988.
14. Greene FL, Page DL, Fleming ID, et al. AJCC Cancer Staging Manual, 6th ed. New York: Springer, 2002.
15. Hoffman HT. Surgical treatment of cervical node metastases from squamous carcinoma of the upper aerodigestive tract: Evaluation of the evidence for modifications of neck dissection. Head Neck 23:907-915, 2001.
16. Jaehne M, Ussmuller J, Kehrl W. [Significance of sternocleidomastoid muscle resection in radical neck dissection]. HNO 44:661-665, 1996.
17. Robbins TK, Medina JE, Wolfe GT, et al. Standardizing neck dissection terminology: Official report of the Academy's Committee for Head and Neck Surgery and Oncology. Arch Otolaryngol Head Neck Surg 117:601-605, 1991.
18. Spiro RH, Strong EW, Shah JP. Classification of neck dissection: Variations on a new theme. Am J Surg 168:415-418, 1994.
19. Suen JY, Goepfert H. Standardization of neck dissection nomenclature [editorial]. Head Neck Surg 10:75-77, 1987.
20. Shah JP. Patterns of lymph node metastases from squamous carcinomas of the upper aerodigestive tract. Am J Surg 160:405-409, 1990.
21. Sharpe DT. The pattern of lymph node metastases in intra-oral squamous cell carcinoma. Br J Plast Surg 34:97-101, 1981.
22. Talmi YP, Hoffman HT, Horowitz Z, et al. Patterns of metastases to the upper jugular lymph nodes (the "submuscular recess"). Head Neck 20:682-686, 1998.
23. Teknos TN, Coniglio JU, Netterville JL. Guidelines to patient management. In Bailey BJ, ed. Head and Neck Surgery: Otolaryngology, 2nd ed. Philadelphia: Lippincott, 1998.
24. Cotter CS, Stringer SP, Landau S, et al. Patency of the internal jugular vein following modified radical neck dissection. Laryngoscope 104:841-845, 1994.
25. Crile G. Excision of cancer of the head and neck. J Am Med Assoc 47:1780-1786, 1906.

29. Scalp and Calvarial Reconstruction

Jason E. Leedy

APPLIED ANATOMY[1-6]

SCALP LAYERS (Fig. 29-1)
- Mnemonic: SCALP
  - **S** *(skin):* Measures 3-8 mm thick
  - **C** *(subcutaneous tissue):* Vessels, lymphatics, and nerves found in this layer
  - **A** *(aponeurotic layer):* Strength layer, continuous with frontalis and occipitalis muscles
  - **L** *(loose areolar tissue):* Also known as *subgaleal fascia* and *innominate fascia;* provides scalp mobility; contains emissary veins
  - **P** *(pericranium):* Tightly adherent to calvarium

CRANIUM LAYERS
- External table
- Diploic space
- Internal table
- Epidural space
- Dura mater
- Subdural space

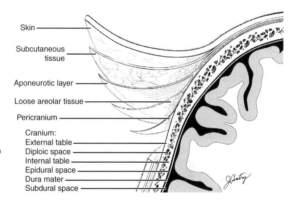

Skin
Subcutaneous tissue
Aponeurotic layer
Loose areolar tissue
Pericranium
Cranium:
External table
Diploic space
Internal table
Epidural space
Dura mater
Subdural space

Fig. 29-1 Layers of scalp and cranium.

VASCULARITY (Fig. 29-2)
Arterial branches and venae comitantes of the **internal and external carotid systems** are divided into **four distinct vascular territories.**

> TIP: Extensive collateralization of these vascular territories allows total scalp replantation based on a single vascular anastomosis.

- **Anterior territory**
  - **Supraorbital and supratrochlear arteries** (terminal branches of the internal carotid system).
  - Supraorbital artery arises through supraorbital notch or groove, which is located in line with the medial limbus.
  - Supratrochlear arteries arise more medially, usually in plane with the medial canthus.
- **Lateral territory** (largest territory)
  - **Superficial temporal artery** (terminal branch of the external carotid system)
  - Bifurcates at the superior helix of the ear into **frontal** and **parietal** branches

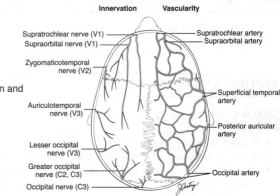

Fig. 29-2   Scalp innervation and vascularity.

- **Posterior territory**
  - Cephalad to the nuchal line: **Occipital arteries**
  - Caudal to the nuchal line: Perforating branches of the trapezius and splenius capitis muscles
- **Posterolateral territory** (smallest territory)
  - **Posterior auricular artery:** A branch of the external carotid system

INNERVATION (see Fig. 29-2)

- **Sensory**

Supplied by branches of the three divisions of the trigeminal nerve, cervical spinal nerves, and branches from the cervical plexus

- **Supraorbital nerve**
  - **Superficial division**
    - Pierces the frontalis muscle on the forehead and supplies the skin of the forehead and anterior hairline region
  - **Deep division**
    - Runs superficial to the periosteum up until the level of the coronal suture where it pierces the galeal aponeurosis, approximately 0.5-1.5 cm medial to the superior temporal line to innervate the frontoparietal scalp
- **Zygomaticotemporal nerve**
  - Branches from the maxillary division of the trigeminal nerve
  - Supplies a small region lateral to the brow up to the superficial temporal crest
- **Auriculotemporal nerve**
  - Branches from the mandibular division of the trigeminal nerve
  - Supplies the lateral scalp territory
- **Greater and lesser occipital nerves**
  - Branch from the dorsal rami of the cervical spinal nerves and the cervical plexus, respectively
  - Innervate the occipital territory
  - Greater occipital nerve shown to emerge from semispinalis muscle approximately 3 cm below occipital protuberance and 1.5 cm lateral to midline[7]
- **Motor**
  - **Frontal branch of facial nerve**
    - Supplies the frontalis
    - See Chapters 37 and 80 for anatomic location

- **Posterior auricular branch of facial nerve**
  - ▶ Supplies the anterior and posterior auricular muscles, occipitalis muscle

SKIN BIOMECHANICS[8]

Skin biomechanics is important for understanding tissue expansion reconstruction of the scalp.
- **Stress relaxation:** Property of the skin that decreases the amount of force necessary to maintain a fixed amount of skin stretch over time.
- **Creep:** Skin property that gives a gain in skin surface area when a constant load is applied.
  - As force is applied to a leading skin edge, tissue thickness decreases from extrusion of fluid and mucopolysaccharides, realignment of dermal collagen bundles, elastic fiber microfragmentation, and mechanical stretching of the skin.

PRINCIPLES OF SCALP RECONSTRUCTION

- **Replace tissue with like tissue.**
  - Use adjacent scalp for reconstruction if possible.
  - Incorporate at least one main-named scalp vessel into flaps.
  - Consider using scalp tissue from the **parietal region** where scalp mobility is the greatest.
  - Only debride devitalized tissue in acute repair of traumatic defects, because robust vascularity of the scalp may allow recovery of marginal tissues.
  - Employ hair micrografting to improve incision lines and subsequent alopecia secondarily.
- **Consider tissue expansion.**[9]
  - It is useful if local tissue rearrangements are inadequate for reconstruction because of the size of the defect, traumatized local tissue, unacceptable rearrangement of hair patterns, or distortion of the hairline.
  - During the expansion process, exposed bone can be covered temporarily with split-thickness skin grafts either after burring of the outer table or coverage with pericranial flaps.
  - Approximately **50%** of the scalp can be reconstructed with tissue expansion before alopecia becomes a significant issue.

TIP: Local anaesthetic with dilute epinephrine decreases intraoperative skin edge bleeding and can be used to hydrodissect the subgaleal plane.

Minimize the use of hemostatic clips and electrocautery on cut edges of the scalp to prevent potential follicular damage and subsequent iatrogenic alopecia.

Score the galea perpendicular to the direction of desired tissue gain, avoiding inadvertent injury to the scalp arteries that lie superficial to the galea.

Closure requires approximation of the galea because it is the strength layer.

GUIDELINES FOR RECONSTRUCTION

Reconstructive options vary depending on the defect's cause, location, and size. An algorithmic approach is useful.

ANTERIOR DEFECTS (Fig. 29-3)

- **Location:** The area posterior to the anterior hairline and anterior to the plane of the superficial temporal vessels that lie in front of the root of the helix
- **Principles:** Recreation of the anterior hairline without derangement of native hairline or creation of dog ears in cosmetically sensitive areas; undermining of forehead for greater tissue gain
- **Small defects (<2 cm²)**
  - Primary closure after undermining
  - Advancement flaps based on subcutaneous pedicles
  - Small rotation advancement flaps
- **Moderate defects (2-25 cm²)**
  - V-Y flaps, V-Y-S flaps, subcutaneous pedicled flaps, rotation advancement flaps
  - Anterior hairline reconstruction: Temporoparietaloccipital flaps or the lateral scalp flap, as described for correction of male pattern baldness
- **Large defects (>25 cm²)**
  - Temporoparietaloccipital flaps
  - Large rotation advancement flaps with back-grafting of the donor site to restore anterior hair and move the defect
  - **Orticochea flaps**
    - ▶ Two flaps for reconstructing the defect, each based off the superficial temporal vessels, and one large flap based off the occipitals to fill the donor defect
    - ▶ Can result in significant alopecia and unnatural hair orientation

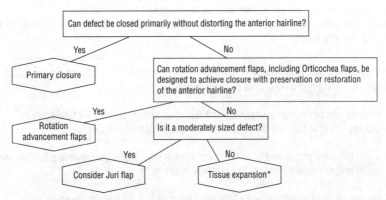

*Rotation advancement flaps can be used to move the defect to a less cosmetically sensitive area, such as the posterior vertex or occiput, with back-grafting and subsequent tissue expansion.

Fig. 29-3   Reconstruction algorithm: Anterior defects.

TIP: Consider tissue expansion in lieu of Orticochea flaps.

PARIETAL DEFECTS (Fig. 29-4)
- **Location:** The parietal scalp territory is supplied by superficial temporal vessels.
- **Principles:** Defects in the parietal scalp are amenable to local tissue rearrangement as a result of high scalp mobility in this region. They are less likely to have exposed bone because of the underlying temporalis muscle. Avoid sideburn displacement.
- **Small defects (<2 cm^2)**
  - Primary closure
  - V-Y flaps, subcutaneous pedicled flaps, and rhomboid flaps possible for temporal sideburn reconstruction
- **Medium defects (2-25 cm^2)**
  - Rotation advancement flaps
  - Bilobed flaps
- **Large defects (>25 cm^2)**
  - Tissue expansion is often the only technique available for satisfactory reconstruction
  - Large bipedicled frontooccipital flaps with large areas of back-grafting have been described but are best reserved for single-stage reconstruction when excellent cosmesis is not required.

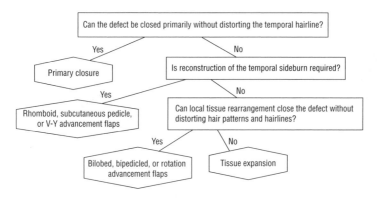

Fig. 29-4   Reconstruction algorithm: Parietal defects.

OCCIPITAL DEFECTS (Fig. 29-5)
- **Location:** Posterior scalp
- **Principles:** Region of moderate scalp mobility amenable to local tissue transfer; may require restoration or preservation of the occipital hairline
- **Small defects (<2 cm^2)**
  - Primary closure
- **Medium defects (2-25 cm^2)**
  - Rotation advancement flaps: Dissection carried over the trapezius and splenius capitis muscles to provide increased tissue gain

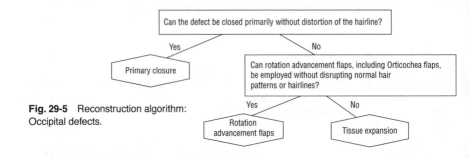

Fig. 29-5 Reconstruction algorithm: Occipital defects.

- **Large defects (>25 cm²)**
  - Larger rotation flaps
  - **Orticochea flaps** (Fig. 29-6)
    - ▸ Classically described for reconstruction of the occipital scalp
    - ▸ Three-flap technique improves flap vascularity over the four-flap technique and decreases postoperative alopecia and wound complications

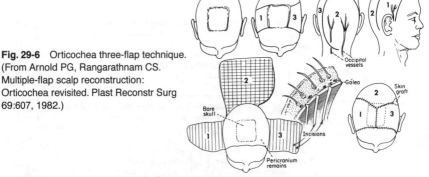

Fig. 29-6 Orticochea three-flap technique. (From Arnold PG, Rangarathnam CS. Multiple-flap scalp reconstruction: Orticochea revisited. Plast Reconstr Surg 69:607, 1982.)

TIP: Tissue expansion routinely gives a superior result.

VERTEX DEFECTS (Fig. 29-7)

- **Location:** Central scalp
- **Principles:** Area of limited scalp mobility; requires extensive undermining and recruitment of tissue from the more mobile regions; characteristic whorl pattern of hair growth should be preserved
- **Small defects (<2 cm²)**
  - Primary closure after subgaleal dissection; up to 4 cm wide described
  - Pinwheel flaps and adjacent rhomboid flaps particularly suited to reconstructing whorl pattern
- **Medium defects (2-25 cm²)**
  - Pinwheel and rhomboid flaps less useful but possible alternatives

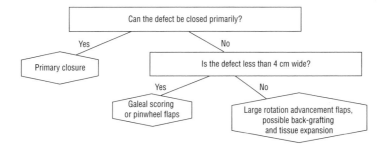

Fig. 29-7   Reconstruction algorithm: Vertex defects.

- Double-opposing rotation advancement flaps with incisions parallel to the hairline to prevent distortion
- Rotation advancement from the occiput with back-grafting of the donor site
- **Large defects (>25 cm²)**
  - Large rotation flaps that require almost complete scalp undermining and galeal scoring and possible back-grafting
  - Orticochea flaps **not** well suited for these defects because location does not allow a large third flap to cover donor site defect
  - Best results with tissue expansion

NEAR TOTAL DEFECTS[10-12]
- **Free tissue transfer:** Latissimus dorsi muscle, omentum, radial forearm fasciocutaneous, anterolateral thigh
  - Muscle flaps atrophy and contour well to skull over time; however, they can thin excessively and may result in exposed bone.
- **Integra** followed by skin grafting
- **Serial tissue expansion**

CALVARIAL RECONSTRUCTION[13-17]

- Goal is to provide protection for the brain and maintain normal calvarial shape

SURGICAL OPTIONS
- **Autogenous tissues**
  - **Split calvarial bone graft:** Parietal bone preferred because of increased thickness and absence of underlying venous sinuses
  - **Split rib graft:** If periosteum left intact the rib should regenerate
- **Alloplastic materials**
  - Methylmethacrylate over titanium mesh

KEY POINTS

- ✔ Scalp avulsions usually occur in the subgaleal plane.
- ✔ The scalp is highly vascularized and can be replanted from a single artery.
- ✔ Most scalp mobility occurs over the parietal region because of the temporoparietal fascia.
- ✔ Consider tissue expansion to achieve coverage with like tissue with acceptable scar placement.

REFERENCES

1. Abdul-Hassan HS, von Drasek Ascher G, Acland RD. Surgical anatomy and blood supply of the fascial layers of the temporal region. Plast Reconstr Surg 77:17-28, 1986.
2. Tolhurst DE, Carstens MH, Greco RJ, et al. The surgical anatomy of the scalp. Plast Reconstr Surg 87:603-612, 1991.
3. Williams PL, Warwick R, eds. Gray's Anatomy, 36th Brit ed. Philadelphia: Saunders, 1980.
4. Anson BJ. Surgical Anatomy, 6th ed. Philadelphia: Saunders, 1984.
5. Anderson JE, ed. Grant's Atlas of Anatomy, 8th ed. Baltimore: Williams & Wilkins, 1983.
6. Last RJ. Anatomy, Regional and Applied, 6th ed. London: Churchill, 1979.
7. Mosser SW, Guyuron B, Janis JE, et al. The anatomy of the greater occipital nerve: Implication for the etiology of migraine headaches. Plast Reconstr Surg 113:693-697, 2004.
8. Jackson IT. General considerations. In Local Flaps in Head and Neck Reconstruction. St Louis: Quality Medical Publishing, 2002.
9. Manders ER, Furrey JA. Skin expansion to eliminate large scalp defects. Plast Reconstr Surg 74:495, 1984.
10. Lutz BS, Wei FC, Chen HC, et al. Reconstruction of scalp defects with free flaps in 30 cases. Br J Plast Surg 51:186-190, 1998.
11. Pennington DG, Stern HS, Lee KK. Free-flap reconstruction of large defects of the scalp and calvarium. Plast Reconstr Surg 83:655-661, 1985.
12. Chicarilli ZN, Ariyan S, Cuono CB. Single-stage repair of complex scalp and cranial defects with the free radial forearm flap. Plast Reconstr Surg 77:577-585, 1986.
13. Freund RM. Scalp, calvarium and forehead reconstruction. In Aston SJ, Beasley RW, Thorne CHM, eds. Grabb and Smith's Plastic Surgery. Philadelphia: Lippincott, 1997, p 473.
14. Shestak KC, Ramasastry SS, Reconstruction of defects of the scalp and skull. In Cohen M, ed. Mastery of Plastic and Reconstructive Surgery, vol 2. Philadelphia: Lippincott, 1994, pp 830-841.
15. Elliott LF, Jurkiewicz MJ. Scalp and calvarium. In Jurkiewicz MJ, Mathes SJ, Krizek TJ, et al, eds. Plastic Surgery: Principles and Practice. St Louis: Mosby, 1990, pp 419-440.
16. Marchac D. Deformities of the forehead, scalp, and cranial vault. In McCarthy JG, ed. Plastic Surgery. Philadelphia: WB Saunders, 1990, pp 1538-1574.
17. Sood R. Scalp and calvarial reconstruction. In Achauer BM, Eriksson E, Kolk CV, et al, eds. Plastic Surgery: Indications, Operations, and Outcomes, vol 3. St Louis: Mosby, 2000.

30. Eyelid Reconstruction

Jason K. Potter

EYELID ANATOMY[1,2]

- The eyelids protect the eye from injury and excessive light and also prevent desiccation of the cornea (Fig. 30-1).
- The eyelids consist of **three lamella:**
  1. Outer lamella: Skin and orbicularis oculi muscle
  2. Middle lamella: Orbital septum
  3. Inner lamella: Tarsal plate, medial/lateral canthal tendons, capsulopalpebul fascia, and conjunctiva

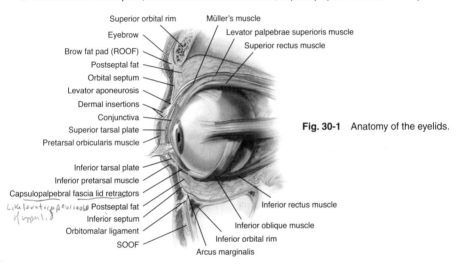

Superior orbital rim
Eyebrow
Brow fat pad (ROOF)
Postseptal fat
Orbital septum
Levator aponeurosis
Dermal insertions
Conjunctiva
Superior tarsal plate
Pretarsal orbicularis muscle

Inferior tarsal plate
Inferior pretarsal muscle
Capsulopalpebral fascia lid retractors
Like levator aponeurosis of upper l. Postseptal fat
Inferior septum
Orbitomalar ligament
SOOF

Müller's muscle
Levator palpebrae superioris muscle
Superior rectus muscle

Inferior rectus muscle
Inferior oblique muscle
Inferior orbital rim
Arcus marginalis

Fig. 30-1 Anatomy of the eyelids.

- Skin or orbicularis oculi
- Tarsoconjunctival layer

SKIN
- **Eyelid skin is the thinnest in the body.**
- Surgical incisions within the skin of the eyelid generally heal with almost imperceptible scarring.

ORBICULARIS OCULI (Fig. 30-2)
- Encircles the periorbital region
- Primary constrictor of the lids
- Innervated by the facial nerve (CN VII)
  - Runs on the deep surface of the muscle
- *Pretarsal fibers:* Lie over region of tarsal plate
  - Responsible for involuntary blink

287

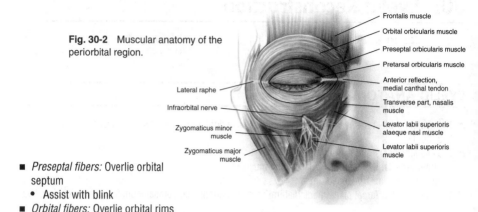

Fig. 30-2 Muscular anatomy of the periorbital region.

Labels:
- Frontalis muscle
- Orbital orbicularis muscle
- Preseptal orbicularis muscle
- Pretarsal orbicularis muscle
- Anterior reflection, medial canthal tendon
- Transverse part, nasalis muscle
- Levator labii superioris alaeque nasi muscle
- Levator labii superioris muscle
- Lateral raphe
- Infraorbital nerve
- Zygomaticus minor muscle
- Zygomaticus major muscle

- *Preseptal fibers:* Overlie orbital septum
  - Assist with blink
- *Orbital fibers:* Overlie orbital rims
  - Produce voluntary, forceful closure

SEPTUM
- Consists of a dense fibrous membrane attached to periosteum of orbital rim and extends through lid to join tarsus
- Separates orbital contents from periorbital soft tissues

TARSUS
- Located adjacent to lid margin
- Approximately 1-2 mm thick
- Laterally, tarsi become joined fibrous condensations, form canthal tendons
- **Upper lid**
  - Approximately 12-15 mm long cephalocaudally
  - Superior margin: Attachment site for Müller's muscle and levator aponeurosis
- **Lower lid**
  - Approximately 9-12 mm long cephalocaudally
  - Inferior margin continuous with capsulopalpebral fascia

CONJUNCTIVA
- Mucosal layer adjacent to the surface of eye
  - **Palpebral portion** lines inner surface of eyelid.
  - **Bulbar portion** lines sclera.

EYELID RETRACTORS
- **Upper lid**
  - **Müller's muscle** is innervated by the **sympathetic nervous system.**
    - This muscle arises from the inferior surface of the levator and inserts onto the superior edge of the tarsus.
    - *Loss of Müller's muscle function results in 2-3 mm of ptosis.*
  - The **levator palpebrae superioris** is innervated by the **superior division of CN III.**
    - This muscle originates from the lesser wing of the sphenoid, above the optic foramen, and extends forward to insert onto the superior edge of the tarsus.

▶ **Whitnall's ligament** serves as a fulcrum to redirect the vector of pull from a horizontal to a superior direction for lid retraction.

■ **Lower lid**
  • The **capsulopalpebral fascia** is a condensation of fibroelastic tissue anterior to Lockwood's ligament, which joins with the inferior tarsus.
  • The **capsulopalpebral fascia** serves as the **lower lid retractor.**
  • Smooth muscle fibers can be found in this condensation.

BLOOD SUPPLY (Fig. 30-3)

■ The **marginal** and **peripheral arcades** provide the primary blood supply to the lids. They are located approximately 2-3 mm from lid margin.
■ Contributions are made from both the **external and internal carotid systems.**
■ The **upper lid** is supplied primarily by **branches of the ophthalmic artery.**
■ The **lower lid** is supplied primarily by **branches of the facial artery.**

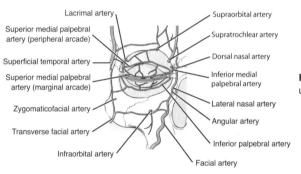

Lacrimal artery

Superior medial palpebral artery (peripheral arcade)

Superficial temporal artery

Superior medial palpebral artery (marginal arcade)

Zygomaticofacial artery

Transverse facial artery

Infraorbital artery

Supraorbital artery

Supratrochlear artery

Dorsal nasal artery

Inferior medial palpebral artery

Lateral nasal artery

Angular artery

Inferior palpebral artery

Facial artery

Fig. 30-3   Arterial supply to the upper lid.

INNERVATION

■ Sensory innervation is provided by the **trigeminal nerve.**
  • The **upper lid** is supplied by the **first division (V_1).**
  • The **lower lid** is supplied by the **second division (V_2).**

GENERAL PRINCIPLES[2-5]

Reconstruction of the eyelids requires a thorough assessment of involved structures and a determination of the amount of missing lid tissue.

■ Selection of appropriate reconstructive technique is based on **partial-** versus **full-thickness loss** and, more importantly, the **amount of missing tissue.**
■ Lid tissue is best reconstructed with lid tissue for optimal aesthetic outcome.

CAUTION: Use techniques that borrow tissue from the upper lid cautiously, because the upper lid makes significant contributions to lid function and protection.

■ Defects up to **35%** of the lid usually can be closed **primarily.**
■ Defects of **35%-50%** usually can be closed with addition of a **canthotomy and cantholysis.**
■ Defects of **50%-75%** usually can be closed with **myocutaneous advancement flaps.**
■ Defects **greater than 75%** generally require bringing **tissue from the opposite lid or adjacent regions** (cheek, temporal, forehead).

DEFECTS

PARTIAL-THICKNESS LOSS
- **Skin**
  - Loss of skin may be closed primarily or replaced with full-thickness skin grafts.
  - **Full-thickness grafts** are indicated to prevent excessive graft contraction.
  - **Skin from the contralateral lid** is the best source for a thickness match. Alternatively, post-auricular skin may be used.

> TIP: It is imperative not to create tension on the lid with primary closure, because this leads to ectropion.

- **Conjunctiva**
  - Losses of conjunctiva are best replaced by **advancement of adjacent conjunctiva.** When this is not possible, grafting is necessary.
    - **Buccal** or **nasal mucosae** are adequate donor grafts.
    - Nasal mucosa tends to contract less (20% versus 50%) than buccal mucosa.
    - Skin grafts are contraindicated because surface characteristics of the graft irritate the cornea.
    - Grafts of conjunctiva are subject to significant contraction and should be avoided.
- **Tarsus**
  - Loss of tarsal structure usually is part of a composite loss.
  - It either should be **repaired primarily** or **replaced with palatal mucosal grafts, cartilage grafts,** or **allografts** (e.g., AlloDerm®; LifeCell Corporation, Branchburg, NJ).

FULL-THICKNESS LOSS
- **Upper lid**
  - **Primary Closure**
    - Defects up to **25%-30%** of the lid may be closed primarily (Fig. 30-4).
    - In older patients with significant laxity, **40%** defects may be closed similarly.
    - When significant tension is present, **lateral canthotomy and cantholysis** may provide additional laxity for closure.
  - **Flap reconstruction**
    - **Tenzel semicircular flap**
      - Combining lateral canthotomy and cantholysis with a laterally based myocutaneous flap allows closure of defects up to **60%** of the upper lid (Fig. 30-5).

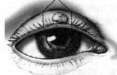
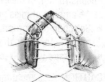

Fig. 30-4   Upper lid full-thickness excisions must be meticulously repaired in layers to avoid postoperative notching. (Modified from DiFrancesco LM, Codner MA, McCord CD. Upper eyelid reconstruction. Plast Reconstr Surg 114:98e-107e, 2004.)

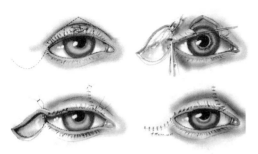

Fig. 30-5 The semicircular rotation flap, or Tenzel flap, is used for defects of 40%-60% of the upper eyelid. Lateral canthotomy is required to rotate the flap and lateral remaining lid margin. (Modified from DiFrancesco LM, Codner MA, McCord CD. Upper eyelid reconstruction. Plast Reconstr Surg 114:98e-107e, 2004.)

▸ **Cutler-Beard flap** (Fig. 30-6)
  • Two-stage procedure
  • Entails advancement of a full-thickness lower lid flap passed beneath the lower lid margin and sutured into the defect
  • Lacks support at the lid margin and requires cartilage grafting between the conjunctiva and muscle layers
  • Flap division performed at 3-6 weeks
▸ **Lid-sharing**
  • This procedure is used for defects of the central upper lid.
  • The flap is divided about week 6 and the donor site closed primarily.
▸ **Temporal forehead flap (Fricke flap)**
  • When adequate lid tissue is unavailable for donor tissue, temporally based flaps may be useful.
  • Tissue quality is thicker and less ideal; it should be reserved for special circumstances (Fig. 30-7).
▸ **Paramedian forehead flap** (Fig. 30-8)
  • This flap is useful for extensive defects.
  • It may be lined with mucosal grafts and cartilage with delayed placement, when needed for lid margin support.

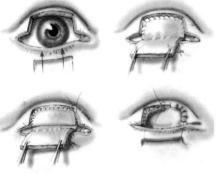

Fig. 30-6 The bridge flap, or Cutler-Beard flap, is used for total upper lid reconstruction. The flap is a biplanar flap passed under the lower lid margin. (Modified from DiFrancesco LM, Codner MA, McCord CD. Upper eyelid reconstruction. Plast Reconstr Surg 114:98e-107e, 2004.)

Fig. 30-7 Temporal forehead flap, or Fricke flap, is a transposition flap, from above the eyebrow, used for total upper lid reconstruction. (Modified from DiFrancesco LM, Codner MA, McCord CD. Upper eyelid reconstruction. Plast Reconstr Surg 114:98e-107e, 2004.)

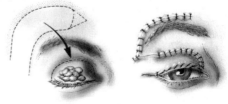

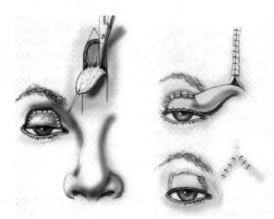

Fig. 30-8 A forehead flap can be used for total upper lid reconstruction, combined with a mucosal graft for a lining against the cornea. (Modified from DiFrancesco LM, Codner MA, McCord CD. Upper eyelid reconstruction. Plast Reconstr Surg 114:98e-107e, 2004.)

- **Lower lid**
  - **Primary closure**
    - ▶ Defects up to **25%-30%** of the lid may be closed primarily.
    - ▶ In older patients with significant laxity, **40%** defects may be closed similarly.

TIP: When significant tension is present, lateral canthotomy and cantholysis may provide additional laxity for closure.

  - **Flap reconstruction**
    - ▶ **Tripier flap** (Fig. 30-9)
      - ◆ This is a musculocutaneous flap used for partial-thickness coverage of the lower lid.
      - ◆ Originally described as a bipedicled flap, it also may be based on a single pedicle.

TIP: Defects extending past the pupil usually require a bipedicle technique to prevent distal necrosis.

Fig. 30-9 Lower eyelid reconstruction with a modified bipedicled musculocutaneous flap from the upper lid. Note that the flap pedicles are incorporated into the wound. (Modified from Levine MI, Leone CR. Bipedicle musculocutaneous flap repair of cicatricial ectropion. Ophthal Plast Reconstr Surg 6:119, 1990.)

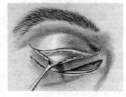 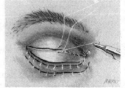

▶ **Tenzel semicircular flap** (Fig. 30-10)
  ♦ As with the upper lid, combining lateral canthotomy and cantholysis with a laterally based myocutaneous flap allows closure of defects up to **60%** of the upper lid.

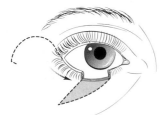

Fig. 30-10   Repair of a lower lid defect with myocutaneous semicircular flap. Outline shows the area of skin-muscle tissue usually needed to be resected to approximate lid edges after the flap has been rotated.

▶ **Hughes tarsoconjunctival flap** (Fig. 30-11)
  ♦ This two-stage procedure transfers conjunctival lining and a small portion of the superior tarsus for subtotal or total lower lid reconstruction.
  ♦ Skin coverage is provided by either flap or full-thickness skin grafting. The flap is divided at 4-6 weeks.

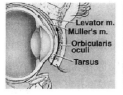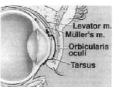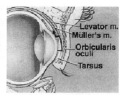

Fig. 30-11   *Left,* The Hughes flap as originally described in 1937. *Center,* The Hughes flap as modified in 1976. The new plane of dissection creates a true transconjunctival flap. *Right,* In this modification the inferior edge of the flap is designed at least 4 mm from the lid margin to ensure that sufficient tarsal plate remains in the donor lid. (Modified from Rohrich RJ, Zbar RIS. The evolution of the Hughes transconjunctival flap for lower eyelid reconstruction. Plast Reconstr Surg 104:518, 1999.)

▶ **Cheek advancement flap**   Mustarde?
  ♦ This flap is useful for total lower lid reconstruction.
  ♦ To prevent lid retraction, it is critical to provide tension-free mobilization of tissue into targeted site.

TIP: Elevation of a thin flap is helpful.

► **Locoregional flaps**
  • If adequate, quality lid tissue is unavailable for reconstruction, regional soft tissues may be used for lower lid reconstruction.
  • These tissues do not provide ideal quality tissue because of thickness (Fig. 30-12).

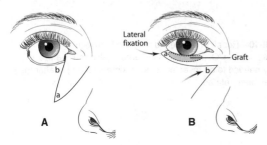

Fig. 30-12   Full-thickness reconstruction of lower lid with transpositional nasolabial flap. **A,** Lower lid defect and outline of transpositional flap for the nasolabial area. **B,** The nasolabial flap has been transposed to form the outer surface of the lower lid. The flap is lined with a free-mucous-membrane–lined graft.

KEY POINTS

✔ Up to 30% of the upper lid or lower lid can be closed primarily.
✔ Lateral canthotomy or cantholysis can permit primary closure of larger defects.
✔ Skin-only defects frequently can be reconstructed with contralateral eyelid skin.
✔ Conjunctival defects are best reconstructed using advancement of adjacent conjunctiva or by buccal or nasal mucosal grafts.
✔ Tarsal defects are best reconstructed with palatal grafts, conchal cartilage, or allografts (e.g., AlloDerm).
✔ Prevention of tension is critical to avoid ectropion.

REFERENCES

1. Hollinshead WH. Anatomy for Surgeons: The Head and Neck. Philadelphia: Lippincott, 1982.
2. DiFrancesco LM, Codner MA, McCord CD. Upper eyelid reconstruction. Plast Reconstr Surg 114:98e-107e, 2004.
3. Putterman AM. Reconstruction of the eyelids following resection for carcinoma. Clin Plast Surg 12:393-410, 1985.
4. Spinelli HM, Gelks GW. Periocular reconstruction: A systematic approach. Plast Reconstr Surg 91:1017-1024, 1993.
5. Rohrich RJ, Zbar RIS. The evolution of the Hughes tarsoconjunctival flap for lower eyelid reconstruction. Plast Reconstr Surg 104:518-522, 1999.

31. Nasal Reconstruction

Melissa A. Crosby

ANATOMY[1] (Fig. 31-1)

- Divided into thirds based on underlying skeletal structure (also called *vaults*)
  - **Proximal:** Lies over nasal bones
  - **Middle:** Lies over upper lateral cartilages
  - **Distal:** Includes nasal tip with paired alae over membranous septum
    - ▶ **Columella:** Supported by the medial crura of alar cartilages

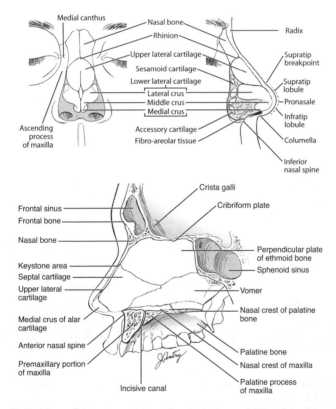

Fig. 31-1 Nasal anatomy. (From Gunter JP, Landecker A, Cochran CS. Nomenclature for frequently used grafts in rhinoplasty. Presented at the Twenty-second Annual Dallas Rhinoplasty Symposium, Dallas, TX, March 2005.)

BLOOD SUPPLY
- **Arterial**
  - **Angular artery** (branch of facial artery): Lateral surface of caudal nose
  - **Superior labial artery:** Nasal sill, nasal septum, and base of columella
  - **Dorsal nasal branch of ophthalmic artery:** Axial arterial network for dorsal and lateral nasal skin
  - **Infraorbital branch of internal maxillary artery:** Dorsum and lateral sidewalls of nose
- **Venous**
  - Venous drainage parallels arterial supply.

INNERVATION
- **Sensory**
  - **Ophthalmic division (V_1) of trigeminal nerve**
    - ▶ Radix, rhinion, and cephalic portion of nasal sidewalls, skin over dorsum to tip
  - **Maxillary division (V_2) of trigeminal nerve**
    - ▶ Lateral tissue on lower half of nose, columella, and lateral vestibule
- **Motor**
  - **Facial nerve VII**
    - ▶ Procerus, depressor septi nasi, and nasalis

SKIN ENVELOPE[2] (Table 31-1)

- **Upper two thirds of nose**
  - Thin, loose, and mobile
  - Few sebaceous glands
- **Lower third of nose**
  - Thick, less mobile
  - Majority of sebaceous glands
- **Zone of thin skin:** Dorsum and columella
- **Zone of thick skin:** Nasal tip and ala

Table 31-1   *Skin Thickness by Location*

Nasal dorsum	1300 μm	Postauricular	800 μm
		Supraclavicular	1800 μm
Nasal lobule	2400 μm	Submental	2500 μm
		Nasolabial	2900 μm

From González-Ulloa M. Restoration of the face covering by means of selected skin in regional aesthetic units. Br J Plast Surg 9:212, 1956.

DEFECT ANALYSIS

ASSESSMENT OF DEFECT
- Location
- Depth
  - Skin and soft tissue coverage

- Cartilage and bone
- Lining

■ Dimensions of defect

GOALS OF RECONSTRUCTION
■ Maintain airway patency
■ Replace missing layers with similar tissue
■ Minimize morbidity
■ Optimize aesthetics

AESTHETIC SUBUNITS OF NOSE (BURGET AND MENICK)[3,4] (Fig. 31-2)

TIP: Not all authors believe in aesthetic subunit reconstruction.

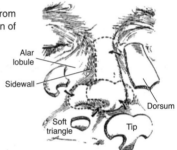

Fig. 31-2   Aesthetic subunits of the nose. (From Burget GC, Menick FJ. Aesthetic Reconstruction of the Nose. St Louis: Mosby, 1994, p 7.)

■ **Rules**
  - If a defect occupies more than 50% of a subunit, enlarge defect to incorporate entire subunit.
  - Use undamaged contralateral subunit as reconstructive model.
  - Divide large defects into multiple defects.

RECONSTRUCTION OF SKIN AND SOFT TISSUE[5,6]

GLABELLA AND MEDIAL CANTHAL DEFECTS
■ Defects ≤ 1 cm heal with best aesthetic result by secondary intention.
■ Larger defects may need flap reconstruction.
■ **Glabellar flap** (McGregor)[7] uses redundant skin in glabella and transfers onto root and upper bridge of nose to repair defects in this area.

NASAL DORSUM AND SIDEWALLS
■ **Banner flap (Elliot)**[8] (Fig. 31-3)
  - Transverse narrow triangular flap of skin from the nasal dorsum adjacent to defect
  - Used for defects 0.7-1.2 cm in diameter
  - Can lengthen and place on side opposite defect, which increases flap reach and elevates nostrils to achieve symmetry

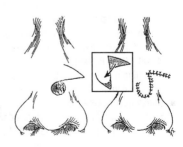

Fig. 31-3   Banner flap. (From Muzaffar AR, English JM. Nasal reconstruction. Sel Read Plast Surg 9[13], 2000.)

- **Bilobed flap (Esser and Zitelli)[9,10]** (Fig. 31-4)
  - Bilobed flap is flap of choice for defects 0.5 to 1.5 cm in **thick-skinned areas.**
  - **Zitelli modification**
    - ▸ Allow no more than 50 degrees of rotation for each lobe (100 degrees total).
    - ▸ Excise a triangle of skin between the defect and the pivot point before rotation (the pivot point lies one radius from the defect); design the flap as large as the nose allows; place the second lobe in thin and loose skin of sidewall or upper dorsum (avoid placing it close to the alar margin or medial canthus).
    - ▸ Undermine widely just above the perichondrium and periosteum.
    - ▸ Make diameter of first lobe equal to that of the defect; reduce width of second flap to allow easy donor site closure (but make sure it closes the defect of the first donor).

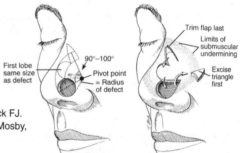

Fig. 31-4 Bilobed flap. (From Burget GC, Menick FJ. Aesthetic Reconstruction of the Nose. St Louis: Mosby, 1994, p 136.)

- Generally, use a laterally based design for defects of the tip, but a medial design for lobule defects.
- Position the pivot away from the alar margin and lower lid to prevent distortion.
- **Dorsal nasal flap (Rieger)[11]**
  - Based laterally and elevated on angular arteries
  - Entire skin of nasal dorsum rotated and advanced caudally
  - For defects of lobule less than 2 cm
  - Can place superior incision across root of nose, concealed in radix crease (Rohrich)[6]
- **Axial frontonasal flap (Marchac and Toth)[12]**
  - Based on vessels emerging at level of inner canthus
  - Pedicle back-cut to a narrow vascular stalk near medial canthus
  - Glabellar portion redundant as flap rotated, and Burow's triangles used to equalize two sides of Y closure
- **Axial nasodorsum flap**
  - Combines pedicle of the nasalis flap with dorsal nasal branches of the ophthalmic artery to encompass territory similar to frontonasal flap
  - Whole nasal dorsal skin elevated and transferred inferiorly for reconstruction of lobule
  - Burow's triangles cut above eyebrows to increase downward mobility
- **Nasalis flap (Rybka)[13]**
  - Sliding nasalis musculocutaneous flap from the upper alar crease with approximately 1.25 cm advancement to repair small defects of lateral tip
- **Cheek advancement flap**
  - Used for replacement of nasal sidewall, especially in elderly patients
  - Up to 2.5 cm^2 of paranasal and cheek areas can be advanced with primary closure of donor site

- **Nasolabial flap** (Fig. 31-5)
  - Superiorly or inferiorly based
  - Good for alar reconstruction and lateral nasal wall
  - May need cartilage graft for alar support
  - Can design as transposition flap in single stage

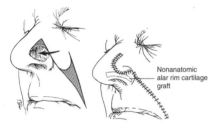

Nonanatomic alar rim cartilage graft

Fig. 31-5   Nasolabial flap. (From Rohrich RJ, Barton FE, Hollier L. Nasal reconstruction. In Aston SJ, Beasley RW, Thorne HM, et al, eds. Grabb and Smith's Plastic Surgery, 5th ed. Philadelphia: Lippincott, 1997, p 518.)

- **Turnover flap (Spear et al)**[14]
  - Flap of nasolabial skin on a subcutaneous pedicle based at piriform aperture
  - Flap turned 180 degrees and rotated at a right angle to its base to furnish lining for nostril
  - Folded on itself to provide external cover
  - Donor site closed primarily
- **Sliding flap**
  - Splitting of dorsal nasal skin from nasal lining and rotation
  - Advancement of nasolabial tissue onto lower nose
  - Incisions placed at junction of aesthetic subunits to hide scars
- **Forehead flap** (Fig. 31-6)
  - Most useful flap for tip, lobule, subtotal, and total nasal reconstruction
  - Midline or paramedian based on **supratrochlear** or **supraorbital** vessels from one or both sides
  - 2.5-3.0 cm can be taken from central forehead with primary closure
  - Can cant obliquely if patient's forehead is less than 3 cm along hairline or into hair-bearing scalp for 1.5 cm; use with caution in smokers

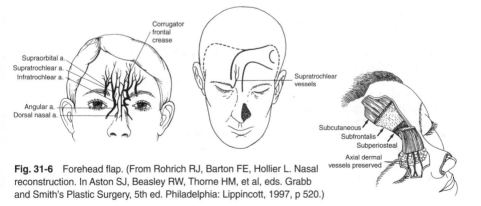

Fig. 31-6   Forehead flap. (From Rohrich RJ, Barton FE, Hollier L. Nasal reconstruction. In Aston SJ, Beasley RW, Thorne HM, et al, eds. Grabb and Smith's Plastic Surgery, 5th ed. Philadelphia: Lippincott, 1997, p 520.)

> TIP: Base forehead flap off vessels contralateral to defect to decrease arc of rotation and subsequent pedicle kinking.

- **Expanded forehead flap**
  - Place expanders and stretch over weeks or intraoperatively.
  - Problems occur with prelaminating nose and unpredictable rebound contraction.
  - Main indication is to expand lateral forehead skin to allow primary closure in large paramedian flaps.
- **Gull winged flap (Millard)**[15]
  - Modification of forehead flap combines generous amount of skin distally for extensive lobular reconstruction; pedicle is only 1 inch wide
  - "Wings" lie transversely on forehead, and scars are hidden in natural skin creases.
- **Up and down flap (Gilles)**[16]
  - Reconstruction of entire nasal lobule is possible.
  - Flap is longer and wider than paramedian forehead flap.
  - Donor site cannot be closed primarily.
- **Scalping flap (Converse)**[17] (Fig. 31-7)
  - Repair of total or near-total defects
  - Elevated through a coronal incision just behind the superficial temporal artery, extending to a skin paddle in the contralateral forehead
  - Frontalis muscle not carried in the distal end of flap, but remainder of pedicle dissected in subgaleal plane
  - Donor site on forehead closed with full thickness skin graft
  - Scalp defect dressed with nondesiccating dressing or interim split-thickness skin graft

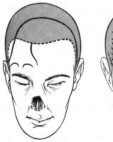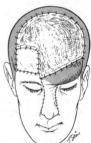

Fig. 31-7 Scalping flap. (From Rohrich RJ, Barton FE, Hollier L. Nasal reconstruction. In Aston SJ, Beasley RW, Thorne HM, et al, eds. Grabb and Smith's Plastic Surgery, 5th ed. Philadelphia: Lippincott, 1997, p 521.)

- **Sickle flap (New)**[18]
  - Donor site in lateral forehead
  - Randomly vascularized so requires delay
  - Problems with pedicle kink and crossing over eyelid
  - Multiple modifications but outcomes poor with any method
- **Frontotemporal flap (Schmid and Meyer)**[19,20]
  - Tubular flap with an internal supraciliary pedicle carrying lateral forehead skin with embedded ear cartilage to tip of nose or ala
  - Narrow horizontal pedicle courses above brow from glabella to temple
  - Young patients with low hairlines
- **Temporomastoid flap (Loeb and Hunt)**[21,22]
  - Also called the **Washio flap**[23]
  - Carries postauricular skin as flap based on superficial temporal arteries
  - Allows thin (auricular) and thick (mastoid) skin transfer
  - Ample hairless skin for complete nasal coverage
  - Auricular cartilage availability

- No flap delay
- No visible facial scars

NASAL TIP AND ALAE

- **Chondrocutaneous composite grafts**
  - Small through-and-through defects of alar rim
  - Donor site ear
  - Maximum safe size is 1.5 cm

SKELETAL/CARTILAGINOUS SUPPORT

BASIC INFORMATION

- Nasal bone widest at nasofrontal suture (14 mm) and narrowest at nasofrontal angle (10 mm)
- Nasal bone thickest superiorly at nasofrontal angle (6 mm) and progressively becomes thinner toward tip
- Screws for fixation placed usually 5-10 mm below nasofrontal angle where bone is 3-4 mm thick

MIDLINE SUPPORT

- **Strut technique (Gilles)[24]**
  - Longitudinal piece of bone or cartilage seated on the nasal radix with extension along the dorsum to the tip where it is bent sharply to rest on the anterior nasal spine
- **Hinged septal flap (Millard)[25]** (Fig. 31-8)
  - L-shaped flap of septum hinged superiorly to augment nasal angle
  - Septal flap carved from remaining septum and hinged on the caudal end of the nasal bones to pivot upward
- **Septal pivot flap (Burget and Menick)[7]**
  - Lining and dorsal skeletal support with a composite flap of septum pivoting anteriorly
  - Entire septum pulled forward out of nasal cavity on narrow pedicle centered over septal branch of superior labial artery
  - Cantilever graft of rib cartilage rongeured through hard tissues of septum and wired to nasal bones
- **Cantilever graft (Converse and Millard)[26,27]**
  - Longitudinal piece of bone extends along dorsum down to tip
  - Graft either secures to frontal bone, nasal bones, or both
  - May use osteocartilaginous rib segment

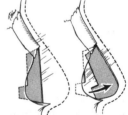

Fig. 31-8   Hinged septal flap. (From Muzaffar AR, English JM. Nasal reconstruction. Sel Read Plast Surg 9[13]:5, 2000.)

ANATOMIC ALAR SUPPORT

- **Anatomic alar grafts**
  - Use autogenous cartilage grafts that are anatomically shaped and bent to resemble normal lateral crura and fixed to the residual medial crura or columella strut.
  - Proposed advantages over extraanatomic grafts are improved alar rim correction with less nostril distortion and columellar retraction.

NONANATOMIC ALAR SUPPORT

Cartilage grafts stiffen nasal ala without compromising patency of airway.

- **Alar batten graft** (Fig. 31-9)
  - Used for alar collapse and external nasal valve obstruction
  - Fashioned to span collapse usually caudal to existing lateral third of lateral crus and extend to piriform aperture
  - Placed cephalad to alar rim and therefore limited in use for correcting alar rim retraction
- **Lateral crural strut graft** (Fig. 31-10)
  - Autogenous cartilage graft placed between the deep surface of the lateral crus and the vestibular skin, and sutured to the crus
  - Measures 3-4 mm wide and 20-25 mm long
  - Lateral end of strut extends to piriform rim and positioned caudal to the alar groove and accessory cartilages
  - Used for alar rim retraction and lateral crural malposition

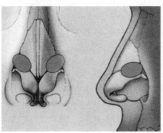

Fig. 31-9   Alar batten graft. (From Gunter JP, Landecker A, Cochran CS. Nomenclature for frequently used grafts in rhinoplasty. Presented at the Twenty-second Annual Dallas Rhinoplasty Symposium, Dallas, TX, March 2005.)

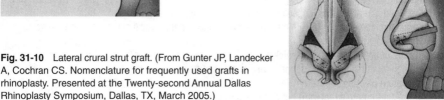

Fig. 31-10   Lateral crural strut graft. (From Gunter JP, Landecker A, Cochran CS. Nomenclature for frequently used grafts in rhinoplasty. Presented at the Twenty-second Annual Dallas Rhinoplasty Symposium, Dallas, TX, March 2005.)

- **Alar spreader graft** (Fig. 31-11)
  - Corrects pinched-tip deformities and alar or internal nasal valve collapse
  - Bar-shaped or triangular graft inserted between the vestibular and the underneath surface of the remaining lateral crura to force the crura apart

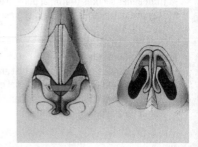

Fig. 31-11   Alar spreader graft. (From Gunter JP, Landecker A, Cochran CS. Nomenclature for frequently used grafts in rhinoplasty. Presented at the Twenty-second Annual Dallas Rhinoplasty Symposium, Dallas, TX, March 2005.)

- **Alar contour graft** (Fig. 31-12)
  - Autogenous cartilage buttress inserted through an infracartilaginous incision into an alar-vestibular pocket inferior and lateral to rim of the crus
  - Reestablishment of a normally functioning external nasal valve and aesthetically pleasing alar contour

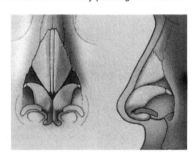

Fig. 31-12 Alar contour graft. (From Gunter JP, Landecker A, Cochran CS. Nomenclature for frequently used grafts in rhinoplasty. Presented at the Twenty-second Annual Dallas Rhinoplasty Symposium, Dallas, TX, March 2005.)

ALLOPLASTS
All used in combination with autogenous tissue.
- **Vitallium or titanium mesh** for dorsal framework
  - Advantages: Pliable, easily stabilized to dorsal and lateral nasal walls, readily accessible
  - Disadvantages: Implant exposure and infection
- **Porous polyethylene** (Medpor®; Porex Surgical, Newnan, GA) available as a strut or sheet
  - Advantages: Incorporated into tissue, readily accessible
  - Disadvantages: Multiple implants required, implant exposure, infection

LINING RECONSTRUCTION

TIP: Lining reconstruction is the most critical aspect of reconstruction.

- **Turn-in nasal flap (Keegan)**[28]
  - Flap hinged on the outer cicatricial edge and flipped over to span defect
- **Folded extranasal flap**
  - Can be forehead, nasolabial, or superiorly based upper lip flap turned in
- **Skin graft to forehead flap**
  - Skin graft applied to undersurface of forehead flap
  - May include cartilage
  - Hard palate mucosa can also be used
- **Septal door flap (deQuervain)**[29] (Fig. 31-13)
  - Septal mucosa is removed ipsilateral to defect and appropriately sized flap of septal cartilage is dissected.
  - Septal door is then made on a dorsal hinge toward the reconstructive side so that septal mucosa on far side bridges the wound and lines the airway.
  - Caudal flap reach is limited to border of upper lateral cartilages.

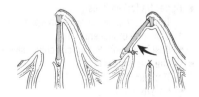

Fig. 31-13 Septal door flap. (From Muzaffar AR, English JM. Nasal reconstruction. Sel Read Plast Surg 9[13]:9, 2000.)

- **Septal mucoperichondrial flap (Gilles[24] and Burget and Menick[30])** (Fig. 31-14)
  - Large rectangle of mucosa or a composite of mucosa and perichondrium is elevated from septum, based on the septal branch of superior labial artery.
  - Flap pivots on an anterior-inferior point near nasal spine and folds outward to furnish lining to nasal domes.

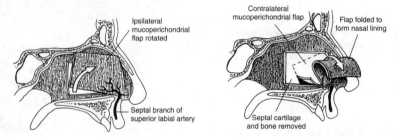

Fig. 31-14   Septal mucoperichondrial flap. (From Burget GC, Menick FJ. Nasal suport and lining: The marriage of beauty and blood supply. Plast Reconstr Surg 84:189, 1989.)

- **Mucosal advancement flap (Burget and Menick)[30]**
  - Bipedicled mucosal advancement flap is based medially on remaining septum and laterally at the piriform aperture.
  - Flap is based on the lateral floor of vestibule and advanced medially to resurface small lining defects of nasal ala.

COLUMELLAR RECONSTRUCTION

NASOLABIAL FLAPS (Fig. 31-15)
- Bilateral flaps are tunneled or rolled inward to line the vestibules and create a central post.

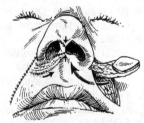

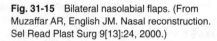

Fig. 31-15   Bilateral nasolabial flaps. (From Muzaffar AR, English JM. Nasal reconstruction. Sel Read Plast Surg 9[13]:24, 2000.)

- **Upper lip forked flaps**
  - Transverse flaps forked from upper lip
  - Unilateral or bilateral
  - Best indication: Superficial columellar loss in an elderly, long-lipped patient
- **Vestibular flaps (Mavili)[31]**
  - Transfer of internal nasal vestibular skin flap combined with bilateral labial mucosa flaps
  - No external scars
- **Forehead flap**
  - Millard prefers extension of forehead flap to reconstruct columella
- **Chondrocutaneous grafts (Paletta and Van Norman)[32]**
  - Auricular composite grafts

TOTAL NASAL RECONSTRUCTION

> TIP: Nose may be prefabricated using cartilage and lining under forehead flap or other large flap.

- **Free flaps:** Used only when forehead flap not available
  - Radial forearm free flap
  - Serratus anterior free flap
  - Dorsalis pedis free flap
  - Postauricular free flap
  - Helix free flap
  - Deltopectoral free flap

RHINOPHYMA

Sebaceous hyperplasia of nasal skin with bulbous enlargement of nose and erythematous skin.
- 12 times more common in men than women
- Typical patient is white male in his sixties.
- Represents a severe form of **acne rosacea** but **has no true association with alcohol intake**
- Malignant degeneration into basal cell carcinoma higher in these patients; reported 15%-30% but likely lower

TREATMENT
- **Nonsurgical**
  - Good skin hygiene
  - Tetracycline
  - Isotretinoin (Accutane®)
  - Metronidazole topical (Metrogel®)
- **Surgical**
  - Tangential excision of skin and hypertrophic appendages using cold knife excision, dermaplaning, or dermabrasion
  - Placement of nondesiccating, bacteriostatic dressings to promote reepithelialization
  - Outcomes similar among excision methods

KEY POINTS
- ✔ It is essential to know blood supply and innervation to various parts of nose.
- ✔ The forehead flap is the workhorse for nasal tip reconstruction.
- ✔ Forehead flap dissection starts subcutaneous to subfrontalis to subperiosteal, from distal to proximal.
- ✔ It is important to follow Zitelli design principles for bilobed flaps.
- ✔ Rhinophyma is 12 times more common in men than women; it is not associated with alcohol.

REFERENCES

1.   Oneal RM, Beil FJ, Schlesinger J. Surgical anatomy of the nose. Clin Plast Surg 23:195, 1996.
2.   González-Ulloa M. Restoration of the face covering by means of selected skin in regional aesthetic units. Br J Plast Surg 9:212, 1956.
3.   Burget GC, Menick FJ. Aesthetic Reconstruction of the Nose. St Louis: Mosby, 1994.
4.   Burget GC, Menick FJ. Nasal support and lining: The marriage of beauty and blood supply. Plast Reconstr Surg 84:189, 1989.
5.   Muzaffar AR, English JM. Nasal reconstruction. Sel Read Plast Surg 9(13), 2000.
6.   Rohrich RJ, Barton FE, Hollier L. Nasal reconstruction. In Aston SJ, Beasley RW, Thorne CHM, eds. Grabb and Smith's Plastic Surgery, 5th ed. Philadelphia: Lippincott, 1997.
7.   McGregor IA. Fundamental Techniques of Plastic Surgery and Their Surgical Application. Edinburgh: Livingston, 1960, p 160.
8.   Elliot RA Jr. Rotation flaps of the nose. Plast Reconstr Surg 44:147, 1969.
9.   Esser JFS. Gestielte lokale nasenplastik mit zweizipfligen lappen, deckung des sekundaren defektes vom ersten zipfel durch den zweiten. Dtsch Z Chir 143:385, 1918.
10. Zitelli JA. The bilobed flap for nasal reconstruction. Arch Dermatol 125:957, 1989.
11. Rieger RA. A local flap for repair of the nasal tip. Plast Reconstr Surg 40:147, 1967.
12. Marchac D, Toth D. The axial frontonasal flap revisited. Plast Reconstr Surg 76:686, 1985.
13. Rybka FJ. Reconstruction of the nasal tip using nasalis myocutaneous sliding flaps. Plast Reconstr Surg 71:40, 1983.
14. Spear SL, Kroll SS, Romm S. A new twist to the nasolabial flap for reconstruction of lateral alar defects. Plast Reconstr Surg 79:915, 1987.
15. Millard DR Jr. Reconstructive rhinoplasty for the lower half of a nose. Plast Reconstr Surg 53:133, 1974.
16. Gilles HD. The development and scope of plastic surgery (The Charles H Mayo Lectureship in Surgery, Fourth Lecture). Bull Northwestern Univ Med Sch 35:1, 1935.
17. Converse JM. New forehead flap for nasal reconstruction. Proc R Soc Med 35:811, 1942.
18. New GB. Sickle flap for nasal reconstruction. Surg Gynecol Obstet 80:497, 1945.
19. Schmid E. Uber die Haut-Knorpel-transplantationen aus der Ohrmuschel und ihre funktionelle und asthetische Bedeutung gei der Dechung von Gesichtsdefekten. Fortschr Kiefer-Gesictschir 7:48, 1961.
20. Meyer R. Aesthetic refinements in nose reconstruction. Aesthetic Plast Surg 24:241, 2000.
21. Loeb R. Temporo-mastoid flap for reconstruction of the cheek. Rev Lat Am Chir Plast 6:185, 1962.
22. Hunt HL. Plastic Surgery of the Head, Face, and Neck. Philadelphia: Lea & Febiger, 1926.
23. Washio H. Retroauricular temporal flap. Plast Reconstr Surg 43:162, 1969.
24. Gilles HD. Plastic Surgery of the Face. London: Oxford, 1920.
25. Millard DR Jr. Hemirhinoplasty. Plast Reconstr Surg 40:440, 1967.
26. Converse JM, ed. Reconstructive Plastic Surgery, vol 2, 2nd ed. Philadelphia: Saunders, 1977.
27. Millard DR Jr. Total reconstructive rhinoplasty and a missing link. Plast Reconstr Surg 37:167, 1966.
28. Ivy RH. Repair of acquired defects of the face. JAMA 84:181, 1925.
29. deQuervain F. Ueber patielle seitliche rhinoplstik. Zentralbl Chir 29:297, 1902.
30. Burget GC, Menick FJ. Nasal reconstruction: Seeking a fourth dimension. Plast Reconstr Surg 78:145, 1986.
31. Mavili ME, Akyurek M. Congenital isolated absence of nasal columella: Reconstruction with an internal nasal vestibular skin flap and bilateral labial mucosa flaps. Plast Reconstr Surg 106:393, 2000.
32. Paletta FX, Van Norman RT. Total reconstruction of the columella. Plast Reconstr Surg 30:322, 1962.

32. Cheek Reconstruction

David W. Mathes
C. Alejandra Garcia

ANATOMY

- **Soft tissue**
  - **Subcutaneous musculoaponeurotic system (SMAS):** Underlies the subcutaneous tissue and skin of the cheek.
- **Muscular**
  - Inferior portion of the orbicular oculi
  - Zygomaticus muscles
  - Masseter muscle
- **Blood supply**
  - End branches of the **external carotid artery**
    - ▶ Facial artery
- **Sensory innervation**
  - Infraorbital nerve
  - Mental nerve
  - Mandibular nerve
  - Great auricular nerve

AESTHETIC UNITS OF THE CHEEK

The cheek is divided into three overlapping aesthetic zones[1] (Fig. 32-1).

ZONE 1: SUBORBITAL
- **Medial boundary:** Nasolabial line
- **Lateral boundary:** Anterior sideburn
- **Inferior boundary:** Gingival sulcus
- **Superior boundary:** Skin of the lower eyelid
- **Can be subdivided into three subunits**
  - **A subunit:** Skin of the malar region up to a line drawn from lateral edge of the eyebrow
  - **B subunit:** Skin lateral to a line drawn perpendicular to the lateral edge of the eyebrow
  - **C subunit:** Skin of the lower eyelid up to its junction with the cheek skin

ZONE 2: PREAURICULAR
- Superolateral junction of the helix and cheek
- Medially across sideburn to malar eminence
- Inferiorly to the mandible

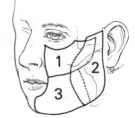

Fig. 32-1　Three overlapping zones of the cheek aesthetic unit. (Modified from Zide BM. Deformities of the lips and cheeks. In McCarthy JR, ed. Plastic Surgery. Philadelphia: WB Saunders, 1990.)

ZONE 3: BUCCOMANDIBULAR
- Includes the lower cheek area and oral lining (in full-thickness defects)
- Inferior to suborbital area
- Anterior to the preauricular zone

TIP:　Zones 1 and 2 can be reconstructed with cervicofacial flaps, whereas zone 3 cannot.

RECONSTRUCTIVE OPTIONS[2]

ZONE 1: SUBORBITAL
- **Primary closure**
  - Smaller lesions can be closed with an elliptical excision in the direction of natural relaxed skin tension lines (RSTLs).
  - Care should be taken not to distort structures such as the lower lid.
- **Skin Grafts**
  - **Full-thickness** skin grafts should be used.
  - **Best harvest sites** include:
    - ▶ Preauricular
    - ▶ Postauricular
    - ▶ Supraclavicular
  - Templates of the defect ensure adequate size and shape. Skin grafts used for lesions with a depth greater than 5 mm often result in a suboptimal result.[3]
- **Local skin flaps** *(lesions less than 4 cm)*
  - **Rhomboid flaps** (Fig. 32-2)
    - ▶ The flap should be designed so that donor site scar is in the direction of the relaxed tension lines.
    - ▶ The flap should be **inferiorly based** when possible to avoid trap-door effect and minimize postoperative edema.

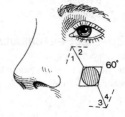

Fig. 32-2　Rhomboid flap. (Modified from Zide BM. Deformities of the lips and cheeks. In McCarthy JR, ed. Plastic Surgery. Philadelphia: WB Saunders, 1990.)

- **Circular flaps**[4] (Fig. 32-3)
  - ▸ The defect does not need to be rhomboid but can be circular (see Fig. 32-2), which increases the versatility of the rhomboid design.
  - ▸ The angle should be **60 degrees.**

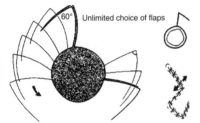

Fig. 32-3 Circular rhomboid flap: Modified rhomboid flap for closure of a circular defect. There is a better distribution of tension across the suture line by using a flap smaller than the defect and allowing the surrounding skin to participate in the closure. (Modified from Zide BM. Deformities of the lips and cheeks. In McCarthy JR, ed. Plastic Surgery. Philadelphia: WB Saunders, 1990.)

- **Bilobed flap** (Fig. 32-4)
  - ▸ The **Zitelli modification** is recommended.
  - ▸ The flap divides the tension between the two advancement lobes.
  - ▸ It is best used for moderate to large central defects where the remaining lateral preauricular skin is used in the primary flap, and posterior auricular or cervical skin is used for secondary flap.
  - ▸ The disadvantage is multiple scars.

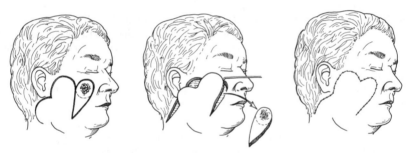

Fig. 32-4 Bilobed flap. (From Baker SR, Swanson NA. Local Flaps in Facial Reconstruction. St Louis: Mosby, 1995.)

TIP: Use a pinch test to make sure the donor defect of the secondary flap can be closed primarily.

- **Local flaps** *(lesions greater than 4 cm)*
  - **Cervicofacial flap**
    - ▸ Large surface defects of the cheek can be repaired.
    - ▸ Flaps bring tissue of excellent color, texture, hair, and contour match to the cheek.

- ▶ The Juri variant carries the dissection posteriorly along the mastoid hairline to create a generous-sized, rotation-advancement flap. Extensive undermining prevents excess tension at the suture lines (Fig. 32-5).

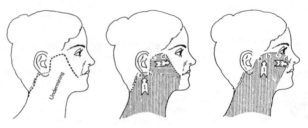

Fig. 32-5   Juri flap.

TIP: To prevent ectropion, anchor sutures to the periosteum along the zygomatic arch and infer-olateral orbital rim.[6]

- ▶ Crow and Crow[7] incorporated platysma into their neck flaps and emphasized the need to design the arc high in the temporal area. Flaps dissected subplatysmally carry the skin anterior to the clavicular border safely and directly.
- ▶ Because of the tenuous vascularity of the distal aspect of cervicofacial flaps, especially in smokers, most authors recommend a **deep-plane cervicofacial advancement** to reconstruct the malar, lateral orbit, and temporal regions. The resulting medial dog-ear is removed with a horizontal blepharoplasty incision.
- • **Inferolateral modification**
  - ▶ This usually requires incisions across the mandible and an extension to the contralateral neck.
  - ▶ Periosteal anchoring is required to avoid ectropion.

TIP: Consider anchoring all advancement flaps on the periosteal surface of the zygoma. It also may be necessary to perform a lateral canthopexy to prevent ectropion.

- ■ **Tissue expansion**
  - • Tissue expansion offers the best match for color and texture with the least number of additional incisions.
  - • Custom-made expanders are often needed for expansion in the cheek.
    - ▶ Two expanders are usually placed and expanded gradually over 6-8 weeks.
  - • Wieslander[8] lists the following guidelines for expansion in the head and neck region.
    - ▶ Orient the incision for expander placement perpendicular to the expander.
    - ▶ Choose an expander with length and width at least as large as the defect.
    - ▶ Fill expander intraoperatively to safest maximum level to reduce hematoma and seroma formation.
    - ▶ Delay expansion for about 2 weeks postoperatively then fill expander at least once per week.
    - ▶ Overexpand to a volume 30% to 50% more than necessary to overcome flap contraction at the second stage of surgery.
    - ▶ Incise the capsule as needed to increase the stretch of the expanded flap, but avoid capsulectomy.

- **Free flaps**
  - Radial forearm
  - Tensor fascia lata
  - Parascapular
  - Anterolateral thigh

ZONE 2: PREAURICULAR

- **Local flaps**
  - Vertical and posterior advancement flaps.
  - Skin laxity in this region allows for advancement as commonly performed for a face lift.
  - Preauricular incision with extension onto the neck can provide well-vascularized tissue for a wide range of defects.
- **Regional flaps**
  - **Anteriorly based cervicofacial flap**[9]
    - ▶ This flap is used for posterior and large anterior defects. The flap is elevated in the subcutaneous plane down to the clavicle, with blood supplied by the facial and submental arteries.
    - ▶ To avoid deep plane dissection, the platysma can be divided 4 cm below the mandible.
    - ▶ Platysma can be incorporated into the flap, which enhances vascularity.
    - ▶ Donor site may require skin grafting.
  - **Cervicopectoral flap**
    - ▶ For larger defects (6-10 cm)
    - ▶ Includes skin from the anterior chest
    - ▶ Platysma muscle, as well as deltoid and pectoral fascia, included
    - ▶ Brings the blood supply from the anterior thoracic perforators from the internal mammary artery
  - **Deltopectoral flap**
    - ▶ Medially based
    - ▶ Provides reliable, well-matched skin from shoulder
    - ▶ May be delayed with previous elevation or division of thoracoacromial vessels
  - **Pectoralis major flap**
    - ▶ May provide both cheek coverage and lining
    - ▶ Flap tends to be bulky
  - **Latissimus dorsi flap**
    - ▶ Flap may be transferred through a tunnel, over or through the pectoralis
    - ▶ Flap can bring bulk from outside a radiated area
- **Tissue expansion** (see earlier section)
- **Free flaps**
  - Radial forearm
  - Tensor fascia lata
  - Parascapular
  - Anterolateral thigh

ZONE 3: BUCCOMANDIBULAR

- Reconstruction may require cheek skin as well as lining and lip.
- If lining is required, this must be completed first to obtain a water-tight closure before skin closure.
- If no lining is required, all options are available.
- **Simple flaps**
  - Transposition flap (e.g., rhomboid flap as mentioned previously)
  - W- or Z-plasty possibly needed if the scar crosses the mandibular border

- **Large flap**
  - Inferiorly based advancement flap[10]
- **Tissue expansion**
- **Lining**
  - Hemitongue flap based on axial lingual artery
  - Turnover or hinge flaps: Donor site must be covered by another tissue source
  - Buccal fat-pad flap
  - Masseter crossover
- **Deep-plane composite flaps**[11]
  - These are for deeper complex defects and high-risk patients.
  - These include deeper subcutaneous fat and SMAS, which augment the blood supply to the flap as well as the mobility.
  - Drawbacks include increased operating time and risk of seventh nerve injury.
- **Free flaps** (defects usually greater than 10 cm or full-thickness): **Fasciocutaneous flaps** are the best option because they are relatively thin and do not atrophy.
  - Radial forearm
  - Tensor fascia lata
  - Parascapular
  - Lateral arm
  - Groin flap
  - Anterolateral thigh

CONTOUR DEFECTS

- **Associated with:**
  - Romberg's disease
  - Scleroderma
  - Facial lipodystrophy
  - First or second branchial arch syndrome
  - Significant facial trauma

RECONSTRUCTIVE OPTIONS

- **Collagen injections**
  - This is a temporary solution because it only lasts 6-12 months or less.
- **Dermal and dermal-fat grafts**[12]
  - Most of the fat is reabsorbed, but 85% percent of the graft bulk persists.
- **Autologous fat grafts**
  - There is a 55% decline in volume 12 months after injection.[13]
  - Fat should be injected in 1 cc aliquots.
  - Fat should be injected subcutaneously.
  - Surgically harvested fat survives better than suction harvested (42% versus 31%).[14]
- **Local deepithelialized flaps**
  - Use of a platysma has been described.
- **Free tissue transfer**
  - Deepithelialized groin flap: Short pedicle but good contour
  - Scapular flap: Longer and larger pedicle, uniform flap thickness

KEY POINTS

✔ Rebuild or resurface entire units.
✔ Use the contralateral as a guide.
✔ Use exact templates to design flaps.
✔ Avoid vertical incisions anterior to a line drawn perpendicular to the lateral canthus.
✔ Hide dog-ears in blepharoplasty incisions or in the nasolabial fold.
✔ Avoid ectropion by anchoring the flap to the underlying periosteum.

REFERENCES

1. Cabrera RC, Zide BM. Cheek reconstruction. In Aston SJ, Beasley RW, Thorne CHM, eds. Grabb and Smith's Plastic Surgery, 5th ed. Philadelphia: Lippincott, 1997.
2. Menick FJ. Reconstruction of the cheek. Plast Reconstr Surg 108:496-505, 2001.
3. Wagner J. Reconstructive considerations in the surgical management of melanoma. Surg Clin of North Am 83:187-230, 2003.
4. Quaba AA, Sommerlad BC. "A square peg into a round hole": A modified rhomboid flap and its clinical application. Br J Plast Surg 40:163-170, 1987.
5. Jelks GW, Jelks EB. Prevention of ectropion in reconstruction of facial defects. Clin Plast Surg 28:297-302, 2001.
6. Juri J, Juri C. Advancement and rotation of a large cervicofacial flap for cheek repairs. Plast Reconstr Surg 64:692-696, 1979.
7. Crow ML, Crow FJ. Resurfacing large cheek defects with rotation flaps from the neck. Plast Reconstr Surg 58:196-200, 1976.
8. Wieslander JB. Tissue expansion in the head and neck. A 6-year review. Scand J Plast Reconstr Hand Surg 25:47-56, 1991.
9. Kaplan I, Goldwyn RM. The versatility of the laterally based cervicofacial flap for cheek repairs. Plast Reconstr Surg 61:390-393, 1978.
10. Kroll SS, Reece GP, Robb G, et al. Deep-plane cervicofacial rotation-advancement flap for reconstruction of large cheek defects. Plast Reconstr Surg 94:88-93, 1994.
11. Al-Shunnar B, Manson PN. Cheek reconstruction with laterally based flaps. Clin Plast Surg 28:283-296, 2001.
12. Leaf N, Zarem HA. Correction of contour defects of the face with dermal and dermal-fat grafts. Arch Surg 105:715-719, 1972.
13. Hörl HW, Feller AM, Biemer E. Technique for liposuction fat reimplantation and long-term volume evaluation by magnetic resonance imaging. Ann Plast Surg 26:248-258, 1991.
14. Kononas TC, Bucky LP, Hurley C, et al. The fate of suctioned and surgically removed fat after reimplantation for soft-tissue augmentation: A volumetric and histologic study in the rabbit. Plast Reconstr Surg 91:763-768, 1993.

33. Ear Reconstruction

Amanda A. Gosman
Edward M. Reece

ANATOMY

CARTILAGINOUS FRAMEWORK: THREE TIERS (Fig. 33-1)
- Conchal complex
- Antihelix-antitragus complex
- Helix-lobule complex

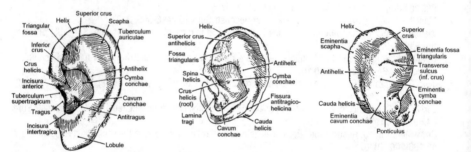

Fig. 33-1 Anatomy of external ear and landmarks of auricular cartilage. (From Hackney FL. Plastic surgery of the ear. Sel Read Plast Surg. 9[16], 2001.)

MUSCULATURE[1]
- **Vestigial intrinsic muscles**
  - Helicis major and minor
  - Tragicus
  - Antitragicus
- **Cranial surface muscles**
  - Intrinsic transverse
  - Intrinsic oblique
- **Extrinsic (auricularis) musculature**
  - Anterior
  - Superior
  - Posterior

BLOOD SUPPLY[2] (Fig. 33-2)
- **Posterior auricular artery** *(dominant blood supply)*
  - Supplies anterior and posterior surface of the auricle
  - Perforators enter ear at medial aspect of triangular fossa, cymba conchae, cavum conchae, helical root, and earlobe

Fig. 33-2 A, The arterial supply of the anterior surface of the ear is supplied by one main subbranch *(●)* of the superficial temporal artery *(STA)* and the perforating branches of posterior auricular artery *(PAA)*. *Up, Md,* and *Lo* designate upper, middle, and lower final branches of the superficial temporal artery, respectively. **B,** Arterial supply of the posterior ear. Arrows show the perforating branches of the posterior auricular artery at the triangular fossa *(Tr)*, helical root *(HR)*, cavum conchae *(CaC)*, and earlobe *(Lb)*. (From Park C, Lineaweaver WC, Rumley TO, et al. Arterial supply of the anterior ear. Plast Reconstr Surg 90:38, 1992.)

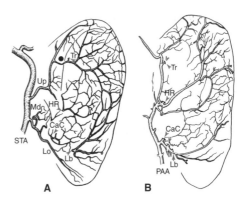

A   **B**

- **Superficial temporal artery**
  - Supplies lateral surface of the auricle
  - Interconnections between posterior auricular and superficial temporal arteries allow perfusion from each system alone
- **Occipital artery**
  - Supplies posterior auricular skin in approximately 7% of population
- **Venous drainage**
  - Posterior auricular veins (drain into external jugular system)
  - Superficial temporal
  - Retromandibular veins

NERVOUS SYSTEM[1,3]

- **Great auricular nerve** (C2-C3)
  - Supplies lower lateral portion and inferior cranial surface of ear
- **Auriculotemporal nerve** (V3)
  - Supplies superior lateral surface and anterior superior surface of external acoustic meatus
- **Lesser occipital nerve** (C2-C3)
  - Supplies superior cranial surface of ear
- **Arnold's nerve** (CN VII, CN XI, CN X)
  - Auricular branch of vagus nerve (CN X) that receives contributions from facial nerve (CN VII) and glossopharyngeal nerve (CN IX)
  - Supplies posterior inferior external auditory canal and meatus, and inferior conchal bowl
  - Mediates clinical phenomena, such as referred otalgia from other structures within the head and neck, and the initiation of coughing during manipulation of the ear canal

LYMPHATIC DRAINAGE[4]

- Drainage correlates with six embryologic hillocks.
- The **tragus, root of the helix,** and **superior helix** arise from **first** branchial arch (anterior hillocks 1-3) and drain to parotid nodes.
- The **antihelix, antitragus,** and **lobule** arise from **second** branchial arch (posterior hillocks 4-6) and drain to cervical nodes.

AESTHETIC RELATIONSHIPS OF THE EAR[5]

- Ear is located one ear-length posterior to lateral orbital rim.
- Height of adult ear is approximately 5.5-6.5 cm.
- Width is approximately 55% of its length.
- Lateral protrusion of the helix is 1-2 cm from the scalp.
- Average incline from the vertical is 21-25 degrees.
- The long axis tilts posteriorly 20 degrees on average, but there is wide variability.
- Projection from mastoid to helix:
  - Superior: 10-12 mm
  - Middle: 16-18 mm
  - Inferior: 20-22 mm

ACQUIRED DEFORMITIES

TRAUMA AND ACUTE MANAGEMENT

- **Human and animal bites**
  - **Dog bites** in children are the **most common** bite injury.
  - **Infection** is the most common complication of bites (1.6%-30%).[6]
  - Treat with conservative debridement and immediate antibiotic prophylaxis.
    - ▸ *Pasteurella multocida* is the most common pathogen in **dog** and **cat bites.**
    - ▸ Viridans group streptococci are most common pathogens in **human bites.**
    - ▸ Both can be treated with amoxicillin/clavulanate.
- **Blunt trauma**
  - **Hematomas** are the most common complication.
    - ▸ **Treat with immediate hematoma evacuation and compressive bolster dressing.**
  - **Cauliflower ear** deformity occurs after a subperichondrial hematoma surrounding devascularized cartilage. This results in fibrosis and the formation of new cartilage is distorted by the scarred and restricting perichondrium.
- **Lacerations, avulsions, and amputations**
  - Cleanse with minimal debridement and use skin-only closure for clean lacerations. Suturing the cartilage is not recommended.
  - Close skin when delayed reconstruction is planned.
  - If immediate closure is not feasible, then clean, debride, and perform frequent dressing changes with silver sulfadiazine (Silvadene®) or bacitracin ointment and with Xeroform (Sherwood Medical Industries, Ontario) to avoid desiccation before definitive reconstruction.
  - Partial skin avulsions can be reattached when underlying perichondrium is present.
  - Small avulsed ear pieces that are clean should be reattached within 6 hours, especially in children.
- **Thermal injury**
  - **Frostbite:** Manage with rapid rewarming, using warm saline-soaked dressings and antibiotics (fluoroquinolones).
    - ▸ Use of heparin or dextran can limit thrombosis and tissue loss.[6]
  - **Burns:** Manage with mafenide acetate (Sulfamylon®) cream, noncompressive dressings, and conservative debridement of eschar after demarcation.
    - ▸ *Pseudomonas* infections are the most common cause of suppurative eschar.

Tumors

- **Benign**
  - **Keloid**
    - ▸ Dense fibrous tissue results from the overaccumulation of collagen in the dermis during healing.
      - ✦ Earlobe is the most common site.
      - ✦ Ear piercing is the most common cause.
    - ▸ **Demographics**
      - ✦ Race: 15 times more frequent in patients with darker skin than those with lighter skin
      - ✦ Age: Highest incidence in the second decade of life
    - ▸ **Treatment**
      - ✦ Simple excision has a recurrence rate of 45%-100%.[6]
      - ✦ Intralesional corticosteroid injections can flatten keloids, but recurrence rates range from 9%-50%.[6]
      - ✦ Corticosteroid injections, combined with surgical excision, have a recurrence rate of 0%-100%.[6]
      - ✦ Radiation alone has a response rate of 10%-94%, but it should be reserved for lesions resistant to other treatment methods because of potential morbidity from radiation.[6]
      - ✦ Excision followed by radiation has a success rate of 25%-100%.[7]
      - ✦ Silicone dressings applied to keloids can decrease the volume of the lesion.
      - ✦ Continuous silicone dressing after surgical excision (24 hours a day for 3 months) can prevent keloid formation in up to 85% of cases.[6]
  - **Chondrodermatitis nodularis chronica helicis**
    - ▸ Painful, chronic inflammatory, papular lesion on helix
    - ▸ More common in men
    - ▸ Frequently resembles malignant skin tumor
    - ▸ Treat with excision of underlying cartilage
    - ▸ Recurrence rate of 10%-30% after excision[8]
- **Malignant**
  - External ear is the site of 6% of all skin cancers and 10% of skin cancers in the head and neck.
  - **Squamous cell carcinomas are the most common** (50%-60%).
    - ▸ The average rate of cutaneous metastasis is 11% compared with 2% from other primary sites.[6]
  - Basal cell carcinomas are the second most common (30%-40%).
  - Melanomas are present in 1%-2% of malignant ear lesions.

RECONSTRUCTIVE ALGORITHM

Auricular Defect Classification

- **Partial-thickness**
- **Full-thickness** defects classified according to location
  - Helical rim
  - Superior, middle, and inferior third of auricle
  - Lobule

Partial-Thickness Defects

- **Perichondrium intact**
  - Cover with skin graft taken from contralateral postauricular region.

■ **Perichondrium missing**
  • Wedge excision is made (<1.5 cm defect).
  • Preauricular or postauricular flaps are rotated, advanced, or tunneled through cartilage into defect.
■ Two bipedicle flap technique, based on posterior skin and advanced anteriorly[9] (Fig. 33-3)

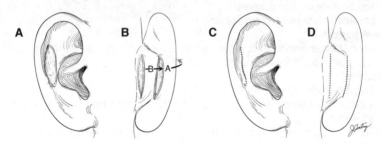

Fig. 33-3 Elsahy's two bipedicle flaps technique. **A,** Defect of the helix. **B,** Design of two bipedicle flaps. Flap *A* is rotated to cover the defect, and flap *B* is advanced to cover the donor area. **C,** Closure of the defect. **D,** Closure of the donor area. (From Elsahy N. Reconstruction of the ear after skin and perichondrium loss. Clin Plast Surg 29:187, 2002.)

FULL-THICKNESS DEFECTS
■ **Helical rim**
  • **Small defects** (<2 cm)
    ▸ Contralateral composite graft made (<1.5 cm defect)
    ▸ **Antia-Buch procedure**[10] (Fig. 33-4)
      1. Incision is made in helical sulcus through anterior skin and cartilage; posteromedial skin is undermined.
      2. Helix is advanced into defect, based on posterior skin flap.
      3. Larger defects (up to 2 cm) are closed by advancing the helix in both directions and creating V-Y advancement of crus helicis.
    ▸ **Chondrocutaneous rotation flaps,** inferiorly based on the antihelix, antitragus, or lobule, are used for defects of the middle and lower helix.[11]

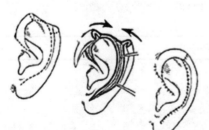

Fig. 33-4 The Antia-Buch procedure of helical rim advancement. (From Antia NH, Buch VI. Chondrocutaneous advancement flap for the marginal defect of the ear. Plast Reconstr Surg 39:472, 1967.)

- **Large defects** (>2 cm)
  - ▸ **Auricular cartilage grafts** are covered by preauricular flap or staged postauricular flap.
  - ▸ **Converse's tunnel technique**[12] (Fig. 33-5): A prefabricated composite flap is created in two stages.
    Stage 1: Contralateral auricular cartilage strut graft is tunneled under postauricular skin adjacent to helical defect.
    Stage 2: After 3 weeks, the anteriorly based skin flap and underlying cartilage strut are inset into helical rim.
  - ▸ **Tubed-pedicle flaps** from the postauricular skin or cervical skin is created and transferred in three stages.
    Stage 1: Elevation and tubing of flap is created in postauricular or cervical skin with direct closure of donor site.
    Stage 2: After 3 weeks, the inferior end of tube is divided and inset into inferior helical rim.
    Stage 3: After 3 more weeks, superior end of tube is divided and transferred to superior helical rim.
    - ◆ Treatment may require delayed insertion of a cartilage graft to support rim and correct drooping flap after transfer and healing are completed.

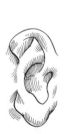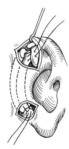

Fig. 33-5 Converse's tunnel technique. Contralateral auricular cartilage strut graft is tunneled under postauricular skin adjacent to helical defect. Anteriorly based skin flap and underlying cartilage strut are inset into helical rim as a composite flap after 3 weeks. (From Aguilar EA. Traumatic total or partial ear loss. In Evans GR, ed. Operative Plastic Surgery. New York: McGraw-Hill, 2000, p 310.)

- ■ **Superior third defects**
  - • **Small defects** (<2 cm)
    - ▸ Auricular reduction is used with Tanzer's excision patterns and primary closure[13] (Fig. 33-6).

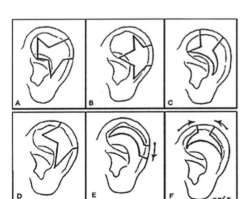

Fig. 33-6 Tanzer's excision patterns for auricular reduction. (From Tanzer RC. Deformities of the auricle. In Converse JM, ed. Reconstructive Plastic Surgery, 2nd ed. Philadelphia: WB Saunders, 1977, pp 1671-1719.)

- **Large defect** (>2 cm)
  - ▶ **Contralateral auricular cartilage graft** is used with preauricular banner flaps.[14]
  - ▶ **Valise handle** technique is used for bipedicled chondrocutaneous flap.[15]
    Stage 1: Contralateral auricular cartilage graft is implanted subcutaneously adjacent to defect.
    Stage 2: After 3 weeks, inferior helix is transposed to cartilage graft.
    Stage 3: After 3 more weeks, bipedicled composite flap is elevated as a "valise handle"; skin graft to posterior sulcus to achieve projection of helix and definition of inferior crus.
  - ▶ **Chondrocutaneous composite flap** is rotated from concha bowl.
    - ✦ Indicated when flap skin unavailable for coverage of cartilage graft
    - ✦ Can be based anteriorly on root of the helix as described by Davis[11] (Fig. 33-7)
    - ✦ Can be based laterally on outer border of helix as described by Orticochea[16] (Fig. 33-8)
  - ▶ **Costal cartilage graft,** covered by temporoparietal or mastoid fascia flap and skin graft, may be needed for very large defects or when residual tissues are inadequate for reconstruction.

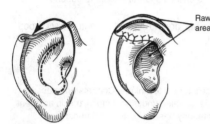

Fig. 33-7 Chondrocutaneous composite flap (as described by Davis) rotated from conchal bowl to reconstruct a defect in superior third of auricle. The flap is based anteriorly on root of helix. The donor site, in the conchal bowl, can be covered with a skin graft. (From Aguilar EA. Traumatic total or partial ear loss. In Evans GR, ed. Operative Plastic Surgery. New York: McGraw-Hill, 2000, p 310.)

Fig. 33-8 Orticochea's composite chondrocutaneous rotation flap for upper and middle third auricular defects. The flap is based on the lateral helical rim. (From Orticochea M. Reconstruction of partial losses of the auricle. Plast Reconstr Surg 46:403, 1970.)

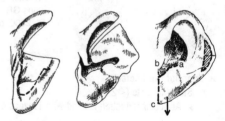

- ■ **Middle third defects**
  - • **Small defects** (<2 cm)
    - ▶ Auricular reduction using Tanzer's excision patterns and primary closure[13] (see Fig. 33-6)
  - • **Larger defects** (>2 cm)
    - ▶ **Contralateral composite graft**
      - ✦ If there is sufficient viable retroauricular skin adjacent to the defect, a contralateral chondrocutaneous composite can be grafted to that retroauricular skin.
      - ✦ Graft take is optimized by removing retroauricular skin and cartilage from composite graft, with preservation of anterior skin and cartilage strut along helical rim.[15]
    - ▶ **Converse's tunnel technique**[12] (see Fig. 33-5)

▸ **Dieffenbach's flap**[12] (Fig. 33-9)
Stage 1: Contralateral auricular cartilage graft is sutured to defect. Postauricular skin is elevated, then advanced over cartilage graft to fill defect.
Stage 2: Postauricular skin flap is divided 3 weeks later.

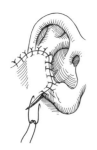

Fig. 33-9 Dieffenbach's flap. A contralateral auricular cartilage graft is sutured to defect and covered with postauricular skin flap. The postauricular skin flap is divided 3 weeks later. (From Aguilar EA. Traumatic total or partial ear loss. In Evans GR, ed. Operative Plastic Surgery. New York: McGraw-Hill, 2000, pp 310-312.)

- **Inferior third defects**
  - Superiorly based flaps are doubled over with subcutaneous cartilage graft for contour and support.
  - "Valise handle" technique for bipedicled chondrocutaneous flaps can be modified for lower defects to achieve definition of posterior conchal wall.[15]
- **Earlobe defects and deformities**
  - Composite graft from contralateral lobule.
  - Postauricular flap is transposed and sutured to superiorly based anterior skin flap.[17]
  - Chondrocutaneous flaps from the postauricular surface can be rotated inferiorly, based on a subcutaneous pedicle, to reconstruct the anterior surface of the lobule. The posterior surface of the lobule can be reconstructed with a local retroauricular skin flap.[18]
    ▸ The inclusion of conchal cartilage prevents scar contracture.
    ▸ The donor defect is closed primarily by advancing retroauricular skin.
  - **Cleft earlobe reconstruction**
    ▸ Make a wedge excision and everted closure.
    ▸ Use a Z-plasty closure to prevent notching.
    ▸ A thin flap from the edge of the cleft can be rolled into superior aspect of wedge repair, to preserve skin-lined channel for earring use, immediately after repair of cleft.[19]

REPLANTATION AND BANKING
- **Replantation**
  - The **superficial temporal artery** or **posterior auricular artery** must be available for microvascular anastomosis to consider replantation.
  - If a venous anastomosis cannot be performed, **leech therapy** can be used.
  - Successful replantation yields a superior aesthetic result compared with secondary reconstruction.
- **Banking of ear cartilage**
  - Traumatized ear cartilage can be banked under temporoparietal fascia, postauricular skin, or volar forearm. The success of banking is inconsistent.
  - **Mladick's "pocket principle" for banking ear cartilage**[20]
    ▸ Dermabrasion is used to remove the epidermis from the avulsed ear.
    ▸ Cartilage is then reapplied to the remaining ear and banked under a postauricular skin pocket.
    ▸ The graft is left in place for 3 weeks and will reepithelialize when exposed.

- **Baudet's fenestration technique**[21]
  - ▸ Posterior skin of the amputated part is removed, and fenestrations made in avulsed auricular cartilage, to increase the vascular recipient area.
  - ▸ The amputated portion is reattached, and exposed cartilage is covered with a postauricular skin flap.
  - ▸ The flap is divided after 3 months, and a skin graft is applied.

TIP: The temporoparietal fascia flap should be preserved for secondary reconstruction; its use for *acute* coverage of replanted cartilage is *not* recommended.

TOTAL EAR RECONSTRUCTION

- Costal cartilage framework is covered with a free or pedicled temporoparietal fascial flap. A skin graft is then placed on top of TP fascia flap.
  - The **contralateral costal synchondrosis (ribs 6-8)** is preferred for construction of the cartilaginous framework.
  - In children the cartilage is flexible, and the helical rim can be created by attaching a separate carved piece of rib cartilage to the framework.
  - In adults the cartilage is stiff, and the framework, including the helical rim, is best carved en bloc because cartilage does not tolerate bending.
  - The framework should be based on a **template from the contralateral ear** to match size and contour.
- Tissue expansion of periauricular skin can also be used for coverage of a costal cartilage framework.
- Successful microvascular reconstruction of the ear, with prefabricated composite flaps, has been reported.[22]

KEY POINTS

- ✔ The blood supply of the auricle is provided by an intercommunicating network from the posterior auricular and superficial arteries. Either artery can perfuse the entire auricle through this network.
- ✔ Arnold's nerve is the auricular branch of the vagus nerve (CN X) and receives contributions from the facial nerve (CN VII) and glossopharyngeal nerve (CN IX). It mediates clinical phenomena, such as the initiation of coughing during manipulation of the ear canal and referred otalgia from other structures within the head and neck.
- ✔ Suturing the cartilage is not recommended when repairing a clean laceration of the ear. Skin-only suturing is sufficient and reduces the risk of secondary deformity.
- ✔ Chondrodermatitis nodularis chronica helicis is a benign tumor that should be completely excised to definitively exclude a malignant skin tumor and reduce the risk of recurrence.
- ✔ The most effective treatment for keloids is excision followed by radiation.
- ✔ To facilitate a logical approach to reconstruction, ear defects should be classified according to location and extent of tissue loss.
- ✔ Replantation of an avulsed auricle yields the best aesthetic result.

REFERENCES

1. Allison, GR. Anatomy of the external ear. Clin Plast Surg 5:419-422, 1978.
2. Park C, Lineaweaver WC, Rumley TO, et al. Arterial supply of the anterior ear. Plast Reconstr Surg 90:38-44, 1992.
3. Brent B. Reconstruction of the auricle, In McCarthy JG, ed. Plastic Surgery, vol 3. Philadelphia: WB Saunders, 1990, pp 2094-2152.
4. Songcharoen S, Smith RA, Jabaley ME, et al. Tumors of the external ear and reconstruction of defects. Clin Plast Surg 5:447-457, 1978.
5. Farkas L. Anthropometry of normal and anomalous ears. Clin Plast Surg 5:401-412, 1978.
6. Elsahy N. Acquired ear defects. Clin Plast Surg 29:175-186, 2002.
7. Lawrence W. In search of the optimal treatment of keloids: Report of a series and a review of the literature. Ann Plast Surg 27:164-178, 1991.
8. Zuber TJ, Jackson E. Chondrodermatitis nodularis chronica helicis. Arch Fam Med 8:445-447, 1999.
9. Elsahy N. Reconstruction of the ear after skin and perichondrium loss. Clin Plast Surg 29:187-200, 2002.
10. Antia NH, Buch VI. Chondrocutaneous advancement flap for the marginal defect of the ear. Plast Reconstr Surg 39:472-477, 1967.
11. Davis JE. Reconstruction of the upper third of the ear with a chondrocutaneous composite flap based on the crus helix. In Milton E, Tanzer RC, eds. Symposium on Reconstruction of the Auricle. St Louis: Mosby, 1974, p 247.
12. Aguilar EA. Traumatic total or partial ear loss. In Evans GR, ed. Operative Plastic Surgery. New York: McGraw-Hill, 2000, pp 308-313.
13. Tanzer R. Deformities of the auricle. In Converse JM, ed. Reconstructive Plastic Surgery, 2nd ed. Philadelphia: WB Saunders, 1977, pp 1671-1719.
14. Crikelair G. A method of partial ear reconstruction for avulsion of the upper portion of the ear. Plast Reconstr Surg 17:438-443, 1956.
15. Brent B. The acquired auricular deformity: A systematic approach to its analysis and reconstruction. Plast Reconstr Surg 59:475-485, 1977.
16. Orticochea M. Reconstruction of partial losses of the auricle. Plast Reconstr Surg 46:403-405, 1970.
17. Larrabee WF, Sherris DA. Ear. In Larrabee WF, Sherris DA, eds. Principles of Facial Reconstruction. Philadelphia: Lippincott-Raven, 1995, pp 150-169.
18. Yotsuyanagi T, Yamashita K, Sawada Y. Reconstruction of the congenital and acquired earlobe deformity. Clin Plast Surg 29:249-255, 2002.
19. Pardue A. Repair of torn earlobe with preservation of the perforation for an earring. Plast Reconstr Surg 51:472-473, 1973.
20. Mladick RA, Horton CE, Adamson JE, et al. The pocket principle: A new technique for the reattachment of a severed ear part. Plast Reconstr Surg 48:219-223, 1971.
21. Baudet J. A propos d'un procede original de reimplantation d'un pavilion de l'oreille totalement separe. Ann Chir Plast 17:67-72, 1972.
22. Zhou G, Teng L, Chang HM, et al. Free prepared composite forearm flap transfer for ear reconstruction: Three case reports. Microsurgery 15:660-662, 1994.

34. Lip Reconstruction

Scott W. Mosser

ANATOMY OF PERIORAL AREA

- **Surface anatomy** (Fig. 34-1)
  - Philtral columns
  - Cupid's bow
  - Tubercle
  - White roll
  - Red line

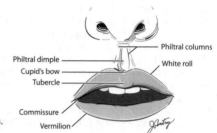

Fig. 34-1 External anatomy of the lips.

TIP: A vermilion mismatch of more than 1 mm during repair can be noticed readily at a conversational distance.

- **Aesthetic units of the lips**[1] (Fig. 34-2)
  - Upper lip
    - Lateral
    - Medial/philtral
  - Lower lip (one unit)

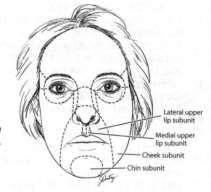

Fig. 34-2 Aesthetic subunits of the face and lips.

- **Muscles of facial expression** (Fig. 34-3, Table 34-1)[2]
  - Sphincteric activity of the lip musculature depends on continuity of the orbicularis oris muscle.
  - Some reconstruction techniques offer better retained innervation for these muscle groups.
  - **Modiolus:** A functional point where muscles attach and act to move the oral commissure.
- **Sensory innervation**
  - *Upper lip* from **maxillary branch of trigeminal nerve** (V_2)
  - *Lower lip* from **mental branch of trigeminal nerve** (V_3)
- **Blood supply**
  - **Superior** and **inferior labial arteries** (branches of the facial artery)
    - Lie within the orbicularis oris, approximately 1 mm deep to the white roll

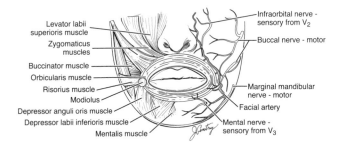

Fig. 34-3   Internal anatomy of the lips.

Table 34-1   *Origins, Insertions, and Actions of Muscles of the Lips*

Muscle	Origin	Insertion	Innervation	Action
Buccinator	Alveolar process of maxilla and mandible, and along pterygo-mandibular raphe	Orbicularis oris	Buccal branch	Compresses the cheeks
Depressor anguli oris	Lateral aspect of mental tubercle of mandible	Modiolus	Mandibular branch	Lowers the angle of the mouth
Depressor labii inferioris	Between mandibular symphysis and mental foramen, along oblique line of mandible	Skin of lower lip	Mandibular branch	Draws lip downward and laterally
Levator anguli oris	Maxilla, inferior to infraorbital foramen	Modiolus	Buccal branch	Elevates the angle of the mouth
Levator labii superioris	Maxilla, medial half of infraorbital margin	Modiolus and orbicularis oris of upper lip	Buccal branch	Elevates the upper lip
Levator labii superioris alaeque nasi	Frontal process of maxilla	Upper lip orbicularis oris, nasal cartilages	Buccal branch	Elevates the upper lip, flares the nostrils
Mentalis	Incisive fossa of mandible	Skin of chin	Mandibular branch	Elevates and protrudes lower lip
Orbicularis oris	Alveolar border of maxilla, mandible	Circumferentially around mouth, inter-digitates with other muscles	Buccal branch	Sphincter of lips, assists in lip protrusion
Platysma	Skin over delto-pectoral region	Mandible and skin of lower face, including lip	Cervical branches	Lowers the lower lip

From Gonzalez-Ulloa M. Restoration of the face covering by means of selected skin in regional aesthetic units. Br J Plast Surg 9:212-221, 1956.   *Continued*

Table 34-1 *Origins, Insertions, and Actions of Muscles of the Lips—cont'd*

Muscle	Origin	Insertion	Innervation	Action
Risorius	Parotid fascia	Modiolus	Buccal branch	Draws angle of mouth laterally
Zygomaticus major	Zygoma, anterior to temporal-zygomatic suture	Modiolus	Buccal branch	Draws angle of mouth supero-laterally
Zygomaticus minor	Zygoma, posterior to zygomatico-maxillary suture	Skin of upper lip	Buccal branch	Elevates the upper lip

From Gonzalez-Ulloa M. Restoration of the face covering by means of selected skin in regional aesthetic units. Br J Plast Surg 9:212-221, 1956.

- **Lymphatic basin**
  - *Upper lip* drains to the preauricular, infraparotid, submandibular, and submental nodes
  - Lymphatics of the upper lip do not cross the midline
  - *Lower lip* drains into the submental and submandibular nodes

ANALYSIS OF THE DEFECT

- **Size**
  - Absolute size (measurement)
  - As percent of the total lip involved
- **Depth**
  - Partial thickness/vermilion only
  - Full thickness
- **Commissure involvement**

REPAIR OF VERMILION DEFECTS[3,4]

- **Volume deficiency alone**
  - A notch or defect in the vermilion can be treated with V-Y advancement.
  - Lip switch uses opposite lip wet and/or dry vermilion to replace identical tissue.

TIP: To avoid chronically dry lips, always replace dry vermilion with dry vermilion.

  - Dermafat grafting can also replace volume.
- **Subtotal vermilion deficiency (up to 50%)**
  - Axial musculovermilion advancement flap (Fig. 34-4)
  - Musculomucosal V-Y advancement flap (Fig. 34-5)
  - Vermilion lip switch flap (Fig. 34-6)

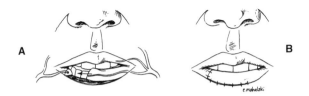

Fig. 34-4 Axial musculovermilion advancement flap. **A,** The flap is elevated deep to the labial artery. The position of the labial artery can be identified at the time of the resection of the lesion. **B,** Forward advancement of the flap permits primary closure of the defect. (From Behmand RA, Rees R. Reconstructive lip surgery. In Achauer BM, Eriksson E, Guyuron B, et al, eds. Plastic Surgery: Indications, Operations, and Outcomes. Philadelphia: Mosby, 2000, pp 1393-1210.)

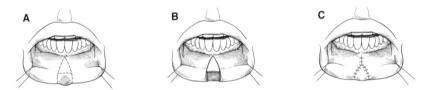

Fig. 34-5 Musculomucosal V-Y advancement flap. **A,** Focal lower lip vermilion deficiency. **B,** V design of the musculomucosal advancement flap. **C,** Local volume increase following V-Y advancement flap.

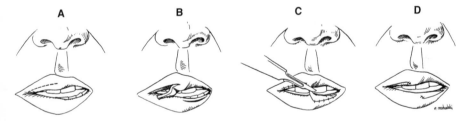

Fig. 34-6 Vermilion lip switch flap. **A,** Left upper and lower lip volume deficiency. **B,** Right upper lip random vermilion pedicle flap is elevated. The transverse incision in the deficient left lower vermilion prepares the recipient bed. **C,** The pedicle is divided at 14 days. **D,** The flap adds volume to the left lower lip vermilion, and the donor site is closed primarily. (From Behmand RA, Rees R. Reconstructive lip surgery. In Achauer BM, Eriksson E, Guyuron B, et al, eds. Plastic Surgery: Indications, Operations, and Outcomes. Philadelphia: Mosby, 2000, pp 1393-1210.)

- **Larger vermilion defects** (more than 50%)
  - Tongue flap, a two-stage procedure to transfer tongue tissue to lip defect
    - ▸ Aesthetics suboptimal compared with reconstruction using vermilion or oral mucosa
- **Total vermilion deficiency**
  - Buccal mucosal advancement: Wet buccal mucosa replaces deficient vermilion (Fig. 34-7).
  - Resultant lip has good color but can be dry and scaly.

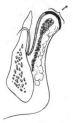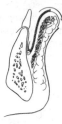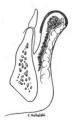

Fig. 34-7   Vermilion reconstruction by advancement of buccal mucosa. (From Behmand RA, Rees R. Reconstructive lip surgery. In Achauer BM, Eriksson E, Guyuron B, et al, eds. Plastic Surgery: Indications, Operations, and Outcomes. Philadelphia: Mosby, 2000, pp 1393-1210.)

GOALS OF LIP RECONSTRUCTION

- **Oral competence**
  - Muscular integrity
  - Oral aperture preservation
  - Reduction to less than 50% of the preoperative stoma produces significant dysfunction, especially for denture wearers

---

TIP: Patients with dentures require special consideration to maintain an adequate oral aperture.

  - Sensation
- **Speech**
- **Cosmesis**
  - Anatomic landmarks
  - Aesthetic proportions and symmetry

FULL-THICKNESS LIP RECONSTRUCTION[5-8]

The **rule of thirds** (Fig. 34-8) has become the standard way to begin analyzing options for lip reconstruction.

PRIMARY CLOSURE (Fig. 34-9)
- **Indication**
  - Up to one third of lip missing
- **Advantage**
  - Single-stage procedure with innervated, muscular continuity
- **Disadvantages**
  - Can only be used for smaller lip defects
  - Does not recreate the cupid's bow or philtral elements in the central upper lip

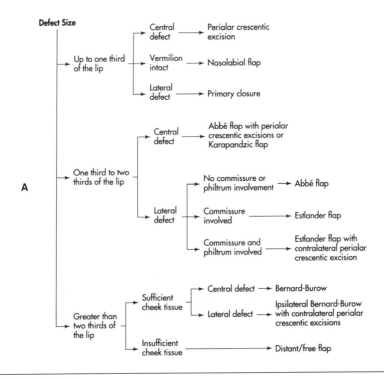

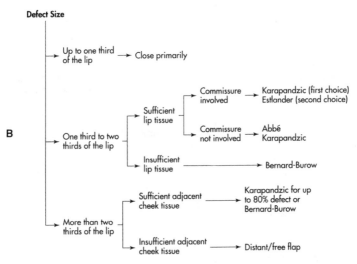

Fig. 34-8   A, Algorithm for **upper lip** reconstruction. **B,** Algorithm for **lower lip** reconstruction. (From Behmand RA, Rees R. Reconstructive lip surgery. In Achauer BM, Eriksson E, Guyuron B, et al, eds. Plastic Surgery: Indications, Operations, and Outcomes. Philadelphia: Mosby, 2000, pp 1393-1210.)

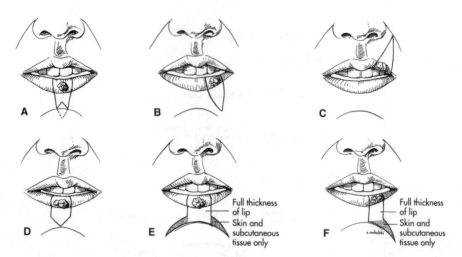

Fig. 34-9   Wedge excision of lesions. **A,** W-shaped excision. **B,** V-shaped excision of the lower lip. **C,** V-shaped excision of upper lip lesion, tapered into the nasolabial fold. **D,** Shield excision. **E,** Double barrel excision. The lesion is excised in full thickness of the lip. Burow's triangles involve only excision of skin and subcutaneous tissue. **F,** Single barrel excision. (From Behmand RA, Rees R. Reconstructive lip surgery. In Achauer BM, Eriksson E, Guyuron B, et al, eds. Plastic Surgery: Indications, Operations, and Outcomes. Philadelphia: Mosby, 2000, pp 1393-1210.)

■ **Technical pearls**
   • Identification and accurate approximation of layers is vital.
   • To medialize a lateral lip element, an **alar crescentic excision** may be indicated. Planning this excision as a crescent within the alar crease significantly decreases its visibility.

ABBÉ LIP SWITCH FLAP (Fig. 34-10)
The flap is pedicled on the lateral side of the donor lip (labial artery) and is designed to be **half the width of the defect.** This flap is left tethered on its pedicle for 2-3 weeks and is then divided in a second stage procedure.[9]
■ **Indication**
   • Replacement of one third to one half of the lip, not involving the commissure
■ **Advantages**
   • Allows continuity of oral musculature
   • Donor site closed primarily
■ **Disadvantages**
   • Two-stage procedure
   • Requires patient compliance
   • Flap is insensate
■ **Technical pearls**
   • Choose flap rotation point to allow greatest opening of mouth while the flap is adherent.
   • Leave a small cuff of muscle around the vascular pedicle.

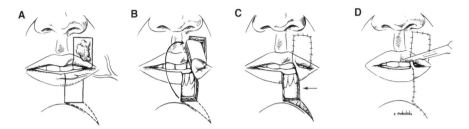

Fig. 34-10 Abbé flap. **A,** Example of a rectangular design of a lip switch flap that fills an upper lip defect. The continuity of the labial artery is maintained in the pivoting portion of the flap. **B,** The flap is elevated in full thickness of lip tissue and rotated into the upper lip defect. **C,** Excision of a Burow's triangle at the base of the donor site allows medial advancement of the lower lateral lip flap and primary closure of the donor site similar to the single barrel excision. **D,** The pedicle is divided and inset at 14-21 days. (From Behmand RA, Rees R. Reconstructive lip surgery. In Achauer BM, Eriksson E, Guyuron B, et al, eds. Plastic Surgery: Indications, Operations, and Outcomes. Philadelphia: Mosby, 2000, pp 1393-1210.)

> TIP: Because the labial artery lies within the orbicularis oris, 1 mm deep to the white roll, an adequate cuff of orbicularis oris should be maintained in the pedicle to safely incorporate the labial artery.

- Test flap viability at 14 days by clamping with a rubber band or injecting local anaesthetic with epinephrine before taking flap down.
- Combine with other procedures such as wedge resections to enable adequate lip advancement (Fig. 34-11).

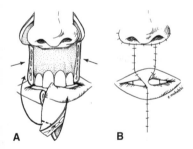

Fig. 34-11 Combination of perialar crescentic excision and central Abbé flap. **A,** Flap elevation and perialar crescentic excisions. **B,** The flap pedicle is divided and inset at about 14 days. (From Behmand RA, Rees R. Reconstructive lip surgery. In Achauer BM, Eriksson E, Guyuron B, et al, eds. Plastic Surgery: Indications, Operations, and Outcomes. Philadelphia: Mosby, 2000, pp 1393-1210.)

> TIP: For the upper lip, an Abbé flap is preferred to a sliding (e.g., Karapandzic, Estlander, or Bernard-Burow) reconstruction, because it can preserve the Cupid's bow and oral commissure/modiolus structures. Both are key structures that are difficult to reconstruct without some aesthetic deficiencies.

ESTLANDER FLAP

Similar to an Abbé flap but performed at the commissure. A full-thickness element of lip is rotated from one lip to another (Figs. 34-12 and 34-13).[10]

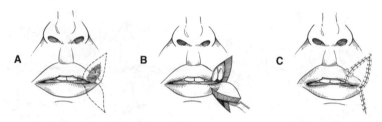

Fig. 34-12　Estlander flap for **upper lip** reconstruction. **A,** The lower lip flap is designed to be no more than one half the size of the upper lip defect. **B,** The flap is rotated about the vermilion, which harbors its blood supply from the contralateral labial artery. **C,** Three-layer closure of the inset flap and donor site. (From Behmand RA, Rees R. Reconstructive lip surgery. In Achauer BM, Eriksson E, Guyuron B, et al, eds. Plastic Surgery: Indications, Operations, and Outcomes. Philadelphia: Mosby, 2000, pp 1393-1210.)

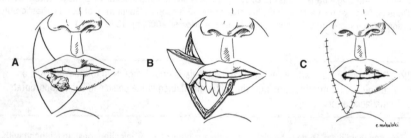

Fig. 34-13　Estlander flap for **lower lip** reconstruction. **A,** The flap is designed to be one third to one half the size of the defect. The commissure must be involved. **B,** Full-thickness upper lateral lip flap is rotated into the lower lip defect. Blood supply to the flap is at the pivot point from the contralateral upper labial artery. **C,** The flap is inset and the donor site is closed primarily. (From Behmand RA, Rees R. Reconstructive lip surgery. In Achauer BM, Eriksson E, Guyuron B, et al, eds. Plastic Surgery: Indications, Operations, and Outcomes. Philadelphia: Mosby, 2000, pp 1393-1210.)

- **Indication**
  - Defects adjacent to the commissure involving one half to two thirds of the lip
- **Advantage**
  - Single-stage procedure
- **Disadvantages**
  - Flap is not innervated
  - Oral animation can be distorted
  - Modiolus area is altered and commissure reconstruction may be necessary later
  - Flap is insensate
  - Vascular supply more tenuous because it comes from the contralateral labial artery
- **Technical pearls**
  - A full-thickness flap of lip tissue is designed to be one third to one half the size of the defect.
  - A cuff of muscle should be preserved at the point of rotation to maintain blood supply to the flap.

KARAPANDZIC FLAP

A rotational flap designed circumorally in which the intramuscular dissection preserves the neurovascular pedicle (Figs. 34-14 and 34-15).[11,12]

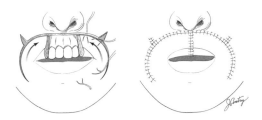

Fig. 34-14   Upper lip Karapandzic flap with Burow's triangles.

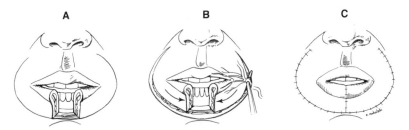

Fig. 34-15   Lower lip Karapandzic flap. **A,** The width of the circumoral incision must be equal to the height of the defect at all points of the flap. **B,** The labial arteries and buccal nerve branches are identified and preserved bilaterally. **C,** Three-layer closure following medial advancement of the flaps. (From Behmand RA, Rees R. Reconstructive lip surgery. In Achauer BM, Eriksson E, Guyuron B, et al, eds. Plastic Surgery: Indications, Operations, and Outcomes. Philadelphia: Mosby, 2000, pp 1393-1210.)

- **Indication**
  - Defect involving one third to two thirds of the lip
- **Advantages**
  - Ensures oral sphincter sensation and competence postoperatively
  - Preserves the philtrum and modiolus
- **Disadvantages**
  - If used for a very large defect (more than two thirds of the lip), can lead to microstomia
  - Upper lip may appear tight after reconstruction
- **Technical pearls**
  - To find the neurovascular pedicle, orbicularis oris muscles are carefully spread longitudinally before division

BERNARD-BUROW
Lateral lip flaps can be dramatically advanced medially with excision of Burow's triangles. In fact, the areas of skin excision are not triangles but are the necessary skin elements to provide final incision placement along anatomic subunit divisions (i.e., the nasolabial fold and labiomental creases) (Fig. 34-16).[13,14]
- **Indication**
  - Defects of two thirds or more of the lip
- **Advantages**
  - Allows adjacent tissue to reconstruct large defects
  - Reconstruction performed in one stage

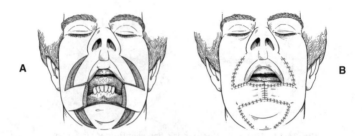

Fig. 34-16 Modified Bernard-Burow procedure. **A,** Excision of lesion does not violate the labiomental fold, but improved resection of the lesion is achieved by widening the base of the resected area. Burow's triangles are resected more laterally along the nasolabial fold and only involve the resection of skin and some subcutaneous tissue. Along the labiomental fold, skin and subcutaneous Burow's triangles are excised to give way for the medial rotation of the lower cheek flaps. **B,** Medial advancement of the lower cheek flaps is followed by three-layer closure at the midline and vermilion reconstruction with buccal mucosa. The nasolabial fold defects are closed in a single layer.

- **Disadvantages**
  - Little or no muscle function
  - Problems with lip competence
- **Technical pearls**
  - After completing the lip excision, Burow's triangles are designed.
  - Lateral flaps are advanced medially, whereas the mucosa from the Burow's triangle excision is used to reconstruct the lateral vermilion.

TOTAL LIP RECONSTRUCTION (Fig. 34-17)[15-17]
Total lip reconstruction with radial forearm free/palmaris longus composite free flap.
- **Indication**
  - Total loss of the lip
- **Advantages**
  - Enables well-vascularized coverage of large defects
  - Can recover sensory innervation if nerve repair is performed

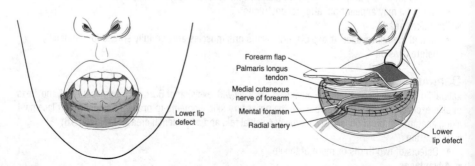

Fig. 34-17 Total lip reconstruction with free radial forearm fasciocutaneous flap with palmaris longus tendon graft to modiolus.

■ **Disadvantages**
  - Flap has no motor innervation
  - May be a poor color match
  - Anatomic landmarks and vermilion not easily reconstructed
■ **Technical pearls**
  - Palmaris longus can be used as sling to maintain lip height
  - Excellent choice if local tissues have been irradiated

POSTOPERATIVE CARE

■ Patients must be educated about obtaining adequate nutrition through small pieces of food or through foods mixed in a blender during the initial perioperative period, especially if they are recipients of the pedicled (Abbé) flap procedure.
■ If patients have oral competence in the early postoperative period, order oral cleaning with swish and spit oral solution. Otherwise gentle intraoral cleaning with swabs can be performed.

KEY POINTS

✔ Meticulous anatomic alignment is critical, because each small mismatch can be noticed easily at conversational distances.
✔ Up to one third of the upper lip and one quarter of the lower lip can be closed primarily.
✔ An Abbé flap is designed to be half the width of the defect.
✔ Estlander flaps are useful if the commissure is involved.

REFERENCES

1. Burget GC, Menick FJ. Aesthetic restoration of one half the upper lip. Plast Reconstr Surg 78:583, 1986.
2. Freilinger G, Gruber H, Happak W, et al. Surgical anatomy of the mimic muscle system and the facial nerve: Importance for reconstructive and aesthetic surgery. Plast Reconstr Surg 80:686, 1987.
3. Kawamoto HK Jr. Correction of major defects of the vermilion with a cross-lip vermilion flap. Plast Reconstr Surg 64:315, 1979.
4. Spira M, Stal S. V-Y advancement of a subcutaneous pedicle in vermilion lip reconstruction. Plast Reconstr Surg 72:562, 1983.
5. Kroll SS. Lip reconstruction. In Kroll SS, ed. Reconstructive Plastic Surgery for Cancer. St Louis: Mosby, 1996, pp 201-209.
6. MacGregor IA. Reconstruction of the lower lip. Br J Plast Surg 36:40, 1983.
7. Webster RC, Coffey RJ, Kelleher RE. Total and partial reconstruction of the lower lip with innervated muscle-bearing flaps. Plast Reconstr Surg 25:360, 1960.
8. Wilson JSP, Walker EP. Reconstruction of the lower lip. Head Neck Surg 4:29, 1981.
9. Abbé RA. A new plastic operation for the relief of deformity due to double harelip. Med Rec 53:477, 1898.
10. Estlander JA. Eine Methode aus der einen Lippe Substanzverluste der anderen zu ersetzen. Arch Kim chir 14:622, 1872.
11. Jabaley ME, Clement RL, Orcutt TW. Myocutaneous flaps in lip reconstruction: Applications of the Karapandzic principle. Plast Reconstr Surg 59:680, 1977.
12. Karapandzic M. Reconstruction of lip defects by local arterial flaps. Br J Plast Surg 27:93, 1974.
13. Freeman BS. Myoplastic modification of the Bernard cheiloplasty. Plast Reconstr Surg 21:453, 1958.

14. Madden JJ Jr, Erhardt WL Jr, Franklin JD, et al. Reconstruction of the upper and lower lip using a modified Bernard-Burow technique. Ann Plast Surg 5:100, 1980.
15. Freedman AM, Hidalgo DA. Full-thickness lip and cheek reconstruction with the radial forearm free flap. Ann Plast Surg 25:287, 1990.
16. Furuta S, Sakaguchi Y, Iwasawa M, et al. Reconstruction of the lips, oral commissure, and full-thickness cheek with a composite radial forearm palmaris longus free flap. Ann Plast Surg 33:544, 1994.
17. Sadove RC, Luce EA, McGrath PC. Reconstruction of the lower lip and chin with the composite radial forearm-palmaris longus free flap. Plast Reconstr Surg 88:209, 1991.

35. Mandibular Reconstruction

Jason K. Potter

With mandibular reconstruction it is important to distinguish bone loss caused by trauma or excision of benign disease processes from excision for malignancy. Treatment of malignancy frequently involves radiation therapy, which significantly affects treatment considerations.

GENERAL PRINCIPLES

- Type of reconstruction determined on individual basis
- Based on **location of defect** and **medical comorbidities**
- Consideration for prognosis
- Consideration for donor site morbidity
- Complication rates increase with size of defect
  - 81% complication rate for defects larger than 5 cm
  - 7% complication rate for defects smaller than 5 cm

SOFT TISSUE FLAPS IN MANDIBLE RECONSTRUCTION

Musculocutaneous flaps support the biology of tissue healing by providing a vascular bulk of tissue into which grafts can be placed with improved success. Soft tissue flaps have also been proposed to decrease the incidence of plate extrusion.

MUSCULOCUTANEOUS FLAPS
- **Pectoralis major**
  - Most common
  - Introduced in 1979 by Ariyan[1]
- **Trapezius**
  - Requires preservation of transverse cervical artery, which in turn requires planning ahead at time of resection
- **Latissimus dorsi**
  - Reserved for large defects
  - Requires repositioning patient

METHODS OF RECONSTRUCTION

COLLAPSE OF MANDIBULAR DEFECT WITHOUT RECONSTRUCTION
- Acceptable for **ascending ramus** and **lateral defects**
- **Advantages**
  - Speech and swallowing are often good
  - Fast

- **Disadvantages**
  - Deviation of chin to affected side
  - Elevation of tongue on affected side

MANDIBULAR RECONSTRUCTION PLATES (MRP)

- In general, mandibular reconstruction plates should be reserved for patients **unable to tolerate longer procedures** and with **short life expectancy.**

TIP: *Anterior* defects have demonstrated high extrusion rates when reconstruction plates are used.

- **Advantages**
  - Shortened OR time
  - No donor site morbidity
  - Theoretical prevention of donor site morbidity in the face of high rates of local recurrence with squamous cell carcinoma
  - Theoretical prevention of delays in diagnosis for recurrence after immediate tissue reconstruction
- **Disadvantages**
  - High extrusion rate when used in anterior mandible
  - Fracture of plate eventually occurs
- **Key studies**
  Schusterman et al[2]
  - 31 patients: 20 AO mandibular reconstruction plates versus 11 osseous free flaps
  - AO plates 75% successful (15/20)
    - 25% extrusion (4/5 anterior defects)
    - Anterior defects: 33% success
    - Lateral defects: 93% success
  - Osseous free flaps 100% successful
  - *Concluded to reserve AO plates for lateral defects*
  Kim and Donoff[3]
  - 37 patients with 41 plates
  - 3 groups by location of defect
    - Anterior mandible (52% failure)
    - Body segment (12.5% failure)
    - Condyle-Ramus (7.7% failure)
  - Dehiscence: 17%
  - *Complications with reconstruction plates are related to high complication rates with plates alone; soft tissue coverage was recommended to reduce rates of extrusion. This has not significantly altered outcome with plate reconstruction of the mandible. Free flaps perform slightly better than pedicled flaps.*
  Kellman and Gullane[4]
  - 17% failure
  - Average retention 8-10 months
  Papazian et al[5]
  - 40% failure with anterior defects
  Blackwell et al[6]
  - 40% failure with lateral defects

Ueyama et al[7]
▸ 28% complication rate
Cordeiro and Hidalgo[8]
▸ 14 patients, 2 groups
▸ Pectoralis flap (n = 9): 44% exposure
▸ Soft tissue free flap (n = 5): 0 exposures
Boyd et al[9]
▸ Failure rate was 35% with anterior plates, 5% with lateral plates.
▸ Most plate failures occurred within first 18 months.
▸ Patients who underwent reconstruction with plate and soft-tissue free flap experienced an aver-
age of **35 days** lost for secondary procedures compared with **4 days** for primary reconstruction
using vascular bone.

BONE GRAFTS

■ **Nonvascular bone grafts**
  • **Indication**
    ▸ Defects smaller than 6 cm long
  • **Contraindications**
    ▸ Radiation therapy: Extrusion, resorption, and infection in at least 50%-80% of cases[10]
    ▸ Anterior mandibular defects

TIP: Nonvascularized bone grafts must be performed in delayed fashion.[11]

  • **Avoid nonvascularized grafts for cancer patients**
    ▸ Nonvascular grafts require temporary stabilization with MRP.
    ▸ Temporary stabilization with MRP or myocutaneous flap is associated with high complication
      rates.
    ▸ Most MRP failures occur within 18 months, with mean time to failure 6-8 months in several
      studies.
    ▸ MRP or flap patients experience significantly more days lost compared with vascularized bone
      grafts.
    ▸ Anterior defects need immediate reconstruction.
■ **Vascularized versus nonvascularized bone grafts**
  • **Nonvascular grafts**
    ▸ Less than 6 cm: 17% failure
    ▸ Greater than 6 cm: 75% failure
  • **Vascularized grafts**
    ▸ Treatment of choice for **irradiated tissues, soft tissue defects, or bone defects larger
      than 9 cm.**[12]
    ▸ Vascularized bone grafts achieved higher incidence of union, with fewer procedures.
      ◆ Implant success rate significantly greater for vascularized bone grafts
■ **Vascularized bone grafts** (Table 35-1)

TIP: Use of vascularized bone has been associated with lower failure rates than reconstruction
      plates.

Table 35-1   *Free Flap Donor Site Comparison for Mandible Reconstruction**

Donor Site	Tissue Characteristics		Donor Site Characteristics		
	Bone	Skin	Pedicle	Location	Morbidity
Fibula	A	C	B	A	A
Ilium	B	D	D	B	C
Scapula	C	B	C	D	B
Radius	D	A	A	C	D

*Ranked in each category from best (A) to worst (D). From Hidalgo DA, Rekow A. Review of 60 consecutive fibula free flap mandible reconstructions. Plast Reconstr Surg 96:585-596, 1995.

- **Fibula flap**
  - ▸ **Blood supply:** Peroneal artery (2 mm diameter)
  - ▸ **Pedicle length:** 6-10 cm
  - ▸ **Bone size:** 25 cm long
  - ▸ **Average cross-section:** 90.2 mm[11]
  - ▸ **Suitability for implants:** Very good
  - ▸ **Soft tissue availability:** Very good
  - ▸ **Donor site disability:** Weight bearing in 10 days to 2 weeks
  - ▸ **Advantages**
    - • Easy simultaneous harvest with two-team approach
    - • Excellent length
    - • Soft tissue size and adaptability
    - • Only choice for long defects
    - • Minimal long-term donor site mobility
    - • Bone suitable for implants
    - • Excellent for edentulous mandible
  - ▸ **Disadvantages**
    - • Lack of vertical height in reconstructed mandible
    - • Skin paddle somewhat thick for implant emergence
  - ▸ **Outcomes**
    - • 93% skin survival when dissected with septomusculocutaneous flap of soleus and flexor hallucis longus versus 33% skin paddle survival when dissected as septocutaneous flap[13]
    - • Increased complication rates with more osteotomies
- **Iliac crest flap**
  - ▸ **Blood supply:** Deep circumflex iliac artery (DCIA) (1-3 mm diameter)
  - ▸ **Pedicle length:** 5-7 cm
  - ▸ **Bone size:** 14 cm maximum length
  - ▸ **Average cross-section:** 262.9 mm[11]
  - ▸ **Suitability for implants:** Excellent
  - ▸ **Soft tissue availability:** Internal oblique muscle can cover intraoral bone; external skin is fat and bulky

- ▶ **Advantages**
  - ✦ Excellent bone height
  - ✦ Internal oblique for intraoral cover
  - ✦ Atrophy of internal oblique allows good bony coverage
  - ✦ Bone very suitable for implants
- ▶ **Disadvantages**
  - ✦ Poor skin for external coverage
  - ✦ Considerable donor defect
  - ✦ Time-consuming
- **Scapula flap**
  - ▶ **Blood supply:** Subscapular artery (3-4 mm diameter)
  - ▶ **Pedicle length:** 4-6 cm, axillary artery to bone
  - ▶ **Bone size:** 14 cm in large men
  - ▶ **Suitability for implants:** 60%-70% have adequate bone for implants
  - ▶ **Soft tissue availability:** Extensive
  - ▶ **Advantage:** Very large soft tissue and fair bone
  - ▶ **Disadvantages**
    - ✦ Difficult to harvest simultaneously with ablation because of patient positioning
    - ✦ Bone quality only fair
- **Radius (osteocutaneous radial forearm flap)**
  - ▶ The radius provides inadequate bone stock for reliable reconstruction of the mandible.

KEY POINTS

- ✔ Reconstructive decisions are based on size and location of defect.
- ✔ Defects 6 cm and larger should be reconstructed with vascularized bone.
- ✔ All defects involving the anterior mandible should be reconstructed immediately.
- ✔ Immediate reconstruction mandates the use of vascularized bone grafts.
- ✔ The fibula is the donor site of choice.

REFERENCES

1. Ariyan S. The pectoralis major myocutaneous flap: A versatile flap for reconstruction in the head and neck. Plast Reconstr Surg 63:73-81, 1979.
2. Schusterman MA, Reece GP, Kroll SS, et al. Use of the AO plate for immediate mandibular reconstruction in cancer patients. Plast Reconstr Surg 88:588-593, 1991.
3. Kim MR, Donoff RB. Critical analysis of mandibular reconstruction using AO reconstruction plates. J Oral Maxillofac Surg 50:1152-1157, 1992.
4. Kellman PM, Gullane PJ. Use of the AO mandibular reconstruction plate for bridging of mandibular defects. Otolaryngol Clin North Am 20:519-533, 1987.
5. Papazian MR, Castillo MH, Campbell JH, et al. Analysis of reconstruction for anterior mandibular defects using AO plates. J Oral Maxillofac Surg 49:1055-1059, 1991.
6. Blackwell KE, Buchbinder D, Urken ML. Lateral mandibular reconstruction using soft-tissue free flaps and plates. Arch Otolaryngol Head Neck Surg 122:672-678, 1996.
7. Ueyama Y, Naitoh R, Yamagata A, et al. Analysis of reconstruction of mandibular defects using single stainless steel AO reconstruction plates. J Oral Maxillofac Surg 54:858-862, 1996.

8. Cordeiro PG, Hidalgo DA. Soft tissue coverage of mandibular reconstruction plates. Head Neck 16:112-115, 1994.
9. Boyd JB, Mulholland RS, Davidson J, et al. The free flap and plate in oromandibular reconstruction: Long-term review and indications. Plast Reconstr Surg 95:1018-1028, 1995.
10. Adamo AK, Szal RL. Timing, results, and complications of mandibular reconstructive surgery: Report of 32 cases. J Oral Surg 37:755-763, 1979.
11. Pogrel MA, Podlesh S, Anthony JP. A comparison of vascularized and nonvascularized bone grafts for reconstruction of mandibular continuity defects. J Oral Maxillofac Surg 55:1200-1206, 1997.
12. Foster RD, Anthony JP, Sharma A, et al. Vascularized bone flaps versus nonvascularized bone grafts for mandibular reconstruction: An outcome analysis of primary bony union and endosseous implant success. Head Neck 21:66-71, 1999.
13. Schusterman MA, Reece GP, Miller MJ, et al. The osteocutaneous free fibula flap: Is the skin paddle reliable? Plast Reconstr Surg 90:787-793, 1992.

36. Pharyngeal Reconstruction

Michael E. Decherd

PHARYNGEAL ANATOMY (Fig. 36-1)

- **Nasopharynx (NP)**
  - From posterior side of nose (choanae) to palatal plane
- **Oropharynx**
  - From hard/soft palate junction to aryepiglottic (AE) folds

NOTE: The tonsils, soft palate, and palatoglossal/palatopharyngeal folds are located in the oropharynx, NOT in the oral cavity. Just as the tongue base and oral tongue have different origins, innervation, function, and tumor behavior, so do the oral cavity and oropharynx.

- **Hypopharynx**
  - From AE folds to esophageal inlet
  - **Subsites**
    - ▸ Postcricoid area
    - ▸ Posterior pharyngeal wall
    - ▸ Piriform sinus

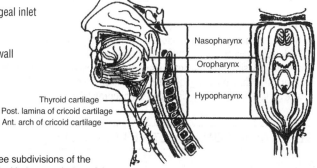

Thyroid cartilage
Post. lamina of cricoid cartilage
Ant. arch of cricoid cartilage

Nasopharynx
Oropharynx
Hypopharynx

Fig. 36-1 Three subdivisions of the pharynx. (Used with the permission of the American Joint Committee on Cancer (AJCC), Chicago, Illinois. The original source for this material is the AJCC Cancer Staging Manual, 6th ed. (2002) published by Springer-Verlag, New York, www.springeronline.com.)

TUMOR BIOLOGY[1-3]

NASOPHARYNGEAL CANCER

- **Subtypes** (World Health Organization)
  - **WHO I:** Keratinizing squamous
  - **WHO II:** Nonkeratinizing squamous
  - **WHO III:** Undifferentiated (lymphoepithelioma)
- **Incidence**
  - 1 in 100,000 in U.S. and European Caucasians
  - Higher incidence in patients serologically positive for Epstein-Barr virus
  - Highest incidence in Guangdong province of China
    - ▸ Incidence higher than average for first-generation immigrants and then becomes normal

343

- **Be suspicious (and examine NP with scope) with:**
  - Unilateral otitis media (especially serous) in an adult
  - Bilateral level V nodes
  - Unknown primary
  - Skull base symptoms (e.g., cranial neuropathies)
- In workup of unknown primary (e.g., a neck node is positive with no obvious primary), random biopsies of bilateral fossae of Rosenmüller are recommended to rule out nasopharyngeal primary

OROPHARYNGEAL CANCER

- **Incidence and etiologic factors**
  - 9100 new cases per year in United States (<1% of new cancers)
  - Mostly in the sixth and seventh decades, predominantly men
  - Squamous cell cancer more than 90% of malignancies
  - Tobacco and alcohol significant risk factors
  - Tonsil cancer can present with:
    - Cystic metastases
    - Unknown primary (perform ipsilateral tonsillectomy)

HYPOPHARYNGEAL CANCER

- This cancer has similar risk factors to other aerodigestive cancers.
- Postcricoid cancer has much higher incidence with Plummer-Vinson syndrome (iron-deficient anemia, glossitis, splenomegaly, esophageal stenosis), especially in women.
- Innervation through pharyngeal plexus can lead to "cortical confusion," and thus tumor can present with otalgia (be especially wary if no ear abnormalities—needs scope).

GENERAL RECONSTRUCTIVE PRINCIPLES

PHARYNGEAL FUNCTION

- Passageway for food and air, including air for middle ear
- Swallowing: Coordinated act that propels a bolus and protects airway
- Speech: Palate, tongue, and lips shape sound generated in larynx to create speech

SWALLOWING PHASES

- **Oral**
  - Preparatory (chewing and preparing the bolus)
  - Motor
- **Pharyngeal**
- **Esophageal**

EVALUATION OF SWALLOWING DYSFUNCTION

- **Barium swallow**
  - Evaluates esophagus for mass only
- **Modified barium swallow**
  - Shows swallowing dysfunction
  - Administered jointly with radiologist and speech pathologist
  - Has barium-enriched substances of different consistencies (e.g., solid, soft, liquid)
  - Evaluates swallowing dynamically; can show subtle abnormalities

- Shows aspiration
- Guides clinical recommendations regarding eating strategies
- **Functional endoscopic evaluation of swallowing with sensory testing (FEEST)**
  - Trained observer watches swallowing through endoscope
  - Can actively test sensation with puffs of air

TRACHEOSTOMY

- Paradoxically increases aspiration risk while providing increased pulmonary toilet
  - Tethers the larynx and prevents its normal elevation, which is one of the first steps in swallowing
  - Helps toilet (when someone is already aspirating) by allowing better suctioning

RECONSTRUCTIVE PRINCIPLES BY SUBSITE[4-16]

NASOPHARYNX

- Almost always treated **nonsurgically**
- Reconstruction rare and usually limited to providing lining, such as with fasciocutaneous flaps or skin/mucosal grafts, or obliterating dead space as with bulkier flaps

OROPHARYNX

- **Soft palate**
  - Thin, pliable flaps have been used but are poorly functional.
  - Total palatal defects may be easier to rehabilitate because these functionally do well with a palatal prosthesis.
- **Base of tongue**
  - If much of the tongue base is sacrificed, then consider performing a laryngectomy, otherwise serious complications of aspiration may ensue.
  - Candidates for laryngeal preservation must have good pulmonary reserve.

> TIP: Clinical test is to observe whether the patient can climb a flight of stairs.

  - **Reconstructive goal is to provide bulk to obliterate dead space during speech and swallowing.**
    - ▶ Regional flaps (e.g., pectoralis)
    - ▶ Free rectus
- **Pharyngeal wall**
  - Thin pliable flaps are needed.
  - Posterior wall may be reconstructed with skin grafts, but if defect involves lateral walls, then free fasciocutaneous flap may be required.

HYPOPHARYNX AND CERVICAL ESOPHAGUS

- Usually requires concomitant laryngectomy
- **Adequate mucosa**
  - Primary closure
- **Inadequate mucosa**
  - Tubed pectoralis flap
  - Radial forearm free flap
    - ▶ Higher rate of stricture than jejunum

- Anterolateral thigh fasciocutaneous flap
- Free jejunum
  - ▶ Orient to keep peristalsis antegrade
  - ▶ May lead to secretory problems
  - ▶ Abdominal morbidity
- **Esophageal defect**
  - Gastric pull up
  - Colonic interposition

KEY POINTS

✔ The pharynx is a shared conduit for speech and swallowing.

✔ Reconstruction of the pharynx generally entails either restoring lining, reestablishing a conduit, or obliterating dead space.

✔ Interference with the normal partitioning between the tracheobronchial tree and the digestive system may lead to aspiration.

REFERENCES

1. Schecter GL, Wadsworth TT. Hypopharyngeal cancer. In Bailey BJ, ed. Head & Neck Surgery: Otolaryngology, 2nd ed. Philadelphia: Lippincott, 1998.
2. Seikaly H, Rassekh CH. Oropharyngeal cancer. In Bailey BJ, ed. Head & Neck Surgery: Otolaryngology, 2nd ed. Philadelphia: Lippincott, 1998.
3. Witte MC, Neel HB III. Nasopharyngeal cancer. In Bailey BJ, ed. Head & Neck Surgery: Otolaryngology, 2nd ed. Philadelphia: Lippincott, 1998.
4. Ariyan S. The pectoralis major myocutaneous flap. Plast Reconstr Surg 63:73, 1979.
5. Chepeha DB, Teknos TN. Microvascular free flaps in head and neck reconstruction. In Bailey BJ, ed. Head & Neck Surgery: Otolaryngology, 3rd ed. Philadelphia: Lippincott, 2001.
6. Baek SM. Two new cutaneous free flaps: The medial and lateral thigh flaps. Plast Reconstr Surg 71:354, 1983.
7. Bakamjian VY. A two-stage method for pharyngoesophageal reconstruction with a primary pectoral skin flap. Plast Reconstr Surg 36:1732, 1965.
8. Daniel RK, Taylor GI. Distant transfer of an island flap by microvascular anastomoses. Plast Reconstr Surg 52:111, 1973.
9. Demergasso F, Piazza MV. Trapezius myocutaneous flap in reconstructive surgery for head and neck cancer: An original technique. Am J Surg 138:533, 1979.
10. Greene FL, Page DL, Fleming ID, et al. AJCC Cancer Staging Manual, 6th ed. New York: Springer, 2002.
11. Panje WR, Bardach J, Krause CJ. Reconstruction of the oral cavity with a free flap. Plast Reconstr Surg 58:415, 1976.
12. Roberts RE, Douglas FM. Replacement of the cervical esophagus and hypopharynx by a revascularized free jejunal autograft: Report of a case successfully treated. N Engl J Med 264:342, 1961.
13. Schusterman MA, Miller JA, Reece GP, et al. A single center's experience with 308 free flaps for repair for head and neck cancer defects. Plast Reconstr Surg 93:472, 1993.
14. Seidenberg B, Rosznak SS, Hurwitt ES, et al. Immediate reconstruction of the cervical esophagus by a revascularized isolated jejunal segment. Ann Surg 149:162, 1959.
15. Taylor G, Corlett RJ, Boyd B. The versatile deep inferior epigastric (inferior rectus abdominis) flap. Br J Plast Surg 37:330, 1984.
16. Urken LM, Weinberg H, Buchbinder D, et al. Microvascular free flaps in head and neck reconstruction. Report of 200 cases and review of complications. Arch Otolaryngol Head Neck Surg 120:633, 1994.

37. Facial Reanimation

Jason E. Leedy

FACIAL NERVE ANATOMY

COMPONENTS
- **Branchial motor:** Voluntary motor control of facial musculature
- **Visceral motor:** Parasympathetic control of lacrimal, submandibular, and sublingual glands
- **General sensory:** Innervation of the external auditory canal
- **Special sensory:** Taste in anterior two thirds of the tongue

THREE SEGMENTS
1. **Intracranial**
   - Facial nucleus cell bodies that give rise to the **frontal branch** receive bilateral cortical input.
   - All other facial nucleus cell bodies receive contralateral cortical input.

> TIP: Ipsilateral supranuclear lesions give contralateral facial paralysis but maintain frontalis function.

2. **Intratemporal**
   - Facial nerve enters the internal auditory canal and travels with the acoustic and vestibular nerves for approximately 8-10 mm.
   - Facial nerve then enters the **fallopian canal** by itself, where it travels for 30 mm.
   - Fallopian canal has **three segments** (Fig. 37-1).
     1. **Labyrinthine segment**
        - 3-5 mm long, from entrance of the fallopian canal to the geniculate ganglion
        - Narrowest segment: 1.42 mm diameter on average, nerve occupies 83% of available space
        - Greater petrosal nerve: First branch of facial nerve, from geniculate ganglion, supplies parasympathetic nerves for lacrimal gland
        - Junction of labyrinthine and tympanic segments formed by an acute angle: Shearing occurs commonly

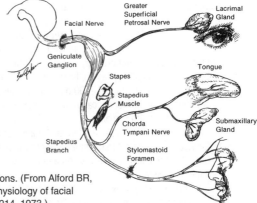

Fig. 37-1   Facial nerve main divisions. (From Alford BR, Jerger JF, Coats AC, et al. Neurophysiology of facial nerve testing. Arch Otolaryngol 97:214, 1973.)

347

2. Tympanic segment
- 8-11 mm long, from geniculate ganglion to bend at lateral semicircular canal
- Midtympanic canal is second region of fallopian canal: Narrowest cross-sectional area

3. Mastoid segment
- 9-12 mm long, from bend at lateral semicircular canal to stylomastoid foramen
- Widest cross-sectional area
- **Three nerve branches**
  - <u>Nerve to stapedius:</u> Motor function for stapedius muscle, allows for dampening of loud sounds; cell bodies of this motor nerve not located in facial nucleus, therefore not affected by Möbius' syndrome
  - <u>Sensory branch to external auditory canal:</u> *Hitselberger's sign:* Hypesthesia of external auditory canal
  - <u>Chorda tympani:</u> Final intratemporal branch, joins lingual nerve to provide parasympathetic innervation to submandibular and sublingual glands; special sensory afferents from anterior two thirds of the tongue travel with chorda tympani

> TIP: In children, the ratio of facial nerve diameter to fallopian canal diameter is less than in adults, which decreases the likelihood of facial nerve entrapment.
>
> The facial nerve in the fallopian canal lacks sufficient identifiable topographic orientation to be clinically useful in selective fascicular nerve grafting.

3. Extratemporal
- Starts where facial nerve exits **stylomastoid foramen;** nerve is protected by mastoid tip, tympanic ring, and mandibular ramus
- **Nerve is superficial in children less than 2 years old**
- Travels along a course anterior to the posterior belly of the digastric muscle and along the styloid process to the posterior edge of the parotid gland
- Facial nerve trunk 1 cm deep, just inferior and medial to the tragal pointer
- Provides motor branches to the posterior belly of the digastric, stylohyoid, superior and posterior auricular muscles, and the occipitalis muscles
- Interconnections between extratemporal facial nerve and trigeminal, glossopharyngeal, vagus, spinal accessory, hypoglossal, and nearby parasympathetic and sympathetic nerves
- **Arborization begins in substance of parotid gland**
  - Nerve first divides into superior and inferior divisions that ultimately give rise to **frontal, zygomatic, buccal, mandibular,** and **cervical branches.**
    - Davis dissected 350 cadaveric halves and identified six branching patterns (Fig. 37-2).[1]
    - Baker and Conley[2] studied 2000 parotidectomies and found facial nerve trunk trifurcation, sometimes with direct buccal branch; the zygomatic was most robust, and the marginal mandibular was the smallest.
    - Frontal branch of nerve is the terminal branch of superior division.
    - Cervical and marginal mandibular branches derive from an inferior division.
    - Buccal branch always receives some innervation from inferior division and occasionally from superior division.
    - Connections exist between major facial nerve divisions in 70%-90% of patients, *except for the frontal and marginal mandibular branches.*
    - Nerves lie just deep to the subcutaneous musculoaponeurotic system (SMAS) layer.

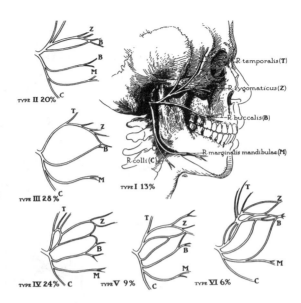

Fig. 37-2 Facial nerve branching patterns. (From Davis RA, Anson BJ, Budinger JM, et al. Surgical anatomy of the facial nerve and parotid gland based upon a study of 350 cervicofacial halves. Surg Gynecol Obstet 102:385, 1956.)

FRONTAL BRANCH ANATOMY

- Frontal branch has consistent course from 0.5 cm below tragus to 1.5 cm above the lateral brow.[3]
- Frontal branch lies within temporoparietal fascia.[4]
- Frontal nerve and superficial temporal artery reside in deep aspects of temporoparietal fascia and the most posterior rami of frontal branch; may be either anterior or posterior to superficial temporal artery.[5]
  - At level of zygomatic arch, frontal branch arborizes into two to four branches.

MARGINAL MANDIBULAR ANATOMY (Fig. 37-3)

- Marginal mandibular is connected to other rami in only 15% of cases.[2]
- Marginal mandibular branch, posterior to facial artery, is located above inferior border of mandible in 81% of cases and below in 19%, and it is above inferior border in 100% of cases if anterior to facial artery.[6]

FACIAL MUSCULATURE (Fig. 37-4, Table 37-1)

- Orbicularis oris and 23 other paired muscles
- **Four layers**[7]
  - Layer 1: Depressor anguli oris, zygomaticus minor, orbicularis oculi
  - Layer 2: Depressor labii inferioris, risorius, platysma, zygomaticus major, levator labii superioris alaeque nasi
  - Layer 3: Orbicularis oris, levator labii superioris
  - Layer 4: Mentalis, levator anguli oris, buccinator

↑ innervated on Ant Surface

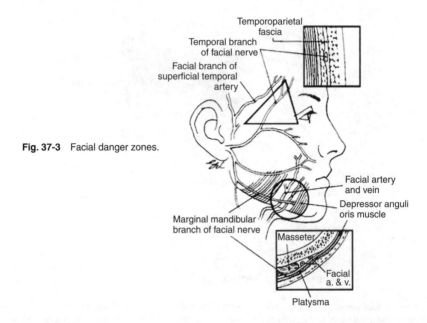

Fig. 37-3   Facial danger zones.

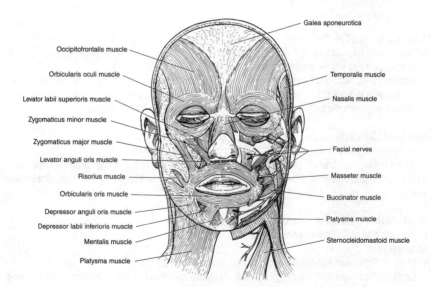

Fig. 37-4   Muscles of the face.

Table 37-1   *Muscle Groups of the Face*

Muscle	Facial Nerve Branch	Action
Corrugator supercilii	Temporal	Moves eyebrow medially and downward
Procerus	Temporal	Moves medial eyebrow downward
Orbicularis oculi	Temporal and zygomatic	Closes eyelids and contracts skin around eye
Zygomaticus major	Zygomatic and buccal	Elevates corner of mouth
Zygomaticus minor	Buccal	Elevates upper lip
Levator labii superioris	Buccal	Elevates upper lip and midportion of nasolabial fold
Levator labii superioris alaeque nasi	Buccal	Elevates medial nasolabial fold and nasal ala
Risorius	Buccal	Aids smile with lateral pull
Buccinator	Buccal	Pulls corner of mouth backward and compresses cheek
Levator anguli oris	Buccal	Pulls angles of mouth upward and medially
Orbicularis oris	Buccal	Closes and compresses lips
Nasalis, dilator	Buccal	Flares nostrils
Nasalis, compressor	Buccal	Compresses nostrils
Depressor anguli oris	Buccal and marginal mandibular	Pulls corner of mouth downward
Depressor labii inferioris	Marginal mandibular	Pulls down lower lip
Mentalis	Marginal mandibular	Pulls skin of chin upward
Platysma	Cervical	Pulls down corner of mouth

From May M, Schaitkin BM. The Facial Nerve, 2nd ed. New York: Thieme Medical, 2000.

TIP: **Layer 4** muscles are innervated on their **superficial** surface; all other muscles receive innervation from their deep surfaces.

■ Subtle movements of normal expression require a delicate balance among all the muscles. However, a few muscles create clinically significant movements that are important when evaluating facial paralysis.
  • **Frontalis:** Raises eyebrows
  • **Orbicularis oculi:** Closes eyelids
  • **Zygomaticus major and minor:** Smiling
  • **Orbicularis oris:** Purses the lips
  • **Lower lip depressor:** Keeps lip from riding up during chewing

DIFFERENTIAL DIAGNOSIS OF FACIAL PARALYSIS

INTRACRANIAL
- Vascular abnormalities, aneurysms
- Central nervous system degenerative disorders
- Tumors of the intracranial cavity
- Trauma to the brain
- Congenital abnormalities and agenesis

INTRATEMPORAL
- Bacterial and viral infections
- Cholesteatoma
- Trauma: Temporal bone fractures, penetrating trauma
- Bell's palsy
- Systemic conditions: Diabetes mellitus, HIV infection

EXTRATEMPORAL
- Malignant parotid tumors
- Trauma: Particularly penetrating
- Primary tumors of the facial nerve
- Malignant tumors of ascending ramus of mandible, pterygoid, and skin

UNILATERAL FACIAL PARALYSIS

BELL'S PALSY[8]
- Idiopathic facial paralysis (Table 37-2)
- Accounts for 85% of all cases of facial paralysis

Table 37-2   *Findings That Rule Out Bell's Palsy*

Symptom/Finding	Diagnosis	Frequency Exclusive of Bell's Palsy
Simultaneous bilateral facial palsy	Guillain-Barré, sarcoidosis, pseudobulbar palsy, syphilis, leukemia, trauma, Wegener's granulomatosis	100%
Unilateral facial weakness slowly progressing beyond three weeks	Facial nerve neuroma, metastatic cancer, adenoid cystic carcinoma	100%
Slowly progressive unilateral facial weakness associated with facial hyperkinesis	Cholesteatoma, facial nerve neuroma	100%
No return of facial nerve function within 6 months after abrupt onset of palsy	Facial nerve neuroma, adenoid cystic carcinoma, basal cell carcinoma	100%
Ipsilateral lateral rectus palsy	Möbius' syndrome	100%
Recurrent unilateral facial palsy	Facial nerve neuroma, adenoid cystic carcinoma, meningioma	30%

From May M, Hardin WB. Facial palsy: Interpretation of neurologic findings. Laryngoscope 88:1352, 1978.

- **Most common** diagnosis in patients with facial paralysis: 15-40 of 100,000/yr
- Associated with **pregnancy:** 17.4 of 100,000/yr in women of child-bearing age versus 45 of 100,000/yr in pregnant women
- **Diagnosis of exclusion** is used to avoid misdiagnosis and delay of treatment.
- **Proposed etiology** is a viral-vascular insult to the facial nerve that causes edema of the nerve within fallopian canal, which disrupts neural microcirculation, thereby impairing conduction of neural impulses.
- *All patients begin to recover function within 6 months of paralysis and none remain totally paretic.*
- Recovery begins within 3 weeks in 85% of patients but not until 3-6 months in 15% of patients.
- 71% of patients with total facial paralysis recover completely without sequela.
- Completeness of recovery decreases with age.
- **Management**
  - Two studies document less denervation and significant improvement of facial grade at recovery if steroids are used within 24 hours.[9,10] The protocol involves prednisone, 60 mg/day for 5 days, tapering to 5 mg/day by the tenth day of treatment.

TRAUMA

Trauma is the **second most common cause of facial paralysis,** usually caused by temporal bone fracture, penetrating wound, or birthing injury.
- **Temporal bone fractures**
  - These are classified as **longitudinal, transverse,** or **mixed** according to the long axis of the temporal bone.
  - Facial paralysis is more likely with **transverse** fractures.
  - Repair requires midcranial fossa or translabyrinthine approach with end-to-end coaptation of the transected nerve.
- **Penetrating wounds**
  - In general, lacerations medial to the lateral canthus do not require repair because of nerve arborization.
  - Repair should be performed **within 72 hours** to allow identification of distal branches by nerve stimulation.

TIP: If soft tissue injury prohibits repair within first 72 hours, the nerve ends should be tagged to allow for delayed repair.

  - Peripheral injuries to the frontal and marginal mandibular branches that have resulted in significant weakness should be repaired, because of low likelihood of spontaneous recovery.

TUMORS

- Paralysis can present variably: Sudden or slow progression, complete or incomplete, recurrent or single episode, possibly hyperkinesis (twitching)
- **High concern for neoplastic causes if:**
  - Unilateral facial weakness, slowly increasing for more than 3 weeks
  - Unilateral facial weakness, onset abrupt with no return of function in 6 months
  - Associated with hyperkinesis (twitching)
- **Types**
  - Primary facial nerve
  - Parotid
  - Acoustic neuroma (Von Recklinghausen's disease)

- Central nervous system
- Cutaneous malignancy
- Metastatic lesion
- Cholesteatoma (benign)
- Hemangiomas (benign)

VIRAL INFECTION
- **Ramsay-Hunt syndrome:** Varicella-zoster virus infection with facial paralysis, ear pain, and varicelliform rash in external auditory canal; accounts for approximately 12% of all cases of facial paralysis.
  - Treatment involves prednisone (1 mg/kg/day divided twice per day) and acyclovir (800 mg, 5 times/day) for 10 days[11]

IATROGENIC
- Postoperative facial paralysis after acoustic neuroma resection: Trauma, thermal injury, devascularization, edema, and reactivation of latent herpes virus infection

BILATERAL FACIAL PARALYSIS

- 0.3%-2% of all cases of facial paralysis
- **Most commonly from Lyme disease** (36% in Teller and Murphy's review)[12]
- **HIV infection** also a common cause

RECURRENT FACIAL PARALYSIS

- **Melkersson-Rosenthal syndrome:** Recurrent facial nerve paralysis, noninflammatory facial edema, and congenital tongue fissures (lingua plicata)
  - Etiology unknown, hereditary factor suspected
  - Treatment usually conservative
- **Bell's palsy** in approximately 10% of patients

PEDIATRIC DIAGNOSES

MÖBIUS' SYNDROME
- Unilateral or bilateral loss of eye abduction
- Unilateral or bilateral, complete or incomplete facial paralysis
- Facial paralysis may be accompanied by other cranial nerve palsies or congenital defects
- Primary developmental defect of central nervous system treatment, usually involves free microneurovascular muscle transfer

HEMIFACIAL MICROSOMIA
- Facial paralysis in small percentage of patients

CONGENITAL UNILATERAL LOWER LIP PALSY (CULLP)
- "Asymmetric crying facies"
- Other major congenital anomalies in 75% of affected children

PATIENT EVALUATION

- History of weakness: Onset, duration, progression
- Grading facial nerve function
  - **House-Brackmann scale**[13]: Gross scale, most commonly used for reporting (Table 37-3)
  - **Burres-Fisch system,**[14] **Sunnybrook scale**[15]: Objective scales, used to limit subjectivity of evaluation
  - **Other scales include**[16]: Botman and Jongkees, May, Stennert, Pietersen, Janssen, and Yanagihara

Table 37-3 *House-Brackmann Scale*

Grade	Description	Characteristics
I	Normal	Normal facial function
II	Mild dysfunction	Gross: Slight weakness on close inspection, normal at rest Motion: *Forehead,* moderate to good; *eye,* complete closure with minimum effort; *mouth,* slight asymmetry
III	Moderate dysfunction	Gross: Obvious but not disfiguring, normal asymmetry and tone at rest Motion: *Forehead,* slight to moderate; *eye,* complete closure with effort; *mouth,* slightly weak with maximum effort
IV	Moderately severe	Gross: Obvious weakness with disfiguring asymmetry at rest Motion: *Forehead,* none; *eye,* incomplete closure; *mouth,* asymmetric with maximum effort
V	Severe dysfunction	Gross: Only barely perceptible motion, asymmetry at rest Motion: *Forehead,* none; *eye,* incomplete closure; *mouth,* slight movement
VI	Total paralysis	No movement

From House JW, Brackmann DE. Facial nerve grading system. Otolaryngol Head Neck Surg 93:146-147, 1985.

DIAGNOSTIC STUDIES

Most cases of facial paralysis are Bell's palsy; therefore a **3-week period of observation** is acceptable before undergoing an extensive diagnostic workup.

TESTS FOR ETIOLOGIC FACTORS
- **Serologic tests:** Syphilis and diabetes
- **CT scan:** Good for evaluating tumors and bony detail of the fallopian canal
- **MRI:** Good for evaluating pathologic and nonpathologic conditions of the nerve

PROGNOSTIC TESTS[8]
- **Nerve excitability test (NET)**
  - Subjective
  - Determines energy required to stimulate the nerve
  - Difference of 3.0 milliamps or more between sides is abnormal
- **Maximal stimulation test (MST)**
  - Assesses facial movement with stimulus level that creates discomfort
  - Becomes positive before NET does in lesions of facial nerve

- **Electroneurography (ENoG)**
  - Apply current to stylomastoid foramen region and record maximal muscle action potentials at nasolabial fold
  - **Most accurate and reproducible test to determine prognosis**
  - When ENoG reveals 75% to 95% degeneration within 2 weeks of onset, facial nerve decompression surgery may preserve the remaining axons.[11]
- **Electromyography (EMG):**
  - Measures muscle activity
  - Does not become positive until 14-21 days after onset of paralysis
  - Useful for late prognosis in complete nerve paralysis

TOPOGRAPHIC TESTS
Attempt to localize the intratemporal site or extent of involvement.
- **Schirmer's test:** Assesses lacrimation
- **Stapedial reflex:** Assesses function of nerve to stapedius muscle
- **Taste testing:** Assesses chorda tympani function

GOALS OF SURGICAL TREATMENT

- Normal appearance at rest
- Symmetry with voluntary motion
- Corneal protection
- Symmetric, dynamic smile
- Restoration of oral, nasal, and ocular sphincter control
- Symmetry with involuntary motion and controlled balance when expressing emotion
- No loss of other significant functions

TREATMENT PLANNING

- Aim for realistic expectations of functional facial movement after intrinsic muscle reinnervation.
- Typically, **3 years** is considered to be the period after which denervation atrophy of facial muscles precludes their usefulness for further reconstruction.[17] However, presence of **fibrillations on EMG** is considered evidence of facial muscle viability and therefore indicates potential for useful function after reinnervation.

TREATMENT TYPES (Table 37-4)

REINNERVATION
- Primary nerve repair (intracranial, intratemporal, extratemporal)
- Interpositional nerve graft
- Cross-facial nerve graft
- Hypoglossal-facial nerve transfer
- Hypoglossal-facial jump graft

Table 37-4   *Algorithm for Management of Facial Paralysis*

Facial Paralysis: Temporal Branch

Deformity	Treatment
Brow ptosis	Brow lift
Dermatochalasis	Upper blepharoplasty
Lagophthalmos	Gold or platinum weight eyelid spring
Lower lid ectropion	Canthoplasty or lid shortening

Facial Paralysis: Zygomatic, Buccal, and Marginal Mandibular Branches

Time From Injury	Treatment
<12 months	• Nerve repair • Ipsilateral nerve graft • Cross-face nerve graft
12-24 months	• Nerve repair • Ipsilateral nerve graft • Hypoglossal-facial transfer • Hypoglossal-facial jump graft
>24 months	• Static reconstruction • Cross-face nerve graft and delayed free-functional muscle transfer • Free-functional muscle transfer with CN XII or V neurotization

Modified from Anderson RG. Facial nerve disorders and surgery. Sel Read Plast Surg 9(20), 2001.

DYNAMIC RECONSTRUCTION

- Regional muscle transfer
  - Temporalis
  - Masseter
- Free-muscle microneurovascular transfer with cross-facial nerve graft
- Free-muscle microneurovascular transfer with coaptation to masseter motor branch

STATIC RECONSTRUCTION[18,19]

- **Indications**
  - Elderly patients with significant comorbidities
  - Massive facial defects secondary to trauma or cancer resection
  - Failed microvascular reanimation
  - Techniques directed to correct functional disabilities (protect cornea, improve nasal airway, and prevent drooling) and improve symmetry at rest
    - ▶ Browlift for brow ptosis
    - ▶ Upper eyelid gold-weight placement, eyelid spring
    - ▶ Lateral and medial tarsorrhaphy, Kuhnt-Szymanowski lower eyelid shortening and suspension, medial canthoplasty, or lateral tarsal strip procedure
    - ▶ Lateral and superior repositioning of nasal alar base with a maxillary periosteal flap
    - ▶ Shortening and thickening of paralyzed upper and lower lips with preservation of oral commissure
    - ▶ Suspension of oral commissure with fascia lata, tendon, or alloplastic materials
    - ▶ Rhytidectomy and stabilization with dermal flaps

ADJUNCT PROCEDURES
- Botulinum toxin to weaken contralateral side to improve symmetry
- Repositioning of the lateral ala to improve airflow resistance
- **Physical therapy:** Neuromuscular rehabilitation critical to success of any treatment

DIRECT NERVE REPAIR AND GRAFTING
- Ideally performed at time of injury
- Better results reported when repair within 1 year, but good results reported up to 3 years after injury
- Nerves regenerate at rate of **1 mm/day**
- **Source of nerve graft**
  - Branches from the cervical plexus, ipsilateral, or contralateral nerves
  - Great auricular nerve
  - Sural nerve

CROSS-FACE NERVE GRAFTING (Fig. 37-5)
- Procedure is indicated when proximal ipsilateral facial nerve stump is unavailable for grafting, a distal stump is present, and facial muscles are capable of useful function after reinnervation.
- Sural nerve grafts are used to connect healthy peripheral nerve branches to corresponding branches of specific muscle groups on paralyzed side.
  - Some recommend using branch that produces maximum zygomaticus major activity for coaptation to cross-facial nerve graft; others recommend using distal buccal branches.
  - **One-stage:** Repair both ends at the same time.[20]

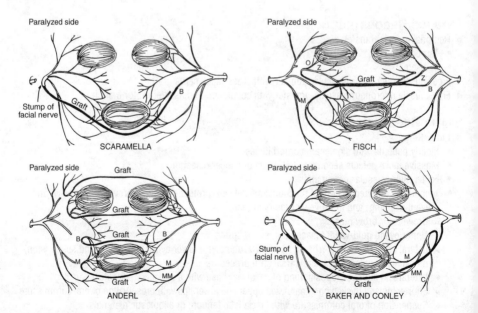

Fig. 37-5   Techniques of cross-face nerve grafting. (From Baker DC, Conley J. Facial nerve grafting: A thirty year retrospective review. Clin Plast Surg 6:343, 1979.)

- **Two-stages:** Repair healthy end, then resect neuroma to verify graft success. Once nerve fascicles grow through graft, repair paralyzed side; perform second stage 9-12 months later, after positive Tinel's sign at distal end.

NERVE CROSSOVER

- Indicated when proximal ipsilateral facial nerve stump is unavailable for grafting, a distal stump is present, and facial muscles are capable of useful function after reinnervation
- Facial nerve stump anastomosed to hypoglossal, glossopharyngeal, accessory, or phrenic nerves
  - Requires only a single suture line: A powerful source of reinnervation
  - Sacrifices donor nerve function and often results in difficulty coordinating facial movement, mass movement, and grimacing

HYPOGLOSSAL NERVE TRANSFER

- Most common
- Best for immediate reconstruction of proximal facial nerve during tumor extirpation
- Provides excellent tone and normal appearance at rest
- Protects eye and permits intentional movement of face, no spontaneous facial expression
- Paralysis and atrophy of the ipsilateral tongue, usually well-tolerated unless ipsilateral low-cranial nerve (CN) dysfunction is present (CNs: IX, X, XI)

HYPOGLOSSAL-JUMP GRAFT

- Same as hypoglossal nerve transfer, except involves partial sectioning of the hypoglossal nerve, thereby preserving ipsilateral hypoglossal function
- Indicated for patients who have ipsilateral low-cranial nerve dysfunction or for those unwilling to accept tongue dysfunction

REGIONAL MUSCLE TRANSFERS

- **Indications**
  - Absence of mimetic muscles after long-standing atrophy with no potential for useful function after reinnervation
  - Adjunct to the mimetic muscles to provide new muscle and myoneurotization
- **Masseter transfer**
  - Suited to give motion to the lower half of face
  - Three muscle slips sutured to dermis of the lower lip, oral commissure, and upper lip
  - During radical parotidectomy, transposing masseter with interdigitation into freshly denervated mimetic muscle provides maximum myoneurotization
- **Temporalis transfer**
  - More frequently performed than masseter transfer because greater excursion of movement and adaptability to orbit
  - Can transfer and suture muscle with its fascial extensions to eyelids, ala of nose, oral commissure, and upper and lower lips

FREE-FUNCTIONAL MUSCLE TRANSFER[21,22]

- Indicated when facial muscles will not provide useful function after reinnervation
- Microneurovascular muscle transfer combined with cross-face nerve graft, ipsilateral nerve graft (facial nerve of motor nerve to masseter)
- Provides new, vascularized muscle that can pull in various directions

- **Ideal donor muscle characteristics**
  - Excursion equal to normal side of face.
  - Reliable vascular and nerve pattern of a size similar to that of recipient.
  - Removal of muscle leaves no functional deficit.
  - Location is distant enough from face to allow two operating teams to work simultaneously.
- **Gracilis muscle most commonly used**
- Other potential muscles: Extensor digitorum brevis, pectoralis minor, serratus anterior, latissimus dorsi, rectus abdominis, and platysma

---

KEY POINTS

✔ Bell's palsy is a diagnosis of exclusion and should be treated empirically during workup.

✔ Successful reanimation involves addressing orbicularis oculi, zygomaticus major, orbicularis oris, and depressor anguli oris function.

✔ Static procedures are useful for restoring facial symmetry in repose, but they do not address dynamic function.

✔ Free-functional muscle transfers are the best option to restore dynamic function.

✔ Successful free functional muscle transfer involves postoperative physiotherapy.

✔ Lower lip depressor function is difficult to achieve; to achieve symmetry, contralateral depressor myomectomy may be beneficial.

REFERENCES

1. Davis RA, Anson BJ, Budinger JM, et al. Surgical anatomy of the facial nerve and parotid gland based upon a study of 350 cervicofacial halves. Surg Gynecol Obstet 102:385-412, 1956.
2. Baker DC, Conley J. Avoiding facial nerve injuries in rhytidectomy. Anatomical variations and pitfalls. Plast Reconstr Surg 64:781-795, 1979.
3. Pitanguy I, Ramos AS. The frontal branch of the facial nerve: The importance of its variations in face lifting. Plast Reconstr Surg 38:352-356, 1966.
4. Stuzin JM, Wagstrom L, Kawamoto HK, et al. Anatomy of the frontal branch of the facial nerve: The significance of the temporal fat pad. Plast Reconstr Surg 83:256-271, 1989.
5. Gosain AK, Sewall SR, Yousif NJ. The temporal branch of the facial nerve: How reliably can we predict its path? Plast Reconstr Surg 99:1224-1233, 1997.
6. Dingman RO, Grabb WC. Surgical anatomy of the mandibular ramus of the facial nerve based on the dissection of 100 facial halves. Plast Reconstr Surg 29:266-272, 1962.
7. Freilinger G, Gruber H, Happak W, et al. Surgical anatomy of the mimetic muscle system and the facial nerve: Importance for reconstructive and aesthetic surgery. Plast Reconstr Surg 80:686-690, 1987.
8. Anderson RG. Facial nerve disorders and surgery. Sel Read Plast Surg 9(20), 2001.
9. Austin JR, Peskind SP, Austin SG, et al. Idiopathic facial nerve paralysis: A randomized double blind controlled study of placebo versus prednisone. Laryngoscope 103:1326-1333, 1993.
10. Shafshak TS, Essa AY, Bakey FA. The possible contributing factors for the success of steroid therapy in Bell's palsy: A clinical and electrophysiological study. J Laryngol Otol 108:940-943, 1994.
11. Adour KK. Medical management of idiopathic (Bell's) palsy. Otolaryngol Clin North Am 24:663-673, 1991.
12. Teller DC, Murphy TP. Bilateral facial paralysis: A case presentation and literature review. J Otolaryngol 21:44-47, 1992.

13. House JW, Brackmann DE. Facial nerve grading system. Otolaryngol Head Neck Surg 93:146-147, 1985.
14. Burres S, Fisch U. The comparison of facial grading systems. Arch Otolaryngol Head Neck Surg 112:755-758, 1986.
15. Ross BG, Fradet G, Nedzelski JM. Development of a sensitive clinical facial grading system. Otolaryngol Head Neck Surg 114:380-386, 1996.
16. Brenner MJ, Neely JG. Approaches to grading facial nerve function. Semin Plast Surg 18:13-21, 2004.
17. Gagnon NB, Molina-Negro P. Facial reinnervation after facial paralysis: Is it ever too late? Arch Otorhinolaryngol 246:303-307, 1989.
18. Seeley BM, To WC, Papy FA. A multivectored bone-anchored system for facial resuspension in patients with facial paralysis. Plast Reconstr Surg 108:1686-1691, 2001.
19. Seiff SR, Chang J. Management of ophthalmic complications of facial nerve palsy. Otolaryngol Clin North Am 25:669-690, 1992.
20. Smith JW. A new technique for facial reanimation. In Hueston JT, ed. Transactions of the Fifth International Congress of Plastic and Reconstructive Surgery. Melbourne: Butterworths, 1971.
21. O'Brien MB, Pederson WC, Khazanchi RK, et al. Results of management of facial palsy with microvascular free-muscle transfer. Plast Reconstr Surg 86:12-22, 1990.
22. Sassoon EM, Poole MD, Rushworth G. Reanimation for facial palsy using gracilis muscle grafts. Br J Plast Surg 44:195-200, 1991.

PART IV

Breast

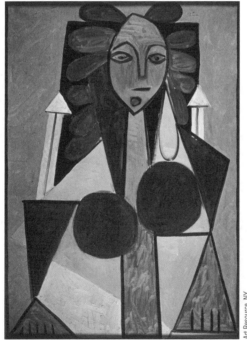

38. Breast Anatomy and Embryology

Melissa A. Crosby

EMBRYOLOGY AND DEVELOPMENT[1]

EMBRYOLOGY

- From the eighth to tenth week of embryologic development, breast growth begins with differentiation of cutaneous epithelium of the pectoral region.
- The milk ridge develops at the sixth week, extending from the axilla to the groin.
- Normal breast development begins in the anterolateral pectoral region at the level of the fourth intercostal space.
- Supernumerary breasts *(polymastia)* and nipples *(polythelia)* can occur along the milk ridge.
  - The most common location for polymastia and polythelia is the left chest wall below the inframammary crease.
  - Polythelia is the most common congenital breast anomaly, occurring in 2% of the population.

DEVELOPMENT

- Puberty begins at age 10-12 years as a result of hypothalamic gonadotropin-releasing hormones secreted into the hypothalamic-pituitary portal venous system.
- The anterior pituitary secretes follicle-stimulating hormone (FSH) and luteinizing hormone (LH).
- FSH causes ovarian follicles to mature and secrete estrogens.
- Estrogens stimulate longitudinal growth of breast ductal epithelium.
- As ovarian follicles become mature and ovulate, the corpus luteum releases progesterone, which, in conjunction with estrogen, leads to complete mammary development.
- **Stages of breast development described by Tanner**[2]
  Stage 1: Preadolescent elevation of nipple but no palpable glandular tissue or areolar pigmentation
  Stage 2: Glandular tissue in the subareolar region; nipple and breast project as single mound
  Stage 3: Further increase in glandular tissue with enlargement of breast and nipple but continued contour of nipple and breast in single plane
  Stage 4: Enlargement of areola and increased areolar pigmentation with secondary mound formed by nipple and areola above level of breast
  Stage 5: Final adolescent development of smooth contour with no projection of areola and nipple

MENSTRUAL CYCLE

- **Follicular phase:** Days 4-14, mitosis and proliferation of breast epithelial cells
- **Luteal phase:** Days 14-28, progesterone levels rise, mammary ductal dilation and differentiation of alveolar epithelial cells into secretory cells, estrogens increase blood flow to breast
- **Premenstrual:** Estrogen peak, breast engorgement, breast sensitivity
- **Menstruation:** Breast involution and decrease in circulating hormones

PREGNANCY AND LACTATION

- Marked ductular, lobular, and alveolar growth occurs under the influence of estrogen, progesterone, placental lactogen, prolactin, and chorionic gonadotropin.

- **First trimester:** Estrogen influences ductular sprouting and lobular formation, early to late breast enlargement ensues, and dilation of superficial veins and increased pigmentation of nipple-areola complex occurs.
- **Second trimester:** Lobular events predominate under the influence of progestins, and colostrum collects within the lobular alveoli.
- **Third trimester:** By parturition, breast size triples because of vascular engorgement, epithelial proliferation, and colostrum accumulation.
- **Delivery:** Withdrawal of placental lactogen and sex hormones results in breast being predominantly influenced by prolactin.
- **Anterior** pituitary secretion of **prolactin** influences **milk production and secretion.**
- **Posterior** pituitary secretion of **oxytocin** leads to breast **myoepithelial contraction** and **milk ejection.**
- Tactile stimulation of nipples by nursing infant results in prolactin and oxytocin secretion.
- Postlactational involution occurs during the 3 months after nursing ceases; regression of extra-lobular stroma is a primary feature.

MENOPAUSE
- Involves loss of glandular tissue and replacement with fat

VASCULAR SUPPLY (Fig. 38-1)

ARTERIAL SUPPLY
- **Skin** receives blood supply from subdermal plexus, which communicates through perforators with underlying deeper vessels supplying breast parenchyma (see following section).
- **Parenchyma** supplied by:
  - Perforating branches of internal mammary artery
  - Lateral thoracic artery
  - Thoracodorsal artery
  - Intercostal perforators
  - Thoracoacromial artery
- **Nipple areolar complex** receives both parenchymal and subdermal blood supply.
- **Venous drainage** follows the arterial supply.

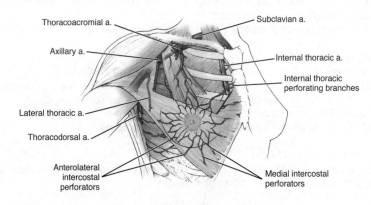

Fig. 38-1

INNERVATION[1,3,4] (Fig. 38-2)

- The process is dermatomal and is derived from the anterolateral and anteromedial branches of the thoracic intercostal nerves T3-T5.
- Supraclavicular nerves from lower fibers of the cervical plexus also provide innervation to upper and lateral portions of the breast.
- Nipple-areola sensation is derived from the anteromedial and anterolateral **T4** intercostal nerve.
- Intercostobrachial nerve travels across axilla to supply upper medial arm.

CAUTION: The intercostobrachial nerve is often injured during axillary dissection, resulting in anaesthesia and paresthesias.

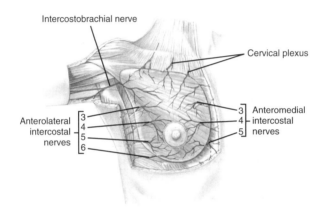

Fig. 38-2

SKIN AND PARENCHYMA

- The adult breast extends from the second to the seventh rib in the midclavicular line, and medially from the sternocostal junction to the midaxillary line laterally.
- The adult breast also extends into the axilla, giving it a teardrop shape *(axillary tail of Spence)*.
- The adult mammary gland is composed of multiple lobules that are connected and drained by 16 to 24 main lactiferous ducts.
- A **lobule** is the functional unit of the breast.
- Lobules are situated in radial distribution (Fig. 38-3).
- Each lobule is composed of hundreds of **acini.**
- Each acinus has secretory potential and is connected to lactiferous ducts by its own interlobular ducts.
- Each main lactiferous duct dilates as it approaches the nipple, forming a sinus *(lactiferous sinus* or *central collecting duct)* that functions as a reservoir for milk storage.
- Nipple contains orifices to drain each lactiferous duct; these may act as conduits for bacteria.
- **Morgagni's tubercles** are located near the periphery of the areola, which has elevations formed by openings of ducts of **Montgomery's glands.**
- **Montgomery's glands** are large sebaceous glands capable of secreting milk. They represent an intermediate stage between sweat and mammary glands and also act to lubricate the areola during lactation.

- Fat content varies but is responsible for most of the bulk, contour, softness, consistency, and shape of the breast.
- Fat content increases as glandular component subsides, such as after lactation or during menopause.
- The breast is supported by layers of **superficial fascia.**
  - **A layer of superficial fascia** is located near the dermis; it is difficult to distinguish unless treating a thin patient.
  - **A deep layer of superficial fascia** is present on the deep surface of the breast; a loose areolar plane exists between this layer and the deep fascial layer that overlies underlying musculature.
- **Cooper's ligaments** penetrate deep layer of superficial fascia into parenchyma breast to dermis; ptosis results from attenuation of these attachments.

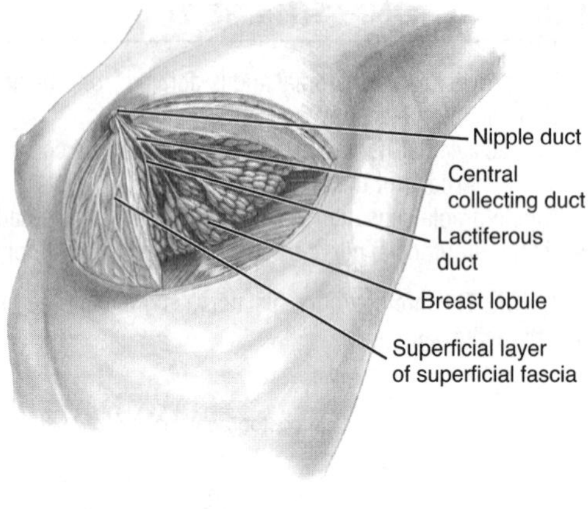

Nipple duct
Central collecting duct
Lactiferous duct
Breast lobule
Superficial layer of superficial fascia

Fig. 38-3

UNDERLYING MUSCULATURE[5] (Fig. 38-4)

PECTORALIS MAJOR

- **Origin:** Medial clavicle, sternum, anterior ribs (second to sixth), external oblique and rectus abdominis fascia
- **Insertion:** Upper humerus, 10 cm from humeral head on lateral side of intertubercular sulcus
- **Function:** Adduction and medial rotation of arm
- **Blood supply:** Internal mammary perforators, thoracoacromial artery, intercostal perforators, lateral thoracic artery

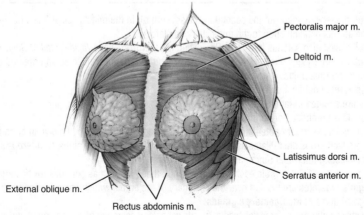

Pectoralis major m.
Deltoid m.
Latissimus dorsi m.
Serratus anterior m.
External oblique m.
Rectus abdominis m.

Fig. 38-4

- **Innervation:** Medial (sternal portion) and lateral (clavicular portion) pectoral nerves *(named for origin in brachial plexus cord)*
- Upper medial portion of breast located over pectoralis major

---

TIP: Absence of sternal head of pectoralis major is seen in Poland's syndrome.

PECTORALIS MINOR
- **Origin:** Anterolateral surfaces of third to sixth ribs
- **Insertion:** Coracoid process of scapula
- **Function:** Draws scapula down and forward
- **Blood supply:** Pectoral branch of thoracoacromial artery, lateral thoracic artery, direct branch of axillary artery
- **Innervation:** Medial pectoral nerve

TIP: The pectoralis minor serves as landmark during axillary dissection because the lateral margin divides superficial from deep axillary nodes.

SERRATUS ANTERIOR
- **Origin:** Anterolateral aspects of upper eight ribs
- **Insertion:** Anterior surface of medial aspect of scapula
- **Function:** Stabilizes scapula against chest wall during abduction and elevation of arm in horizontal direction; also pulls scapula forward and laterally
- **Blood supply:** Lateral thoracic artery, branches of thoracodorsal artery
- **Innervation:** Long thoracic nerve

RECTUS ABDOMINIS
- **Origin:** Pubic line
- **Insertion:** Third to seventh costal cartilages
- **Function:** Flexes the vertebral column and tenses abdominal wall
- **Blood supply:** Superior and inferior epigastric artery and vein, subcostal and intercostal perforators
- **Innervation:** Segmental motor nerves from seventh to twelfth intercostal nerves

EXTERNAL OBLIQUE
- **Origin:** External surface of lower anterior and lateral ribs
- **Insertion:** Iliac crest and medial abdominal fascial aponeurosis
- **Function:** Compression of abdominal contents
- **Blood supply:** Inferior eight intercostal arteries
- **Innervation:** Seventh to twelfth intercostal nerves

LYMPHATIC DRAINAGE[6]

- There is an extensive network of both **superficial** and **deep** lymphatic drainage.
- **Superficial lymphatic drainage** originates from a periareolar lymphatic plexus that accompanies venous drainage.

- **Deep lymphatic drainage** begins as individual lymphatic channels that drain each lactiferous duct and lobule and then penetrate through the deep fascia of underlying musculature.
- Lymphatic drainage from the upper outer quadrant passes around pectoralis major to deep pectoral nodes or directly to subscapular nodes.
- Lymphatic efferent of breast travels to central axillary nodes, then to apical axillary nodes and to supraclavicular nodes.
- Medial lymphatic channels follow internal mammary perforating vessels and drain to parasternal nodes.
- **Most of breast drains into axillary nodes, with three levels identified.**
    Level I: Lateral to lateral border of pectoralis minor
    Level II: Behind pectoralis minor and below axillary vein
    Level III: Medial to medial border of pectoralis minor
- **Rotter's nodes** are between pectoralis major and minor.

KEY POINTS

- ✔ The nipple-areola complex is innervated by the anterolateral branch of the fourth intercostal nerve.
- ✔ Supernumerary nipples and breasts can occur along the milk line from axilla to groin.
- ✔ Attenuation of Cooper's ligaments leads to ptosis and increased breast mobility.
- ✔ Injury to the intercostobrachial nerve results in paresthesias or anaesthesia of the upper medial arm.
- ✔ Three levels of axillary lymph nodes exist.
- ✔ Poland's syndrome results in the absence of sternal head of pectoralis major.

REFERENCES

1. Bostwick J III. Anatomy and Physiology, vol 1, 2nd ed. St Louis: Quality Medical Publishing, 2000, pp 77-123.
2. Tanner JM. Growth at Adolescence. Oxford: Blackwell Scientific, 1962.
3. Hanna MK, Nahai F. Applied anatomy of the breast. In Nahai F, ed. Art of Aesthetic Surgery: Principles and Techniques, vol 3. St Louis: Quality Medical Publishing, 2005.
4. August DA, Sondak VK. Breast. In Greenfield LJ, Mulholland MW, Oldham KT, et al, eds. Surgery: Scientific Principles and Practice, 2nd ed. Philadelphia: Lippincott-Raven, 1997, pp 1357-1416.
5. Mathes SJ, Nahai F. Reconstructive Surgery: Principles, Anatomy, and Technique, vols 1 and 2. New York: Quality Medical Publishing/Churchill Livingston, 1997.
6. Haagensen CD. Diseases of the Breast, 3rd ed. Philadelphia: WB Saunders, 1986.

39. Breast Augmentation

Thornwell Hay Parker III
Michael E. Decherd

BACKGROUND

- Breast augmentation is the second most common cosmetic surgery (after liposuction).[1]
- Silicone implants were first introduced in 1964.
- Saline implants were introduced in 1970s as an alternative to silicone.
- The U.S. Food and Drug Administration (FDA) placed a moratorium on silicone implants in 1992 for primary augmentation because of concerns about autoimmune and connective tissue disease.
  - In 1999, the **NIH Institute of Medicine and the National Academy of Sciences reviewed 17 epidemiologic studies and were unable to detect any link between silicone and systemic, autoimmune, or prenatal disease.**
  - Studies found silicone in local macrophages, lymph nodes, and breast tissue.
  - Studies did **not** demonstrate elevated systemic levels (normal liver, lung, and spleen).[2]
- Saline implants increased in popularity during the 1990s because of silicone scare.
- Silicone implants have evolved through different generations.
  - First: Thick shell and thick filler
  - Second: Thin shell and thin filler—less palpable, but higher rupture rate
  - Current: Thicker shell with barrier coating and cohesive gel filler (form stable)
  - NOTE: Some consider the introduction of textured surfaces and anatomic shapes to represent fourth or fifth generations
- Cohesive gel implants are considered the gold standard.
  - In Europe since 1995
  - In Canada since 2000
  - Advantages: More natural, less rippling, maintains integrity after rupture
  - Disadvantages: Larger incision, more expensive, stiffer
- Silicone implants are currently approved in the United States for:
  - Breast reconstruction
  - Silicone implant exchange
  - Replacement of saline implant if complications
- Silicone implants appear likely to be approved by the FDA for primary breast augmentation in the future.

INDICATIONS[3]

- Enhance breast shape and volume
- Improve body image, symmetry, and balance
- Help clothes fit better
- Provide the appearance of a breast lift and increased cleavage
- Rejuvenation after postpartum deflation

CONTRAINDICATIONS

- Body dysmorphic disorder
- Psychological instability
- Responding to peer, spousal, or parental pressure
- Attempting to salvage marriage or relationship, or to find husband
- Patient less than 18 years old
- Significant breast disease (severe fibrocystic disease, ductal hyperplasia, high-risk breast cancer)
- Collagen vascular disease

PATIENT EVALUATION

MEDICAL HISTORY
- Personal history of breast disease or cancer
- Family history of breast disease or cancer
- Pregnancy history: Breast size before, during, and after; plans for future children
- Mammography
  - Screening mammogram by age 35 years, if planning to operate on breast
  - General public: Every 2 years starting at age 40, every year from age 50 onward[4]
- Current breast size
- Desired breast size

PHYSICAL EXAM
- **Cancer screening:** Masses, dimpling, discharge, and lymph nodes
- **Skin quality**
  - Tone
  - Elasticity
  - Striae
- **Asymmetries:** Chest wall, scoliosis, and breast
  - Difference in breast volume
  - Difference in inframammary fold (IMF) height
  - Difference in nipple-areola complex (NAC) height
- **Ptosis** (see Chapter 40)
  - Mild ptosis is improved by augmentation.
  - Moderate to severe ptosis may require mastopexy.
- **Measurements** (patient sitting up straight)
  - Height, weight, body frame (small to large)
  - Sternal notch to nipple (SN:N)
  - Nipple to inframammary fold (N:IMF) during stretch
  - Base width (width of breast base)
  - Parenchymal coverage (pinch test)
    - ▸ Superior pole
    - ▸ Lower pole
  - Anterior pull skin stretch (centimeters of stretch with pull at edge of areola)
  - Parenchymal fill (percentage of skin envelope filled by parenchyma)

IMPLANT CHOICE

VOLUME
- **Patient preference**
  - Sizers put in bra to establish desired volume (not recommended)
  - Photos of other women
  - Digital imaging
- **Surgeon's experience**
  - 125-150 ml to increase by one cup size
  - Larger body frames require larger implant volumes to increase cup size
- **Breast analysis**
  - *High Five system*[5]
    - ▶ Objective measures to determine optimal implant and volume
    - ▶ Volume based on breast base width
    - ▶ Add or subtract volume based on skin stretch, breast envelope fill, and N:IMF
- **Intraoperative breast sizers**
- **Pitfalls of large implant volume**
  - Stretch and stress tissues
  - Atrophy and thinning of parenchyma and skin
  - Increased palpability
  - Traction rippling

CAUTION: Large implants (larger than 350-400 ml) can have detrimental effects.

FILLER
- **Saline**
  - **Advantages**
    - ▶ Low contracture rates
    - ▶ Adjusts quickly to body core temperature
    - ▶ Leaks are safely absorbed by body
    - ▶ Easier to adjust for size and correct breast asymmetry
  - **Disadvantages**
    - ▶ Wrinkling
    - ▶ Leaks lead to complete deflation
  - **Construction**
    - ▶ Silicone shell filled with physiologic saline solution
- **Silicone**
  - **Advantage**
    - ▶ More natural feel than saline
  - **Disadvantages**
    - ▶ High contracture rates
    - ▶ Slow to adjust to body core temperature (e.g., implants remain cold after swimming)
    - ▶ Rupture may cause local inflammation and granulomas
  - **Construction**
    - ▶ Silicone shell with silicone filler
    - ▶ Silicone: Polymer of dimethylsiloxane; longer chains lead to increased viscosity

- **Double-lumen (Becker implant)**
  - **Advantages**
    - ▸ Natural feel of silicone
    - ▸ Able to make postoperative adjustments to inner-lumen saline volume
    - ▸ Useful for asymmetry or if patient uncertain of desired size
  - **Disadvantages**
    - ▸ Fill port temporarily implanted, requiring second procedure to remove
    - ▸ Possible fill valve failure
  - **Construction**
    - ▸ Outer and inner silicone shell, but **outer lumen filled with silicone, and adjustable inner lumen filled with saline**
- **Polyvinylpyrrolidone (PVP) hydrogel[6] (not recommended)**
  - **Advantages**
    - ▸ Higher viscosity than saline
    - ▸ PVP not metabolized; excreted by kidneys after leak
  - **Disadvantages**
    - ▸ **Increased size after implantation because of osmotic gradient**
    - ▸ High contracture rates
  - **Construction**
    - ▸ Developed as alternative to gel following moratorium on silicone
    - ▸ Filler: Hydrocolloid bio-oncotic gel of low-molecular-weight polymers
    - ▸ Misti Gold PVP (Novamed Medical Products, Inc., Minneapolis, MN)
    - ▸ Misti Gold PVP II
      - ◆ Decreased osmotic gradient, but still reports of increased size
- **Triglyceride**
  - **Advantage**
    - ▸ Higher viscosity than saline gives more natural feel
  - **Disadvantages**
    - ▸ Oil oxidizes, becomes rancid, bleeds from shell
    - ▸ Inflammation, pain, foul smell
  - **Construction**
    - ▸ Another alternative to gel following moratorium
    - ▸ Filler: Soybean oil
    - ▸ Trilucent implant
    - ▸ Medical Devices Agency (MDA) recommendation to remove all Trilucent implants

SURFACE
- **Textured**
  - **Advantages**
    - ▸ Lower contracture rates (surface disorients collagen deposition)
    - ▸ Less migration and implant rotation
  - **Disadvantages**
    - ▸ Thicker shells
    - ▸ More palpable
    - ▸ Traction rippling
  - **Technique**
    - ▸ Intraoperative positioning of implant is critical, because textured surface resists migration or movement in pocket; base must be properly oriented along IMF

- **Smooth**
  - **Advantages**
    - ▸ Thinner capsule formed
    - ▸ Less palpable: Preferable for patients with thin coverage
  - **Disadvantage**
    - ▸ Slightly higher contracture rates
- **Polyurethane (PU)-covered**
  - **Advantage**
    - ▸ Dramatically low contracture rates (less than 1% over 10 years)
  - **Disadvantage**
    - ▸ Pulled from U.S. market because PU breaks down as a carcinogenic compound (although levels likely insignificant)
  - **Construction**
    - ▸ PU coating separates over weeks to months and becomes incorporated into the capsule, helping to disperse contractile forces.
    - ▸ Textured implants were developed to mimic the effect of PU on the capsule.

DIMENSION/SHAPE

- **Round (circular implant)**
  - Low-profile
  - Moderate-profile
  - Moderate-plus-profile
  - High-profile
    - ▸ Increased projection for given base width
    - ▸ Increased projection with less volume
    - ▸ Advantage with a constricted lower pole or a narrow breast base width
- **Anatomic (implant height different than width)**
  - Designed to give more natural breast shape
  - Increased implant height and projection for a given base width
  - Upper pole tapered; fuller lower pole, reducing upper pole collapse and filling out lower pole of breast
  - Disadvantage: Must be oriented properly and symmetrically
  - Most textured to maintain position

INCISION CHOICE (Table 39-1)

INFRAMAMMARY FOLD

- **Advantages**
  - Well hidden with mild ptosis or well-defined IMF
  - Best control
- **Disadvantage**
  - Visible scar on breast
- **Technique**
  - Place incision at planned IMF location, keep majority (two thirds) of incision lateral to nipple because more visible when placed medially.

Table 39-1   *Incision Options for Breast Augmentation*

Factor	Axillary	Periareolar	Inframammary	Transumbilical*
Implant Plane				
Submuscular	+	+	+	−
Subglandular	−	+	+	+
Implant Type				
Saline, round	+	+	+	+
Saline, shaped	−	+	+	−
Silicone, round or shaped	−	+	+	−
Preoperative Breast Volume				
High (>200 g)	+	+	+	+
Low (<200 g)	+	+	−	+
Preoperative Breast Base Position				
High	+	+	+	+
Low	−	+	+	+
Breast Shape				
Tubular	−	+	−	−
Glandular ptosis	+	+	+	+
Ptosis (grades I and II)	−	+	−	−
Areola Characteristics				
Small diameter	+	−	+	+
Light or indistinct	+	−	+	+
Inframammary Fold				
None	+	+	−	+
High	+	+	−	+
Low	+	+	+	+
Secondary Procedure	−	+	+	−

From Hidalgo DA. Breast augmentation: Choosing the optimal incision, implant, and pocket plane. Plast Reconstr Surg 105:2202-2206, 2000.
+, Applicable; −, not generally recommended.
*Included for completeness, but generally not recommended.

PERIAREOLAR

- **Advantages**
  - Well hidden at interface of NAC and skin
  - Good access if areola diameter greater than 3.5 cm
- **Disadvantages**
  - May traverse and scar a cancer-prone organ
  - White or hypopigmented scar when placed within areola
  - Potential for visible hypertrophic scarring
- **Technique**
  - Place around the lower half of the areola precisely at the junction of areola and breast skin
  - Dissection options
    - ▶ **Direct dissection**
      - ⬩ Through breast parenchyma
      - ⬩ Discouraged because of possible bacterial contamination from ducts and may scar breast parenchyma
    - ▶ **Stair-step dissection**
      - ⬩ After cutting through the skin, dissect inferiorly following the subcutaneous plane to the inferior edge of the breast mound, then create a pocket.
      - ⬩ This technique is preferred because less parenchyma is disrupted.

TRANSAXILLARY

- **Advantages**
  - No breast scar
- **Disadvantages**
  - Potential scar visibility when sleeveless and raising arms
  - Difficult to insert silicone implants
- **Technique**
  - Blind procedure in the early 70s, now significantly advanced by endoscopic technique[7]
  - 2-3 cm horizontal incision at highest point of axilla, 1 cm behind border of pectoralis; dissect medially in superficial subcutaneous plane, and continue to posterolateral border of pectoralis, incising vertically to enter subpectoral or subglandular plane

> TIP: Avoid deep dissection in axilla; intercostobrachial and median brachial cutaneous nerves are vulnerable.

TRANSUMBILICAL

- **Advantages**
  - Scar hidden and distant from breast
- **Disadvantages**
  - Difficult, blind dissection
  - High or asymmetric placement
  - Difficult to make adjustments or corrections
- **Technique**
  - **Blind dissection** from superior umbilical incision through inferomedial breast; expander or implant sizer inflated to create pocket, then replaced with permanent implant

POCKET PLANE AND DISSECTION (Fig. 39-1)

SUBGLANDULAR

- **Advantages**
  - Good projection and shape
  - Avoids distortion in muscular or active patients
- **Disadvantages**
  - High contracture rate
  - Implant edges may be palpable
  - Interference with mammography
- **Contraindication:** Thin parenchymal coverage (upper pole pinch test less than 2 cm)
- **Technique**
  - Dissection on top of pectoralis major, below gland

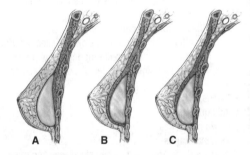

Fig. 39-1 Implant location. **A,** Subglandular augmentation. **B,** Submusculofascial augmentation. **C,** Biplanar augmentation.

SUBPECTORAL

- **Advantages**
  - Low contracture rates (<10%)
  - Thick soft tissue coverage
  - Good preservation of nipple sensation
- **Disadvantages**
  - "Dancing breasts" during pectoralis contraction
  - Lateral displacement of implant over time
  - Difficult to control upper pole fill
- **Relative contraindication**
  - Muscular or active patient
- **Technique**
  - Dissection below pectoralis major but above pectoralis minor
  - Does not disrupt inferior attachments of pectoralis if "total subpectoral"

BIPLANAR (DUAL PLANE)[8]

- **Advantages**
  - Subpectoral coverage of upper pole
    - ▸ Thick soft tissue coverage
    - ▸ Low contracture rate
  - Less implant displacement at rest and during pectoralis contraction
  - Allows implant to sit along IMF
  - Increases implant-parenchymal interface, which expands lower pole and prevents double-bubble deformity

- **Disadvantage**
  - Usually restricted to IMF incision when performing dual plane II and III
- **Contraindication**
  - IMF pinch test less than 0.4 cm
- **Rationale**
  - Complete muscle coverage restricts expansion of inferior pole, forcing implant superiorly and laterally.
  - Especially with ptotic and loose breast parenchyma, breast tissue may slide inferior to the axis of the implant while implant remains fixed higher on the chest wall, causing a type-A double-bubble deformity.
  - Dual plane techniques release inferior pectoralis attachments, allowing some pectoralis retraction superiorly. This maximizes implant contact with lower pole breast parenchyma, with the advantage of upper pole coverage by the pectoralis.
- **Types**
  - *Dual plane I*
    - ▶ Pectoralis released along IMF in addition to subpectoral dissection
    - ▶ Used for most typical breasts
    - ▶ Criteria
      - ◆ All breast above IMF
      - ◆ Tight attachment of parenchyma to pectoralis
      - ◆ Minimally stretched lower pole (4-6 cm from NAC to IMF)
  - *Dual plane II*
    - ▶ In addition to pectoralis release along IMF and subpectoral dissection, the pectoralis is separated from breast parenchyma **to level of inferior NAC**
    - ▶ Criteria
      - ◆ Most breast above IMF
      - ◆ Loose parenchymal-pectoral attachments
      - ◆ Moderate lower pole stretch (5.5-6.5 cm from NAC to IMF)
  - *Dual plane III*
    - ▶ Released as for dual plane II, but separation of pectoralis from parenchyma is continued **to level of superior NAC**
    - ▶ For glandular ptotic or constricted breasts
    - ▶ Criteria
      - ◆ At least one third of breast below IMF
      - ◆ Very loose parenchymal-pectoral attachments
      - ◆ Marked lower pole stretch (7-8 cm from NAC to IMF)
      - ◆ Lower pole constricted
    - ▶ Constricted breast
      - ◆ Use radial and concentric scoring through breast parenchyma

TREATMENT OF INFRAMAMMARY FOLD

- Appropriate IMF height centers the axis of the implant behind or just below the nipple-areolar complex.
- N:IMF length should correspond to implant volume.
  - Approximately 7 cm at 250 cc, 8 cm at 300 cc, 8.5 cm at 350 cc, 9 cm at 375 cc, 9.5 cm at 400 cc
  - Areola to inframammary fold distance: Should approximate radius of implant and half of breast base width

> TIP: IMF can be carefully lowered when a significant discrepancy exists between implant size and N:IMF distance, or when asymmetry exists.

TECHNICAL POINTS[9]

- Perioperative antibiotics (first-generation cephalosporin 30 minutes before incision)
- Precise dissection
- Meticulous hemostasis
- Hand-switched monopolar cautery
- Talc-free gloves
- Triple antibiotic solution (TAB)[10]
  - Mix 50,000 units bacitracin, 80 mg gentamicin, and 1 gm cefazolin in 500 cc normal saline solution (soak pocket 5 minutes).
  - In 2000, FDA banned povidone iodine (Betadine) from contacting implants because of complications when used **intraluminally** (implant delamination and leakage), but there is **no scientific evidence that extraluminal contact is harmful.**
- Deep closing sutures placed before implant inserted, with knots away from implant
- Skin wiped with antibiotic solution
- Gloves changed before insertion of permanent implant
- "No-touch technique": Prevents implant contamination from skin[11]
- Sterile saline injected through closed system

POSTOPERATIVE CARE

MEDICATIONS
- Acetaminophen preferred for routine pain control
- Narcotics only as needed for severe pain
- Carisoprodol (Soma®, Vanadom): Helps pectoralis relax
- Antibiotics: No proven benefit, but usually given for 3 days

BRASSIERE AND DRESSING
- Steri-Strips™ (3M Corporation, St. Paul, MN) for 6 weeks
- Brassiere optional; avoid underwire or push-up bras for 6 weeks

ACTIVITY
- Implant displacement exercises
  - Push implant medially and superiorly
  - Begin postoperative day 3 or when not painful for patient
  - 10 pushes, 3 times a day for 1 month, then once daily
- Aerobic exercise after 2 weeks
- Heavy lifting after 6 weeks

COMPLICATIONS AND CONSENT

CAPSULAR CONTRACTURE

The body naturally forms capsules around all implants. Capsular contracture *is when the capsule tightens, compresses, and distorts the implant.*

- **Baker classification system**
  - I: **Normal,** soft, nonpalpable implant
  - II: **Palpable,** minimally firm, not visible
  - III: **Visible,** easily palpated, and moderately firm
  - IV: **Painful,** hard, and breast distorted
- **Etiologic factors**
  - Subclinical infection[12-16]
    - ▸ Correlation well-established, but causal relationship uncertain
    - ▸ *Staphylococcus epidermidis* most common, but many other types of bacteria implicated
  - Hypertrophic scar hypothesis
- **Time course**
  - Most contractures occur within 1 year.
  - Late occurrence may be secondary to systemic bacterial seeding or capsular maturation.
- **Historical rates and risk factors**
  - **Pocket location[17]**
    - ▸ Subglandular: 32% contracture rate
    - ▸ Subpectoral: 12% contracture rate
  - **Filler[18]**
    - ▸ Silicone: 50% contracture rate
    - ▸ Saline: 16% contracture rate
  - **Implant surface[19,20]** (Fig. 39-2)
    - ▸ Smooth: 58% contracture rate
    - ▸ Textured: 11% contracture rate

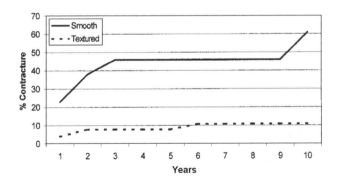

Fig. 39-2   Ten-year development of subglandular capsular contracture in smooth versus textured implants. (From Collis N, Coleman D, Foo IT, et al. Ten-year review of a prospective randomized controlled trial of textured versus smooth subglandular silicone gel breast implants. Plast Reconstr Surg 106:786-791, 2000.)

- **Recent data**
  - ▸ With significantly low contracture rates, data have shown less correlation between implant texture, filler, or pocket choice
  - ▸ Saline trial: 2001, Mentor Corporation[21]
    - ✦ 9% contracture rate with primary augmentation
    - ✦ 30% contracture rate with reconstruction
  - ▸ Saline trial: 2001, Inamed Corporation[22]
    - ✦ 9% contracture rate with primary augmentation
    - ✦ 25% contracture rate with reconstruction
  - ▸ Silicone Gel Premarket Approval trial: 2003, Inamed Corporation and 2005, Mentor Corporation[23]
    - ✦ 8%-9% contracture rate with primary augmentation
- ■ **Treatment**
  - **Capsulectomy**
    - ▸ **Indications**[24]
      - ✦ Baker III or IV classification
      - ✦ Calcified or thick capsule
      - ✦ Ruptured silicone implant
      - ✦ Silicone granulomas
      - ✦ Infection around implant
      - ✦ Polyurethane implant
      - ✦ Previous implant needs to be replaced with larger-volume implant
      - ✦ New plane needed (e.g., subglandular changes to subpectoral)
    - ▸ **Advantages**
      - ✦ Low contracture recurrence
      - ✦ Removal of potential contaminants
    - ▸ **Disadvantages**
      - ✦ Hemostasis more difficult
      - ✦ Anteriorly: Thins soft tissue coverage
      - ✦ Posteriorly: Risk of pneumothorax (if previous subpectoral implant)
    - ▸ **Technique**
      - ✦ Complete capsulectomy is preferred in the subglandular plane, but caution is needed anteriorly with thin soft tissue coverage.
      - ✦ Anterior capsulectomy alone, if in the subpectoral plane and posterior capsule is densely adherent to chest wall, to avoid entering chest cavity.
  - **Open capsulotomy**
    - ▸ Controlled scoring through capsule, concentric and radial
    - ▸ 37%-89% recurrence
  - **Closed capsulotomy**
    - ▸ Manual external compression attempts to break capsule
    - ▸ Generally condemned because risks implant rupture and bleeding
    - ▸ 31%-80% recurrence
  - **Breast massage and displacement exercises**
  - **Exercise** (early, less than 2 weeks postoperative)
  - **Pharmacotherapy**
    - ▸ Leukotriene inhibitors (e.g., zafirlukast [Accolate®]): Potential for rare liver toxicity
    - ▸ Papaverine hydrochloride (Pavabid)

▸ Oral vitamin E
▸ Intraluminal steroids: Reduced contracture, but higher rate of implant rupture, skin erosion, atrophy, and ptosis
▸ Cyclosporine (Neoral®, Sandimmune®), mitomycin C (Mutamycin)

LEAK OR RUPTURE

■ **Rupture rates**
  • Saline: 1% per year
  • Silicone[20]
    ▸ 30% at 5 years
    ▸ 50% at 10 years
    ▸ 70% at 17 years
■ **Etiologic factors**
  • Fold flaw
  • Underfilling
  • Manufacturing flaws
  • Technical errors
  • Higher problem rates with thin-shell implants (second generation)
■ **Diagnosis**
  • Examination
    ▸ Asymmetry
    ▸ Obvious deflation (less obvious with silicone)
  • Radiographs
    ▸ Mammogram
      ✦ Low sensitivity
      ✦ Moderate specificity
      ✦ Expense low
    ▸ Ultrasound
      ✦ Findings: Snowstorm, stepladder appearance
      ✦ Moderate sensitivity
      ✦ Moderate specificity
      ✦ Expense moderate
    ▸ MRI
      ✦ Findings: **Linguine sign,** silicone extrusion
      ✦ High sensitivity
      ✦ High specificity
      ✦ Expense high
■ **Treatment**
  • Treat as soon as possible to prevent further distortion of the deflated breast, contraction of the capsules, and local inflammation and granulomas with silicone leak.
  • Remove implant and residual implant material.
  • Perform capsulotomy (or capsulectomy) as needed.
  • Possible replacement of implants.

CAPSULAR CALCIFICATION[25]
- Related to implant age
- 0% occurrence for implants less than 10 years old
- 100% occurrence for implants more than 23 years old
- Remove by capsulectomy

NIPPLE SENSATION
- Permanent sensory change: 15% of patients

HEMATOMA
- Rare: 0.5% of patients

CLINICAL INFECTION OF IMPLANT
- Rare: Less than 1% of patients
- Usually requires implant removal

ASYMMETRY

MIGRATION AND TISSUE CHANGES
- Bottoming out
  - Increased nipple to IMF distance, greater than half of base width
  - Related to poor tissue characteristics, large implant size, and overdissection of IMF
- Double-bubble deformity *type A* (waterfall deformity)
  - *Implant is A bove* breast mound.
  - Implant is held high on chest wall by total pectoral coverage or contracture, and loose parenchyma slides off pectoral muscles inferior to axis of the implant.
- Double-bubble deformity *type B*
  - *Implant is B elow* breast mound.
  - With significant overdissection of IMF, implant can slide caudally to the breast mound and create a second IMF below the native IMF and breast mound.

REOPERATION
- Large-scale prospective studies (2004 FDA hearings about Inamed Corporation data)[21-23]
- Current 3-year reoperation rate: 13% for saline and 21% for silicone

CANCER SURVEILLANCE
- Implants do cause interference with normal mammogram imaging.
- **Eklund mammogram views** displace breast and implant to increase parenchymal imaging after breast augmentation.
- With appropriate imaging, no increased risk for cancer is found; diagnosis not later; no difference in survival or recurrence.[26,27]

KEY POINTS

✔ Silicone is not currently approved in the United States for primary augmentation unless patient is enrolled in a study.

✔ Early mammograms are recommended for patients undergoing breast surgery (by age 30 to 35 years).

✔ Eklund mammographic views improve radiographic imaging of breast tissue following augmentation.

✔ It is important to note asymmetries during preoperative evaluations and discuss these with the patient. If there are asymmetries before surgery, there will be asymmetries afterward.

✔ Mild ptosis is improved with augmentation. However, when the N:IMF distance is more than 9.5 cm, the patient should undergo mastopexy.

✔ Subglandular augmentation is not recommended with thin upper pole coverage (superior pole pinch test is less than 2 cm).

✔ Larger implants increase long-term detrimental effects on the breast.

✔ Historically, higher contracture rates occur with smooth implants, silicone implants, and subglandular placement.

✔ Textured implant surfaces disorient collagen deposition, thereby reducing contracture.

✔ Subglandular placement potentially increases risk of implant contamination, subclinical infection, and subsequent contracture.

✔ Use of antibiotic irrigation, and other techniques, dramatically reduces contracture rates.

✔ Dual plane (biplanar) technique takes advantage of extra upper pole pectoralis coverage while maximizing the implant-parenchymal interface in the lower pole.

✔ MRI is the most sensitive and specific test for implant rupture or leak.

REFERENCES

1. American Society of Plastic Surgeons. Procedural statistics trends 1992-2004. Available at *www.plasticsurgery.org/public_education/Statistical-Trends.cfm.*

2. Barnard JJ, Todd EL, Wilson WG, et al. Distribution of organosilicon polymers in augmentation mammaplasties at autopsy. Plast Reconstr Surg 100:197-203, 1997.

3. Nahai F, ed. The Art of Aesthetic Surgery: Principles and Techniques. St Louis: Quality Medical Publishing, 2005.

4. National Breast Cancer Foundation. Early detection. Available at *www.nationalbreastcancer.org/early_detection/index.html.*

5. Tebbetts JB, Adams WP. Five critical decisions in breast augmentation using five measurements in 5 minutes. The high five decision support process. Plast Reconstr Surg 116:2005-2016, 2005.

6. Hoover SJ, Kenkel JM. Augmentation Mammoplasty. Sel Read Plast Surg 9(30), 2002.

7. Price CI, Eaves FF, Nahai F, et al. Endoscopic transaxillary subpectoral breast augmentation. Plast Reconstr Surg 94:612-619, 1994.

8. Tebbetts JB. Dual plane breast augmentation: Optimizing implant-soft-tissue relationships in a wide range of breast types. Plast Reconstr Surg 107:1255-1272, 2001.

9. Rohrich RJ, Kenkel JM, Adams WP. Preventing capsular contracture in breast augmentation: In search of the Holy Grail. Plast Reconstr Surg 103:1759-1760, 1999.

10. Adams WP, Rios JI, Smith SJ. Enhancing patient outcomes in aesthetic and reconstructive breast surgery using triple antibiotic breast irrigation: Six-year prospective clinical study. Plast Reconstr Surg 117:30-36, 2006.

11. Mladick RA. "No-touch" submuscular saline breast augmentation technique. Aesthetic Plast Surg 17:183-192, 1993.
12. Virden CP, Dobke MK, Stein P, et al. Subclinical infection of the silicone breast implant surface as a possible cause of capsular contracture. Aesthetic Plast Surg 16:173-179, 1992.
13. Dobke MK, Svahn JK, Vastine VL, et al. Characterization of microbial presence at the surface of silicone mammary implants. Ann Plast Surg 34:563-569, 1995.
14. Burkhardt BR, Dempsey PD, Schnur MD, et al. Capsular contracture: A prospective study of the effect of local antibacterial agents. Plast Reconstr Surg 77:919-932, 1986.
15. Burkhardt BR. Effects of povidone iodine on silicone gel implants in vitro: Implications for clinical practice. Plast Reconstr Surg 114:711-712, 2004.
16. Adams WP, Conner WC, Barton FE Jr, et al. Optimizing breast pocket irrigation: The post-betadine era. Plast Reconstr Surg 107:1596-1601, 2001.
17. Biggs TM, Yarish RS. Augmentation mammoplasty: A comparative analysis. Plast Reconstr Surg 85:368-372, 1990.
18. Gylbert L, Asplund O, Jurell G. Capsular contracture after breast reconstruction with silicone gel and saline-filled implants: A 6-year follow-up. Plast Reconstr Surg 85:373-377, 1990.
19. Collis N, Coleman D, Foo IT, et al. Ten-year review of a prospective randomized controlled trial of textured versus smooth subglandular silicone gel breast implants. Plast Reconstr Surg 106:786-791, 2000.
20. Marotta JS, Widenhouse CW, Habal MB, et al. Silicone gel breast implant failure and frequency of additional surgeries: Analysis of 35 studies reporting examination of more than 8000 explants. J Biomed Mater Res 48:354-364, 1999.
21. Mentor Corporation. Saline implant premarket approval information, 2001. Available at *www.fda.gov/cdrh/breastimplants*.
22. Inamed Corporation. Saline implant premarket approval information, 2001. Available at *www.fda.gov/cdrh/breastimplants*.
23. Inamed Corporation. Silicone breast implant premarket approval information, 2003 and 2005. Available at *www.fda.gov/cdrh/breastimplants*.
24. Young VL. Guidelines and indications for breast implant capsulectomy. Plast Reconstr Surg 102:884-891, 1998.
25. Peters W, Smith D. Calcification of breast implant capsules: Incidence, diagnosis, and contributing factors. Ann Plast Surg 34:8-11, 1995.
26. Hoshaw SJ, Klein PJ, Clark BD, et al. Breast implants and cancer: Causation, delayed detection, and survival. Plast Reconstr Surg 107:1393-1408, 2001.
27. Jakubietz M, Janis JE, Jakubietz R, et al. Breast augmentation: Cancer concerns and mammography: A review of the literature. Plast Reconstr Surg 113:117e-122e, 2004.

40. Mastopexy

Joshua A. Lemmon
Jose L. Rios

TERMINOLOGY

PTOSIS
- *Ptosis* from Greek, meaning "falling"
- Describes descended breast parenchyma that occurs with aging

MASTOPEXY
- Surgical procedure designed to correct breast ptosis
- Often referred to as "breast lift"

NATURAL HISTORY AND CLASSIFICATION[1,2]

BREAST CHANGES WITH AGE
- The amount of breast parenchyma changes with body weight, pregnancy, and hormonal changes.
  - The skin envelope is stretched when the parenchyma enlarges.
  - Supporting ligaments and ductal structures are also stretched.
  - Ptosis results when the parenchymal volume decreases and the skin envelope and supporting structures do not retract.
- The breast assumes a lower position on the chest wall; youthful breast contour is lost.

REGNAULT CLASSIFICATION[1] (Fig. 40-1)
Ptosis is described by the relative positions of the nipple-areola complex and the inframammary fold.
Grade I ptosis (mild ptosis)
  - The nipple-areola complex is at the level of the inframammary fold.
Grade II ptosis (moderate ptosis)
  - Nipple-areola complex lies below the level of the inframammary fold, but remains above the most dependent part of the breast parenchyma.
Grade III ptosis (severe ptosis)
  - Nipple-areola complex lies well below the inframammary fold and is at the most dependent part of the breast parenchyma along the inferior contour of the breast.
Pseudoptosis or glandular ptosis
  - Nipple-areola complex is above or at the level of the inframammary fold, but the majority of the breast parenchyma has descended below the level of the fold.
  - Nipple to inframammary fold distance has increased.

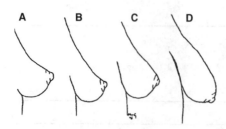

Fig. 40-1 Classification of breast ptosis. **A,** Pseudoptosis. **B,** Grade I ptosis. **C,** Grade II ptosis. **D,** Grade III ptosis. (From Kirwan L. Augmentation of the ptotic breast: Simultaneous periareolar mastopexy/breast augmentation. Aesth Surg J 19:34-39, 1999.)

PREOPERATIVE EVALUATION[2,3]

HISTORY
- Age
- Breast history: Lactation, pregnancy changes, size changes with weight loss or gain, tumors, previous procedures, family history of breast cancer, recent mammogram

MEASUREMENTS
- Sternal notch to nipple distance: Allows detection of asymmetry in nipple position
- Nipple to inframammary fold distance: Measures redundancy of the lower pole skin envelope
- Classification of ptosis severity (as in previous section)

OTHER CONSIDERATIONS
- Skin quality: Presence of striae reflects inelastic quality of affected skin
- Parenchymal quality: Fatty, fibrous, or glandular parenchyma
- Areolar shape and size: Areola are often stretched, large, and asymmetrical.

PHOTOGRAPHS
- Obtain anteroposterior, lateral, and oblique photographs.

PATIENT EXPECTATIONS
- **Breast size**
  - Mastopexy techniques combine small amounts of parenchymal resection and redistribution with reduction of the skin envelope; this can result in a reduction of breast size.
  - Many patients seek restoration of upper pole fullness, which may necessitate simultaneous placement of an implant (see Augmentation-Mastopexy later in this chapter).
- **Scar position**
  - Mastopexy procedures trade scars for improved contour.
  - Inform patients in detail, preoperatively, about scar placement and quality.
- **Other considerations**
  - Thorough patient education regarding procedural complications, use of drains, and recurrence of ptosis are essential components of preoperative preparation.

GOALS OF MASTOPEXY SURGERY

- Reliable nipple-areolar transposition to an aesthetic position on the breast mound
- Obtain pleasing breast shape
- Produce optimal scar quality: Short-scar techniques preferred when possible

TIP: Breast shape should not be compromised to reduce scar burden.

MASTOPEXY TECHNIQUES

PERIAREOLAR TECHNIQUES
- **General**
  - Incisions are made and closed around the areola.
  - Scars are therefore camouflaged at the areola-skin junction.
- **Patient selection**
  - Useful for mild and moderate ptosis.
  - Skin quality should be reasonable without striae, and parenchyma should be fibrous or glandular.
- **Techniques**
  - **Simple periareolar deepithelialization and closure**
    - Breast parenchyma is not repositioned, therefore only useful with mild ptosis.
    - This technique permits nipple repositioning.
    - Limited elliptical techniques can elevate the nipple-areola complex approximately 1-2 cm.[2]
  - **Benelli technique[4]** (Fig. 40-2)
    - This periareolar technique is used for patients with larger degrees of breast ptosis.
    - Technique allows for parenchymal repositioning.

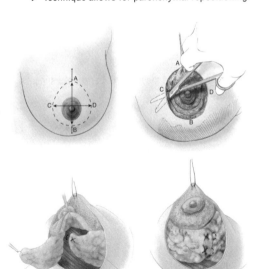

Fig. 40-2 Benelli periareolar mastopexy. Markings, undermining, and parenchymal coning. (Modified from Benelli L. A new periareolar mammaplasty: The "round block" technique. Aesth Plast Surg 14:99, 1990; and Grotting JC, Chen SM. Control and precision in mastopexy. In Nahai F, ed. The Art of Aesthetic Surgery: Principles & Techniques. St Louis: Quality Medical Publishing, 2005, pp 1907-1950.)

- ▸ Areolar sizers are used to mark a new areolar diameter, and a wider ellipse is marked to reposition nipple-areola complex and resect redundant skin envelope.
- ▸ Undermining separates the breast gland from overlying skin.
- ▸ Breast parenchyma is incised, leaving the nipple-areola complex on a superior pedicle.
- ▸ Medial and lateral parenchymal flaps are mobilized and crossed or invaginated at midline, narrowing breast width and coning the breast shape.
- ▸ Periareolar incision is closed in "purse-string" fashion with permanent sutures.
- • **Other periareolar techniques**
  - ▸ Variations on the previous technique include use of mesh to support parenchyma[5] or use of breast implant to reduce amount of skin resection required.[6,7]
- ■ **Advantages**
  - • Short scar
  - • Scar camouflaged at border of areola
- ■ **Disadvantages**
  - • Scar and areolar widening occur frequently.
  - • Breast projection can be flattened.
  - • Purse-string closure results in skin pleating that takes several months to resolve.

TIP: If periareolar purse-string suture remains palpable, it can be removed with simple office-based procedure after 6 weeks.

VERTICAL SCAR TECHNIQUES
- ■ **General**
  - • Vertical mastopexy techniques are variations of vertical reduction mammaplasty techniques.
  - • Incisions are closed around the areola and inferiorly toward the inframammary fold.
  - • Techniques rely on parenchymal support inferiorly to narrow and cone the breast.
- ■ **Patient selection**
  - • Techniques can be applied to patients with all degrees of ptosis.
- ■ **Techniques:**
  - • **Vertical mastopexy without undermining (Lassus)**[8] (Fig. 40-3)
    - ▸ Skin is incised as shown in Fig. 40-4.
    - ▸ Inferior, ptotic skin, fat, and gland are resected en bloc, and the nipple is transposed superiorly without undermining.
    - ▸ Medial and lateral breast pillars are closed.

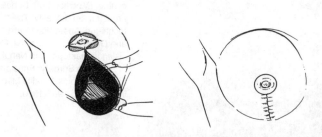

Fig. 40-3 Vertical mastopexy without undermining. Inferior skin, fat, and gland resected en bloc. Nipple transposed to desired position. Vertical closure of medial and lateral breast pillars. (From Lassus C. A 30-year experience with vertical mammaplasty. Plast Reconstr Surg 97:373-380, 1996.)

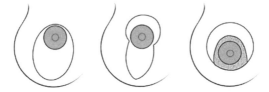

Fig. 40-4 Vertical scar mastopexy techniques. Lassus *(left)*, Lejour *(center)*, Hammond *(right)*. (From Rohrich RJ, Thornton JF, Jakubietz RG, et al. The limited scar mastopexy: Current concepts and approaches to correct breast ptosis. Plast Reconstr Surg 114:1622-1630, 2004.)

- **Vertical mastopexy with undermining and liposuction (Lejour)[9]**
  - Skin is incised as shown in Fig. 40-4.
  - Liposuction is performed in larger breasts to reduce parenchymal volume and add mobilization of superior dermal-parenchymal pedicle.
  - Inferior skin, fat, and gland are resected.
  - Wide undermining is performed, and medial and lateral breast pillars are closed inferiorly.
  - Skin is closed in a single vertical line, with redundant skin remaining as fine wrinkles between inferior sutures.
- **Short-scar periareolar inferior-pedicle reduction mammaplasty/mastopexy (Hammond)[10]**
  - Skin is incised as shown in Fig. 40-4.
  - Nipple-areola complex is transposed to desired location based on an inferior pedicle.
  - Nipple is transposed and supported with parenchymal suspension sutures.
  - Inferior skin is "tailor-tacked" to create desired contour and closed in a vertical pattern.
- **Medial-pedicle vertical mammaplasty/mastopexy (Hall-Findlay)[11]**
  - Medial pedicle is designed to carry the nipple-areola complex.
  - Lateral and inferior tissues are removed or repositioned superiorly.
  - Nipple is transposed to desired position.
  - Breast pillars are closed inferiorly to provide parenchymal support.
  - Skin is closed in vertical fashion.
  - Redundant skin is gathered along vertical closure.

■ **Modifications**
- Inferior-chest-wall–based flap[12]
  - Vertical mastopexy technique is performed, but inferior dermoglandular flap is tunneled superiorly under a sling of pectoralis major muscle to secure it in place.
  - Technique designed to restore upper pole fullness and increase breast projection.

■ **Advantages**
- Limited vertical scar is achieved without horizontal inframammary fold incision.
- Inferior parenchymal closure provides additional support to limit recurrent ptosis.

■ **Disadvantages**
- Immediate postoperative result often displays pronounced upper pole fullness that settles over time.
- Inferior skin redundancy occasionally does not retract, requiring horizontal excision later.

TIP: To limit redundancy in inferior pole skin, the vertical closure is brought obliquely lateral (creating an L-shape). This eliminates excessive inferior skin redundancy and still prevents a medial horizontal scar.

INVERTED-T SCAR TECHNIQUES

- **General**
  - Incisions are closed around the areola, vertically to the vertical limbs, and horizontally to the infra-mammary fold.
- **Patient selection**
  - Inverted-T used for severe ptosis
  - Considered for mastopexy in patients with both very poor skin quality and fatty parenchyma
- **Principles**
  - Frequently, Wise-pattern skin incision technique is used because this breast reduction technique is popular.
  - Other skin excision patterns exist that attempt to reduce the length of the horizontal scar (Fig. 40-5).
  - Parenchymal resection is indicated for breast hypertrophy.
  - In most mastopexy patients, parenchymal support is obtained by inferior closure of the medial and lateral breast pillars.

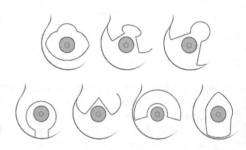

Fig. 40-5   Several skin incision patterns for inverted-T mastopexy techniques. (From Rohrich RJ, Thornton JF, Jakubietz RG, et al. The limited scar mastopexy: Current concepts and approaches to correct breast ptosis. Plast Reconstr Surg 114:1622-1630, 2004.)

  - The inferior parenchyma is repositioned superiorly to restore superior pole fullness or used to support the inferior pole of the breast.
    - ▶ Tunneled under a pectoralis sling[12]
    - ▶ Folded under superior pedicle and secured to pectoralis fascia[13]
    - ▶ Folded over to create supportive sling for lower pole[14]

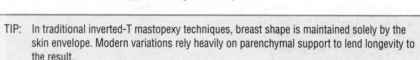

TIP: In traditional inverted-T mastopexy techniques, breast shape is maintained solely by the skin envelope. Modern variations rely heavily on parenchymal support to lend longevity to the result.

- **Advantages**
  - Surgeons familiar with technique because of widespread use in reduction techniques[15]
  - Predictable results
- **Disadvantages**
  - Scar burden
  - Recurrent ptosis probable if parenchymal support not used

POSTOPERATIVE CARE

- Drains, when used, are removed within the first 1-3 days postoperatively.
- Postoperative pain is treated with oral analgesics.
- A supportive bra is required for 6 weeks postoperatively to ensure full support during the healing process.

- Scar treatment begins 3 weeks postoperatively using the surgeon's preferred technique.
- Scar revisions, when necessary, are performed 1 year after initial surgery.

COMPLICATIONS[2,3]

HEMATOMA
- Relatively infrequent
- Patients should abstain from aspirin and antiplatelet medications for 10 days preoperatively.
- Tight hematomas require urgent reoperation for evacuation, hemostasis, and closure.

INFECTION
- Uncommon problem
- Perioperative antibiotics used routinely to reduce risk of infection[16]

WOUND HEALING PROBLEMS
- Mostly present in inverted-T procedures
- More common among smokers: Mastopexy not performed on active smokers for this reason

NIPPLE AND BREAST ASYMMETRY
- Counsel patients preoperatively that breast symmetry never will be perfectly achieved.
- Large asymmetries in nipple position, areola size, and breast shape require revision surgery.

SCAR DEFORMITIES
- Periareolar scar widening and medial horizontal inframammary fold scars are the source of frequent patient dissatisfaction.
- Scar revisions can be performed 1 year following initial surgery.

RECURRENT PTOSIS
- Gravity and aging continue to affect the breast following mastopexy.
- Inferior parenchymal (not dermal) support is thought to decrease the likelihood of recurrent ptosis.
- Ultimately, mastopexy is a temporary solution, and long-term results usually reveal some recurrence of the deformity.[2]

SPECIAL CONSIDERATIONS

AUGMENTATION-MASTOPEXY
- Loss of upper pole fullness with breast ptosis leads many surgeons to advocate placement of sub-glandular or subpectoral breast implants at the time of mastopexy.[2,3,7]
- Unfortunately, augmentation and mastopexy techniques work against each other.[17]
  - Mastopexy is designed to reposition the nipple, reshape the breast without tension to limit scarring, and reduce the size of the redundant skin envelope.
  - Augmentation increases the size of the skin envelope, the mass of the breast (subjecting it more to the force of gravity), and the tension of wound closure.
- Surgeons should consider staging augmentation and mastopexy in patients with moderate or severe ptosis.

MASTOPEXY AFTER EXPLANTATION
- Many patients with previously placed silicone gel implants seek explantation for various reasons, including rupture, fear of rupture, and capsular contracture.
- Often these patients benefit from simultaneous breast contouring procedures at the time of capsulectomy and implant exchange.[18]
  - Preexplantation ptosis is rarely corrected without formal mastopexy.
  - Good candidates are nonsmokers with mild to moderate ptosis, and adequate soft tissue coverage (>4 cm) over the implant.
  - In patients with sparse soft tissue coverage or severe ptosis, mastopexy should be staged 3 months following explantation.

TIP: Avoid mastopexy in all smokers.

- Choice of mastopexy technique depends on preoperative classification of ptosis (Table 40-1).

Table 40-1 *Breast Contouring at Time of Explantation and Choice of Technique*

Ptosis Type	Characteristics	Technique
Pseudoptosis	• Adequate volume • Good nipple position • Nipple to inframammary fold: 6 cm	Inframammary fold wedge-excision
Grade I	• Nipple repositioned ≤2 cm • Areola: ≤50 mm diameter	Periareolar mastopexy Vertical mastopexy
Grade II	• Nipple repositioned 2-4 cm	Wise-pattern mastopexy
Grade III	• Nipple repositioned >4 cm • <4 cm breast thickness	Delayed mastopexy (3 months, smoker)

From Rohrich RJ, Beran SJ, Restifo RJ, et al. Aesthetic management of the breast following explanation: Evaluation and mastopexy options. Plast Reconstr Surg 101:827-837, 1998.

TUBEROUS BREAST DEFORMITY[19]
- **Definition**
  - Spectrum of deformity with variable severity[20]
  - Deficient breast development in vertical and horizontal dimensions
    - ▶ Constricted (narrowed) breast base
    - ▶ High inframammary fold
    - ▶ Breast parenchyma herniation into the areola resulting in disproportionately large areola
- **At a consultation, these patients often seek mastopexy or augmentation.**

TIP: It is essential to distinguish and counsel these patients. They often are unaware of their anatomic abnormalities and that typical mastopexy techniques are not adequate.

- **Treatment goals[21]**
  - Expand breast circumference
  - Expand skin envelope in the lower pole

- Release constriction at the breast-areola junction
- Lower the inframammary fold
- Increase breast volume (when appropriate)
- Reduce areola size and correct herniation
- Correct nipple location and breast ptosis

- **Treatment options**[20]
  - Periareolar mastopexy techniques are used to reduce areola size and reposition the nipple-areola complex on the breast mound.
  - The breast parenchyma usually requires modification with inferior pole radial scoring, mobilization, or division.
  - Augmentation with permanent implants or expandable permanent implants usually is required to restore parenchymal volume.

> TIP: Tissue expansion is necessary if there is severe inferior pole skin deficiency.

KEY POINTS

✔ Classification of breast ptosis is determined by the nipple-areola position relative to the inframammary fold.

✔ Modern mastopexy techniques rely on inferior parenchymal support to elevate the gland on the chest wall and limit recurrent ptosis.

✔ Mild ptosis can be corrected with periareolar techniques alone.

✔ Moderate and severe ptosis require vertical, or vertical and horizontal, skin excision.

✔ Mastopexy and augmentation procedures have conflicting properties and should be combined cautiously.

✔ It is important to identify patients with tuberous breast deformities, because specific techniques are required for treatment.

REFERENCES

1. Regnault P. Breast ptosis. Definition and treatment. Clin Plast Surg 3:193-203, 1976.
2. Bostwick J III. Mastopexy. In Bostwick J III, ed. Plastic and Reconstructive Breast Surgery, 2nd ed. St Louis: Quality Medical Publishing, 1999, pp 499-579.
3. Grotting JC, Chen SM. Control and precision in mastopexy. In Nahai F, ed. The Art of Aesthetic Surgery: Principles & Techniques. St Louis: Quality Medical Publishing, 2005, pp 1907-1950.
4. Benelli L. A new periareolar mammaplasty: The "round block" technique. Aesthetic Plast Surg 14:93-100, 1990.
5. Goés JCS. Periareolar mammaplasty: Double skin technique with application of polyglactin or mixed mesh. Plast Reconstr Surg 97:959-968, 1996.
6. Spear S, Giese SY, Ducic I, et al. Concentric mastopexy revisited. Plast Reconstr Surg 107:1294-1299, 2001.
7. Kirwan L. Augmentation of the ptotic breast: Simultaneous periareolar mastopexy/breast augmentation. Aesthetic Surg J 19:34-39, 1999.
8. Lassus C. A 30-year experience with vertical mammaplasty. Plast Reconstr Surg 97:373-380, 1996.
9. Lejour M. Vertical mammaplasty and liposuction of the breast. Plast Reconstr Surg 94:100-114, 1994.

10. Hammond DC. Short scar periareolar inferior pedicle reduction (SPAIR) mammaplasty. Plast Reconstr Surg 103:890-901, 1999.
11. Hall-Findlay EJ. A simplified vertical reduction mammaplasty: Shortening the learning curve. Plast Reconstr Surg 104:748-759, 1999.
12. Graf R, Biggs TM, Steely RL. Breast shape: A technique for better upper pole fullness. Aesthetic Plast Surg 24:348-352, 2000.
13. Flowers RS, Smith EM Jr. "Flip-flap" mastopexy. Aesthetic Plast Surg 22:425-429, 1998.
14. Svedman P. Correction of breast ptosis utilizing a "fold over" deepithelialized lower thoracic fasciocutaneous flap. Aesthetic Plast Surg 15:43-47, 1991.
15. Rohrich RJ, Gosman AA, Brown SA, et al. Current preferences for breast reduction techniques: A survey of board-certified plastic surgeons in 2002. Plast Reconstr Surg 114:1724-1733, 2004.
16. Platt R, Zucker JR, Zalesnik DF, et al. Perioperative antibiotic prophylaxis and wound infection following breast surgery. J Antimicrob Chemother 31(Suppl B):43-48, 1993.
17. Spear S. Augmentation/mastopexy: "Surgeon, beware." Plast Reconstr Surg 112:905-906, 2003.
18. Rohrich RJ, Beran, SJ, Restifo RJ, et al. Aesthetic management of the breast following explantation: Evaluation and mastopexy options. Plast Reconstr Surg 101:827-837, 1998.
19. Rees TD, Aston SJ. The tuberous breast. Clin Plast Surg 3:339-347, 1976.
20. von Heimburg D, Exner K, Kruft S, et al. The tuberous breast deformity: Classification and treatment. Br J Plast Surg 49:339-345, 1996.
21. Versaci AD, Rozzelle AA. Treatment of tuberous breasts utilizing tissue expansion. Aesthetic Plast Surg 15:307-312, 1991.

41. Breast Reduction

Jose L. Rios
Jason K. Potter

ANATOMY

ARTERIAL BLOOD SUPPLY
(Fig. 41-1)
- **Provided by several arterial systems**
  - Internal thoracic
  - Thoracoacromial
  - Intercostals
  - Thoracodorsal
  - Lateral thoracic
- **Clinical Correlation**
  - **Inferior**
    - ▸ Consistent vessel enters 2-4 cm above inframammary fold (IMF)
    - ▸ Supplies inferior and central pedicles
  - **Medial**
    - ▸ Branches of internal thoracic artery, providing main blood supply to breast
    - ▸ Supplies medially based pedicles
  - **Superior**
    - ▸ Travels near breast meridian
    - ▸ Superficial location (about 1 cm deep)
    - ▸ Allows thin superior pedicles
  - **Lateral**
    - ▸ Superficial location

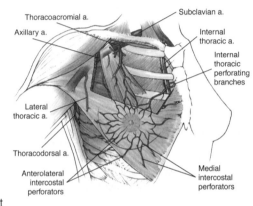

Fig. 41-1

VENOUS DRAINAGE
- Veins rarely accompany arteries.
- Most venous drainage is provided by superficial venous system.

INNERVATION (Fig. 41-2)
- Third to fifth anteromedial intercostal nerves
- Fourth and fifth anterolateral intercostal nerves
- **Lateral cutaneous branch of fourth intercostals:** A "unique nerve" to the nipple-areola complex (NAC); provides primary innervation[1]

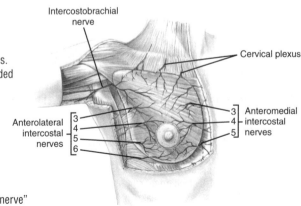

Fig. 41-2

> TIP: Pectoralis fascia dissection is avoided to preserve maximum number of nerves.

AESTHETICS

NIPPLE-AREOLA COMPLEX
- Normal NAC: 38-45 mm diameter
- Placement at Pitanguy's point (transposition of IMF to anterior breast)

CLASSIC PENN NUMBERS
- Notch to nipple distance: 21 cm
- Nipple to IMF distance: 6.9 cm

> TIP: Many patients need numbers in the 22-24 cm (notch to nipple) or 10-12 cm (nipple to IMF) range for optimal shape.

PATHOPHYSIOLOGY

- Abnormal excessive growth in response to circulating estrogens
- Normal estrogen levels and number of receptors
- Primarily an increase in fibrous tissue and fat, relatively smaller increase in glandular tissue

INDICATIONS FOR SURGERY

SYMPTOMS
- Back pain
- Neck pain
- Shoulder grooving
- Chronic headaches
- Intertriginous infections, rashes, maceration
- Cervical or thoracic degenerative joint disease (DJD) in extreme cases
- Difficulty with wardrobe

GIGANTOMASTIA (JUVENILE VIRGINAL HYPERTROPHY OF THE BREAST)
- Cause is unknown; endocrine studies are usually normal.
- At least 1800 g is removed per breast.
- Condition mostly occurs in girls 11-14 years old.
- Regression is rare.
- Once growth ceases, early intervention may be warranted for severe symptoms.
- Surgical reduction is standard therapy.
- Repeat reduction is standard treatment for recurrences.

EVIDENCE

- **Netscher et al[2]**
  - Symptomatic hypermastia is better defined by symptom complex than volume of tissue removed.
  - There is no correlation between patient's weight and symptoms.
- **Kerrigan et al[3,4]**
  - Symptoms are more important than volume.
  - Weight loss, special bras, and medical treatments are not successful.

SURGICAL OPTIONS

A vast number of breast reduction pedicles and techniques have been described; only the more common are mentioned here.

SUCTION LIPECTOMY

- **Indications and general points**
  - Used alone or with excisional techniques
  - Areolas in ideal location (may elevate slightly with decreased breast weight, but not reliable)
  - Older patients with heavy breasts and less concern for cosmesis
  - Patients must understand that breast shape not affected
    - ▸ Tendency toward flatter breast with residual ptosis
- **Benefits**
  - Smaller scars
  - Preserve NAC vascularity and innervation
- **Evidence**
  - **Courtiss[1,5]**
    - ▸ Up to 835 cc removed per breast
    - ▸ No calcifications on mammogram up to 2 years postoperatively
    - ▸ Pathologic examination of aspirate difficult
  - **Gray[6]**
    - ▸ Up to 2250 cc removed
    - ▸ Improvement of all grades of ptosis
    - ▸ No complications
- **Technique highlights**
  - Infiltrate with liposuction wetting solution (500-1000 cc).
  - Access through medial and lateral IMF incisions.
  - Use 2.4-5 mm cannulas.
  - Postoperative garment is worn day and night for 6 weeks.
  - Postoperative edema and firmness may take months to resolve.

ULTRASOUND-ASSISTED LIPECTOMY

- Indications are similar to those for suction-assisted lipectomy.
- Extensive counseling and informed consent are required because of unknown effects of ultrasonic energy on breast tissue.

PEDICLE DESIGNS
- **Inferior pedicle technique** (Fig. 41-3)
  - Safely remove up to 2500 g
  - Milk secreted postpartum by 72% of patients
  - Pedicle width
    - ▸ 3:1 ratio recommended by Georgiade et al[7]
    - ▸ 6-8 cm adequate for most reductions

TIP: N:IMF distances greater than 18 cm may result in bulky pedicles, which may limit extent of reduction.

- **Superior pedicle** (Fig. 41-4)
  - Perceived to result in less ptosis because of inferior tissue excision
  - Must thin pedicle to allow inset
  - NAC based on dermal pedicle (not dermoglandular), therefore poor breast feeding potential
- **Central pedicle/mound** (Fig. 41-5)
  - Modification of inferior pedicle
  - Same blood supply as inferior pedicle but depends on arterial and venous flow through glandular component, not through dermal component
- **Medial pedicle** (Fig. 41-6)
  - Modified from horizontal bipedicle (Strombeck) techniques
  - Dermal or dermoglandular pedicle

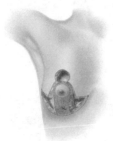 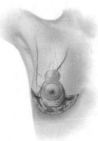 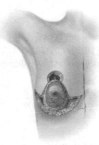 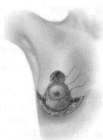

Fig. 41-3   Fig. 41-4   Fig. 41-5   Fig. 41-6

SKIN RESECTION PATTERNS
In general, patterns of skin resection are independent of pedicle design.
- **Inverted-T pattern** (Fig. 41-7)
  - Most commonly associated with inferior pedicle
  - Relies on integrity of skin to shape and hold breast parenchyma
  - Allows for removal of large areas of skin
  - Best suited for large breasts or poor quality skin that cannot be remodeled

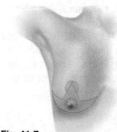

Fig. 41-7

- **Vertical pattern** (Fig. 41-8)
  - Usually associated with superior or medial pedicle techniques
  - Relies on parenchyma to shape skin
  - Up to 1400-2000 g per reduction
  - Eliminates horizontal scar
  - Requires healthy skin (elasticity) for remodeling
  - Dog-ear revision necessary in 10%-15% of patients
- **Circumareolar pattern** (Fig. 41-9)
  - Not recommended for breast reduction or ptosis greater than 2 cm
  - Tendency toward widening of NAC

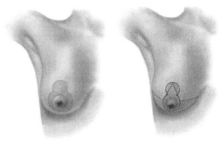

Fig. 41-8

FREE-NIPPLE GRAFTING

- **Indications**
  - Patients with very long N:IMF distances (>18 cm) seeking small postoperative breast size (B or small C cup)
  - Patients with significant systemic diseases that may impair blood flow
  - Patients requiring short anaesthesia times
- **Disadvantages**
  - Possible depigmentation in blacks
  - Loss of nipple sensation
  - Loss of lactation potential

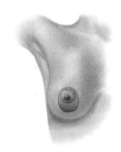

Fig. 41-9

TECHNIQUES

- **Inferior pedicle with inverted-T skin resection**
  - **Markings**
    1. Place patient in an upright position.
    2. Mark the midline.
    3. Mark the position of IMF, elevating mark a few millimeters onto the breast. This keeps the IMF scar on the breast and not on the chest, because the base of the breast is narrowed during reduction.
    4. Mark the vertical nipple location (Pitanguy's point) by transposition of IMF to front of breast.
    5. Measure bilaterally from notch to nipple and from midline to assure symmetry.

TIP: Large pendulous breasts demonstrate recoil of superior skin flap following elevation of the flap; it is important to plan for this when marking the new nipple location.

---

6. Mark the breast meridian to determine a new horizontal nipple position.
7. Mark the vertical limbs, which should measure approximately 7-8 cm under tension.
   - Long limbs always can be shortened on the operating table; short limbs may result in closure under tension, which may compromise shape and skin viability.
   - The angle of divergence determines amount of skin resection.

8. Mark the pedicle approximately 10-12 cm from the midline.
9. Mark the areola at 42 mm; replace at 38 mm to minimize traction and distortion on the areola.
10. Mark any areas to be liposuctioned.
- **Technical Tips:**
  - ▸ Develop the pedicle before raising skin flaps. To avoid undercutting, bevel away from pedicle.
  - ▸ Sit the patient up and tailor-tack, as needed, to achieve desired shape.
- **Medial pedicle with vertical skin resection**
- **Markings**
  1. Place patient in an upright position.
  2. Mark the midline.
  3. Mark the position of the IMF.
  4. Mark the vertical nipple location by transposing IMF to front of breast. Measure bilaterally from notch to nipple and from midline to assure symmetry.
  5. Mark the breast meridian to determine a new horizontal nipple position.
  6. Mark the vertical limbs by rotating the breast medially and laterally.
  7. Mark the inferior extent of the resection above the IMF.
  8. Mark the areolar opening.
  9. Design the pedicle.
  10. Mark areas to be liposuctioned.
- **Technical Tips:**
  - ▸ Following excision of parenchyma, breast pillars are approximated, NAC is inset, and vertical incision is closed in a gathering fashion, as needed.
  - ▸ Refer to Hall-Findlay's article for an excellent review of this technique.[8]

BREAST REDUCTION IN ADOLESCENTS

- Stabilization of breast size for 12-24 months preferred
- Surgery earlier only if severe physical or psychological symptoms
- **McMahan et al[9]**
  - The study included 48 women, an average of 17.8 years old at time of reduction.
  - 94% reported satisfaction (i.e., would recommend the surgery to a friend).
  - 60% complained of a prominent scar.
  - 35% reported changes in nipple sensation.
  - About 80% experienced relief of pain.
  - 72% had some regrowth of tissue; only one had reoperation for hypermastia.

SECONDARY BREAST REDUCTION

- Use same pedicle as for first reduction, if known.
- Data demonstrate mixed outcomes from use of transected pedicles.
  - **Hudson and Skoll[10]**
    - ▸ Two patients had previous pedicle transected; both developed NAC compromise.
    - ▸ One out of five developed healing complications when pedicle was not transected.
    - ▸ Authors recommended free-nipple graft if primary pedicle was unknown.

- **Losee et al**[11]
  - Two thirds of patients with transected pedicles had a complication that healed conservatively.
  - Authors concluded it was safe to change pedicles.

REDUCTION OF IRRADIATED BREASTS

- **Spear et al**[12]
  - No complications in three cases
  - Waited 6 months between cessation of radiation and surgery
  - Minimized pedicle length and flap undermining

BREAST INFILTRATION

- Infiltration with dilute epinephrine-containing solutions (e.g., liposuction wetting solution) reduces operative blood loss.
  - Wilmink et al[13]
  - Samdal et al[14]

POSTOPERATIVE DRAINS

- Use of a single drain in each breast for 24 hours is typical.
- Studies do not demonstrate lower complication or hematoma rates attributable to drain use.
  - **Wrye et al**[15]
    - 49 consecutive patients with inferior pedicle reductions
    - One drained and undrained breast, per patient, chosen by randomization
    - No difference in complications or hematomas

OUTCOME STUDIES

- **Miller et al**[16]
  - 93% of patients reported decrease in symptoms.
  - 62% of patients reported increase in activity.
- **Dabbah et al**[17]
  - 97% of patients reported symptom improvement (59% had no symptoms).
- **Davis et al**[18]
  - Patients reported 87% overall satisfaction rate.

COMPLICATIONS AND CONSENT

- **Nipple-areola compromise:** 4%-7% of patients
  - Monitoring options: Clinical exam, laser Doppler flowmeter
- **Altered nipple sensation:** 9%-25% of patients
  - Increased rates with increased amounts of resection
  - Improved sensation in patients with gigantomastia
- **Unsatisfactory scarring:** 4% of patients
- **Wound healing complications:** Up to 19% of patients
- **Breast feeding**
  - **Aboudib et al**[19]
    - 91% of patients reported normal lactation postoperatively.
  - **Sandsmark et al**[20]
    - 65% of patients could breast feed.
    - Supplemental feeding was needed in all cases.
- **Other:** Fat necrosis, hypertrophic scarring, asymmetry, insufficient reduction, persistent pain, over-reduction, infection, change in breast shape over time

CANCER DETECTION

- Recommendations for preoperative mammography vary widely.
  - At a minimum, follow American Cancer Society guidelines.
  - Many surgeons recommend mammography for reduction patients more than 25 years old.[21]
- Send all specimens to a pathologist.
  - Incidence of cancer in reductions is reported at 0.16%-1%.
- Obtain baseline mammograms 3-6 months postoperatively.

WHAT TO DO IF THE NIPPLE TURNS BLUE OR DIES

- **During flap elevation or pedicle formation:**
  1. Cease dissection.
  2. Ensure patient has adequate BP, urinary output, and temperature.
  3. Observe for 10-15 minutes for red bleeding from areolar or pedicle borders.
  4. Convert to free-nipple graft if nonviable; be sure nonviable parenchyma underlying nipple is also resected.
- **During closure:**
  1. Open flaps and inspect.
  2. Evacuate hematoma if present.
  3. Check pedicle for kinking.
  4. Ensure patient has adequate BP, urinary output, and temperature.
  5. May need to resect more tissue to decrease pressure on pedicle with flap closure.
  6. If nipple returns to normal color, close.
  7. Options are available if nipple is compromised with reclosure.
     - Convert to free-nipple graft.
     - Loosely approximate, allow 2-3 days for edema resolution; then attempt closure.

- **Postoperative:**
  1. If hematoma is obvious, release periareolar suture and return to operating room.
  2. If no hematoma is obvious, release periareolar suture(s)
     ‣ If nipple returns to pink, leave wound open and close when edema resolves.
     ‣ If nipple remains blue, return to operating room and use previous algorithms.

KEY POINTS

✔ Choice of procedure is based on needs and concerns of the patient. There is no single best procedure.
✔ Liposuction alone does not allow control of breast projection or nipple position.
✔ Inverted-T skin resection patterns are best suited for large breasts or those with significant skin excess.
✔ Vertical patterns use remodeled parenchyma to reshape skin.
✔ Accurate preoperative markings are key to the success of all procedures.
✔ **Regardless of technique, the patient must have a thorough understanding of the extent of breast scarring to clarify patient expectations.**

REFERENCES

1. Courtiss EH, Goldwyn RM. Breast sensation before and after plastic surgery. Plast Reconstr Surg 58:1-13, 1976.
2. Netscher DT, Meade RA, Goodman CM, et al. Physical and psychosocial symptoms among 88 volunteer subjects compared with patients seeking plastic surgery procedures to the breast. Plast Reconstr Surg 105:2366-2373, 2000.
3. Kerrigan CL, Collins ED, Kneeland TS, et al. Measuring health state preferences in women with breast hypertrophy. Plast Reconstr Surg 106:280-288, 2000.
4. Kerrigan CL, Collins ED, Striplin D, et al. The health burden of breast hypertrophy. Plast Reconstr Surg 108:1591-1599, 2001.
5. Courtiss EH. Reduction mammaplasty by suction alone. Plast Reconstr Surg 92:1276-1284, 1993.
6. Gray LN. Liposuction breast reduction. Aesthetic Plast Surg 22:159-162, 1998.
7. Georgiade NG, Serafin D, Morris R, et al. Reduction mammaplasty utilizing an inferior pedicle nipple-areolar flap. Ann Plast Surg 3:211-218, 1979.
8. Hall-Findlay EJ. A simplified vertical reduction mammaplasty: Shortening the learning curve. Plast Reconstr Surg 104:748-759, 1999.
9. McMahan JD, Wolfe JA, Cromer BA, et al. Lasting success in teenage reduction mammaplasty. Ann Plast Surg 35:227-231, 1995.
10. Hudson DA, Skoll PJ. Repeat reduction mammaplasty. Plast Reconstr Surg 104:401-408, 1991.
11. Losee JE, Cladwell EH, Serletti JM. Secondary reduction mammaplasty: Is using a different pedicle safe? Plast Reconstr Surg 106:1004-1008, 2000.
12. Spear SL, Burke JB, Forman D, et al. Experience with reduction mammaplasty following breast conservation surgery and radiation therapy. Plast Reconstr Surg 102:1913-1916, 1998.
13. Wilmink H, Spauwen PH, Hartman EH, et al. Preoperative injection using a diluted anesthetic/adrenaline solution significantly reduces blood loss in reduction mammaplasty. Plast Reconstr Surg 102:373-376, 1998.
14. Samdal F, Serra M, Skolleborg KC. The effects of infiltration with adrenaline on blood loss during reduction mammaplasty: An early survey. Scand J Plast Reconstr Hand Surg 26:211-215, 1992.

15. Wrye SW, Banducci DR, Mackay D, et al. Routine drainage is not required in reduction mammaplasty. Plast Reconstr Surg 111:113-117, 2003.
16. Miller AP, Zacher JB, Berggren RB, et al. Breast reduction for symptomatic macromastia: Can objective predictors for operative success be identified? Plast Reconstr Surg 95:77-83, 1995.
17. Dabbah A, Lehman JA Jr, Parker MG, et al. Reduction mammaplasty: An outcome analysis. Ann Plast Surg 35:337-341, 1995.
18. Davis GM, Ringler SL, Short K, et al. Reduction mammaplasty: Long-term efficacy, morbidity, and patient satisfaction. Plast Reconstr Surg 96:1106-1110, 1995.
19. Aboudib JH Jr, de Castro CC, Coelho RS, et al. Analysis of late results in postpregnancy mammoplasty. Ann Plast Surg 26:111-116, 1991.
20. Sandsmark M, Amland PF, Abyholm F, et al. Reduction mammaplasty: A comparative study of the Orlando and Robbins methods in 292 patients. Scand J Plast Reconstr Hand Surg 26:203-209, 1992.
21. Adams WP Jr, ed. Reduction mammaplasty and mastopexy. Sel Read Plast Surg 9(29), 2002.

42. Gynecomastia

Jose L. Rios

DEFINITION

Excessive development of male mammary glands

DEMOGRAPHICS

- Most males experience some degree of gynecomastia during their lives, but definition and reporting are inconsistent.
- Overall incidence is 32%-36% (up to 40% in autopsy series).
- Up to 65% of adolescent boys are affected.
- Up to 75% of cases are bilateral.

ETIOLOGIC FACTORS AND CLASSIFICATION[1]

Primary causes are a relative or absolute excess of circulating estrogens, or a decrease in circulating androgens.

CLINICAL CLASSIFICATION
- **Idiopathic** *(most common)*
- **Physiologic**
  - **Neonatal:** Circulating maternal estrogens via placenta
  - **Pubertal:** Relative excess of plasma estradiol versus testosterone
  - **Elderly:** Decreases in circulating testosterone, peripheral aromatization of testosterone to estrogen
- **Pathologic:** Cirrhosis, adrenal tumors, hyperthyroidism, adrenal hyperplasia, congenital or acquired hypogonadism, testicular tumors
- **Pharmacologic:** Marijuana, calcium channel blockers, spironolactone (Aldactone®, Spironol), cimetidine (Tagamet®), ketoconazole (Nizoral®), anabolic steroids

HISTOLOGIC CLASSIFICATION[2]
- Degrees of stromal and ductal proliferation
  - **Florid:** Increased budding ducts and cellular stroma; seen in gynecomastia that is present for approximately 4 months
  - **Intermediate:** Overlapping florid and fibrous patterns
  - **Fibrous:** Extensive stromal fibrosis, minimal ductal proliferation; seen in gynecomastia that is present for more than 1 year

RISK OF MALIGNANT TRANSFORMATION

- **No increased cancer risk for patients without Klinefelter's syndrome**
- **Klinefelter's syndrome:** Risk increases **60-fold** (1:1000 increases to 1:400)

PREOPERATIVE WORKUP

HISTORY
- Age of onset
- Duration
- Symptoms
- Medications
- Recreational drug use
- Medical history

PHYSICAL EXAMINATION
- Breast: Fat versus glandular predominance, ptosis, skin excess, masses
- Testicular exam
- Thyroid, liver, or other abdominal masses
- Lack of male hair distribution
- Feminizing characteristics
- Additional diagnostic tests indicated by history and findings from physical examination
  - **Small, firm testes:** Karyotyping, because this is hallmark finding in cases of 47,XXY.
  - **Abnormal testicular exam or mass:** Testicular ultrasound, β-human chorionic gonadotropin (β-HCG), follicle-stimulating hormone (FSH), luteinizing hormone (LH), serum testosterone or estradiol

STAGING[3]

- **Grade I:** Minimal hypertrophy (<250 g) with no ptosis
- **Grade II:** Moderate hypertrophy (250-500 g) with no ptosis
- **Grade III:** Severe hypertrophy (>500 g) with grade I ptosis
- **Grade IV:** Severe hypertrophy with grade II or III ptosis

MANAGEMENT

IDIOPATHIC
- Observation
  - Gynecomastia often regresses after 3-18 months of enlargement.
  - Gynecomastia present for more than 12 months rarely regresses, because of tissue fibrosis.
- Weight reduction if obese
- Surgery

PHYSIOLOGIC
- Tamoxifen (Nolvadex®) is particularly useful for "lump"-type gynecomastia.
- Testosterone, antiestrogen treatments have limited success.

PATHOLOGIC
- Removal of testicular tumors
- Correction of underlying causes or disease

PHARMACOLOGIC
- Removal of offending agent
- Change of medication

SURGICAL OPTIONS

TECHNIQUES
- Periareolar or intraareolar incisions
- All types of dermal and glandular pedicles for nipple relocation
- Free-nipple grafting
- Traditional and ultrasound-assisted liposuction (UAL)
  - Basic tenets of UAL treatment
    - Super-wet infiltration
    - Stab incisions at inferolateral aspects of intramuscular fat (IMF)
    - Radial pattern across entire chest
    - Disruption of IMF
    - Avoid upper lateral pectoral region
  - Dressing: 2 layers of Topifoam® (3M Corporation, St. Paul, MN); compression vest for 4 weeks continuously, then 4 more weeks at night

RESULTS AND COMPLICATIONS

EXCISION (COURTISS)[4]
- Overresection in 18.7% of cases
- Poor scarring in 18.7% of cases
- Hematomas in 16% of cases
- Seromas in 9% of cases
- Underresection in 22% of cases

UAL (GINGRASS AND SHERMAK)[5]
- No hematomas, skin necrosis, or other complications
- Results uniformly good to excellent at 4-year follow-up

UAL (ROHRICH ET AL)[3]
- Overall, 87% of patients required only UAL
- Staged skin excision required by 33% of stage III and 57% of stage IV patients

UAL WITH EXCISION (HAMMOND ET AL)[6]

- No nipple-areola complex (NAC) necrosis, hematoma, or infection
- One patient each with scar retraction, seroma, access port skin burn, epidermolysis, or decreased NAC sensation
- All patients pleased with results

SUCTION-ASSISTED LIPOSUCTION (SAL) WITH EXCISION (BABIGIAN AND SILVERMAN)[7]

- Treated 20 patients who used anabolic steroids
- Found 2 hematomas, 2 seromas, 3 recurrences

KEY POINTS

- ✔ Gynecomastia is most commonly idiopathic.
- ✔ Most adolescent males (65%) experience transient gynecomastia.
- ✔ The risk of malignant transformation increases only in those patients with Klinefelter's syndrome.
- ✔ A testicular exam is mandatory in patients with gynecomastia to rule out testicular tumors.
- ✔ Some medications and drug abuse are associated with the development of gynecomastia.
- ✔ UAL is the mainstay of initial treatment in most cases.

REFERENCES

1. Wise GJ, Roorda AK, Kalter R. Male breast disease. J Am Coll Surg 200:255-269, 2005.
2. Banyan GA, Hajdu SI. Gynecomastia: Clinicopathologic study of 351 cases. Am J Clin Pathol 57:431-437, 1972.
3. Rohrich RJ, Ha RY, Kenkel JM, et al. Classification and management of gynecomastia: Defining the role of ultrasound-assisted liposuction. Plast Reconstr Surg 111:909-923, 2003.
4. Courtiss EH. Gynecomastia: Analysis of 159 patients and current recommendations for treatment. Plast Reconstr Surg 79:740-753, 1987.
5. Gingrass MK, Shermak MA. The treatment of gynecomastia with ultrasound-assisted lipoplasty. Perspect Plast Surg 12:101, 1999.
6. Hammond DC, Arnold JF, Simon AM, et al. Combined use of ultrasonic liposuction with the pull-through technique for the treatment of gynecomastia. Plast Reconstr Surg 112:891-895, 2003.
7. Babigian A, Silverman RT. Management of gynecomastia due to anabolic steroids in bodybuilders. Plast Reconstr Surg 107:240-242, 2001.

43. Breast Reconstruction

Michel Saint-Cyr
Jose L. Rios

BREAST CANCER

INCIDENCE[1]
- The American Cancer Society estimated 211,000 cases of breast cancer in 2003.
- The lifetime risk for developing breast cancer is **12%.**
- Breast cancer is the **second leading cause** of cancer deaths in women (lung cancer is the first leading cause).

GENETICS[2]
- 80% of cases are sporadic
- 15% are familial, without evidence of autosomal dominant inheritance pattern
- 5% are from genetic germ line mutations (BRCA1/BRCA2)
- 85% lifetime risk of developing breast cancer if BRCA1 or BRCA2 positive

CHOOSING BREAST RECONSTRUCTION

- Why women choose breast reconstruction[3]
  - Eliminates need for external breast prosthesis
  - Allows ability to wear different types of clothing
  - Helps regain feelings of femininity and wholeness
- Why women avoid breast reconstruction
  - Fear of complications
  - Belief they are too old
  - Fear it will interfere with cancer treatment and surveillance

INSURANCE COVERAGE

- Women's Health and Cancer Rights Act of 1988
  - Mandates coverage of breast reconstruction
  - Includes contralateral breast-matching procedures

TIMING

IMMEDIATE RECONSTRUCTION
- **Advantages**
  - Potential psychological benefit and immediate return of body image
  - Single-stage procedure with lower overall socioeconomic cost

- Noncontracted and nonscarred mastectomy skin flaps easy to manage
- Preserves skin envelope
- Natural breast landmarks optimize final aesthetic results
- Easier access and dissection of recipient vessels
- Used for stage I and stage II breast cancer patients not expected to receive postoperative radiation therapy
- **Disadvantages**
  - Risk of postoperative radiation therapy requirements must be carefully evaluated to prevent flap fat necrosis and deformity (30% risk).
  - Postoperative complications can delay postoperative adjuvant chemotherapy.

DELAYED RECONSTRUCTION

- **Advantages**
  - No delay in postoperative chemotherapy/radiation therapy as a result of reconstructive complications
  - Allows careful monitoring of patients with advanced carcinomas (stages III and IV) over time before performing definitive reconstruction
- **Disadvantages**
  - Loss of breast skin envelope and natural landmarks (e.g., the inframammary fold)
  - Recipient vessel dissection more tedious because of scarred axilla and chest wall
  - Higher rate of recipient vessel conversion because of unusable vessels
  - Flap size requirement usually greater than with immediate reconstruction

CONSIDERATIONS

- Patient selection
- Need for adjuvant chemotherapy/radiation therapy
- Donor site availability
- Surgeon experience and preference
- Size and shape of contralateral breast
- Anticipated skin defect

IMPLANTS AND TISSUE EXPANDERS

- **Prerequisite:** Healthy mastectomy skin flaps to avoid prosthesis exposure

ADVANTAGES

- Lower initial cost compared with autologous reconstruction[4]
- Technical ease (no specialized equipment required)
- No additional scar or donor site morbidity
- Shorter operative time and recovery compared with autologous tissue reconstruction

DISADVANTAGES

- Early cost advantage of implant-based reconstruction over autologous tissue reconstruction disappears over time as a result of additional revision surgeries[5]
- Potential capsular contracture (30% in the Mentor Saline Prospective Study)
- Potential implant rupture or valve failure

- Potential infection requiring implant removal
- Higher risk of multiple long-term operative procedures being needed
- Harder to recreate inframammary fold and natural breast ptosis
- Difficult to achieve symmetry in unilateral reconstruction compared with bilateral reconstruction

Two-Stage Immediate Reconstruction With Tissue Expander and Implant

- Minimizes tension and stress on skin flaps at time of mastectomy
- Increases flexibility in choosing final breast volume

Implant and Tissue Expander Size and Shape

- Consider base diameter of breast to be reconstructed (use contralateral breast in delayed cases)
- Consider tissue expander height based on amount of upper pole expansion needed
- Consider projection, volume, and shape of preoperative or contralateral breast

Principles

- Ensure that placement of tissue expander is submuscular (i.e., under pectoralis major muscle anteriorly and under slips of serratus anterior muscle laterally) or partially submuscular (i.e., upper pole of tissue expander covered by the pectoralis muscle and lower pole covered by subcutaneous tissue of lower mastectomy skin flap).
- Ensure that the inferior portion of the expander is placed precisely at the inframammary fold.
- Close lateral dead space by suturing skin flap to chest wall to prevent lateral migration of implant and tissue expander. Tissue expander may also be covered with slips of serratus muscle to prevent lateralization.
- Tissue expander can be filled intraoperatively 50-200 cc or more based on mastectomy skin flap quality and perfusion.
- Continue expansion 2 weeks postoperatively, injecting 50-100 cc weekly or biweekly.
- Remove saline if there is blanching of skin or patient discomfort.
- Overexpand 20%-40% above final breast volume to allow for anticipated contracture and breast ptosis.
- Maintain tissue expander in place at final volume for 3-6 months to allow capsule maturation before definitive implant placement.

Long-Term Results[6]

- 86% of results are acceptable at 2 years, 54% are acceptable at 5 years.
- Asymmetry is caused by differences between implant and natural-breast aging

Variation for Large or Ptotic Breasts[7]

- Reduction pattern can be designed
- Perform deepithelialization of inferior skin that is normally discarded
- Result is skin flap–muscle pocket for implant with double skin coverage at the point of the inverted "T"

LATISSIMUS DORSI FLAP

Advantages

- Potential autologous reconstruction of small- or medium-sized breasts[8]
- Increases soft tissue coverage when used with tissue expander and implants, thus improving aesthetic result

- Reliable pedicle and large-diameter thoracodorsal artery and vein
- Allows versatile skin paddle design
- Minimal long-term donor site morbidity

DISADVANTAGES
- High seroma rate: Formation in up to 79% of patients; use of progressive tension sutures can significantly reduce seroma formation[9,10]
- Often requires tissue expander and implant for increased breast projection and volume

VARIATIONS
- Extended latissimus dorsi musculocutaneous flap[8,11]
- Muscle-sparing latissimus dorsi flap[12]
- Thoracodorsal artery perforator flap[13]

PEDICLED TRANSVERSE RECTUS ABDOMINIS MUSCLE (TRAM) FLAP

ADVANTAGES
- Allows complete autologous reconstruction in most patients
- Avoids disadvantages of prosthetic-only reconstruction
- Good long-term result
- Allows contouring of the abdominal area

DISADVANTAGES
- Donor site morbidity: Hernia/bulge, scarring, seroma, etc.
- Long recovery time
- Abdominal weakness
- Mesh reinforcement of rectus fascia often required
- Higher fat necrosis rate than free TRAM

PERFUSION ZONES[14]
- **I:** Ipsilateral to pedicle, overlying the rectus muscle
- **II:** Contralateral to pedicle, overlying contralateral rectus muscle
- **III:** Ipsilateral to pedicle, lateral to the rectus muscle
- **IV:** Contralateral to pedicle, lateral to contralateral rectus muscle
  - Reevaluation of perfusion zones (Holm et al)[15]
    - According to these authors, the ipsilateral TRAM flap side has an axial pattern of blood supply, and the contralateral side has a random blood supply.
    - *Their conclusion: Hartrampf's zone III should be replaced by zone II and vice versa.*

SURGICAL DELAY
- Optimal delay is 7-14 days
- Division of the deep inferior epigastric artery and vein
- Increases perfusion pressure from 13.3 to 40.3 mm Hg[16]
- Significant increases in perfusion pressure noted by end of 1 week
- No benefit if time of delay extended further (e.g, 2+ weeks)

> TIP: Dissect deep inferior epigastric artery (DIEA) and vein (DIEV) as lifeboat during pedicled TRAM flap harvest. Supercharge with DIEA or enhance venous outflow with DIEV if needed once flap is transferred.

COMPLICATIONS[17-21]

- **Fat necrosis:** 1.6%-28%
- **Abdominal hernia:** 0.8%-10%
- **Flap necrosis:** 0.6%-5%
- **Partial skin loss:** 3%-25%

FREE TRAM FLAP

ADVANTAGES

- Robust blood supply
- No pedicle bulge from tunneling
- Ease of breast-mound shaping

RECIPIENT VESSEL OPTIONS

- **Internal mammary (IM)**
  - **Advantages[22]**
    - Easier access for microsurgery and better positioning for assistant
    - Avoids dissection in the axilla
    - Allows more medial placement of the flap with reduced lateral fullness compared with using thoracodorsal vessels as the recipient vessels
    - Less axillary dissection–related morbidity (lymphedema, shoulder stiffness, brachial plexus injury)
    - Less lateral fullness than thoracodorsal vessels
  - **Disadvantages**
    - Dissection and exposure can be tedious.
    - Vessels are thin walled and more fragile, especially veins. The left IM vein also tends to be smaller than the right IM vein.
    - There may be loss of focus during microsurgery because of respiratory movements.
    - Future use of IM artery for coronary artery bypass grafting is compromised.
    - There is a small but potential risk for pneumothorax.
- **Thoracodorsal**
- **Alternate recipient artery and vein (A&V):** Internal mammary A&V perforators, thoracoacromial A&V, circumflex scapular A&V, lateral thoracic A&V, axillary A&V, external jugular vein, cephalic vein

COMPLICATIONS[23,24]

- **Fat necrosis:** 6%-9%
- **Partial flap loss:** 0%-7%
- **Abdominal hernia:** 1.6%-6.3%
- **Total flap loss:** 0%-3%

> TIP: Dissect the superficial inferior epigastric vein (SIEV) as lifeboat for additional venous outflow. The superficial venous system sometimes is dominant over the deep inferior epigastric system.

TRAM FLAP RECONSTRUCTION IN OBESE PATIENTS
- Increased rates of total flap loss, hematoma, seroma, mastectomy skin flap loss, donor site infection, and hernia.[24]

OTHER FREE TRAM OPTIONS
- Muscle-sparing free TRAM flap[25]

PERFORATOR FLAPS

TYPES OF PERFORATOR FLAPS
- Deep inferior epigastric artery perforator (DIEP)
- Periumbilical artery perforator (PUAP)
- Superior gluteal artery perforator (S-GAP)
- Inferior gluteal artery perforator (I-GAP)
- Thoracodorsal artery perforator (TDAP)
- Anterolateral thigh (ALT) (rare)

ADVANTAGES
- Less donor site morbidity
- Complete muscle sparing with reduced risk of abdominal hernia and bulging
- Reduced postoperative pain
- Accelerated recovery time

DISADVANTAGES
- Steep learning curve
- Meticulous dissection with increased operating time (dissection time significantly decreases with increasing experience)

ALTERNATE FLAPS

TYPES OF ALTERNATE FLAPS
- Superficial inferior epigastric artery (SIEA)
- Transverse upper gracilis myocutaneous (TUG)
- Rubens (based on cutaneous perforators of the deep circumflex iliac artery and vein)

ADVANTAGES
- Minimal abdominal donor site morbidity (SIEA)
- No functional donor site morbidity caused by harvesting the gracilis flap
- Valuable alternative for autologous breast reconstruction for patients with small or medium-sized breasts and inadequate soft tissue bulk in the lower abdomen and gluteal region (TUG)

DISADVANTAGES

- Available in only 30% of cases (SIEA)
- The SIEA can be small
- Small to medium-sized breasts only (SIEA)
- Hemi-abdomen only
- Potential contour deformity and wound dehiscence when skin paddle is wider than 10 cm (TUG)

NIPPLE-AREOLA RECONSTRUCTION

- **Nipple sharing**
  - Can be used for patients willing to sacrifice about 50% of their nipple height
  - Excellent color texture match
- **C-V flap**[26]
- **Skate flap**[27]
- **Free skin-fat graft**
- **Areolar tattooing**[28]
  - 60% report fading over time
  - 84% overall satisfaction

ADJUVANT RADIATION

PROSTHETIC RECONSTRUCTION[29]

- 48% need autologous tissue in addition or as replacement
- 33% capsular contracture rate

TRAM RECONSTRUCTION[30]

- 88% immediate versus 9% delayed late complication rate
- 28% of immediate reconstruction group required second flap for correction of contour deformities

---

KEY POINTS

- ✔ **Immediate Breast Reconstruction**
  - Establish good communication with the oncologic surgeon.
    - Stress the importance of preserving internal mammary perforators (potential recipient vessels and blood supply to the mastectomy skin flaps).
    - Ease of reconstruction is also dictated by the quality of the mastectomy performed.
    - A good-quality skin-sparing mastectomy that does not violate the breast's natural landmarks yields the best aesthetic results.
- ✔ **Tissue Expanders**
  - Avoid using tissue expanders in previously irradiated breasts. The complication rate and capsular contracture rate are higher than those in nonirradiated breasts.
  - Partial submuscular coverage is best with adequate subcutaneous tissue at the inframammary fold and inferior pole, and in patients with uncompromised mastectomy skin flaps.

Continued

KEY POINTS—cont'd

- Partial submuscular tissue expansion usually results in less upper pole fullness than commonly seen with complete muscle coverage.
- ✔ **Pedicled TRAM Flap**
  - The superior epigastric vessels can be very superficial in the rectus muscle; care must be taken to elevate the rectus fascia without injuring the underlying rectus muscle and pedicle.
  - Always harvest a portion of the deep inferior epigastric vessels with the pedicled TRAM flap to allow for additional arterial supercharging or venous outflow, if needed.
  - Ensure that the subcutaneous tunnel is wide enough to avoid compressing the TRAM pedicle.
  - Avoid bilateral pedicled TRAM flaps because of the significant abdominal donor site morbidity (i.e., weakness, abdominal bulge, and hernia formation).
- ✔ **Free TRAM flap**
  - Always try to harvest a portion of the SIEA and SIEV when performing a free TRAM flap.
  - In case of venous congestion (e.g., damage to perforators, dominant superficial venous system), the SIEV can be used for additional venous outflow.
  - Discard zone IV of the TRAM flap when performing unilateral reconstructions, especially when performing a DIEP flap or pedicled TRAM flap.
  - When performing an SIEA flap, use only the ipsilateral abdominal donor tissue, and avoid crossing the midline.
  - When using the thoracodorsal vessels as recipient vessels, the anastomosis should be performed proximal to the serratus takeoff from the thoracodorsal vessel. This preserves the latissimus dorsi flap for future reconstruction, if needed, via retrograde flow through the serratus branch.
  - Most free TRAM flap failures can be linked to a technical error performed by the surgeon.
    - Always make sure that pedicle kinking, twisting, or compression is avoided during flap insetting.
    - Avoid large vessel mismatches between recipient and donor vessels.
  - The DIEA and DIEV are usually well matched in size to the thoracodorsal or IM vessels.
  - The smaller SIEA pedicle can produce a mismatch with the thoracodorsal or IM vessels and is usually better matched with the IM perforator vein and artery.
- ✔ **Abdominal Donor Site Closure**
  - Close Scarpa's fascia to avoid a trapdoor deformity and step-off along the lower abdominal incision line.
  - Use of an abdominal On-Q pump for pain control has been proven to decrease overall postoperative pain medication intake.

REFERENCES

1. Bostwick J III. Plastic and Reconstructive Breast Surgery. St Louis: Quality Medical Publishing, 1990.
2. Couch FJ, Weber BL. The Genetic Basis of Human Cancer. New York: McGraw Hill, 1988.
3. Reaby LL. Reasons why women who have mastectomy decide to have or not to have breast reconstruction. Plast Reconstr Surg 101:1810, 1998.
4. Spear SL, Mardini S, Ganz JC. Resource cost comparison of implant-based breast reconstruction versus TRAM flap breast reconstruction. Plast Reconstr Surg 112:101, 2003.
5. Kroll SS, Evans GR, Reece GP, et al. Comparison of resource costs between implant-based and TRAM flap breast reconstruction. Plast Reconstr Surg 97:364, 1996.

6. Clough KB, O'Donoghue JM, Fitoussi AD. Prospective evaluation of late cosmetic results following breast reconstruction: I. Implant reconstruction. Plast Reconstr Surg 107:1702, 2001.

7. Hammond DC, Capraro PA, Ozolins EB, et al. Use of a skin-sparing reduction pattern to create a combination skin-muscle flap pocket in immediate breast reconstruction. Plast Reconstr Surg 110:206, 2002.

8. Heitmann C, Pelzer M, Kuentscher M, et al. The extended latissimus dorsi flap revisited. Plast Reconstr Surg 111:1697, 2003.

9. Delay E, Gounot N, Bouillot A, et al. Autologous latissimus breast reconstruction: A 3-year clinical experience with 100 patients. Plast Reconstr Surg 102:1461, 1998.

10. Rios JL, Pollock T, Adams WP. Progressive tension sutures to prevent seroma formation after latissimus dorsi harvest. Plast Reconstr Surg 112:1779, 2003.

11. Chang D, Youssef A, Cha S, et al. Autologous breast reconstruction with the extended latissimus dorsi flap. Plast Reconstr Surg 110:751, 2002.

12. Schwabegger A, Harpf C, Rainer C. Muscle-sparing latissimus dorsi myocutaneous flap with maintenance of muscle innervation, function, and aesthetic appearance of the donor site. Plast Reconstr Surg 111:1407, 2003.

13. Hamdi M, Van Landuyt K, Monstrey S, et al. Pedicled perforator flaps in breast reconstruction: A new concept. Br J Plast Surg 57:531, 2004.

14. Hartrampf CR, Scheflan M, Black PW. Breast reconstruction with a transverse abdominal island flap. Plast Reconstr Surg 69:216, 1982.

15. Holm C, Mayr M, Hofter E, et al. Perfusion zones of the DIEP flap revisited: A clinical study. Plast Reconstr Surg 117:37, 2006.

16. Codner MA, Bostwick J III, Nahai F. TRAM flap vascular delay for high-risk breast reconstruction. Plast Reconstr Surg 96:1615, 1995.

17. Saint-Cyr M, Youssef A, Bae HW, et al. Changing trends in recipient vessel selection for microvascular autologous breast reconstruction: An analysis of 1483 cases. Plast Reconstr Surg (in press).

18. Bunkis J. Experience with the transverse lower rectus abdominis operation for breast reconstruction. Plast Reconstr Surg 72:819, 1983.

19. Scheflan M, Dinner MI. The transverse abdominal island flap: Part I. Indications, contraindications, results, and complications. Ann Plast Surg 10:24, 1983.

20. McGraw JB. An early appraisal of the methods of tissue expansion and the transverse rectus abdominis musculocutaneous flap in reconstruction of the breast following mastectomy. Ann Plast Surg 18:93, 1987.

21. Hartrampf CR Jr. The transverse abdominal island flap for breast reconstruction. A 7-year experience. Clin Plast Surg 15:703, 1988.

22. Baldwin BJ. Bilateral breast reconstruction: Conventional versus free TRAM. Plast Reconstr Surg 93:1410, 1994.

23. Schusterman MA. The free transverse rectus abdominis musculocutaneous flap for breast reconstruction: One center's experience with 211 consecutive cases. Ann Plast Surg 32:234, 1994.

24. Chang DW, Wang BG, Robb GL. Effect of obesity on flap and donor site complications in free transverse rectus abdominis myocutaneous flap breast reconstruction. Plast Reconstr Surg 105:1640, 2000.

25. Nahabedian M, Tsangaris T, Momen B. Breast reconstruction with the DIEP flap or the muscle-sparing (MS-2) free TRAM flap: Is there a difference? Plast Reconstr Surg 115:436, 2005.

26. Jones G, Bostwick J III. Nipple-areolar reconstruction. Op Tech Plast Reconstr Surg 1:35, 1994.

27. Little JW. Nipple-areolar reconstruction. In Habal MB, ed. Advances in Plastic and Reconstructive Surgery, vol 3. Chicago: Yearbook Medical, 1987, p 43.

28. Spear SL, Arias J. Long-term experience with nipple-areola tattooing. Ann Plast Surg 35:232, 1995.

29. Spear SL, Onyewu C. Staged breast reconstruction with saline-filled implants in the irradiated breast: Recent trends and therapeutic implications. Plast Reconstr Surg 105:930, 2000.

30. Tran NV, Chang DW, Gupta A. Comparison of immediate and delayed free TRAM flap breast reconstruction in patients receiving postmastectomy radiation therapy. Plast Reconstr Surg 108:78, 2001.

PART V

Trunk and Lower Extremity

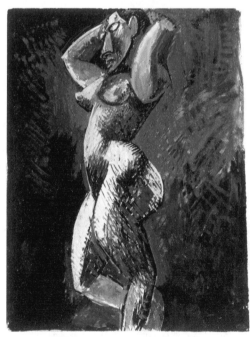

44. Chest Wall Reconstruction

Jeffrey E. Janis

ANATOMY

PLEURAL CAVITY
- Visceral pleura
- Parietal pleura

NOTE: Separate embryologic origins result in anatomic differences between the visceral pleura and the parietal pleura, including arterial supplies, venous and lymphatic drainage patterns, and innervations.[1]

THORACIC SKELETON (Fig. 44-1)
- **Purposes**
  - Provides stable skeletal support
  - Protects vital organs (e.g., heart, lungs, great vessels, and some abdominal organs)
  - Contributes to respiratory function
  - Supports the upper extremities
- **Structures**
  - **12 paired ribs**
    - **True ribs,** or *vertebrosternal ribs (1-7, sometimes 8)*
      - Articulate directly with the sternum through costal cartilages
    - **False ribs,** or *vertebrochondral ribs (8-12)*
      - Connect with the costal cartilages superior to them rather than connecting directly to the sternum
    - **Floating ribs,** or *vertebral ribs (11 and 12)*
      - Do not communicate directly with either the sternum or the ribs superior to them
      - Articulate only with their own vertebral bodies
  - **Sternum**
    - Large, elongated, flat bone that measures approximately 15-20 cm in length

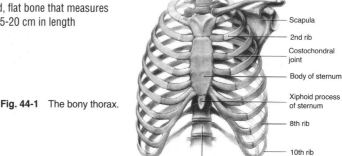

Fig. 44-1   The bony thorax.

1st thoracic vertebra
1st rib
Clavicle
Scapula
2nd rib
Costochondral joint
Body of sternum
Xiphoid process of sternum
8th rib
10th rib
12th thoracic vertebra

- ▶ **Divisions**
  - ✦ **Manubrium**
    - Wider and thicker than the other two parts of the sternum
    - Articulates with the clavicles and the first costal cartilage
    - The *angle of Louis* represents the junction of the manubrium and body of the sternum—corresponds to the articulation with the second rib
  - ✦ **Body**
    - Longest of the three parts
    - Located anterior to T5 to T9
  - ✦ **Xiphoid**
    - Smallest and most variable portion
    - Usually ossifies and unites with the sternal body around age 40 years
- • **Clavicles**
- • **Thoracic vertebrae**

THORACIC SOFT TISSUES (Fig. 44-2)
- ■ Bony thorax is covered by muscle, subcutaneous tissue, and skin
- ■ Subdivisions of thoracic muscles
  - • **Primary muscles of respiration**
    - ▶ Diaphragm
    - ▶ Intercostal muscles (external, internal, and innermost)
      - ✦ Neurovascular bundles run between the **internal** and **innermost** intercostals.
      - ✦ The bundles are positioned behind the costal groove inferior to the rib, with the vein positioned most superiorly, followed by the artery and the nerve in descending order (VAN).
      - ✦ All 11 intercostal spaces are wider anteriorly, and each intercostal bundle falls away from the rib posteriorly to become more central within each space.
  - • **Secondary muscles of respiration**
    - ▶ Sternocleidomastoid
    - ▶ Serratus posterior (superior and inferior heads)
    - ▶ Levatores costarum

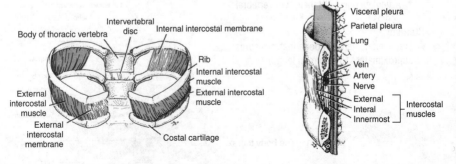

Fig. 44-2   The neurovascular bundle and the intercostal musculature. (From Moore KL. Clinically Oriented Anatomy, 3rd ed. Baltimore: Williams & Wilkins, 1992.)

- **Muscles that attach the upper extremities to the body**
  - ▸ Help secure scapulae to bony thorax
  - ▸ Superficial muscles
    - ✦ Pectoralis major
    - ✦ Pectoralis minor (anterior)
    - ✦ Trapezius
    - ✦ Latissimus dorsi (posterior)
  - ▸ Deep muscles
    - ✦ Serratus anterior and posterior
    - ✦ Levatores costarum
    - ✦ Rhomboideus major
    - ✦ Rhomboideus minor

NOTE: In cases of respiratory distress, the pectoralis major and the serratus anterior act as accessory muscles of respiration. They do so when a person holds onto a table to fix their pectoral girdles (clavicles and scapulae), allowing these muscles to act on their attachments to the ribs.

- ■ **Internal mammary vessels**
  - Serve as important and useful recipient sites for microvascular tissue transfer, although rarely needed in chest wall reconstruction
  - **Anatomic studies**
    - ▸ According to Shaw,[2] when the mammary vessels are dissected at the fifth intercostal space, approximately 42% of the internal mammary veins are unsuitable for use.
    - ▸ Clark et al[3] discovered that the internal mammary veins gradually become smaller distally and often bifurcate, making them unsuitable for use as recipient vessels below the fourth intercostal space.
      - ✦ They concluded that the most consistent interval to find suitable recipient vessels was the **third intercostal space,** where 40% of the veins on the left and 70% of the veins on the right were 3 mm in diameter or larger.
      - ✦ Furthermore, 90% of veins on the left and 40% of veins on the right bifurcated by the third rib.

CHEST WOUNDS

ETIOLOGIC FACTORS
- ■ Trauma
- ■ Tumor
- ■ Infection
- ■ Radiation
- ■ Congenital

PATIENT EVALUATION
- ■ **History**
  - See Chapter 1 for general principles for the management of complex wounds.
  - Evaluate for underlying pulmonary disease.
    - ▸ Need preoperative pulmonary function tests (PFTs)
    - ▸ May help determine whether small defects require reconstruction
  - Obtain specific surgical history.
    - ▸ Previous thoracotomy may compromise latissimus dorsi and serratus muscles.
    - ▸ Previous subcostal incision may compromise rectus abdominis.

- ▶ Previous axillary dissection may compromise thoracodorsal pedicle.
- ▶ Previous coronary artery bypass graft may have used the internal mammary artery, thereby compromising the rectus abdominis or pectoralis major turnover.

> TIP: When in doubt, obtain an arteriogram or magnetic resonance arteriogram, and always read previous operation reports.

- **Physical examination**
  - See Chapter 1 for general principles for the management of complex wounds.
  - Evaluate congenital disorders that may influence reconstructive options.
    - ▶ Poland's syndrome (pectoralis, latissimus dorsi)
    - ▶ Pectus excavatum (repair may have compromised vascular pedicles in the area)
    - ▶ Pectus carinatum (repair may have compromised vascular pedicles in the area)

RECONSTRUCTION GOALS[4]

- Debride devitalized tissue and hardware, and obtain healthy wound bed.
- Restore stability and structure.
  - Reconstruct the skeleton if **more than four ribs are resected** or if the **defect is greater than 5 cm.**
  - Restore normal respiratory mechanics.
  - Protect vital structures and organs.
- Obliterate dead space.
- Provide durable coverage.
- Achieve aesthetic results.

> TIP: There is no substitute for early and aggressive debridement of all devitalized tissue. It is the cornerstone of treatment, and if it is not performed adequately, then all reconstructive efforts will be sabotaged.

RECONSTRUCTION OF PLEURAL CAVITY

- Defect is usually secondary to complications of tumor resection (pulmonary or esophageal).
- Defect is usually present as bronchopleural or tracheoesophageal fistulas.
  - High morbidity and mortality rate

GOALS

- Eradicate infection.
- Obtain airtight pleural cavity.

TREATMENT

- Obliterate pleural space with local muscle flaps or omentum.
  - Latissimus dorsi
  - Serratus anterior
  - Pectoralis major
  - Rectus abdominis
  - Omentum

- Access muscle flaps or omentum through a previous thoracotomy incision, or create a second incision.
- To prevent ischemic failure it is imperative that the flap pedicle is not kinked or twisted.

RECONSTRUCTION OF THORACIC SKELETON

DEFECT CAUSES

- Usually caused by postoperative infection after cardiac surgery
- Can also occur after resection of chest wall tumors, trauma, or radiation
- **Sternotomy wound infections** (Table 44-1)[5]
  - **Incidence**[6]
    - ▶ Most common defect, likely after sternotomy wound infection/osteomyelitis
    - ▶ Occurs in up to **5%** of cardiac procedures
    - ▶ Can be life threatening
    - ▶ More common when IMA is harvested
      - ✦ **0.3%** with **unilateral** IMA harvest, **2.4%** with **bilateral** IMA harvest
  - **Classification**
    - ▶ Pairolero[7]
      - ✦ **Type 1:** Serosanguinous drainage within first 3 days, negative cultures, no cellulitis or osteomyelitis
        - Treatment: Reexplore, debride, reclose
      - ✦ **Type 2:** Purulent mediastinitis occurring within first 3 weeks, positive cultures, and cellulitis and/or osteomyelitis
        - Treatment: Reexplore, debride, flap
      - ✦ **Type 3:** Draining sinus tract from chronic osteomyelitis months to years after procedure
        - Treatment: Reexplore, debride, flap

Table 44-1 *Starzynski Classification of Sternal Defects*

Defect	Physiologic Deficit
Loss of upper sternal body and adjacent ribs	Minimal
Loss of entire sternal body and adjacent ribs	Moderate
Loss of manubrium and upper sternal body with adjacent ribs	Severe

From Starzynski TE, Snyderman RK, Beattie BJ. Problems of major chest wall reconstruction. Plast Reconstr Surg 44:525, 1969.

INDICATIONS FOR RECONSTRUCTION

- **Defect affects more than four contiguous ribs or is greater than 5 cm.**[8,9]
  - **Purpose:** Stabilize paradoxical motion and protect vital organs
  - May reconstruct smaller defect if underlying pulmonary disease (less tolerance for loss of respiratory mechanical efficiency)
  - May not reconstruct larger defects if previous radiation therapy
    - ▶ *Radiation stiffens chest wall through ischemic fibrosis, which leads to less paradoxical motion and loss of respiratory mechanical efficiency for a same-sized defect*
- **If defect is located posteriorly and/or superiorly (shielded by the scapula), then a larger defect is tolerated.**

RECONSTRUCTIVE OPTIONS

- **Alloplastic reconstruction**
  - **Mesh**[9-11]
    - ▶ **Polypropylene (Marlex®)**
      - ✦ Semirigid
      - ✦ Reduces ventilator dependence and overall hospital stay
      - ✦ Can fragment or cause seroma formation
      - ✦ Can become infected
      - ✦ Forms fibrous capsule
    - ▶ **e-PTFE (Gore-Tex®)**
      - ✦ Semirigid
      - ✦ Malleable and flexible
      - ✦ Does not become incorporated but forms a fibrous capsule
      - ✦ Prone to seroma formation
      - ✦ Expensive
  - **Methylmethacrylate**
    - ▶ Exothermic reaction
    - ▶ Rigid
    - ▶ Higher infection and extrusion rates
  - **Bone grafts**
- **Autogenous tissue reconstruction**
  - **Locoregional flaps (most common)** (Table 44-2)
    - ▶ Pectoralis major
      - ✦ Advancement

Table 44-2 *Commonly Used Locoregional Flaps for Chest Wall Reconstruction*

Flap	Mathes/Nahai Flap Type	Origin	Insertion	Dominant Pedicle
Pectoralis major	V	Clavicle, sternum, upper seven ribs	Humerus	Pectoral branch of thoracoacromial artery
Latissimus dorsi	V	Spinous processes of lower six thoracic vertebrae, thoracolumbar fascia, iliac crest	Humerus	Thoracodorsal artery
Serratus anterior	III	Upper eight ribs	Scapula	Lateral thoracic artery and the serratus branch of thoracodorsal artery
Rectus abdominis	III	Pubic symphysis and crest	Costal cartilages of ribs 5-7	Superior and inferior epigastric artery
Omentum	III	Stomach, duodenum, gastrosplenic ligament	Transverse colon and gastrocolic ligament	Right and left gastroepiploic artery

- Turnover
  - Composite myocutaneous
- ▸ Latissimus dorsi
- ▸ Rectus abdominis
- ▸ Serratus anterior
- ▸ Omentum

RECONSTRUCTION OF THORACIC SOFT TISSUES

PARTIAL-THICKNESS DEFECTS
- Reconstruct with split-thickness skin grafts if wound bed well perfused

FULL-THICKNESS DEFECTS
- Usually reconstruct with locoregional flaps (as with partial-thickness defects) or free flaps in rare cases

CHEST WALL DEFORMITIES

There are various congenital chest wall abnormalities. Although most of them result in no noticeable physiologic impairment, some can be severe or even life threatening.

CHEST WALL ABNORMALITIES

Depression deformities (pectus excavatum)
Protrusion deformities (pectus carinatum)
Poland's syndrome
Sternal defects
Cervical ectopia cordis
Thoracic ectopia cordis
Thoracoabdominal ectopia cordis
Bifid sternum

POLAND'S SYNDROME
- **Incidence**
  - Occurs in approximately 1:30,000 births[12]
  - No gender prevalence
  - Right side is affected twice as much as left side
- **Current theory** postulates syndrome caused by hypoplasia of subclavian artery secondary to kinking during week 6 of gestation
- **Components**[13-15]
  - Absence of sternal head of pectoralis major muscle
  - Absence of costal cartilages
  - Hypoplasia or aplasia of breast and subcutaneous tissue, including the nipple complex

- Deficiency of subcutaneous fat and axillary hair
- Syndactyly or hypoplasia of ipsilateral extremity

■ **Additional findings**
- Absence or hypoplasia of pectoralis minor muscle
- Shortening and hypoplasia of forearm
- Variable deformities of the serratus, infraspinatus, supraspinatus, latissimus dorsi, and external oblique muscles
- Total absence of anterolateral ribs with herniation of the lung
- Symphalangism with syndactyly and hypoplasia or aplasia of middle phalanges
- Occasionally associated with Möbius' syndrome (facial palsy and abducens oculi palsy) or childhood leukemia

■ **Indications for treatment**
- Patients with absent ribs
- Female patients with breast asymmetry

■ **Timing of surgery**
- Delayed in females until after puberty to allow full development of the contralateral breast

■ **Surgical techniques**
- The ipsilateral latissimus dorsi is mobilized over a customized breast implant. The insertion of the latissimus dorsi is moved anteriorly on the humerus to establish an anterior axillary fold.[13]
- Alloplastic meshes and custom-fabricated silicone moulages can also be used to correct the deformity.

DEPRESSION DEFORMITIES (PECTUS EXCAVATUM)

■ Also called *funnel chest*

■ **Incidence**
- **Most common chest wall deformity**
  ▶ Occurs in 1:400 children
  ▶ Approximately ten times more common than pectus carinatum
- Affects males more than females (4:1)
- More than 30% have family history, although research has not proved genetic factors[16]
- Approximately 20% associated with other musculoskeletal abnormalities such as scoliosis (15%) and Marfan's syndrome
- Congenital heart disease observed in 1.5%[17]

■ **Pathophysiology**
- Results from excessive growth of the lower costal cartilages, causing a posterior sternal depression
- Rotation of sternum can result if depression is deeper on right side than left side
- Usually recognized within first year of life and progressively worsens as the child grows older
- Usually begins asymptomatically but eventually can result in significant pulmonary abnormalities
- May result in a spectrum of severity, ranging from a mildly depressed sternum to sternal depression abutting the vertebral column

■ **Indications for reconstruction**
- Cosmesis
- Psychosocial factors
- Presence of respiratory or cardiovascular insufficiency

- **Timing of reconstruction**
  - Poor self-image is an important concern for many patients, particularly children and young adults or adolescents who are teased by peers. Because of these concerns, early repair is supported, with the best results being reported between the ages of 2 and 5 years.[18]
- **Surgical techniques**
  - Requires multiple osteotomies of the sternum and the affected rib segments to help reposition the sternum and restore a normal contour
  - **Procedures**
    - ▸ Sternal osteotomy to reposition the sternum anteriorly
    - ▸ A modification that involves using a posterior strut (sternal strut) to support the repositioned sternum (Ravitch technique)[19]
    - ▸ Removing the sternum and repositioning it in a front-to-back rotated position before stabilization (sternum turnover procedure)
    - ▸ Creating a silastic mold that is implanted into the subcutaneous space to fill the defect without altering the thoracic cage[20]

PROTRUSION DEFORMITIES (PECTUS CARINATUM)

- Also called *pigeon chest*
- Defect characterized by an anterior protrusion deformity of the sternum and costal cartilages
- **Incidence**
  - Affects males more than females (4:1)
  - Family history (30%)
  - Associated with scoliosis (15%) and congenital heart disease (20%)[21]
- **Pathophysiology**
  - Defect typically not recognized until after first decade of life
  - Physiologic symptoms uncommon
  - **Types of defects**
    - ▸ *Chondrogladiolar protrusion*
      - ✦ Anterior displacement of the body of the sternum and symmetrical concavity of the costal cartilages
      - ✦ Most common of the three variants
    - ▸ *Lateral depression of the ribs on one or both sides of the sternum*
      - ✦ Poland's syndrome frequently associated with this type
    - ▸ *Pouter pigeon breast*
      - ✦ Upper or chondromanubrial prominence with protrusion of the manubrium and depression of the sternal body
      - ✦ Least common of the three variants
- **Surgical techniques**
  - Similar to pectus carinatum with resection of abnormal costal cartilages, repositioning of the sternum, and possible use of struts

KEY POINTS

✔ A complete history and physical examination is mandatory before embarking on chest wall reconstruction, because the presence of significant comorbidities and previous surgeries can impact the outcome.

✔ Debridement of devitalized bone and cartilage is the cornerstone of treatment for infected sternal wounds.

✔ Remove all foreign bodies (e.g., sternal wires).

✔ Reconstruct skeletal stability if the defect affects more than four contiguous ribs or is greater than 5 cm in dimension, or if the defect causes significant pulmonary complications (e.g., flail chest with paradoxical movement).

✔ Restoration of skeletal stability is less likely in posteriorly located defects as a result of shielding by the scapula, and in patients with a history of radiation therapy, which causes stiffening of the chest wall.

✔ Locoregional flaps, particularly muscle flaps, are the workhorses of reconstruction.

✔ It is rare for congenital deformities to significantly impact cardiorespiratory function. The indications for treatment are largely aesthetic.

REFERENCES

1. Satterfield TS. The thorax. In Moore KL, ed. Clinically Oriented Anatomy, 3rd ed. Baltimore: Williams & Wilkins, 1992, pp 33-125.
2. Shaw WW. Breast reconstruction by superior gluteal microvascular free flaps without silicone implants. Plast Reconstr Surg 72:490-501, 1983.
3. Clark CP III, Rohrich RJ, Copit S, et al. An anatomic study of the internal mammary veins: Clinical implications for free-tissue-transfer breast reconstruction. Plast Reconstr Surg 99:400-404, 1997.
4. Cohen M, Ramasastry SS. Reconstruction of complex chest wall defects. Am J Surg 172:35-40, 1996.
5. Starzynski TE, Snyderman RK, Beattie EJ Jr. Problems of major chest wall reconstruction. Plast Reconstr Surg 44:525-535, 1969.
6. Cosgrove DM, Lytle BW, Loop FD, et al. Does bilateral internal mammary artery grafting increase surgical risk? J Thorac Cardiovasc Surg 95:850-856, 1988.
7. Pairolero PC, Arnold PG. Management of infected median sternotomy wounds. Ann Thorac Surg 42:1-2, 1986.
8. Dingman RO, Argenta LC. Reconstruction of the chest wall. Ann Plast Surg 32:202-208, 1981.
9. McCormack PM. Use of prosthetic materials in chest wall reconstruction: Assets and liabilities. Surg Clin North Am 69:965-976, 1989.
10. Hurwitz DJ, Ravitch M, Wolmark N. Laminated Marlex-methyl methacrylate prosthesis for massive chest wall resection. Ann Plast Surg 5:486-490, 1980.
11. Kroll SS, Walsh G, Ryan B, et al. Risks and benefits of using Marlex mesh in chest wall reconstruction. Ann Plast Surg 31:303-306, 1993.
12. Freire-Maia N, Chautard EA, Opitz JM, et al. The Poland syndrome—clinical and genealogical data, dermatoglyphic analysis, and incidence. Hum Hered 23:97-104, 1973.
13. Hester TR Jr, Bostwick J III. Poland's syndrome: Correction with latissimus muscle transposition. Plast Reconstr Surg 69:226-233, 1982.
14. Ohmori K, Takada H. Correction of Poland's pectoralis major muscle anomaly with latissimus dorsi musculocutaneous flaps. Plast Reconstr Surg 65:400-404, 1980.

15. Ravitch MM. Poland's syndrome: A study of an eponym. Plast Reconstr Surg 59:508-512, 1977.
16. Shamberger RC, Welch KJ. Surgical repair of pectus excavatum. J Pediatr Surg 23:615-622, 1988.
17. Shamberger RC, Welch KJ, Castaneda AR, et al. Anterior chest wall deformities and congenital heart disease. J Thorac Cardiovasc Surg 96:427-432, 1988.
18. Shamberger RC, Welch KJ. Chest wall deformities. In Ashcraft KW, Holder TM, eds. Pediatric Surgery, 2nd ed. Philadelphia: WB Saunders, 1993, p 146.
19. Ravitch MM. Congenital deformities of the chest wall and their operative correction. Philadelphia: WB Saunders, 1977.
20. Crump HW. Pectus excavatum. Am Fam Physician 46:173-179, 1992.
21. Shamberger RC, Welch KJ. Surgical correction of pectus carinatum. J Pediatr Surg 22:48-53, 1987.

45. Abdominal Wall Reconstruction

Jeffrey E. Janis

ANATOMY (Fig. 45-1)

- **The anterior/anterolateral abdominal borders are:**
  - **Superiorly:** Xiphoid process and costal cartilage of the seventh and twelfth ribs
  - **Inferiorly:** Pubic tubercle and inguinal ligament
  - **Laterally:** Midaxillary line

LAYERS

- Skin
- Subcutaneous tissue
- Scarpa's fascia
- Rectus sheath
  - **Above the arcuate line:**
    - ▶ Anterior rectus sheath: Aponeuroses of the external oblique and anterior leaf of the internal oblique
    - ▶ Posterior rectus sheath: Posterior leaf of the internal oblique aponeurosis, transversus abdominis muscle, and transversalis fascia
  - **Below the arcuate line:**
    - ▶ Anterior rectus sheath: Aponeuroses of the external and internal obliques and transversus abdominis
    - ▶ Posterior rectus sheath: Transversalis fascia only

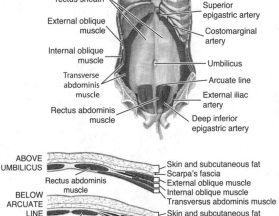

Fig. 45-1

NOTE: The arcuate (semicircular) line is approximately at the level of the anterior superior iliac spines.

- Preperitoneal fat
- Peritoneum

MUSCLES

- **Rectus abdominis**
  - **Origin:** Pubic ramus
  - **Insertion:** Xiphoid process and fifth, sixth, and seventh ribs
- **External oblique**
  - **Origin:** Lower eight ribs
  - **Insertion:** Linea alba through aponeurosis

- **Internal oblique**
  - **Origin:** Thoracolumbar fascia, iliac crest, and inguinal ligament
  - **Insertion:** Costal margin and linea alba, through its aponeurosis
- **Transversus abdominis**
  - **Origin:** Costal cartilages of ribs 6-12, thoracolumbar fascia, anterior iliac crest, and inguinal ligament
  - **Insertion:** Linea alba through aponeurosis
- **Pyramidalis**
  - Functionally insignificant triangular muscle
  - Not present in everyone

VASCULAR SUPPLY
- Superior and inferior epigastrics
- Superficial and deep circumflex iliacs
- Superficial external pudendals
- Intercostals
- Lumbar vessels

INNERVATION
- Ventral rami of T7 through L4
- Iliohypogastric
- Ilioinguinal

PATIENT EVALUATION (see Chapter 1)

HISTORY
- Comorbidities
- Surgical history
- Medications
- Social history (including tobacco, alcohol, and drug use)
- Radiation

PHYSICAL EXAMINATION
- Acute or chronic
- Partial or full-thickness defect
- Size and location
  - Measure at **superior, middle,** and **inferior** thirds of the abdomen
- Wound contamination
- Presence of ostomy
- Presence of enterocutaneous fistulas
  - Must be controlled before flap coverage
  - Can be associated with electrolyte imbalances and nutritional deficiencies

PREOPERATIVE STUDIES
- **Laboratory tests**
  - Albumin/prealbumin
  - Electrolytes (especially with fistula or open wound)

- **Imaging**
  - CT or MRI
    - ▸ Aids in evaluation of size and extent of defect, including integrity of adjacent muscles that may be used in reconstruction
  - Fistulogram

ABDOMINAL WALL DEFECTS

ETIOLOGIC FACTORS
- Trauma
- Tumor
- Infection
- Prior surgery (hernia)
- Congenital (gastroschisis, omphalocele)
- Radiation

GOALS OF RECONSTRUCTION
- Debride all devitalized/infected/irradiated tissue.
- Obtain tumor-free status, if applicable.
- Restore integrity of abdominal wall when initial problem and associated complications are addressed and resolved.
  - Protect abdominal viscera.
  - Prevent herniation.
- Address aesthetic considerations.

TIMING OF RECONSTRUCTION[1-3]
- **Immediate**
  - Hernia repair
  - After tumor resection
- **Delayed**
  - Patient instability
  - Infected or contaminated wound
  - Extensive injury that has not fully declared itself

PREOPERATIVE CONSIDERATIONS
- Bowel preparation in case of enterotomy
- General surgery notification
- Backup plan in case of inability to achieve closure
- Nasogastric tube (decompress stomach)
- No nitrous oxide (prevent intestinal dilation) (notify anaesthesiologist)
- Watch for increased peak inspiratory pressures and decreased urinary output

RECONSTRUCTION OF ABDOMINAL WALL DEFECTS

RECONSTRUCTION OPTIONS

- **Healing by secondary intention**
  - Used only for small defects
  - Can use standard normal saline wet-to-dry dressing changes or potentially negative-pressure wound therapy[4]
- **Primary closure**
  - Used for small- to moderate-sized defects
    - ► Layered complex closure
    - ► Must be tension free or will be prone to dehiscence and necrosis

CAUTION: Watch for respiratory compromise and/or abdominal compartment syndrome from too tight a closure.

  - ► Possible need to perform relaxing incisions of the external oblique muscle or muscles (not recommended)
- **Prosthetic (alloplastic) materials**[5,6]
  - **Polyglactin 910 (Vicryl®) or polyglycolic acid (Dexon™)**
    - ► Absorbable meshed alloplastic material
    - ► Provides excellent temporary coverage and support
    - ► No need for removal because it is absorbable
    - ► Will eventually result in hernia because of lack of permanence
  - **Polypropylene (Marlex®)**
    - ► Nonabsorbable meshed alloplastic material
    - ► Durable and strong
    - ► Resistant to bacterial contamination
    - ► Promotes fibrous ingrowth through its interstices
    - ► Can extrude, especially if thin soft tissue coverage
    - ► Can cause enterocutaneous fistulas, especially if not placed under mild tension (bowel erosion caused by folds)
  - **Polypropylene fiber (Prolene™)**
    - ► Nonabsorbable mesh alloplastic material
    - ► More pliable than Marlex
    - ► Comes in "soft" form, as well
    - ► More easily removed
  - **Expanded polytetrafluoroethylene (ePTFE) (Gore-Tex®)**
    - ► Nonabsorbable, nonmeshed alloplastic sheet
    - ► Allows no fibrous ingrowth (not meshed)
      - ◆ Makes for easier removal
    - ► Soft and pliable
    - ► Causes fewer adhesions
    - ► Less adherent to bacteria
    - ► Does not allow egress of fluid

CAUTION: Without fluid egress, problems can develop in open abdominal wounds; therefore Gore-Tex should be used with discretion.

> TIP:　If using mesh, be sure to use a large piece, preferably on the undersurface of the peritoneum, with wide margins on each side.

- **Skin grafts[7]**
  - Generally used as temporary coverage over exposed bowel and visceral contents
  - Underlying wound bed must be vascular and not be grossly contaminated
  - Difficult to remove once healed
    - ▶ Deepithelialization suggested, leaving deep dermis behind

> TIP:　Because of the increased chance of enterotomy when peeling skin grafts off of bowel, it is wise for these patients to undergo bowel preparation before surgery and to notify general surgery that they may be needed.

- **Tissue expanders[8-10]**
  - Can be used underneath the skin/subcutaneous tissue to create additional tissue
  - Can also be placed between external and internal oblique muscles, or between internal oblique and transversus abdominis muscles to create additional muscle and fascia
  - Can be inserted using an open approach or endoscopically
- **Local flaps**
  - **Rectus abdominis**
    - ▶ Muscle transposition or turnover
      - ✦ Superiorly based
      - ✦ Inferiorly based
    - ▶ Transverse rectus abdominis myocutaneous (TRAM) or vertical rectus abdominis myocutaneous (VRAM) flap
  - **External oblique**
  - **Components separation[11,12]**
    - ▶ Rectus muscle peeled off the posterior rectus sheath
    - ▶ External oblique muscle separated from internal oblique at linea semilunaris
    - ▶ Can obtain advancement of composite flap (rectus, anterior rectus sheath, attached internal oblique, and transversus abdominis muscles) for variable distances:
      - ✦ **Epigastrium:** 5 cm
      - ✦ **Waist:** 10 cm
      - ✦ **Suprapubic region:** 3 cm

NOTE: Components separation can be performed unilaterally or bilaterally. If bilateral, figures can be doubled (Fig. 45-2).

- **Regional flaps**
  - Latissimus dorsi
  - Groin flap
  - Tensor fascia lata
  - Rectus femoris
  - Vastus lateralis
  - Gracilis
  - Anterolateral thigh
  - Omentum

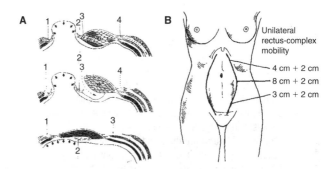

Fig. 45-2 **A,** Dissection of the abdominal wall musculature into components for medial advancement of separate muscle layers. (From Ramirez OM, Ruas E, Dellon AL. "Components separation" method for closure of abdominal-wall defects: An anatomic and clinical study. Plast Reconstr Surg 86:519, 1990.) **B,** Unilateral advancement distances for components separation. (From Shestak KC, Edington HJ, Johnson RR. The separation of anatomic components technique for the reconstruction of massive midline abdominal wall defects: Anatomy, surgical technique, applications, and limitations revisited. Plast Reconstr Surg 105:731, 2000.)

■ **Free tissue transfer**
- Donor vessels may be an issue
- Tensor fascia lata
- Latissimus dorsi
- Anterolateral thigh

■ **Other choices**
- AlloDerm®
  ▸ Freeze-dried cadaveric dermis
  ▸ Undergoes replacement after fibrous ingrowth (host tissue remodeling)
  ▸ Comes in various sizes that can be used off the shelf with no donor site morbidity
  ▸ Comparable to tensor fascia lata, if not stronger, by preliminary data

BASIC ALGORITHM[13]

■ If **acute and contaminated**—place mesh (Vicryl), allow to granulate, skin graft, and consider for delayed reconstruction
■ For **noncontaminated wounds or delayed reconstruction**
- Components separation
- Tissue expansion and closure
- Permanent mesh with or without relaxing incisions and/or flap coverage
  ▸ Prolene or Marlex
- AlloDerm
- Tensor fascia lata (pedicled or free)

POSTOPERATIVE CARE

■ Multiple drains
■ Abdominal binder
■ Antiemetics to prevent vomiting, which may disrupt repair
■ Early ambulation
■ Aggressive respiratory care
■ Avoidance of strenuous activity or heavy lifting for at least 6 weeks

KEY POINTS

- ✔ If the wound is contaminated or the patient has significant comorbidities, place VAC or Vicryl mesh and allow bed to granulate. Then perform skin graft and repair subsequent hernia in delayed (but controlled) fashion.
- ✔ Be sure to correct malnutrition and electrolyte imbalances before undertaking reconstruction.
- ✔ Control all enterocutaneous fistulas before repair.
- ✔ Components separation is an extremely useful technique that allows for repairing sizeable defects with autogenous tissue.
- ✔ Prolene and Marlex are the standard meshes used in abdominal wall reconstruction because of their strength, durability, pliability, and ability to allow tissue ingrowth.
- ✔ Tissue expansion can be used to create additional skin, subcutaneous tissue, muscle, and fascia, depending on where it is placed.
- ✔ AlloDerm holds promise for reconstructing abdominal wall defects. More data and experience will be required before its role is completely defined.

REFERENCES

1. Gottlieb JR, Engrav LH, Walkinshaw MD, et al. Upper abdominal defects: Immediate or staged reconstruction? Plast Reconstr Surg 86:281, 1990.
2. Yeh KA, Saltz R, Howdieshell TR. Abdominal wall reconstruction after temporary abdominal wall closure in trauma patients. South Med J 89:497, 1996.
3. Mansberger A, Kang JS, Beebe HJ, et al. Repair of massive acute abdominal defects. J Trauma 13:766, 1973.
4. Argenta LC, Morykwas MJ. Vacuum-assisted closure: A new method for wound control and treatment: Clinical experience. Ann Plast Surg 38:563, 1997.
5. Brown GL, Richardson JD, Malangoni MA, et al. Comparison of prosthetic materials for abdominal wall reconstruction in the presence of contamination and infection. Ann Surg 201:705, 1985.
6. Mathes SJ, Steinwald PM, Foster RD. Complex abdominal reconstruction: A comparison of flap and mesh closure. Ann Surg 232:586, 2000.
7. Millard DR, Pigott R, Zies P. Free skin grafting of full-thickness defects of the abdominal wall. Plast Reconstr Surg 43:569, 1969.
8. Byrd HS, Hobar PC. Abdominal wall expansion in congenital defects. Plast Reconstr Surg 84:347, 1989.
9. Livingston D, Sharma P, Galntz A. Tissue expanders for abdominal wall reconstruction following severe trauma: Technical note and case report. J Trauma 32:82, 1992.
10. Jacobsen WM, Potty PM, Bite U, et al. Massive abdominal wall reconstruction with expanded external/internal oblique and transversalis musculofascia. Plast Reconstr Surg 100:326, 1997.
11. Ramirez OM, Ruas E, Dellon AL. "Components separation" method for closure of abdominal-wall defects: An anatomic and clinical study. Plast Reconstr Surg 86:519, 1990.
12. Lowe JB, Garza JR, Bowman JL, et al. Endoscopically assisted "components separation" for closure of abdominal wall defects. Plast Reconstr Surg 105:720, 2000.
13. Fabian TC, Croce MA, Pritchard FE, et al. Planned ventral hernia: Staged management for acute abdominal wall defects. Ann Surg 219:643, 1994.

46. Genitourinary Reconstruction

Melissa A. Crosby

EMBRYOLOGY

- **Germ layers:**
  - **Mesoderm:** Nephric system, gonads, wolffian ducts (mesonephric ducts), müllerian ducts (paramesonephric ducts)
  - **Endoderm:** Cloaca and membrane
  - **Ectoderm:** External genitalia[1]
- Gonads start as genital ridges, which begin male or female differentiation at **6 weeks of embryological life.** The testes precede differentiation of the ovaries by 1 week.
- Both mesonephric duct (i.e., the primary duct of the male) and paramesonephric ducts (i.e., the primary ducts of the female) are present in the developing fetus.
- **Differentiation of the ductal system:**
  - Influenced by the **müllerian inhibiting substance**
    - ▸ Produced by **Sertoli cells**
    - ▸ Causes regression of the paramesonephric ducts
  - Influenced by the **testosterone analog**
    - ▸ Produced by the **interstitial cells of Leydig**
    - ▸ Stimulates masculine development of mesonephric ducts
- The **mesonephric duct** develops into the epididymis, vas deferens, and seminal vesicles.
- The **paramesonephric ducts** develop into the fallopian tubes, uterus, and upper portion of the vagina.

CONGENITAL VAGINAL DEFECTS

VAGINAL AGENESIS (MAYER-ROKITANSKY-KÜSTER-HAUSER SYNDROME)
- Congenital absence of vagina: Occurs in **1:5000 births**
- Defect in paramesonephric duct development or fusion of urogenital sinus with paramesonephric duct

NOTE: A developmental defect in the mesonephric duct can cause both vaginal agenesis and renal abnormalities.

- Urinary abnormalities including ectopy, duplication, and agenesis occur 25%-50% of the time
- **Clinical findings**
  - Genetic female with or without functioning uterus, with absent vagina who is otherwise normal
  - Genetic female with or without functioning uterus, with absent vagina and anomalies of skeletal, urinary, or digestive system
  - True hermaphrodite or male hermaphrodite of masculinizing or feminizing type
- **Diagnosis**
  - Pelvic/rectal examination
  - Intravenous pyelogram (IVP) to rule out urinary abnormalities
  - Karyotype screening
  - Spinal radiographs to rule out associated vertebral abnormalities

441

■ **Reconstruction**
  • **Frank's technique:** Nonsurgical autodilation
  • **Malaga flap:** Vulvoperineal fasciocutaneous flaps
  • **McIndoe procedure:** Dissect tunnel in perineum above rectum and below bladder to peritoneal reflection; cavity lined with split- or full-thickness skin grafts; patients wear stent for years; stenosis and fistulas common
  • **Vascularized bowel segment:** Problems with mucus secretion and bleeding with intercourse
  • **Other flaps:** Rectus abdominis flap, gracilis flap, pudendal thigh flap, ureter method, and inferior abdominal wall skin flap

ADDITIONAL ANOMALIES AND CORRECTION (Table 46-1)[1]

Table 46-1   *Corrective Technique for Vaginal Anomalies*

Imperforate hymen	Perforate, trim, oversew edges
Double vagina	Incise septum transversely
Introitus obstructed by perineal skin	Cut-back on flap; vaginoplasty; perineal approach if vagina enters low; pull-through vaginoplasty using an abdominal approach if vagina enters high (proximal to the external urethral sphincter)
Deformed cloaca	Initial decompressive colpotomy followed by identification of anatomic structures and decompressive vaginoplasty

From Kelton PL. Genitourinary repair and reconstruction. Sel Read Plast Surg 8(40), 1999.

CONGENITAL PENILE/SCROTAL DEFECTS

HYPOSPADIAS (Fig. 46-1)[2]
*The congenital development of the male urethra is incomplete. The meatus exits **ventrally** anywhere from the corona to the perineum.*
■ **Characteristics**
  • **The more proximal, the more severe the curvature and deformity**
  • Occurs in **1:350 males**
  • Surgery performed between **6 and 18 months of age**
  • Ventral curvature of penis with prominent dorsal hood

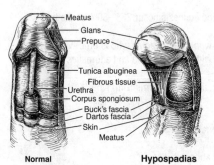

Normal   **Hypospadias**

Fig. 46-1   (From Horton CE, Devine CJ. Hypospadias. In Converse JM, ed. Reconstructive Plastic Surgery, vol 7. Principles and Procedures in Correction Reconstruction and Transplantation, 2nd ed. Philadelphia: WB Saunders, 1977, pp 3845-3861.)

- **Meatus location**
  - ▶ **Distal third (50%):** Glanular, coronal, subcoronal
  - ▶ **Middle third (30%):** Distal penile, shaft, proximal penile
  - ▶ **Proximal third (20%):** Penoscrotal, scrotal, perineal
- **Reconstruction**
  - **Goals**
    - ▶ Release chordee
    - ▶ Creation of new urethra
    - ▶ Advancement of urethral meatus to tip of penis
  - **Techniques**
    - ▶ **Meatal advancement and glanuloplasty (MAGPI)**
      - • Indicated for coronal and glanular variants
      - • Vertical incision of the transverse mucosal bar distal to hypospadias meatus, which is closed transversely
      - • Glanuloplasty achieved by midline approximation of lateral glanular wings, which are freed from corporal tunica
      - • No urethral lengthening achieved; does not correct chordee
    - ▶ **Urethral advancement**
      - • Indicated for glanular, coronal, and distal cases with minimal chordee
      - • Meatus and distal urethra freed from tunica albuginea of cavernous bodies and then from ventral skin for 1-2 cm
      - • Distal urethra pulled through the tunneled glans and secured to tip of glans penis
      - • Avoids urethral reconstruction, so fistula formation should not occur
    - ▶ **Tubularized incised plate (TIP) urethroplasty (i.e., Snodgrass)**
      - • Indicated for most variants, especially midshaft
      - • Longitudinal incision made through midline epithelium of urethral plate, extending from hypospadiac meatus to end of glans
      - • Urethral plate tubularized on itself
      - • Dorsal prepuce mobilized and rotated ventrally to cover urethroplasty
      - • Glans wings closed over urethroplasty in midline
    - ▶ **Flip-flap technique**
      - • Indicated for distal variants without chordee and large meatal opening
      - • Parallel incisions on each side of lateral plate to tip of glans form dorsal urethral wall
      - • Meatal-based flip flap of ventral shaft skin makes up ventral wall
      - • Lateral glans wings approximated over flip-flap urethroplasty after extension of meatus onto tip of glans
    - ▶ **Full-thickness graft urethroplasty**
      - • Indicated for proximal variants
      - • Ventral curvature corrected first by careful removal of chordee tissue
      - • Skin graft harvested from inner surface of prepuce and rolled around catheter to form tube
      - • Graft sutured in oblique fashion to normal urethra proximally and sutured to edges of triangular flap raised from the glans distally
      - • Ventral defect may need coverage with prepuce flaps
    - ▶ **Preputial flap urethroplasty**
      - • Indicated for proximal variants
      - • Island flap from skin of prepuce brought to ventral surface of penis and its inner surface used for urethral reconstruction in form of a tube

* Outer surface of flap used to cover ventral surface defect
► **Onlay grafts of bladder/buccal mucosa**

EPISPADIAS

*A severe congenital anomaly in which the urethral opening is on the **dorsal** aspect of the penis.*

■ **Characteristics**
  • Usually occurs in combination with **bladder exstrophy**
  • Occurs in **1:30,000 males**
  • Classified as **glanular, penile,** or **penopubic,** depending on location of urethral opening
  • Penis is short, wide, and stubby with flat and cleft glans and dorsal curvature

■ **Reconstruction**
  • **Goals**
    ► Penile lengthening
    ► Correction of dorsal chordee
    ► Urethroplasty
    ► Penile skin coverage
  • **Techniques**
    ► **Young technique**
      ✦ Penile skin used to construct longitudinal mucosal strip in shape of tube from neourethra
    ► **Cantwell-Ransley technique**
      ✦ Circumcising incision performed and shaft degloved down to base
      ✦ Urethral plate outlined with lateral incisions and tubularized
    ► **W-flap technique**
      ✦ For secondary epispadias
      ✦ W-shaped incision to produce bilateral, superiorly based groin flaps, with apex of each flap extending below penoscrotal junction
      ✦ Dorsal chordee corrected and urethra reconstructed with full-thickness grafts
      ✦ Dorsal defect covered with preputial skin flaps

ACQUIRED VAGINAL/VULVAR DEFECTS[3,4]

VAGINAL DEFECTS

■ Classification system proposed by Cordeiro based on anatomic location[5] (Fig. 46-2)
■ Algorithm proposed based on the Cordeiro classification[5] (Fig. 46-3)
■ **Reconstruction flaps**
  • **Modified Singapore fasciocutaneous flap**
  • **Vertical rectus flap**
  • **Rolled rectus flap**
  • **Bilateral gracilis flap**

VULVAR DEFECTS

■ **Causes**
  • Oncologic
  • Infectious
  • Traumatic
■ **Reconstruction**
  • Skin grafts

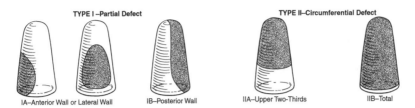

TYPE I –Partial Defect

IA–Anterior Wall or Lateral Wall   IB–Posterior Wall

TYPE II–Circumferential Defect

IIA–Upper Two-Thirds   IIB–Total

Fig. 46-2   (From Cordeiro PG, Pusic AL, Disa JJ. A classification system and reconstructive algorithm for acquired vaginal defects. Plast Reconstr Surg 110:1058-1065, 2002.)

Vaginal Defect

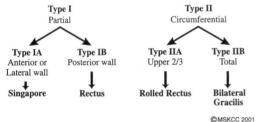

Type I
Partial

Type II
Circumferential

Type IA
Anterior or
Lateral wall
↓
Singapore

Type IB
Posterior wall
↓
Rectus

Type IIA
Upper 2/3
↓
Rolled Rectus

Type IIB
Total
↓
Bilateral
Gracilis

©MSKCC 2001

Fig. 46-3   (From Cordeiro PG, Pusic AL, Disa JJ. A classification system and reconstructive algorithm for acquired vaginal defects. Plast Reconstr Surg 110:1058-1065, 2002.)

- Fasciocutaneous medial thigh flaps
- Gracilis myocutaneous V-Y advancement flaps

ACQUIRED PENILE/SCROTAL DEFECTS[3,4]

PEYRONIE'S DISEASE
A disorder of the penis involving connective tissue that affects 1% of the male population 40-60 years old.

- **Characteristics**
  - Painful erections
  - Penile curvature during erection
  - Firm palpable nodule or inelastic plaque on penile shaft
  - 10% also have Dupuytren's contracture of palmar fascia
- **Reconstruction**
  - **Plication procedure**
    - Males with minimal penile curvature (30-45 degrees) and relatively long erect penis
    - Circumcising incision with degloving of penile shaft
    - Tunica albuginea opposite area of maximum curvature identified and ellipse excised from each corporal body
    - Tunica defects closed primarily
    - Slightly shortens penis
  - **Dermal graft procedure**
    - Curvature greater than 45 degrees
    - Circumcising incision with complete degloving of penile shaft

- ▸ Incisions made through Buck's fascia and mobilized off tunica albuginea
- ▸ Diseased tunica albuginea excised (plaque)
- ▸ Dermal graft used to cover corporal defects

OTHER PENILE/SCROTAL DEFECTS

- **Reconstruction**
  - **Goals**
    - ▸ One-stage operation, often microvascular technique
    - ▸ Reproducible with predictable results
    - ▸ Creation of competent neourethra that allows voiding while standing
    - ▸ Restore penis with tactile and erogenous sensibility
    - ▸ Bring enough bulk to permit insertion of prosthesis if necessary
    - ▸ Achieve aesthetic result
  - **Techniques** (most require penile implant)
    - ▸ Radial forearm flap (with or without radius)
    - ▸ Scapular flap
    - ▸ Groin flap
    - ▸ Gracilis flap
    - ▸ Free fibula osteocutaneous flap
    - ▸ Ulnar forearm flap
    - ▸ Lateral arm flap
    - ▸ Dorsalis pedis flap
    - ▸ Abdominal flaps (rectus abdominis myocutaneous or DIEP flaps)
    - ▸ Urethral reconstruction with split- and full-thickness grafts taken from inner thigh, abdomen, or scrotum, and grafts of saphenous vein, appendix, ileum, or bladder
- **Subtotal defects**
  - Reconstruction technique depends on defect and missing components
  - Reconstructive options include skin grafts and more complex repairs with free tissue transfer
- **Traumatic amputation**
  - Attempt microvascular replantation
  - Preservation: Rinse amputated part in saline, wrap in saline-soaked gauze, place in sterile bag, and place bag in ice slush
  - Reports of successful replantation after 16 hours cold ischemia

FOURNIER GANGRENE

Perineal tissue necrosis caused by polymicrobial infection is seen in patients with suppressed immune systems. Fournier gangrene is primarily seen in diabetics, renal transplant recipients, postchemotherapy or postradiation cancer patients, and patients who have undergone medical or surgical perineal manipulation.

- **Treatment**
  - Wide debridement to control infection
  - Broad-spectrum antibiotics
  - Local wound care
  - Testes in thigh pouches (temporary)
- **Reconstruction**
  - Meshed/unmeshed split-thickness skin graft
  - Thigh flaps

UROLOGIC DEFECTS

BLADDER EXSTROPHY

A congenital anomaly in which a portion of the lower abdominal wall and anterior bladder wall is absent, with eversion of the posterior bladder wall through the defect, an open pubic arch, and widely separated ischia connected by a fibrous band. Its cause is related to the failure of the cloaca membrane to allow ingrowth of the mesoderm, leading to its premature rupture. The severity depends on the developmental stage at which the rupture occurs.

- **Incidence**
  - 1:25,000 to 1:40,000 live births
  - 2:1 M/F ratio
- **Reconstruction**
  - Diversion of urinary stream
  - Closure of exstrophic bladder
  - Reconstruction of external genitalia

TRANSGENDER SURGERY

TRANSSEXUALISM

Characterized by a sense of discomfort and inappropriateness with one's anatomic sex; a desire to be rid of one's own genitals and live as a member of the opposite sex; a continuous disturbance for at least 2 years; and an absence of physical, psychological, intersex, or chromosomal abnormalities.

The Harry Benjamin International Gender Dysphoria Association has set standards of care and internationally accepted guidelines for treatment for transgender surgery.

- **Reconstruction**
  - **Goals**
    - ▶ Single stage
    - ▶ Aesthetically pleasing
    - ▶ Erogenous sensibility
    - ▶ Minimal morbidity
  - **Male to female**
    - ▶ Hormonal therapy and introduction into society as female for at least 2 years
    - ▶ Surgical interventions
      - ✦ Breast augmentation
      - ✦ Rhinoplasty
      - ✦ Male pattern hair removal
      - ✦ Reduction of thyroid cartilage
      - ✦ Feminizing genital surgeries (penectomy, penile inversion, skin grafts, and intestinal substitution)
  - **Female to male**
    - ▶ Hormonal therapy and introduction into society as male for at least 2 years
    - ▶ Surgical interventions
      - ✦ Breast amputation or reduction
      - ✦ Hysterectomy and oophorectomy
      - ✦ Phallus construction (pedicled flaps, free flaps, phalloplasty, and urethral lengthening)
      - ✦ Neoscrotum (perineal advancement flaps, labia majora flaps, and testicular prosthesis)

KEY POINTS

✔ Patients with Peyronie's disease may also have Dupuytren's contracture of hands.
✔ The mesonephric duct develops into the epididymis, vas deferens, and seminal vesicles.
✔ The paramesonephric ducts develop into the fallopian tubes, uterus, and upper portion of the vagina.
✔ The goals for epispadias repair include penile lengthening, correction of dorsal chordee, urethroplasty, and penile skin coverage.
✔ The goals for hypospadias repair include release of chordee, creation of new urethra, and advancement of urethral meatus to the tip of the penis.

REFERENCES

1. Kelton PL. Genitourinary repair and reconstruction. Sel Read Plast Surg 8(40), 1999.
2. Horton CE, Devine CJ. Hypospadias. In Converse JM, ed. Reconstructive Plastic Surgery, vol 7. Principles and Procedures in Correction Reconstruction and Transplantation, 2nd ed. Philadelphia: WB Saunders, pp 3845-3861, 1977.
3. Ninkovic M, Dabernig W. Flap technology for reconstructions of urogenital organs. Curr Opin Urol 13:483-488, 2003.
4. Sievert K. Vaginal and penile reconstruction. Curr Opin Urol 13:489-494, 2003.
5. Cordeiro PG, Pusic AL, Disa JJ. A classification system and reconstructive algorithm for acquired vaginal defects. Plast Reconstr Surg 110:1058-1065, 2002.

47. Pressure Sores

Jeffrey E. Janis

EPIDEMIOLOGY[1]

PREVALENCE[2-5]
- **General acute setting:** 10%-18% (average approximately 15%)
- **Long-term care facilities:** 2.3%-28% (average approximately 15%)
- **Home care setting:** 0%-29% (average approximately 15%)

INCIDENCE[6-9]
- **General acute setting:** 0.4%-38%
- **Long-term care facilities:** 2.2%-23.9%
- **Home care setting:** 0%-17%
- **Highest incidences**
  - Elderly patients with femoral neck fractures (66%)
  - Quadriplegic patients (60%)
  - Neurologically impaired young
  - Chronic hospitalization

MORTALITY[1]
- Combined data support the conclusion that pressure sores are not directly the cause of increased mortality, but rather these patients succumb to their overall disease burden, which leads to severe malnutrition, immobility, and decreased tissue perfusion that allow pressure sores to form.

COSTS[10,11]
- National Pressure Ulcer Advisory Panel has estimated a cost of **$30,000 per patient** to treat and heal ulcers acquired in hospitals.
- Total estimated costs for surgical and nonsurgical management are **$3.5-7 billion annually.**

SUSCEPTIBLE AREAS[1]
- **Bony prominences**
  - Ischial tuberosity (28%)
  - Trochanter (19%)
  - Sacrum (17%)
  - Heel (9%)
  - Scalp

ETIOLOGIC FACTORS[12]

EXTRINSIC FACTORS
- Environment exerts a mechanical force on soft tissues
  - **Shear:** Mechanical stress parallel to plane

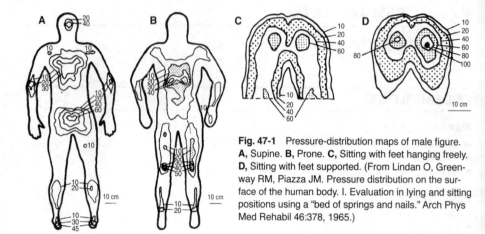

Fig. 47-1 Pressure-distribution maps of male figure. **A,** Supine. **B,** Prone. **C,** Sitting with feet hanging freely. **D,** Sitting with feet supported. (From Lindan O, Greenway RM, Piazza JM. Pressure distribution on the surface of the human body. I. Evaluation in lying and sitting positions using a "bed of springs and nails." Arch Phys Med Rehabil 46:378, 1965.)

- ▸ Causes superficial necrosis
- ▸ Stretches or compresses muscle perforators to the skin resulting in ischemic necrosis
- **Pressure:** Perpendicular force per unit area (Fig. 47-1)
  - ▸ Causes deep necrosis
  - ▸ Leads to tissue deformation, mechanical damage, blockage of vessels
- **Friction:** Resistance to movement between two surfaces
  - ▸ Outermost skin layer lost, resulting in increased water loss
  - ▸ Most often incurred during **patient transfers**
- **Moisture**
  - ▸ Leads to skin maceration and breakdown
  - ▸ Most often the result of **incontinence**

INTRINSIC FACTORS
- Native elements of the patient or wound that can cause soft tissue effects
  - **Ischemia/sepsis**
    - ▸ Causes decreased tissue perfusion and predisposes to necrosis
  - **Decreased autonomic control**
    - ▸ Can lead to excess perspiration, spasms, lack of bowel and bladder control
  - **Infection**
    - ▸ *Staphylococcus aureus, Streptococcus spp., Corynebacterium* (skin), *Proteus mirabilis, Escherichia coli, Pseudomonas aeruginosa,* or *Enterococcus spp.*
  - **Increased age**
    - ▸ Decreased skin moisture, tensile strength
    - ▸ Increased friability
  - **Sensory loss**
    - ▸ Unable to experience discomfort from prolonged sitting or other position, leading to tissue ischemia
  - **Small vessel occlusive disease**
    - ▸ Diabetes, peripheral vascular disease, and smoking decrease tissue perfusion and predispose to necrosis

- **Anemia**
  - ▸ Decreased wound healing capabilities
  - ▸ Weakness or fatigue that leads to prolonged immobilization
- **Malnutrition**
  - ▸ Diminished ability to heal wounds
  - ▸ Vitamin supplementation only effective if truly deficient
- **Altered level of consciousness**
  - ▸ Loss of protective reflexes or voluntary movements to offload pressure

RISK ASSESSMENT[13-15]

BRADEN SCALE
- Most commonly used
- **Subscales**
  - Sensory perception
  - Skin moisture
  - Activity
  - Mobility
  - Friction and shear
  - Nutritional status
- **Minimum** value of **6**
- **Maximum** value of **23**
- *Lower scores indicate increased risk for developing pressure ulcers*
- **Threshold scores for pressure sore development**
  - ▸ Tertiary care facilities: **16**
  - ▸ Veteran's hospitals: **19**
  - ▸ Skilled nursing care facilities: **18**

CLASSIFICATION[11]

- **Stage I:** Nonblanchable erythema of intact skin
  - Can be seen within 30 minutes
  - Usually resolves after 1 hour
- **Stage II:** Partial-thickness skin loss presenting clinically as a blister, abrasion, or shallow crater
  - 2-6 hours of pressure
  - Erythema lasts more than 36 hours
- **Stage III:** Full-thickness tissue loss down to, but not through, fascia
- **Stage IV:** Full-thickness tissue loss with involvement of underlying muscle, bone, tendon, ligament, or joint capsule

PREVENTION[16-19]

- Proper **skin care** to minimize moisture
- Care during **transfers**

- **Address spasticity**
  - Diazepam
  - Baclofen
  - Dantrolene sodium
- **Pressure dispersion**
  - Padding of pressure points (OR, ICU, hospital bed)
  - Pressure-relief behavior or alternate weight-bearing surfaces
    - ▸ **Kosiak's principle:** Tissue tolerates increased pressure if interspersed with pressure-free periods
      - ✦ Seated patients must lift up for 10 seconds every 10 minutes.
      - ✦ Supine patients must be turned every 2 hours.
- **Proper mattresses**
  - **Static pads**
    - ▸ At least **4 inches** of foam required to provide modest protection
  - **Alternating air cell mattresses**
    - ▸ Composed of air cells oriented perpendicularly to the patient
    - ▸ Available as overlays and as replacement mattresses
    - ▸ May facilitate dispersal of accumulated metabolites through the vascular and lymphatic channels
  - **Low-airloss mattresses**
    - ▸ Facilitate drying of the skin
    - ▸ Exert less than 25 mm Hg of pressure on any one point of the body
  - **Air-fluidized beds**
    - ▸ Patient floats on ceramic beads while warm regulated air is forced through, eliminating skin moisture
    - ▸ Maintains pressure less than 20 mm Hg (capillary arterial pressure)
- **Minimize head-of-bed elevation** to reduce sacral sheer and pressure (less than 45 degrees)
- Attention to **incontinence** (urinary and fecal)
- Proper **nutrition**
- **Optimization** of underlying comorbidities
  - Blood glucose control
  - Smoking cessation

TIP: Careful attention to preventive measures helps decrease incidence and recurrence of pressure sores. It is critical to take a multidisciplinary approach to treat the whole patient, with significant input from an experienced physical medicine and rehabilitation physician.

PATIENT EVALUATION

- **History and physical examination**
  - Determine etiologic factors for pressure sores.
  - See Chapter 1.
- **Laboratory studies and imaging**
  - Complete blood count
    - ▸ White blood cell count with differential
    - ▸ Hemoglobin/hematocrit
  - Glucose/HgbA$_1$C
  - Erythrocyte sedimentation rate/C-reactive protein

- Albumin/Prealbumin
- MRI[20]
  - ▶ Evaluates extent of osteomyelitis
    - ✦ **97% sensitive**
    - ✦ **89% specific**

TIP: All medical comorbidities should be documented and optimized before embarking on reconstruction.

If the extent of osteomyelitis is unknown or underappreciated, reconstruction is destined to fail.

MEDICAL MANAGEMENT[1,21]

- **Relieve pressure**
  - Positional changes
  - Proper mattress, cushion, or wheelchair
- Control **infection**
- Control **extrinsic factors** (shear, moisture, friction)
- **Debridement**
- **Dressings**
  - DuoDerm® (ConvaTec, Princeton, NJ)
  - Wet-to-dry saline dressing changes
  - Dakin's solution if *Pseudomonas* suspected

TIP: Dakin's solution (sodium hypochlorite and boric acid) is toxic to healthy tissue and should be used in dilute form (quarter strength) only for a limited period (e.g., 3 days).

- Silver sulfadiazine
- Other topicals (e.g., hydrogels, absorbant foams) (Fig. 47-2)
- Negative pressure wound therapy (VAC)

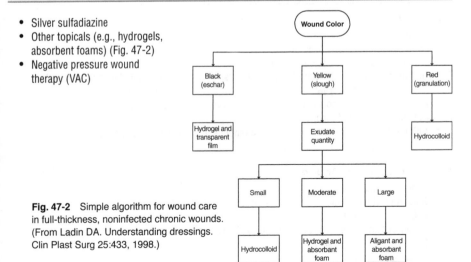

Fig. 47-2 Simple algorithm for wound care in full-thickness, noninfected chronic wounds. (From Ladin DA. Understanding dressings. Clin Plast Surg 25:433, 1998.)

SURGICAL GUIDELINES[22]

- **Stage I** and **II** pressure ulcers usually can be managed **nonsurgically.**
- **Stage III** and **IV** pressure ulcers frequently require **surgical intervention.**
  - Consider the patient's **ambulatory status** to help with proper flap selection.
  - **Design flaps as large as possible** with suture lines away from area of direct pressure.
  - **Do not violate adjacent flap territories** for possible future flap coverage.

RECONSTRUCTION GOALS
- Debridement of all devitalized tissue
- Complete excision of pseudobursa
- Ostectomy of all devitalized or infected bone to clinically hard, healthy, bleeding bone
- Excellent hemostasis
- Obliteration of dead space with well-vascularized tissue
- Selection and creation of flaps that do not jeopardize future flap coverage
- Tension-free closure
- Pressure offloading of reconstructed area

TIP: Infiltration of the peribursal area with wetting solution (1000 ml normal saline solution, plus 30 ml 1% plain lidocaine, plus one ampoule of 1:1000 concentration epinephrine) using a liposuction infiltration cannula can help decrease blood loss and help hydrodissect the bursal tissues from the surrounding tissues.[23]

Coating the bursa with methylene blue dye before excision can help verify that all bursal tissue has been completely excised.

RECONSTRUCTION BY ANATOMIC SITE

SACRAL ULCERS
- **Common options**
  - **Lumbosacral flap (fasciocutaneous)**
    - ▸ Requires backgrafting at donor site
  - **Unilateral or bilateral gluteal fasciocutaneous flap versus musculocutaneous rotation flap**
    - ▸ Can be segmental or full flap depending on patient's ambulatory status
    - ▸ Consider muscle flap if deep ulcer requires obliteration of dead space
    - ▸ Can be rerotated if recurrence
  - **Unilateral or bilateral gluteal musculocutaneous V-Y advancement flap**
    - ▸ Can be readvanced if recurrence

ISCHIAL PRESSURE SORES
- **Common options**
  - **Gluteal fasciocutaneous flap versus musculocutaneous rotation flap**
    - ▸ Can be segmental or full flap depending on patient's ambulatory status
  - **Posterior hamstring musculocutaneous V-Y advancement flap**
  - Posterior thigh flap (fasciocutaneous)
  - Tensor fascia lata flap

TROCHANTERIC PRESSURE SORES
■ **Common options**
  • **Tensor fascia lata**
  • Tensor fascia lata and vastus lateralis
  • **Girdlestone procedure** (proximal femurectomy and obliteration of dead space with vastus lateralis)

MULTIPLE PRESSURE SORES
■ **Common options**
  • Treat with single stage if possible
  • If significant bony involvement, may require hip disarticulation, hemipelvectomy, or hemicorporectomy
  • Total or subtotal thigh flaps

> TIP: Consider raising fasciocutaneous flaps with sharp scissors dissection rather than electrocautery to avoid thermal injury to the suprafascial vasculature.
>
> It is unnecessary to completely undermine all rotation flaps. Instead, check excursion constantly until a tension-free closure is possible. Any further undermining only jeopardizes blood supply.

POSTOPERATIVE MANAGEMENT[22,24,25]

■ Pressure relief bed for 3-6 weeks
■ Culture-directed antibiotics
■ Spasm control
■ Bowel regimen or ostomy care
■ Aggressive nutritional repletion
■ Active or passive range of motion of the uninvolved extremity
■ Seat mapping
■ Sitting protocol
■ Education

COMPLICATIONS

■ Hematoma
■ Infection
■ Wound dehiscence
■ Recurrence
  • **Relander and Palmer**[26]: Cutaneous flaps (43%), musculocutaneous flaps (33%) (follow-up 2-12 years)
  • **Disa et al**[27]: 69% recurrence rate at 1 year (mean 9.3 months)
    ▸ **Young posttraumatic paraplegic:** 79% recurrence rate at mean 10.9 months
    ▸ **Cerebrally compromised elderly:** 69% recurrence rate at mean 7.7 months
    ▸ *Reconstruction in these subgroups may not be warranted*

- **Evans et al**[28]: 82% recurrence rate at same location at mean 18.2 months for paraplegic patients
  - 64% developed new pressure sore at different site
  - Nonparaplegic: 0% recurrence rate
- **Kierney et al**[29]: Mean postoperative follow-up 3.7 years
  - **Overall** recurrence rate: 19%
  - **Fasciocutaneous** reconstruction recurrence rate: 15%
  - **Musculocutaneous** reconstruction recurrence rate: 13%
  - **Primary** pressure sore recurrence rate: 22%
  - **Secondary** pressure sore recurrence rate: 15%
- **Tavakoli et al**[30]: Mean follow-up 62 months for ischial pressure sores reconstructed with musculocutaneous flap coverage
  - **Overall** ulcer recurrence rate: 41.4%

KEY POINTS

✔ Proper and thorough evaluation of the patient with pressure sores is critical. Taking the patient to the OR is the last thing to do. Uncovering the etiologic factors and addressing them is the key to a successful outcome.

✔ A multidisciplinary team consisting of a physical medicine and rehabilitation physician, infectious disease specialist, nutritionist, physical therapist, psychiatrist, and plastic surgeon can help optimize outcomes.

✔ Vitamin supplementation is not helpful for patients who do not have a true deficiency.

✔ Elderly patients with hip fractures, quadriplegics, and chronically hospitalized patients are at the highest risk for developing pressure sores.

✔ Stage I and II pressure sores usually can be managed nonsurgically.

✔ Stage III and IV pressure sores frequently require flap surgery.

✔ Segmental muscle flaps or fasciocutaneous flaps should be used for ambulatory patients to decrease morbidity.

✔ Adhere to surgical principles when selecting flaps. Given the overall high rates of recurrence, favor rotation or advancement flaps that can be rerotated or readvanced.

✔ Be sure to seat-map the patient after reconstruction in case pressure dynamics have changed, especially after ostectomies.

✔ Prevention is key and education is critical.

REFERENCES

1. Janis JE, Kenkel JM. Pressure sores. Sel Read Plast Surg 9(39), 2003.
2. O'Brien SP, Wind S, Van Rijswijk L, et al. Sequential biannual prevalence studies of pressure ulcers at Allegheny–Hahnemann University Hospital. Ostomy Wound Manage 44(Suppl 3A):S78, 1998.
3. Langemo DK, Olson B, Hunter S, et al. Incidence and prediction of pressure ulcers in five patient care settings. Decubitus 4:25, 1991.
4. Baker J. Medicaid claims history of Florida long-term care facility residents hospitalized for pressure ulcers. J Wound Ostomy Continence Nurs 23:23, 1996.
5. Oot-Giromini BA. Pressure ulcer prevalence, incidence and associated risk factors in the community. Decubitus 6:24, 1993.

6. O'Sullivan KL, Engrav LH, Maier RV, et al. Pressure sores in the acute trauma patient: Incidence and causes. J Trauma 42:276, 1997.
7. Lyder CH, Yu C, Stevenson D, et al. Validating the Braden scale for the prediction of pressure ulcer risk in blacks and Latino/Hispanic elders: A pilot study. Ostomy Wound Manage 44(Suppl 3A):S42, 1998.
8. Berlowitz DR, Bezerra HQ, Brandeis GH, et al. Are we improving the quality of nursing home care: The case of pressure ulcers. J Am Geriatr Soc 48:59, 2000.
9. Bergstrom N, Braden B, Kemp M, et al. Predicting pressure ulcer risk: A multisite study of the predictive validity of the Braden scale. Nurs Res 47:261, 1998.
10. Granick MS, McGowan E, Wong CD. Outcome assessment of an in-hospital cross-functional wound care team. Plast Reconstr Surg 101:1243, 1998.
11. National Pressure Ulcer Advisory Panel (NPUAP). Pressure ulcers prevalence, cost and risk assessment: Consensus development conference statement. Decubitus 2:24, 1989.
12. Enis J, Sarmiento A. The pathophysiology and management of pressure sores. Orthop Rev 2:26, 1973.
13. Whitfield MD, Kaltenthaler EC, Akehurst RL, et al. How effective are prevention strategies in reducing the prevalence of pressure ulcers? J Wound Care 9:261, 2000.
14. Bergstrom N, Braden BJ, Laguzza A, et al. The Braden scale for predicting pressure sore risk. Nurs Res 36:205, 1987.
15. Braden NJ, Bergstrom N. Predictive validity of the Braden scale for pressure sore risk in a nursing home population. Res Nurs Health 17:459, 1994.
16. Reuler JB, Cooney TG. The pressure sore: Pathophysiology and principles of management. Ann Intern Med 94:661, 1981.
17. Krouskop TA. The role of mattress and beds in preventing pressure sores. In Lee BY, Ostrander LE, Cochran GVB, et al, eds. The Spinal Cord Injured Patient: Comprehensive Management. Philadelphia: Saunders, pp 244-250, 1991.
18. McLeod AG. Principles of alternating pressure surfaces. Adv Wound Care 10:30, 1997.
19. Goetz LL, Brown GS, Priebe MM. Interface pressure characteristics of alternating air cell mattresses in persons with spinal cord injury. J Spinal Cord Med 25:167, 2002.
20. Huang AB, Schweitzer ME, Hume E, et al. Osteomyelitis of the pelvis/hips in paralyzed patients: Accuracy and clinical utility of MRI. J Comput Assist Tomogr 22:437, 1998.
21. Wooten MK. Management of chronic wounds in the elderly. Clin Fam Med 3:1, 2001.
22. Conway H, Griffith BH. Plastic surgery for closure of decubitus ulcers in patients with paraplegia: Based on experience with 1000 cases. Am J Surg 91:946, 1956.
23. Han H, Fen J, Fine NA. Use of the tumescent technique in pressure ulcer closure. Plast Reconstr Surg 110:711, 2002.
24. Vasconez LD, Schneider WJ, Jurkiewicz MJ. Pressure sores. Curr Probl Surg 24:23, 1977.
25. Hentz VR. Management of pressure sores in a specialty center: A reappraisal. Plast Reconstr Surg 64:683, 1979.
26. Relander M, Palmer B. Recurrence of surgically treated pressure sores. Scand J Plast Reconstr Surg 22:89, 1988.
27. Disa JJ, Carlton JM, Goldberg NH. Efficacy of operative cure in pressure sore patients. Plast Reconstr Surg 89:272, 1992.
28. Evans GR, Dufresne CR, Manson PN. Surgical correction of pressure ulcers in an urban center: Is it efficacious? Adv Wound Care 7:40, 1994.
29. Kierney PC, Engrav LH, Isik FF, et al. Results of 268 pressure sores in 158 patients managed jointly by plastic surgery and rehabilitation medicine. Plast Reconstr Surg 102:765, 1998.
30. Tavakoli K, Rutkowski S, Cope C, et al. Recurrence rates of ischial sores in para- and tetraplegics treated with hamstring flaps: An 8-year study. Br J Plast Surg 52:476, 1999.

48. Lower Extremity Reconstruction

Jeffrey E. Janis

LOWER EXTREMITY WOUNDS

ETIOLOGIC FACTORS
- Trauma or open fractures
- Postsurgical dehiscence
- Compartment syndrome
- Tumor (e.g., sarcoma)
- Infection or osteomyelitis
- Radiation
- Vascular insufficiency
  - Arterial
  - Venous
- Diabetes

RECONSTRUCTION GOALS
- Debride devitalized tissue and obtain healthy wound bed
- Restore stability, structure, vascularity, and function
- Obliterate dead space
- Provide durable coverage of vital structures
- Aesthetic result

EVALUATION
- ABCs
- Assessment of size, depth, and exposure of vital structures
- Vascular examination (e.g., palpable pulses, Doppler examination)
- Neurologic examination
- Evaluation of radiographs

NOTE: See Chapter 1 for evaluation of complex wounds.

OPEN TIBIAL FRACTURES

CLASSIFICATION[1,2] (Tables 48-1 and 48-2; Fig. 48-1)
- The **severity of soft tissue damage** is the foremost predictor of the clinical course and likelihood of eventual healing.

Table 48-1 *Gustilo Classification of Open Fracture*

Type	Criteria
I	Open fracture with clean laceration <1 cm long
II	Open fracture with clean laceration >1 cm long without extensive soft tissue injury, flaps, or avulsions
III	Open fracture with extensive damage to soft tissue, including muscle, skin, and neurovascular structures
A	Adequate coverage available despite extensive damage
B	Extensive injury with periosteal stripping, bone exposure, and/or massive contamination
C	Open fracture with arterial injury requiring repair

From Gustilo RB, Anderson JT. Prevention of infection in the treatment of one thousand and twenty-five open fractures of long bones. J Bone Joint Surg Am 58:453, 1976; and from Gustilo RB, Mendoza RM, Williams DN. Problems in the management of type III (severe) open fractures: A new classification of type III open fractures. J Trauma 24:742, 1984.

Table 48-2 *Byrd Classification of Lower Extremity Trauma*

Type	Criteria
I	Low-energy forces causing a spiral or oblique fracture pattern with skin lacerations <2 cm and a relatively clean wound.
II	Moderate-energy forces causing a comminuted or displaced fracture pattern with skin laceration >2 cm and moderate adjacent skin and muscle contusion but *without* devitalized muscle.
III	High-energy forces causing a significantly displaced fracture pattern with severe comminution, segmental fracture, or bone defect with extensive associated skin loss and devitalized muscle.
IV	Fracture pattern as in type III but with extreme-energy forces as in high-velocity gunshot or shotgun wounds, a history of crush or degloving, or associated vascular injury requiring repair.

From Byrd HS, Spicer TE, Cierny G III. Management of open tibial fractures. Plast Reconstr Surg 76:719, 1985.

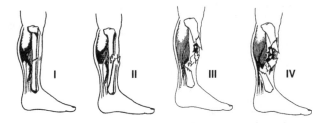

Fig. 48-1 Byrd classification of lower extremity trauma. (From Byrd HS, Spicer TE, Cierny G III. Management of open tibial fractures. Plast Reconstr Surg 76:719, 1985.)

PROGNOSTIC FACTORS
- **Keller**[3]
  - Reviewed 10,000 tibial shaft fractures and found risk of systemic complications increased with presence of the following:
    - Comminution
    - Displacement
    - Bone loss
    - Distraction
    - Soft tissue injury
    - Infection
    - Polytrauma

NOTE: Fracture location or configuration and concomitant fibular fracture have NO prognostic significance.

ORDER OF ACUTE TREATMENT
1. Stabilization of fracture (usually external fixator)
2. Restoration of inflow, if required
3. Four compartment fasciotomies, if required
4. Debridement and washout of wound
   - If vascular exposure, then immediate coverage
   - If no exposed vital structures, then repeat scheduled debridement

> TIP: The most important factor for the management of any open, lower extremity fracture is thorough debridement of devitalized tissue.

TIMING OF RECONSTRUCTION
- **Byrd et al**[4] (Table 48-3)
  - Advocated radical bone and soft tissue debridement with flap coverage in the **first 5-6 days** after injury for type III and IV fractures
    - Muscle flap coverage during acute phase: Fewest complications and shortest hospitalization

Table 48-3   *Biologic Phases of the Open-Fracture Wound*

Category	Clinical Features	Time Since Injury
Acute	Contaminated but not infected Hemorrhagic and edematous Presence of ischemic and devitalized soft tissue and bone Serosanguinous drainage	1-5 days
Subacute	Colonized and infected wound Seropurulent drainage Erythema, increased swelling, cellulitis Exudative wound surfaces late	1-6 weeks
Chronic	Infection limited to scar and sequestra in fracture Granulating, contracting wound Soft tissues stuck to healthy bone outside of fracture	More than 6 weeks

From Byrd HS, Spicer TE, Cierny G III. Management of open tibial fractures. Plast Reconstr Surg 76:719, 1985.

- Fractures not treated during the acute phase predictably entered a subacute, colonized, infected phase from **1 to 6 weeks** after injury
  - *Increased complication rate during subacute phase attributed to difficulty in establishing adequate borders for bony debridement*
- Chronic phase (more than 6 weeks after injury) characterized by granulating wound, adherent soft tissue, and local areas of infection
  - Limits of bony debridement become well demarcated during chronic phase
  - Can identify devitalized and infected bone when cortical surfaces have nonadherent soft tissue and medullary bone is pale and fibrotic
- Incidence of infection for **type III fracture:** 5%
- Incidence of infection for **type IV fracture:** 15%
- Time to full-weight-bearing status: **Average 6 months** for types III and IV
- **Yaremchuk et al[5]**
  - Reviewed patients with flap coverage at average of **17 days** after injury with infection rate at 14%
  - **Key difference:** *Complete removal of all bone fragments*
- **Godina[6]**
  - **Group I:** Free flap within 75 hours
    - Failure rate: 0.75%
    - Postoperative infection rate: **1.5%**
    - Time to union: 6-8 months
  - **Group II:** Flap between 3 days and 3 months
    - Failure rate: 12%
    - Postoperative infection rate: **17.5%**
    - Time to union: 12.3 months
  - **Group III:** Flap between 3 months and 12.6 years
    - Failure rate: 9.5%
    - Postoperative infection rate: **6%**
    - Time to union: 29 months

BONY RECONSTRUCTION

- Performed to promote bone healing
- **Essential elements** for osseous healing of opposed fracture fragments are **blood supply** and **stabilization**
  - **Blood supply[7,8]** (Fig. 48-2)
    - **Nutrient artery**
      - Enters groove on posterior tibia and extends as a nutrient channel within the cortex (vulnerable to injury); then enters the medulla, where it divides into network of vessels supplying the cortex from the endosteal surface
        - **Endosteal circulation:** Supplies inner two thirds of the cortex

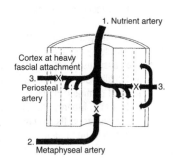

1. Nutrient artery

Cortex at heavy fascial attachment

3. Periosteal artery

2. Metaphyseal artery

Fig. 48-2 Blood supply to the tibia. (From Byrd HS, Cierny G, Tebbetts JB. The management of open tibial fractures with associated soft-tissue loss: External pin fixation with early flap coverage. Plast Reconstr Surg 68:73, 1981.)

- ▶ **Metaphyseal vessels**
- ▶ **Periosteal vessels**
  - ✦ Derive from the primary limb vessels and run down to the long axis of the bone
  - ✦ **Periosteal circulation:** Supplies outer third of the cortex

NOTE: When a long bone is fractured, the nutrient vessels are disrupted and the distal fragment is rendered avascular up to the point where the metaphyseal vessels enter the bone. However, because periosteal vessels run transversely, the blood supply to the periosteum is maintained.

- ■ Types of osseous callus
  - • **Medullary**
    - ▶ First noted on **day 4**
    - ▶ Blood supply solely from **medulla**
    - ▶ Stable, nondisplaced fractures heal with this type of callus, and time to union is the shortest
  - • **Periosteal**
    - ▶ Callus appears **day 3**
    - ▶ Provides ancillary external support to the fracture and always contains a zone of fibrocartilage
    - ▶ Blood supply initially from **surrounding soft tissues** and **periosteum**
    - ▶ Once endosteal circulation reconstituted, blood supply assumed by endosteal route

NOTE: The periosteal callus is extremely important in the union of displaced and comminuted fractures.

  - • **Intracortical**
    - ▶ Composed of woven bone
    - ▶ Blood supply is intraosseous, extraosseous, or both
    - ▶ May be absent if bone fragments are too closely apposed for blood vessels to grow between them (e.g., compression plate fixation)
    - ▶ Fewer progenitor cells in adults than in children (so limited in amount of repair capability)
      - ✦ The periosteum is believed to be the origin of these cells.
      - ✦ Studies suggest that overlying soft tissues are important for osseous healing, because they provide an immediate source of blood supply to the fracture.
- ■ Options for stabilizing opposed fractures
  - • Plaster immobilization enclosing open wound (Trueta technique)
  - • Internal fixation with plates, rods, and screws
  - • External fixation
- ■ Options for bone gap reconstruction
  - • **Nonvascularized bone grafting**
    - ▶ Some authors state that cancellous bone grafts can be used beneath vascularized muscle flaps for defects **up to 10 cm.**[9]
    - ▶ An intact fibula facilitates bone grafting of longer defects by acting as a strut to keep the extremity at length. (If the fibula is not intact, then other reconstruction methods may be necessary, particularly with defects larger than 8 cm.)
  - • **Free osseous or osteocutaneous flap transfer**
    - ▶ Usually necessary for patients with long bone gaps
    - ▶ **Most common:** Fibula, iliac crest, scapula
    - ▶ **Weiland, Moore, Daniel**[10]: Concluded that vascularized bone grafts are indicated for segmental defects **larger than 6 cm**
    - ▶ May take up to 15 months for stable union after vascularized bone grafts

- **Distraction osteogenesis (Ilizarov technique)**[11,12] (Fig. 48-3)
  - ▸ May be used for **bone gaps larger than 10 cm**
  - ▸ Involves radical debridement of the fractured bone ends and transection of the cortical bone outside the zone of injury, leaving the medullary bone and blood supply intact
  - ▸ Once corticotomy performed, insert Ilizarov pins near bone ends on either side of gap and apply distraction apparatus
  - ▸ Wait **7 days** before beginning distraction
  - ▸ Distract at **1 mm/day** until defect spanned
  - ▸ Frame usually kept on for **1 year**
  - ▸ **Advantages**
    - ◆ The amount of bone generated is anatomically correct for the size of the defect.
    - ◆ Soft tissue defects can be closed by the docking method during the same process.
    - ◆ Blood transfusions are usually not required.

NOTE: **Patient cooperation and compliance are key to success.**

  - ▸ **Contraindications**
    - ◆ **Defects larger than 12 cm**
    - ◆ Compromised or deficient residual bone stock that cannot support two or three serial corticotomies
  - ▸ **Complications**
    - ◆ Pin-tract infection
    - ◆ Stiffness of adjacent joints
    - ◆ Severe pain

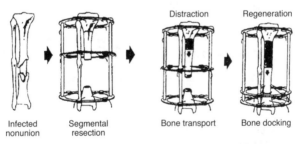

Infected nonunion   Segmental resection   Distraction / Bone transport   Regeneration / Bone docking

Fig. 48-3   The Ilizarov technique for bony reconstruction. (From Cierny G III, Zorn KE, Nahai F. Bony reconstruction in the lower extremity. Clin Plast Surg 19:905, 1992.)

OPEN JOINT INJURIES

- In acute injury, obtain preoperative and intraoperative cultures, and use broad spectrum antibiotic agents, early and copious irrigation, debridement of joint and injured soft tissues, and first-stage closure of wounds without drains.[13]
- The most common pathogens are *Pseudomonas* and *Klebsiella.*
- Soft tissue closure alone over chronically contaminated and open joints likely leads to **septic joint.**
- Studies of Trueta's closed plaster method have shown that joints allowed to remain open while patients ambulate eventually heal without the loss of the cartilaginous interface and without infection.[4]
- Second-stage muscle or soft tissue cover without water-seal closure can be performed.

SOFT TISSUE RECONSTRUCTION

GOALS
- Stable wound coverage
- Acceptable appearance
- Minimal donor site morbidity

PRINCIPLES
- Adequate and thorough wound debridement
  - May require multiple serial debridements
- Control of any wound colonization or infection
  - Base antibiotic coverage on wound cultures
- Flap donor tissues should be harvested outside zone of injury

LOCAL FLAPS
- **Thigh**
  - Extensive flap reconstruction not required because of large amounts of muscle tissue that can be advanced locally into wound and because of coverage with split thickness skin graft, if necessary
  - Tensor fascia lata, gracilis, rectus femoris, vastus lateralis, biceps muscle flaps
- **Leg**
  - **Upper third** (in order of preference)
    - ▶ **Medial head of gastrocnemius**
      - ✦ Single, proximal neurovascular pedicle
      - ✦ Broad belly (larger than lateral head)
      - ✦ No functional deficit

> TIP: Score the fascia of the gastrocnemius to obtain greater muscular coverage of larger surface area defects.

- ▶ **Lateral head of gastrocnemius**
  - ✦ Smaller
  - ✦ No functional deficit
- ▶ **Proximally based soleus**
  - ✦ Can be reliably carried to a point approximately 5 cm above its tendinous insertion
  - ✦ Responsible for the venous pump
  - ✦ "Slow" muscle used for posture stabilization and slow gait
  - ✦ No functional deficit
- ▶ **Bipedicled tibialis anterior** (Fig. 48-4)
  - ✦ Extremely important for dorsiflexion of foot and should not be entirely sacrificed
  - ✦ Muscle function preserved when raised as a bipedicled flap
  - ✦ Transfer requires detaching dense anterior tibial connections while retaining segmental blood supply from anterior tibial artery
  - ✦ Can use muscle-splitting approach and use tibialis anterior for coverage of middle third
    - No functional deficit ensues
- **Middle third**
  - ▶ **Common options:**
    - ✦ **Proximally based soleus**

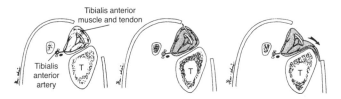

Fig. 48-4 Technique of longitudinal splitting of the tibialis anterior muscle. (From Hirshowitz B, Moscona R, Kaufman T, et al. External longitudinal splitting of the tibialis anterior muscle for coverage of compound fractures of the middle third of the tibia. Plast Reconstr Surg 79:407, 1987.)

- ✦ **Medial head of gastrocnemius**
- ✦ **Lateral head of gastrocnemius**
- ✦ **Flexor digitorum longus (FDL) for lower portion of middle third**
  - Can be transferred without significant functional loss
  - Used for small defects
  - Neurovascular pedicle usually enters at junction of proximal and middle third
- ✦ **Extensor digitorum longus (EDL)**
  - Supplied by anterior tibial artery
  - Used for closure of small wounds (<5 cm)
  - Incision made 2 cm lateral to tibia
  - Located lateral to tibial artery
  - Preserve superficial peroneal nerve
  - If entire muscle used, then there is permanent loss of toe extension
- ✦ **Extensor digitorum hallucis (EDH) for lower portion of middle third**
  - Very narrow, so can only be used for small defects or to augment other flaps
  - To prevent great toe drop, distal tendon should be attached to EDL when dividing the muscle for transfer
- ✦ **Flexor hallucis longus (FHL) for lower portion of middle third**
  - Primary function is providing push-off for the great toe, so consider patient's occupation before using (e.g., athlete)
- ✦ **Tibialis anterior**
- • **Lower third**
  - ▸ **Local flaps**
    - ✦ **Medial lower third:** Consider FHL, FDL, tibialis anterior, abductor hallucis, and extensor digitorum brevis muscle island flap
    - ✦ **Lateral lower third:** Peroneus brevis or tertius (very small; usually transferred with other flap) and lateral supramalleolar flap
  - ▸ **Distant flaps**
    - ✦ **Cross leg flap**[14]
      - Can use if free flap is not an option
      - Local flap necrosis in **40%**
      - Infection in **28%**
      - Transferred as fasciocutaneous tissue units with length/width ratio 3:1 or 4:1
      - Can base on the axial blood supply of the posterior descending subfascial cutaneous branch of the popliteal artery

- **Reverse turndown sural artery flap**[15,16]
  - Can be used for adults and children
  - Include the sural nerve and lesser saphenous vein in the flap
  - Avoid compression of the pedicle
  - Local flap necrosis in **21%**
- **Foot**
  - **Split thickness skin graft (STSG)**
    - ▶ Can use STSG even on calcaneus and first metatarsal head
      - ◆ Postoperative ink pad recordings have shown that patient's gait patterns change to enhance graft protection despite weight.[17]
  - Island instep fasciocutaneous or musculocutaneous flap that preserves sensation
  - Toe fillet
  - Plantar digital web space island flap (for distal sole)

FREE TISSUE TRANSFER

- Particularly useful for **distal third** defects (the gold standard)
- **Use free flap when defect has the following characteristics:**
  - Large
  - Sacrifice of local tissue not desirable
  - Dead space after bony irrigation and debridement
  - Local tissues or vessels damaged
  - Local flaps have failed
- **Usual flaps**
  - Latissimus dorsi
  - Rectus abdominis
  - Serratus anterior
  - Gracilis
  - Scapular or parascapular
  - Anterolateral thigh perforator flap
- Perform anastomosis outside of and proximal to the zone of injury
- Can perform end-to-end or end-to-side anastomoses
- Can use vein grafts if necessary

> TIP: Give strong consideration to performing end-to-side anastomoses to preserve blood flow to the distal lower extremity, especially when there is less than three-vessel runoff.

NOTE: Integra (bilaminate neodermis) (Integra NeuroSciences, Plainsboro, NJ) can be used for any area of the lower extremity when there is a clean, vascular wound bed.

TISSUE EXPANSION IN THE LOWER EXTREMITY[18]

- Primary application for lower extremity is to resurface areas of unstable soft tissue or unsightly scar
- Better results in the thigh and buttocks

- High complication rates if placed below the knee
  - **Infection rates:** 5%-30%

TIP: One of most common causes of implant exposure is an inadequately dissected pocket.

AMPUTATION

- Consider amputation if two or more of the following factors are present:
  - Three or more fascial compartments involved
  - Two or more injured tibial vessels
  - Failed vascular reconstruction
  - Cadaveric foot at initial examination
  - Severe muscle crush injury or muscle tissue loss

COMPARTMENT SYNDROMES

See Chapter 65 for more detail.
- **Incidence** of compartment syndrome with tibial shaft fracture is **9.1%.**
- *An open tibial fracture does not allow adequate compartmental decompression* (fasciotomies may still be required).

SIGNS AND SYMPTOMS
- Pain disproportionate to injury
- Palpably swollen compartments
- Pain during passive stretching of involved muscles
- Diminished simple touch perception
  - Loss of sensation over the saphenous nerve distribution should not be expected, because this nerve lies outside the compartments of the lower leg.
- Decreased strength of involved compartment muscles
- Hyperesthesia or anaesthesia in the involved compartment

NOTE: Distal pulses may or may not be palpable.

SIGNS OF DEVELOPING COMPARTMENT SYNDROME

> **Anterior compartment:** Pain during passive plantar flexion, especially of the big toe, and foot eversion
> **Lateral compartment:** Pain during passive dorsiflexion and foot inversion
> **Superficial posterior compartment:** Pain during passive dorsiflexion with knee extended and ankle flexed
> **Deep posterior compartment:** Pain during passive ankle dorsiflexion, foot eversion, and toe extension (especially the big toe)

Modified from Hyde GC, Peck O, Powell DC. Compartment syndromes. Early diagnosis and a bedside operation. Am Surg 49:563, 1983.

OSTEOMYELITIS

CAUSES[19]
- Retained necrotic and infected bone
- Avascular or infected scar
- Dead space at the surgical site
- Inadequate skin cover
- Most common pathogen is *Staphylococcus aureus*

INCIDENCE[20]
- Type III and IV open tibial fractures
  - **24%** infection rate without antibiotics
  - **4%** infection rate with prophylactic cephalosporin and aminoglycoside for 3 days

TREATMENT
- Aggressive debridement of all necrotic and infected bone and poorly vascularized and scarred soft tissues
- Dead space obliteration
- Stable, vascularized soft tissue coverage

CHRONIC WOUNDS OF THE LOWER EXTREMITY[21]

ETIOLOGIC FACTORS
- Diabetic wounds
- Vascular insufficiency
- Venous stasis disease
- Lymphedema
- Osteomyelitis
- Cancer
- Radiation
- Vasculitis

PATIENT EVALUATION
- History
  - Comorbidities
    - Diabetes
    - Claudication
    - Rest pain
  - Onset, location, and drainage
  - Ambulatory status
  - Shoewear
  - Prior trauma
  - Prior ulcer
  - Prior treatment

PHYSICAL EXAMINATION

- Size and depth
- Location
- Atrophic skin changes (hair or skin texture)
- Pulse examination
- Sensation
- Skin temperature
- Hemosiderin deposition
- Edema
- Ankle/brachial index

LABORATORY STUDIES

- Glucose or hemoglobin A_1C
- Radiographs (for osteomyelitis, calcification of vessels, etc.)
- Culture and sensitivities
- Biopsy

DIAGNOSIS AND TREATMENT FOR ULCER TYPES

- **General goals of treatment**
  - Complete healing of ulcer
  - Return to ambulatory status
  - Prevention of recurrence
- **Diabetic ulcers**
  - History of peripheral neuropathy
    - ▸ Greater than 40% incidence after 20 years of diabetes
  - Examination reveals decreased sensation
    - ▸ Protective sensation lost if patient cannot feel 5.07 Semmes-Weinstein filament (i.e., cannot appreciate 10 grams of pressure)
- **Vascular insufficiency (arterial ulcers)**
  - History of claudication and/or rest pain
  - Abnormal pulses
  - Cool extremity with cyanosis and/or rubor and shiny hairless skin
  - Appear "punched out" and are painful
  - Check with transcutaneous O_2, duplex, MRA, or arteriogram
  - **Requires revascularization** by vascular surgeon
- **Venous stasis disease (venous ulcers)**
  - Chronic edema
  - Varicosities
  - Lipodermatosclerosis
  - History of deep venous thrombosis
  - Generally located in the "gaiter region," between the malleoli and gastrocnemius musculotendinous junction ("bootstrap distribution")
  - Treat with **compression**
  - Can also attempt varicose vein stripping

- **Lymphedema**
  - Chronic edema with massively swollen leg and decreased skin blood flow
  - May have concomitant arterial disease
  - Treat with lymph-press pumps and leg wrapping techniques
  - Can surgically excise to fascia and skin graft (Charles procedure)
- **Osteomyelitis**
  - History of prior trauma
  - History of hardware placement
  - Chronic draining sinus tract that fails to close despite appropriate local wound care
  - MRI
  - Culture
  - Aggressive debridement of infected bone
  - Culture-directed antibiotics
  - Appropriate reconstruction (usually muscle-based flap)
- **Cancer**
  - Unusual ulcer appearance
  - History of coexisting malignancy
  - Biopsy
    - **Marjolin's ulcer:** Malignant SCC from transformation of chronic wounds (years)
  - Resection or amputation with margins
  - Reconstruction
- **Radiation**
  - History of prior radiation
  - Damaged vascularity to the affected area
  - Can pretreat with hyperbaric oxygen to stimulate angiogenesis at wound periphery
  - Requires resection of irradiated tissue and free flap reconstruction
    - Local flaps are frequently ineffective because they are within the zone of radiation injury
- **Vasculitis**
  - History of systemic inflammatory disease
    - Rheumatoid arthritis
    - Lupus
    - Scleroderma
  - Disproportionate pain
  - Confirmation by histopathology
  - Treatment by calcium channel blockers, steroids, and antineoplastic drugs
  - Should be overseen by a rheumatologist

KEY POINTS

✔ Debridement of all devitalized tissue (soft tissue and bone) is the key to a successful outcome in posttraumatic situations.

✔ Obtain stable soft tissue coverage early to help decrease the incidence of complications.

✔ VAC may help decrease edema, decrease bacterial counts, and stimulate blood flow to wounds before definitive coverage.

✔ The medial head of the gastrocnemius is the workhorse for proximal third lower extremity reconstruction.

✔ The soleus is the workhorse for middle third lower extremity reconstruction.

✔ Free tissue transfer is the workhorse for distal third lower extremity reconstruction.

✔ Integra can be used in any location as long as there is a clean, healthy wound bed (even if there is exposed bone).

✔ Tissue expansion historically has not been reliably successful below the knee.

✔ Watch out for compartment syndrome with lower extremity trauma.

✔ Amputation is an option in select cases and can result in a functional outcome for the patient.

✔ Know the characteristics of the various chronic wounds of the lower extremity so that the proper diagnosis can be made and appropriate treatment selected.

REFERENCES

1. Gustilo RB, Anderson JT. Prevention of infection in the treatment of one thousand and twenty-five open fractures of long bones. J Bone Joint Surg Am 58:453, 1976.

2. Gustilo RB, Mendoza RM, Williams DN. Problems in the management of type III (severe) open fractures: A new classification of type III open fractures. J Trauma 24:742, 1984.

3. Keller CS. The principles of the treatment of tibial shaft fractures. Orthopaedics 6:993, 1983.

4. Byrd HS, Spicer TE, Cierny G III. Management of open tibial fractures. Plast Reconstr Surg 76:719, 1985.

5. Yaremchuk MJ, Brumback RJ, Manson PN, et al. Acute and definitive management of traumatic osteocutaneous defects of the lower extremity. Plast Reconstr Surg 80:1, 1987.

6. Godina M. Early microsurgical reconstruction of complex trauma of the extremities. Clin Plast Surg 13:619, 1986.

7. Rhinelander FW. Tibial blood supply in relation to fracture healing. Clin Orthop Relat Res 105:34, 1974.

8. Macnab I, De Haas WG. The role of periosteal blood supply in the healing of fractures of the tibia. Clin Orthop Relat Res 105:27, 1974.

9. Christian EP, Bosse MJ, Robb G. Reconstruction of large diaphyseal defects without free fibular transfer in Grade IIIb tibial fractures. J Bone Joint Surg Am 71:994, 1989.

10. Weiland AJ, Moore JR, Daniel RK. Vascularized bone autografts: Experience with 41 cases. Clin Orthop Relat Res 174:87, 1983.

11. Ilizarov GA, Devyatov AA, Kamerin VK. Plastic reconstruction of longitudinal bone defects by means of compression and subsequent distraction. Acta Chir Plast 22:32, 1980.

12. Cierny G III, Zorn KE, Nahai F. Bony reconstruction in the lower extremity. Clin Plast Surg 19:905, 1992.

13. Patzakis MJ, Dorr LD, Ivler D, et al. The early management of open joint injuries: A prospective study of one hundred and forty patients. J Bone Joint Surg Am 57:1065, 1975.

14. Dawson RLG. Complications of cross-leg flap operation. Proc R Soc Med 65:2, 1972.
15. Almeida MF, da Costa PR, Okawa RY. Reverse-flow island sural flap. Plast Reconstr Surg 109:583, 2002.
16. Suga H, Oshima Y, Harii K, et al. Distally-based sural flap for reconstruction of the lower leg and foot. Scand J Plast Reconstr Surg 38:16, 2004.
17. Woltering EA, Thorpe WP, Reed JK Jr, et al. Split thickness skin grafting of the plantar surface of the foot after wide excision of neoplasms of the skin. Surg Gynecol Obstet 149:229, 1979.
18. Manders EK, Oaks TE, Au VK, et al. Soft tissue expansion in the lower extremities. Plast Reconstr Surg 81:208, 1988.
19. Ger R, Efron G. New operative approach in the treatment of chronic osteomyelitis of the tibial diaphysis. A preliminary report. Clin Orthop Relat Res 70:165, 1970.
20. Patzakis MJ, Wilkins J, Moore TM. Use of antibiotics in open tibial fractures. Clin Orthop Relat Res 178:31, 1983.
21. Smith APS. Etiology of the problem wound. In Sheffield PJ, Smith APS, Fife CE, eds. Wound Care Practice. Flagstaff, AZ: Best Publishing Company, 2004, pp 3-49.

PART VI

Hand, Wrist, and Upper Extremity

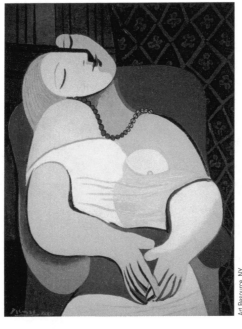

49. Hand Anatomy and Biomechanics

David S. Chang

ABBREVIATIONS

DIGITS
- **IF:** Index finger
- **MF:** Middle finger
- **RF:** Ring finger
- **LF** or **SF:** Little finger or small finger

JOINTS
- **IPJ:** Interphalangeal joint
- **DIPJ:** Distal interphalangeal joint
- **PIPJ:** Proximal interphalangeal joint
- **MPJ:** Metacarpophalangeal joint
- **CMCJ:** Carpometacarpal joint
- **DRUJ:** Distal radioulnar joint

MUSCLES
- **FCR/FCU:** Flexor carpi radialis/flexor carpi ulnaris
- **FPL/FPB:** Flexor pollicis longus/flexor pollicis brevis
- **FDS:** Flexor digitorum superficialis
- **FDP:** Flexor digitorum profundus
- **ECRL/ECRB:** Extensor carpi radialis longus/extensor carpi radialis brevis
- **ECU:** Extensor carpi ulnaris
- **EDC:** Extensor digitorum communis
- **EIP:** Extensor indicis proprius
- **EDM** or **EDQ:** Extensor digiti minimi or extensor digiti quinti
- **EPL/EPB:** Extensor pollicis longus/extensor pollicis brevis
- **PL:** Palmaris longus
- **PT:** Pronator teres
- **PQ:** Pronator quadratus
- **AdP:** Adductor pollicis
- **APL/APB:** Abductor pollicis longus/abductor pollicis brevis

TERMINOLOGY

FOREARM AND HAND
- *Radial* and *ulnar, dorsal* and *volar* (or *palmar*) used more commonly than medial/lateral, anterior/posterior.

475

DIGITS

- Thumb
- Index finger
- Long or middle finger
- Ring finger
- Small or little finger

PALM

- Thenar eminence
- Hypothenar eminence
- Midpalm: Area between thenar and hypothenar eminences

HAND MOTION

- **Thumb**
  - **Abduction:** Movement out of plane of palm (i.e., palmar abduction) or in plane of hand (i.e., planar or radial abduction)
- **Fingers** (reference point is sagittal line through third ray)
  - **Abduction:** Movement is **away** from the long finger
  - **Adduction:** Movement is **toward** the long finger

ANATOMY OF THE HAND[1-6]

SKIN

- **Palmar** skin is **thicker, less mobile,** and has **papillary ridges** for grasping.
- Fingertips have specialized nerve endings (e.g., **Meissner's corpuscles**) for sensory perception.

RETINACULAR SYSTEM

- **Palmar fascia**
  - Anchors palmar skin to bone for grasping, in contrast to loose skin on dorsum
  - **Midpalmar fascia:** Triangular-shaped fascia attached proximally to PL tendon or transverse carpal ligament; composed of longitudinal fibers, vertical fibers, transverse fibers, and natatory ligaments
- **Retaining ligaments of fingers** (Fig. 49-1)
  - Stabilize skin and extensor mechanism of digits and support neurovascular bundles
    - ▶ **Grayson's ligament:** Passes transversely from palmar aspect of flexor tendon sheath to skin
      - ✦ Prevents bowstringing of neurovascular bundle during finger flexion

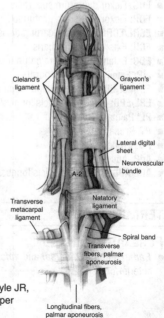

Cleland's ligament
Grayson's ligament
Lateral digital sheet
Neurovascular bundle
A-2
Natatory ligament
Transverse metacarpal ligament
Spiral band
Transverse fibers, palmar aponeurosis
Longitudinal fibers, palmar aponeurosis

Fig. 49-1   Distal palmar and digital fascia. (From Doyle JR, Botte MJ, eds. Surgical Anatomy of the Hand and Upper Extremity. Philadelphia: Lippincott, 2003, p 597.)

- ▶ **Cleland's ligament** (dorsal digital septum): Passes from juncture of periosteum and flexor tendon sheath to skin laterally
  - ◆ Lies dorsal to neurovascular bundle
- ▶ **Transverse retinacular ligament:** Lateral side of PIPJ, superficial to collateral ligament
  - ◆ Prevents dorsomedial displacement of lateral bands
- ▶ **Oblique retinacular ligament:** Part of extensor apparatus inserting on base of distal phalanx
  - ◆ Helps prevent hyperextension at PIPJ during extension

DEEP FASCIAL SPACES

- ■ **Potential spaces,** can be sites of infection
- • **Midpalmar space**
  - ▶ **Boundaries**
    - ◆ **Dorsal:** Palmar interossei
    - ◆ **Volar:** Palmar aponeurosis and flexor tendons of ring, long, and small fingers
    - ◆ **Ulnar:** Hypothenar septum
    - ◆ **Radial:** Midpalmar oblique septum
- • **Thenar space**
  - ▶ **Boundaries**
    - ◆ **Dorsal:** AdP
    - ◆ **Volar:** Index flexor tendon
    - ◆ **Ulnar:** Oblique septum
    - ◆ **Radial:** Adductor insertion and thenar muscle fascia
- • **Hypothenar space**
  - ▶ **Boundaries**
    - ◆ **Dorsal:** Hypothenar muscles
    - ◆ **Volar:** Small finger flexor tendon
    - ◆ **Ulnar:** Hypothenar muscles
    - ◆ **Radial:** Hypothenar septum
- • **Interdigital web space**
  - ▶ Location of *collar button abscess*
  - ▶ **Boundaries**
    - ◆ **Dorsal:** Dorsal fascia and skin
    - ◆ **Volar:** Palmar fascia extensor mechanism and metacarpophalangeal joint (MPJ) capsule
    - ◆ **Ulnar:** Extensor mechanism and MPJ capsule
    - ◆ **Radial:** Extensor mechanism and MPJ capsule
- • **Parona's space**
  - ▶ Infections can spread to this space from radial or ulnar bursa
  - ▶ **Boundaries**
    - ◆ **Dorsal:** Pronator quadrators
    - ◆ **Volar:** Digital flexors
    - ◆ **Ulnar:** FCU
    - ◆ **Radial:** Radial bursa

MUSCLES AND TENDONS OF FOREARM, WRIST, AND HAND (Fig. 49-2)

Fig. 49-2 Cross section of the wrist illustrating basic anatomic relations of major structures. Note the configuration of the flexor tendons (flexor digitorum superficialis *[FDS]* and flexor digitorum profundus *[FDP]* groups). *APL,* Abductor pollicis longus; *BR,* brachioradialis; *ECRB,* extensor carpi radialis brevis; *ECRL,* extensor carpi radialis longus; *ECU,* extnesor carpi ulnaris; *EDC,* extensor digitorum communis; *EDM,* extensor digiti minimi; *EIP,* extensor indicis proprius; *EPB,* extensor pollicis brevis; *EPL,* extensor pollicis longus; *FCR,* flexor carpi radialis; *FCU,* flexor carpi ulnaris; *FPL,* flexor pollicis longus; *PL,* palmaris longus; *PQ,* pronator quadratus. (From Beasley RW, ed. Beasley's Surgery of the Hand. New York: Thieme, 2003.)

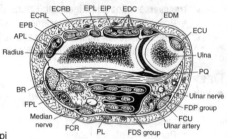

EXTRINSIC MUSCLES
- **Extensors**
  - Finger extensors extrinsic, *except interossei* and *lumbricals,* which aid in interphalangeal extension
  - All extensors innervated by **radial nerves**
  - **Extensor zones of hand** (Fig. 49-3)
    - ▸ **Nine zones:** Odd numbers are over joints starting with zone I over DIPJ, even numbers between joints
    - ▸ **Thumb** has only **two zones**

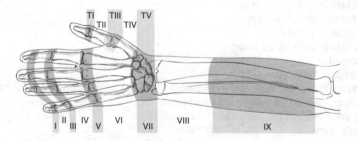

Fig. 49-3 Extensor zones of the hand and forearm. Note that the thumb has only two zones.

- **Dorsal wrist compartments** (Table 49-1)
  - ▸ Synovial-lined tunnels at wrist through which extensor tendons pass, covered by extensor retinaculum
- **Forearm muscles**
  - ▸ Common origin from mobile wad at lateral epicondyle of humerus
  - ▸ **Superficial layer:** EDC, EDM, and ECU
  - ▸ **Deep:** APL, EPB, EPL, and EIP
  - ▸ **Lateral:** Brachioradialis, ECRL, and ECRB

Table 49-1   *Muscles of the Dorsal Wrist Compartments*

Compartment	Muscle	Insertion	Action
First	APL	Base of first metacarpal	Extensor of first metacarpal and aids in abduction of thumb
	EPB	Base of proximal phalanx of thumb	Combines with EPL to extend thumb IPJ
Second	ECRL	Base of second metacarpal	Primarily radial deviation of wrist and secondarily wrist extension
	ECRB	Base of third metacarpal	Prime wrist extensor
Third	EPL	Passes around Lister's tubercle of radius and inserts on distal phalanx of thumb	Extends thumb IPJ
Fourth	EDC	No direct bony attachment to proximal phalanx (see Extensor mechanism below)	Extends MPJs and, with intrinsic muscles, extends IPJs; EDC to small finger absent in 50% of population
	EIP	Tendon lies ulnar to EDC tendon; functionally independent	Extends index finger while others are flexed
Fifth	EDM	Tendon lies ulnar to EDC tendon	Prime extensor of fifth MPJ, allows independent small finger extension Also abducts small finger
Sixth	ECU	Inserts on base of fifth metacarpal	Primarily ulnar deviation of wrist, secondarily wrist extension

APL, Abductor pollicis longus; *ECRB,* extensor carpi radialis brevis; *ECRL,* extensor carpi radialis longus; *ECU,* extensor carpi ulnaris; *EDC,* extensor digitorum communis; *EDM,* extensor digiti minimi; *EIP,* extensor indicis proprius; *EPB,* extensor pollicis brevis; *EPL,* extensor pollicis longus; *IPJ,* interphalangeal joint; *MPJ,* metacarpophalangeal joint.

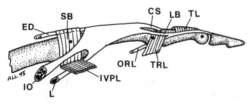

Fig. 49-4   Extensor mechanism. *CS,* central slip; *ED,* extensor digitorum; *IO,* interosseus; *IVPL,* intervolar plate ligament (deep transverse metacarpal ligament); *L,* lumbrical; *LB,* lateral band; *ORL,* oblique retinacular ligament of Landsmeer; *SB,* sagittal band; *TL,* triangular ligament; *TRL,* transverse retinacular ligament. (From Lluch AL. Repair of the extensor tendon system. In Aston SJ, Beasley RW, Thorne CH, eds. Grabb and Smith's Plastic Surgery, 5th ed. Philadelphia: Lippincott, 1997, p 885.)

- **Juncturae tendinum**
  - ▶ Interconnections of fascia between EDC tendons on dorsum of hand
  - ▶ Prevents independent action of extensors on single digit
  - ▶ Can also transmit MPJ extension to a finger even if its tendon is cut
- **Extensor mechanism** (Fig. 49-4)
  - ▶ EDC tendons insert onto extensor aponeurosis over the MPJ, then continue as central and two lateral slips.

> ▸ The central slip inserts on the base of middle phalanx and, with interossei, causes PIPJ extension.
> ▸ The lateral slips join interossei and lumbricals to become conjoined lateral bands and insert on the base of distal phalanx, causing DIPJ extension.
> ▸ Sagittal bands arise from the volmar plate and help stabilize the extensor tendon over the MPJ.

- **Flexors**
  - Consist of three wrist flexors and muscles that allow thumb and finger flexion at IPJ
  - **Forearm muscles**
    - ▸ **Superficial** (Table 49-2)
      - ✦ Originate from medial epicondyle of humerus
    - ▸ **Intermediate** (Table 49-3)
      - ✦ Originate from three separate heads: Humeral, ulnar, and radial
    - ▸ **Deep** (Table 49-4)
      - ✦ Origin from ulna
      - ✦ Tendons for long, ring, and small fingers share origin
      - ✦ Lumbricals originate from radial side of FDP tendon in palm

Table 49-2 *Superficial Muscles of Forearm*

Muscle	Insertion	Action	Innervation
Pronator teres (PT)	Midlateral radius	Pronates forearm, wrist, hand	Median nerve
Flexor carpi radialis (FCR)	Base of third metacarpal	Prime wrist flexor	Median nerve
Palmaris longus (PL)	Attaches to palmar aponeurosis	Ancillary wrist flexor Absent in 10%-15% Expendable as tendon graft	Median nerve
Flexor carpi ulnaris (FCU)	Pisiform and base of fifth metacarpal, and variably on fourth metacarpal and hook of hamate	Primarily ulnar deviator of wrist	Ulnar nerve

Table 49-3 *Intermediate Muscles of Forearm*

Muscle	Insertion	Action	Innervation
Flexor digitorum superficialis (FDS)	Four tendons to index, long, ring, and small fingers Splits into radial and ulnar bands and passes dorsal to FDP tendon in finger and inserts on middle phalanx	Flexes proximal interphalangeal joint (PIPJ)	Median nerve

Table 49-4 *Deep Muscles of Forearm*

Muscle	Insertion	Action	Innervation
Flexor digitorum profundus (FDP)	Distal phalanx after passing through Camper's chiasm (decussation of FDS)	Flexes distal interphalangeal joints (DIPJs), fingers	Median nerve (radial half) Ulnar nerve (ulnar half)
Flexor pollicis longus (FPL)	Distal phalanx of thumb	Flexes DIPJs, thumb	Median nerve

INTRINSIC MUSCLES
- Located completely within the hand
- Allow fine movements
- **Thenar**
  - **Divisions** (divided by FPL tendon)
    - ▶ **Radial group** (Table 49-5)
      - ◆ Positions thumb pad toward tips of index and long fingers for precision pinch
      - ◆ **Median** innervated (recurrent motor branch)
      - ◆ Overlapping ulnar innervation in 35%-40% of patients
    - ▶ **Ulnar group** (Table 49-6)
      - ◆ **Median** innervated

Table 49-5   *Radial Group Thenar Muscles*

Muscle	Origin	Insertion	Action
Abductor pollicis brevis (APB)	Flexor retinaculum and tubercles of scaphoid and trapezium	Lateral side of base of proximal phalanx of thumb	Palmar abduction, slight metacarpophalangeal (MP) flexion and interphalangeal (IP) extension
Opponens pollicis	Flexor retinaculum and tubercle of trapezium	Lateral side of first metacarpal bone	Rotates thumb pinch with index finger
Flexor pollicis brevis (FPB) superficial portion	Flexor retinaculum and tubercle of trapezium	Medial side of base of proximal phalanx of thumb	Flexes and stabilizes MPJ

Table 49-6   *Ulnar Group Thenar Muscles*

Muscle	Origin	Insertion	Action
Adductor pollicis (AdP)	Oblique head: Bases of second and third metacarpals, capitate and adjacent carpal bones Transverse head: Anterior surface of body of third metacarpal bone	Lateral side of base of proximal phalanx of thumb	Adducts thumb and flexes metacarpophalangeal (MPJ)
Flexor pollicis brevis (FPB) (deep portion)	Flexor retinaculum and tubercle of trapezium	Medial side of base of proximal phalanx of thumb flexes MP joint	Flexes MPJ

- **Hypothenar** (Table 49-7)
  - Clustered around fifth metacarpal
  - **Ulnar** innervated
- **Interossei** (Table 49-8)
  - Pass volar to MPJ and dorsal to PIPJ
  - Flexes MPJ and extends PIPJ
  - Ulnar innervated

Table 49-7   *Hypothenar Muscles*

Muscle	Origin	Insertion	Action
Opponens digiti minimi	Hook of hamate and flexor retinaculum	Medial border of fifth metacarpal	Rolls fifth metacarpal toward thumb Flexes fourth and fifth metacarpal joints for better thumb opposition
Flexor digiti minimi	Hook of hamate and flexor retinaculum	Medial side of base of proximal phalanx of small finger	Flexes metacarpophalangeal joint (MPJ)
Abductor digiti minimi	Pisiform bone	Medial side of base of proximal phalanx of small finger	Abducts small finger Flexes fifth MPJ Extends interphalangeal joints (IPJs) when MPJ is stabilized
Palmaris brevis	Flexor retinaculum and palmar aponeurosis	Skin on medial side of palm	Pulls skin to help cup palm Rudimentary muscle Occasionally absent

Table 49-8   *Interosseous Muscles*

Muscle	Origin	Insertion	Action
Palmar interossei (3)	Palmar surfaces of third, fourth, and fifth metacarpals	Distal fibers of the metacarpophalangeal joint (MPJ) capsule	Adduct the index, ring, and small fingers
Dorsal interossei (4)	Adjacent sides of two metacarpals	Distal fibers of the MPJ capsule	Abduct the index, long, ring, and small fingers

TIP: Think PAD (*P*almar interossei *AD*duct) and DAB (*D*orsal interossei *AB*duct)

- **Lumbricals**
  - Flexes MPJ and extends PIPJ
  - **Radial** two lumbricals **median** innervated
  - **Ulnar** two lumbricals **ulnar** innervated
  - Four muscles on radial sides of index fingers through small fingers
  - **Origin:** FDP tendons
  - **Insertion:** Extensor apparatus at proximal phalanx

TENDONS
- **Wrist** (see Fig. 49-2)
  - Carpal tunnel contains **median nerve** and **nine tendons** (4 FDS, 4 FDP, 1 FPL)
  - Long and ring finger FDS tendons superficial to index and small finger FDS tendons
  - FDP tendons are deep to FDS tendons

TIP: Think "34 over 25," the configuration of FDS tendons at the wrist.

Fig. 49-5   Flexor zones of the hand. (From Zidel P. Tendon healing and flexor tendon surgery. In Aston SJ, Beasley RW, Thorne CH, eds. Grabb and Smith's Plastic Surgery, 5th ed. Philadelphia: Lippincott, 1997, p 876.)

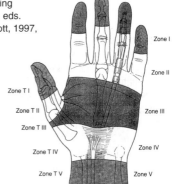

Zone I

Zone II

Zone T I

Zone T II

Zone T III

Zone III

Zone IV

Zone T IV

Zone T V

Zone V

- **Hand**
  - **Flexor zones:** Used to describe level of injury; determines treatment and prognosis (Fig. 49-5)
    Zone I: Distal to FDS
    Zone II: A1 to FDS (called *"no-man's land"* because of historically poor results with primary repair)
    Zone III: Distal carpal tunnel to A1
    Zone IV: Carpal tunnel
    Zone V: Proximal to carpal tunnel
- **Digits**
  - **Flexor sheaths:** From metacarpal heads to distal phalanges, tendons encased in fibroosseous sheaths lined with synovium that act as pulleys (Fig. 49-6)[7-9]
    - **Pulley function**
      - Allows smooth excursion of tendons
      - Keeps flexor tendons close to axis of rotation of joints
      - Prevents bowstringing and decreases arm movement
      - Increases mechanical advantage of flexor tendons
    - **Annular pulleys** (A1-A5)
      - **Odd** numbers arise from **volar plates** of MPJ, PIPJ, and DIPJ
      - **Even** numbers arise from **periosteum** of proximal and middle phalanges
      - **A2 and A4 pulleys most important and should be preserved**[6-9]
    - **Cruciate pulleys** (C1-C3)
      - Thin with crisscrossing fibers
      - C1 between A2 and A3, C2 between A3 and A4, and C3 between A4 and A5
    - **Thumb**
      - A1 and A2 pulleys are over MPJ and IPJ
      - **Oblique pulley** is continuation of AdP insertion and is **most important to preserve**

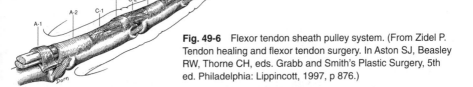

Fig. 49-6   Flexor tendon sheath pulley system. (From Zidel P. Tendon healing and flexor tendon surgery. In Aston SJ, Beasley RW, Thorne CH, eds. Grabb and Smith's Plastic Surgery, 5th ed. Philadelphia: Lippincott, 1997, p 876.)

VASCULATURE

ARTERIAL (Fig. 49-7)

- **Radial artery**
  - Runs between brachioradialis and FCR tendons at wrist
  - Splits into larger dorsal branch that courses through anatomic snuffbox to supply deep palmar arch
  - Smaller palmar branch joins superficial palmar arch
- **Ulnar artery**
  - Lateral to ulnar nerve at the wrist and medial to FCU tendon as it runs through Guyon's canal
  - Splits into larger palmar branch that forms superficial palmar arch (dominant in 88% of the population)
  - Smaller dorsal branch that joins deep palmar arch

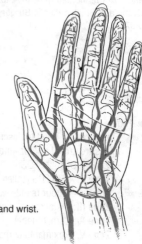

Fig. 49-7 Arterial anatomy of the hand and wrist.

TIP: *Kaplan's cardinal line* is a line drawn across the palm from the first web space to the hook of hamate. It approximates location of the superficial palmar arch; deep arch is 1 cm proximal to this line.

- **Superficial arch**
  - Gives rise to **common digital arteries** in interspaces
    - Lie **volar to nerves** and bifurcate in distal palm into radial and ulnar digital arteries, which lie **dorsal to nerves in fingers**
    - Digital arteries bifurcate at **DIPJ**
    - At IPJs, digital arteries give off branches that pass under flexor tendons and anastomose with branch from other side to form vincular blood supply
    - **Blood supply to thumb is princeps pollicis artery,** from deep palmar arch

VENOUS DRAINAGE

- **Superficial:** Larger system; runs on dorsal surface of hand
- **Deep:** Small system; has random pattern
- Veins of hand drain into **cephalic** and **basilic** veins in forearm

---

NERVES (Fig. 49-8)

MEDIAN

- Mainly involved in precision manipulation
- Enters forearm between two heads of PT
- Lies between FDS and FDP in forearm
  - **Motor innervation**
    - **Anterior interosseous branch** supplies FPL, FDP to index finger, and PQ

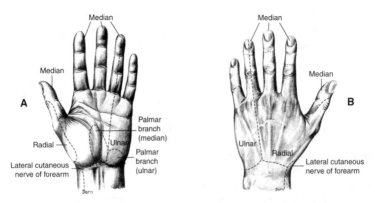

Fig. 49-8 Sensory distribution. **A,** Palmar. **B,** Dorsal. (From Beasley RW, ed. Beasley's Surgery of the Hand. New York: Thieme, 2003.)

- ▸ **Main nerve** innervates FCR, PT, FDS, PL, FDP to long finger, and lumbricals to index and long fingers
- ▸ **Recurrent motor branch** innervates intrinsic muscles of the thumb: APB, FPB (superficial portion), and opponens pollicis

---

TIP: Thumb opposition is a quick test to determine nerve function (i.e., have the patient gesture "OK").

- • **Sensory innervation**
  - ▸ **Palmar cutaneous branch** arises **5 cm** proximal to wrist crease; innervates thenar eminence
  - ▸ Also sensory to thumb and the index, long, and ring (radial side) fingers

---

TIP: Determining sensation at the tip of the index finger is a quick test to determine nerve function.

ULNAR
- ■ Essential for power grasp by innervating the intrinsic muscles of the small and ring fingers, and thumb adductors
- ■ Enters forearm between two heads of FCU
- ■ Lies under FCU in forearm and enters **Guyon's canal** (bounded by pisiform, hook of hamate, volar carpal ligament, and transverse carpal ligament) at the wrist
- • **Motor innervation**
  - ▸ **Forearm:** FCU and FDP to ring and small fingers
  - ▸ **Main nerve** innervates hypothenar muscles (palmaris brevis, adductor digiti minimi, opponens digiti minimi, and flexor digiti minimi), lumbricals to ring and small fingers, interossei, FPB (deep portion), and AdP

TIP: Finger abduction and adduction are quick tests to determine nerve function.

- **Sensory innervation**
  - ▸ **Dorsal sensory branch** originates 5-7 cm proximal to ulnar styloid process
  - ▸ Innervates skin on ulnar aspect of hand and small finger and ulnar side of ring finger

---

TIP: Determining sensation of the small finger is a quick test to determine nerve function.

RADIAL

- Motor branch innervates muscles that position and stabilize the hand
- Enters forearm between two heads of supinator muscle
- Lies between brachioradialis and ECRL and ECRB
  - **Motor innervation**
    - ▸ **Forearm:** Innervates brachioradialis and ECRL
    - ▸ **Posterior interosseous branch** innervates wrist and finger and thumb extensors (i.e., EDC, EDM, ECU, APL, EPL, EPB, and EIP)

TIP: Finger and thumb extension are quick tests to determine nerve function.

- **Sensory innervation**
  - ▸ **Superficial branch** passes between tendons of brachioradialis and ECRL
  - ▸ Becomes superficial at musculotendinous junction of brachioradialis and runs toward anatomic snuffbox
  - ▸ Supplies sensibility to dorsoradial aspect of hand and dorsum of thumb and index and long fingers to the IPJ
  - ▸ **Lateral antebrachial cutaneous nerve** (continuation of musculocutaneous nerve) has overlapping innervation with radial nerve at radial aspect of wrist

---

TIP: Determining first dorsal web space sensation is a quick test to determine nerve function.

ANASTOMOSES
- **Martin-Gruber anastomosis**
  - Motor fiber connection between median and ulnar nerves in forearm
  - Affects 10%-25% of population
- **Riche-Cannieu anastomosis**
  - Motor fiber connection between median and ulnar nerves in the hand

BONES AND JOINTS

BASIC ARCHITECTURE
- **Bones**
  - **27 bones** arranged into four basic units: three mobile and one fixed
  - **Fixed unit** is composed of second and third metacarpals and carpal bones
  - **Mobile units** in descending order of mobility are thumb, index finger, and fourth and fifth metacarpals with long, ring, and small fingers

HAND
- **Bones**
  - 5 metacarpals
  - 14 phalanges
  - Thumb only has proximal and distal
- **MPJs**
  - Relatively loose-fitting joints
  - Collateral ligaments pass obliquely from metacarpal neck to base of proximal phalanx
  - Collateral ligaments provide greatest stability when MPJs are flexed and allow lateral movement with MPJ in extension
  - When MPJ extended stability provided by interosseous muscles
- **IPJs**
  - Tight-fitting joints with collateral ligaments providing same lateral stability throughout range of motion
  - **Volar plates:** Fibrocartilaginous part of joint capsule that provide additional stability and limits hyperextension

WRIST
- **Bones**
  - **Proximal** (scaphoid, lunate, triquetrum, and pisiform)
  - **Distal** (trapezium, trapezoid, capitate, and hamate)
  - *Pisiform is sesamoid and is not functional*
  - Scaphoid links proximal and distal rows; makes it vulnerable to fracture
- **Ligaments**
  - Capsules of radiocarpal and midcarpal joints are reinforced by series of ligaments (i.e., **dorsal, palmar,** and **interosseous**).
  - All ligaments are **intracapsular** and interosseous ligaments are **intraarticular.**
  - Integrity of ligaments is essential for normal wrist motion because **no tendons insert directly on carpal bones.**
- **Carpometacarpal joints (CMCJs)**
  - **Thumb CMCJ** (basal) is **saddle joint,** designed for maximal mobility stabilized primarily by radiopalmar (beak) ligament.
  - Second and third CMCJs have no mobility.
  - Fourth and fifth CMCJs have about 30 degrees of flexion or extension important for power grip.
- **Biomechanics**
  - Movements are complex interactions between carpal bones and radius.
  - Main movements are flexion-extension and radioulnar deviation with axis through capitate.
  - Radiocarpal and midcarpal joints participate equally in flexion-extension; radiocarpal joint more important for radioulnar deviation.
  - Scaphoid is primary rotational element during radial deviation; triquetrum is primary rotational element during ulnar deviation.

DRUJ

- Sigmoid notch and head of ulna articulate
- **Triangular fibrocartilage complex (TFCC) ligament** most important stabilizer; consists of articular disk, distal radioulnar ligaments, ulnocarpal ligaments, and ECU tendinous subsheath
  - Originates from radius, attaches to base of ulnar styloid, and transmits 18% of load across wrist
  - Central 80% of TFCC is avascular; tears in this ligament problematic
- DRUJ provides forearm rotation

KEY POINTS

✔ All finger extensors are extrinsic, except the interossei and lumbricals, and are innervated by the radial nerve.

✔ The FDS flexes the PIPJ. To test its function, hold the remaining fingers in extension and ask the patient to flex the affected finger.

✔ The FDP flexes the DIPJ. To test its function, hold the PIPJ in extension and ask the patient to flex the finger tip.

✔ Anastomoses between the median and ulnar nerves in the forearm and hand can mask an ulnar nerve injury.

REFERENCES

1. Beasley RW. Surgical anatomy of the hand. In Beasley RW, ed. Beasley's Surgery of the Hand. New York: Thieme Medical Publishers, 2003, p 5.
2. Monaghan BA. Anatomy. In Beredjiklian PK, Bozentka DJ, eds. Review of Hand Surgery. Philadelphia: WB Saunders, 2004, p 1.
3. Naam NH. Anatomy, function, and biomechanics of the hand and wrist. In Achauer BM, Elof Eriksson E, Vander Kolk C, eds. Plastic Surgery, Indications, Operations, and Outcomes. St Louis: Mosby, 2000, p 1627.
4. Seiler JG III. Essentials of Hand Surgery. Philadelphia: Lippincott, 2002.
5. Young DM, Mankani M, Alexander JT, et al. Hand Surgery. In Way LW, Doherty GM, eds. Current Surgical Diagnosis and Treatment. New York: McGraw-Hill, 2003, p 1270.
6. Moore KL. Clinically Oriented Anatomy, 3rd ed. Philadelphia: Williams & Wilkins, 1992.
7. Peterson WW, Manske PR, Bollinger BA, et al. Effect of pulley excision on flexor tendon biomechanics. J Orthop Res 4:96, 1986.
8. Lin GT, Amadio PC, An KN, et al. Functional anatomy of the human digital flexor pulley system. J Hand Surg 14:949, 1989.
9. Lin GT, Cooney WP, Amadio PC, et al. Mechanical properties of human pulleys. J Hand Surg 15:429, 1990.

50. Basic Hand Examination

Jeffrey E. Janis

HISTORY

TRAUMA
- Determine age, occupation, and other pursuits.
- Determine whether the dominant hand is injured.
- Is there any history of previous trauma to the extremity?
- *When* did the injury occur?
- *Where* did the injury occur?
- *How* did the injury occur?
- *What* previous treatment has been administered?

NONTRAUMA
- When did the pain, swelling, sensory change, or other symptoms begin?
- Is there a progression of symptoms, and in what order did they occur?
- How is function impaired?
- Are other joints or digits affected?
- What makes the pain (swelling, tingling) worse or better?
- Is it worse at some particular time (day or night)?

PHYSICAL EXAMINATION[1,2]

- **Initial examination of the injured hand in the emergency room must establish the following:**
  - Is the injured hand or digit viable?
  - Is there a vascular injury?
  - Is there ischemic compartment syndrome?
  - Is there tendon damage?
  - Is there nerve injury?
  - Is the skeleton stable?
  - Is there actual or threatened skin loss?

OVERVIEW
- **Skin**
  - Uncover the entire upper extremity.
  - Examine for swelling or edema.
  - Evaluate color.

- Evaluate moisture and papillary ridges.
- Examine, characterize, and document any wounds.
- **Compare with the contralateral extremity.**
- Note any atrophy (thenar or other muscle groups).
- **Motor function**
  - Determine active and passive range of motion.
  - Instruct patient to "make a fist."
  - Instruct patient to "straighten out your fingers."
  - Pain disproportionate to the injury or significant pain with passive motion may suggest serious underlying pathology, such as ischemic compartment syndrome or suppurative flexor tenosynovitis.
  - Observe cascade of the fingers.
  - Determine whether patient can fully extend and flex each joint of the hand and wrist.
- **Sensation**
  - **Static two-point discrimination (2PD)** of digits should approach **6 mm.**
  - **Dynamic 2PD** should be approximately **3 mm.**
  - **Sweating ability is lost** concomitant with the distribution of digital nerve interruption, as is **loss of papillary ridges.**
  - Glabrous skin will wrinkle after immersion in water for 5 minutes, *denervated skin will not.*
- **Vascular**
  - Palpate radial and ulnar pulses.
  - Capillary refill should occur in less than 2 seconds.
  - **Allen's test** may be performed on the hand, as well as on individual digits.
  - Use Doppler test when any question of vascular compromise remains.
- **Skeleton**
  - Swelling
  - Deformity
  - Abnormal range of motion
  - Decreased range of motion
  - Increased range of motion (possible ligamentous injury)
  - Tenderness
- **Radiographs**
  - Carefully review all radiographs.
  - Take posteroanterior and lateral views at the least.
  - Reorder when inadequate, or add additional views as indicated.

> TIP: Obtain comparison views of the contralateral side, particularly in children or when the wrist is involved.

- Pay particular attention to insertion points of ligaments or tendons and to articular surfaces.

ANATOMY (Figs. 50-1, 50-2, and 50-3)

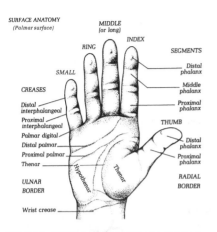

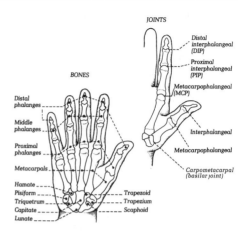

Fig. 50-1 Surface anatomy of the hand. (From American Society for Surgery of the Hand. The Hand: Examination and Diagnosis, 3rd ed. Philadelphia: Churchill Livingstone, 1990, pp 13-56.)

Fig. 50-2 Skeleton of the hand and wrist. (From American Society for Surgery of the Hand. The Hand: Examination and Diagnosis, 3rd ed. Philadelphia: Churchill Livingstone, 1990, pp 13-56.)

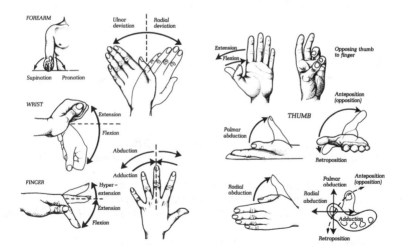

Fig. 50-3 Terminology of the hand and digit motion. (From American Society for Surgery of the Hand. The Hand: Examination and Diagnosis, 3rd ed. Philadelphia: Churchill Livingstone, 1990, pp 13-56.)

SPECIFIC MOTOR EXAMINATIONS

- **Flexor pollicis longus (FPL)**
  - Test the function of FPL by instructing patient, *"Bend the tip of your thumb"* (Fig. 50-4).
  - Test motor strength by adding resistance supplied by the examiner.
- **Flexor digitorum profundus (FDP)**
  - Test the function of FDP by instructing patient, *"Bend the tip of your finger"* (Fig. 50-5).
  - The examiner stabilizes proximal interphalangeal (PIP) joint while actively flexing distal interphalangeal (DIP) joint.

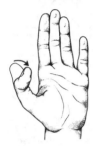

Fig. 50-4   Test for FPL musculotendinous function. (From American Society for Surgery of the Hand. The Hand: Examination and Diagnosis, 3rd ed. Philadelphia: Churchill Livingstone, 1990, pp 13-56.)

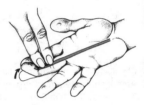

Fig. 50-5   Test for FDP musculotendinous function. (From American Society for Surgery of the Hand. The Hand: Examination and Diagnosis, 3rd ed. Philadelphia: Churchill Livingstone, 1990, pp 13-56.)

- **Flexor digitorum superficialis (FDS)**
  - Test the function of each FDS individually by instructing patient, *"Bend your finger at the middle joint"* (Fig. 50-6).
  - The examiner must block other fingers in extension.

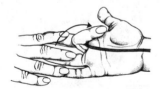

Fig. 50-6   Test for FDS musculotendinous function. (From American Society for Surgery of the Hand. The Hand: Examination and Diagnosis, 3rd ed. Philadelphia: Churchill Livingstone, 1990, pp 13-56.)

- **Abductor pollicis longus (APL) and extensor pollicis brevis (EPB)**
  - Test the function of APL and EPB by instructing patient, *"Bring your thumb out to the side"* (Fig. 50-7).
  - The examiner then palpates the taut tendons over the radial side of the wrist.
- **Extensor carpi radialis longus (ECRL) and extensor carpi radialis brevis (ECRB)**
  - Test the function of ECRL and ECRB by instructing patient, *"Make a fist and strongly bring your wrist back"* (Fig. 50-8).
  - The examiner then palpates the tendons over dorsoradial aspect of wrist.
- **Extensor pollicis longus (EPL)**
  - Test the function of EPL by placing hand flat on the table and instructing patient, *"Lift only the thumb off the table"* (Fig. 50-9).

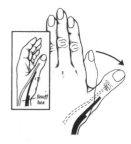

Fig. 50-7   Test for EPB and APL musculotendinous function. (From American Society for Surgery of the Hand. The Hand: Examination and Diagnosis, 3rd ed. Philadelphia: Churchill Livingstone, 1990, pp 13-56.)

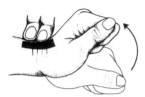

Fig. 50-8   Test for ECRL and ECRB musculotendinous function. (From American Society for Surgery of the Hand. The Hand: Examination and Diagnosis, 3rd ed. Philadelphia: Churchill Livingstone, 1990, pp 13-56.)

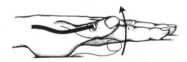

Fig. 50-9   Test for EPL musculotendinous function. (From American Society for Surgery of the Hand. The Hand: Examination and Diagnosis, 3rd ed. Philadelphia: Churchill Livingstone, 1990, pp 13-56.)

- **Extensor digitorum communis (EDC), extensor indicis proprius (EIP), and extensor digiti minimi or extensor digiti quinti (EDM or EDQ)** (Fig. 50-10).
  - Test the function of EDC by instructing patient, *"Straighten your fingers."*
  - Test the function of EIP by instructing patient, *"Stick out your index finger with the others in a fist."*
  - Test the function of EDM or EDQ by instructing patient, *"Stick out your small finger with the others in a fist."*
- **Extensor carpi ulnaris (ECU)**
  - Test the function of ECU by instructing patient, *"Pull your hand up and out to the side"* (Fig. 50-11).
  - Then palpate the tendon over the ulnar side of the wrist.

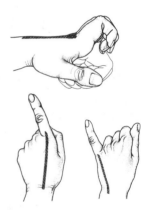

Fig. 50-10   Test for EDC, EIP, and EDM musculotendinous function. (From American Society for Surgery of the Hand. The Hand: Examination and Diagnosis, 3rd ed. Philadelphia: Churchill Livingstone, 1990, pp 13-56.)

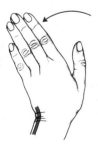

Fig. 50-11   Test for ECU musculotendinous function. (From American Society for Surgery of the Hand. The Hand: Examination and Diagnosis, 3rd ed. Philadelphia: Churchill Livingstone, 1990, pp 13-56.)

- **Thenar muscles**
  - The thenar muscles include the **abductor pollicis brevis** (APB), **opponens pollicis** (OP), and **flexor pollicis brevis** (FPB).
  - Test these muscles by instructing patient, *"Touch the thumb to the small finger"* (Fig. 50-12).
- **Adductor pollicis (AdP)**
  - Test the function of adductor pollicis by having patient forcibly grasp a piece of paper between the thumb and radial side of the index P1 (Fig. 50-13).
  - This is *Froment's sign;* a positive response is shown in Fig. 50-13.
- **Interosseous muscles**
  - Test the interosseous muscle by instructing patient, *"Spread your fingers apart,"* while the examiner applies resistance to the index and small finger (Fig. 50-14).
- **Hypothenar muscles**
  - The hypothenar muscles include the **abductor digiti minimi** (ADM), **flexor digiti minimi** (FDM), and **opponens digiti minimi** (ODM).
  - Test these muscles by instructing patient, *"Bring your little finger away from the others"* (Fig. 50-15).

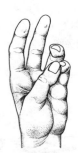

Fig. 50-12 Test for thumb opposition. (From American Society for Surgery of the Hand. The Hand: Examination and Diagnosis, 3rd ed. Philadelphia: Churchill Livingstone, 1990, pp 13-56.)

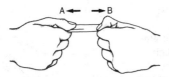

Fig. 50-13 Froment's sign. Test is positive in *B* (compensatory flexion at IP joint). (From American Society for Surgery of the Hand. The Hand: Examination and Diagnosis, 3rd ed. Philadelphia: Churchill Livingstone, 1990, pp 13-56.)

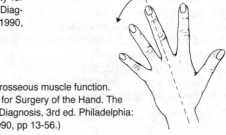

Fig. 50-14 Test for interosseous muscle function. (From American Society for Surgery of the Hand. The Hand: Examination and Diagnosis, 3rd ed. Philadelphia: Churchill Livingstone, 1990, pp 13-56.)

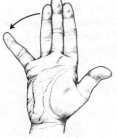

Fig. 50-15 Test for hypothenar muscle function. (From American Society for Surgery of the Hand. The Hand: Examination and Diagnosis, 3rd ed. Philadelphia: Churchill Livingstone, pp 13-56, 1990.)

SENSORY EXAMINATION

ULNAR NERVE INNERVATION (Fig. 50-16)
- Ulnar half of ring finger
- All of small finger

ULNAR NERVE

Fig. 50-16   Muscles innervated by the ulnar nerve in the forearm and hand. (From American Society for Surgery of the Hand. The Hand: Examination and Diagnosis, 3rd ed. Philadelphia: Churchill Livingstone, 1990, pp 13-56.)

Flexor carpi ulnaris

Flexor digitorum profundus

MEDIAN NERVE INNERVATION (Fig. 50-17)
- Volar surface of thumb
- Index finger
- Middle finger
- Radial side of ring finger
- Volar wrist capsule (terminal branch of **anterior** interosseous nerve)

Adductor pollicis
Deep head of flexor pollicis brevis
Palmaris brevis
Abductor
Opponens
Flexor } Digit minimi
Little lumbrical
Ring lumbrical
Interossei

* Profundus muscle is also supplied by median nerve

RADIAL NERVE INNERVATION (Fig. 50-18)
- Radial three fourths of the dorsum of hand
- Dorsum of thumb
- Dorsum of index finger to PIP joint
- Dorsum of middle finger to PIP joint
- Dorsoradial half of ring finger to PIP joint
- **Dorsal** wrist capsule through terminal branch of **posterior** interosseous nerve

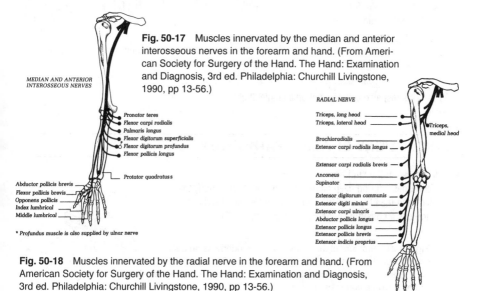

Fig. 50-17   Muscles innervated by the median and anterior interosseous nerves in the forearm and hand. (From American Society for Surgery of the Hand. The Hand: Examination and Diagnosis, 3rd ed. Philadelphia: Churchill Livingstone, 1990, pp 13-56.)

MEDIAN AND ANTERIOR INTEROSSEOUS NERVES

Pronator teres
Flexor carpi radialis
Palmaris longus
Flexor digitorum superficialis
Flexor digitorum profundus
Flexor pollicis longus

Protator quadratuss

Abductor pollicis brevis
Flexor pollicis brevis
Opponens pollicis
Index lumbrical
Middle lumbrical

* Profundus muscle is also supplied by ulnar nerve

RADIAL NERVE

Triceps, long head
Triceps, lateral head
Triceps, medial head

Brachioradialis
Extensor carpi radialis longus

Extensor carpi radialis brevis
Anconeus
Supinator

Extensor digitorum communis
Extensor digiti minimi
Extensor carpi ulnaris
Abductor pollicis longus
Extensor pollicis longus
Extensor pollicis brevis
Extensor indicis proprius

Fig. 50-18   Muscles innervated by the radial nerve in the forearm and hand. (From American Society for Surgery of the Hand. The Hand: Examination and Diagnosis, 3rd ed. Philadelphia: Churchill Livingstone, 1990, pp 13-56.)

DERMATOMAL DISTRIBUTION (Fig. 50-19)

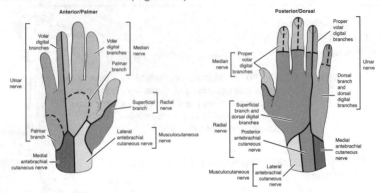

Fig. 50-19 Dermatomal distribution of the hand and wrist. (From American Society for Surgery of the Hand. The Hand: Examination and Diagnosis, 3rd ed. Philadelphia: Churchill Livingstone, 1990, pp 13-56.)

VASCULAR TESTS

ALLEN'S TEST
- This test is used to determine **patency** of the ulnar and radial arteries (Fig. 50-20).
    1. Occlude both arteries.
    2. Exsanguinate the hand.
    3. Release the radial artery.
    4. Examine palm for pink color/capillary refill.
    5. Repeat for ulnar artery.

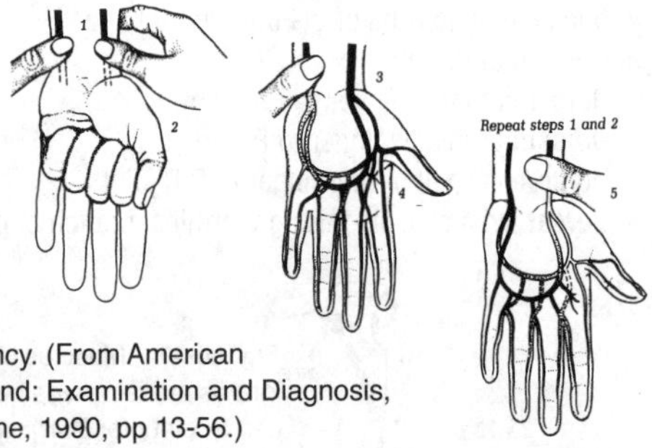

Fig. 50-20 Allen's test for arterial patency. (From American Society for Surgery of the Hand. The Hand: Examination and Diagnosis, 3rd ed. Philadelphia: Churchill Livingstone, 1990, pp 13-56.)

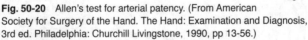

TIP: This test also can be used on a single digit.

CLINICAL SIGNS OF ACUTE PATHOLOGY

- **Tenderness in the snuffbox**
    - Tenderness during deep palpation of the anatomic snuffbox (between the EPL and EPB, just distal to the radial styloid) suggests a **possible scaphoid fracture** (Fig. 50-21).

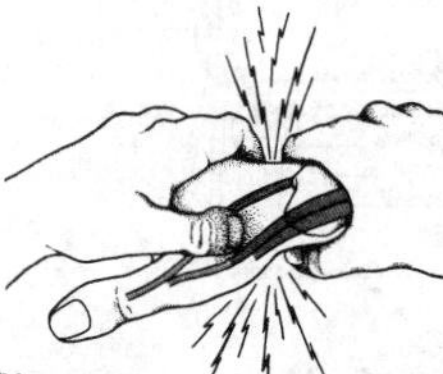

Fig. 50-21 Fracture of the scaphoid with tenderness on deep palpation in the snuffbox area. (From American Society for Surgery of the Hand. The Hand: Examination and Diagnosis, 3rd ed. Philadelphia: Churchill Livingstone, 1990, pp 13-56.)

- **"Grind test"**
  - Test **degenerative arthritis** of the thumb metacarpophalangeal (MP) joint by compression and adduction (Fig. 50-22, *A*), or by compression and rotation (Fig. 50-22, *B*).

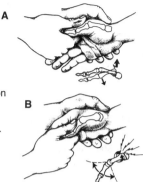

A

B

Fig. 50-22   A, Axial compression-adduction test; **B,** Axial compression-rotation test. (From American Society for Surgery of the Hand. The Hand: Examination and Diagnosis, 3rd ed. Philadelphia: Churchill Livingstone, 1990, pp 13-56.)

- **Finkelstein's test**
  - Use Finkelstein's test for *de Quervain's disease* (tenosynovitis of APL and EPB tendons) (Fig. 50-23).
  - Grasp the thumb and deviate the wrist ulnarly.
- **Tinel's sign**
  - Tinel's sign is **positive** if tapping over the course of the median nerve in the carpal tunnel creates paresthesias in the hand (Fig. 50-24). This suggests **carpal tunnel syndrome.**
  - Test the cubital and radial tunnels similarly.
- **Phalen's maneuver**
  - Perform by positioning the wrists in complete flexion for 1 minute (Fig. 50-25).
  - Paresthesias in the hand constitute a positive test and suggest **carpal tunnel syndrome.**

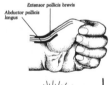

Extensor pollicis brevis
Abductor pollicis longus

Fig. 50-23   Finkelstein's test for de Quervain's disease. (From American Society for Surgery of the Hand. The Hand: Examination and Diagnosis, 3rd ed. Philadelphia: Churchill Livingstone, 1990, pp 13-56.)

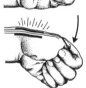

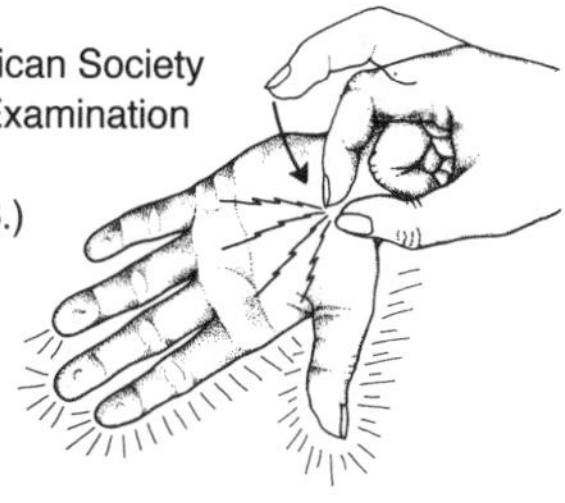

Fig. 50-24   Tinel's sign. (From American Society for Surgery of the Hand. The Hand: Examination and Diagnosis, 3rd ed. Philadelphia: Churchill Livingstone, 1990, pp 13-56.)

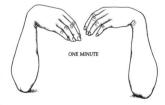

ONE MINUTE

Fig. 50-25   Phalen's sign (wrist flexion test). (From American Society for Surgery of the Hand. The Hand: Examination and Diagnosis, 3rd ed. Philadelphia: Churchill Livingstone, 1990, pp 13-56.)

> ## KEY POINTS
>
> ✔ It is imperative to obtain a thorough and proper history to design the most appropriate treatment.
> ✔ An organized approach to a physical examination will help prevent inadvertent omissions.
> ✔ A static 2PD should be less than or equal to 6 mm whereas the dynamic 2PD should be less than or equal to 3 mm.
> ✔ The immersion test helps test innervation in children.
> ✔ Allen's test can be performed on digits as well as on the hand.
> ✔ Comparison of contralateral radiographs can be very helpful.
> ✔ Know key diagnostic maneuvers to test for abnormal pathology.

REFERENCES

1. American Society for Surgery of the Hand. The Hand: Examination and Diagnosis, 3rd ed. New York: Churchill Livingstone, 1990.
2. American Society for Surgery of the Hand. The Hand: Primary Care of Common Problems, 2nd ed. New York: Churchill Livingstone, 1990.

51. Congenital Hand Anomalies

Ashkan Ghavami

GENERAL PRINCIPLES[1,2]

- Thorough history
  - Problems during pregnancy
  - Details of newborn period
  - Family history of congenital deformities
- Total body examination is always necessary—looking for a range of craniofacial to toe deformities.
- **Always address parental concerns.** Parents go through a grieving process not unlike mourning a loss of the "perfect baby" that was expected.[1,3]
- Timing is critical.
  - Anaesthesia risks are increased in children less than 6 months old.
  - Prioritize other medical and surgical problems.
  - Optimal hand size: Hand size doubles in the first 2-2½ years of life.
    - Important for any microsurgery
  - Consider child's maturity level (e.g., for rehabilitation and cooperation with splinting regimens).
  - Time operation(s) before child starts school (4-5 years old).
- Use of meticulous dressing and a cast that cannot be removed is imperative (often an above-elbow full cast is necessary).

> TIP: Use toys and gadgets, and visually observe the child's hand function while he or she is engaged in playing with the toys.
>
> Do not assume that someone else has diagnosed other anomalies such as a sacral dimple, duplicate toes, or an unusual facial appearance, all of which may warrant a more extensive workup and can point to a syndromic disorder.

EMBRYOLOGY[1,4]

Upper limbs develop between 5 and 8 weeks.

APICAL ECTODERMAL RIDGE (AER)
- Transient ectodermal thickening at leading edge of bud
- Induces underlying mesoderm to differentiate
- Mesoderm produces morphogens (apical ectodermal ridge maintenance factor [AERMF]) that maintain the AER

ZONE OF POLARIZING ACTIVITY
- Cluster of mesenchymal cells along postaxial border of limb bud
- Provides stimulus to AER

THREE MAIN INTERACTIONS GUIDE FORMATION

1. **Proximal to distal progression**
   - Mesenchyme interacts with AER
2. **Dorsal to palmar axis**
   - Dorsal ectoderm
   - *Example:* Fingernails versus pulp; flexor versus extensor tendon
3. **Anteroposterior axis cell differentiation**
   - *Example:* Thumb differentiated from little finger and other digits in anteroposterior plane

HOX GENES

- HoxA, HoxB, HoxC, and HoxD
- Regulate patterning during limb development
- Important proteins that assist in Hox expression:
  - Sonic hedgehog (Shh), FGFs, and Wnt-7a

APOPTOSIS

Programmed cell death that is vital to organization and differentiation during embryogenesis

- All hands begin as a hand plate (38 days) with webs and gradual recession of interdigit spaces.
  - Cells at periphery of webs cease AERMF.
  - Once AERMF ceases, webs recess by apoptosis—beginning distally and progressing proximally.
  - By **day 50,** individual digits and web spaces are well defined.
    - *Syndactyly thought to be failure of proper apoptosis between digits*

CLASSIFICATION OF ANOMALIES

NOTE: Classification systems are less commonly used today because there are many confounding variables.

I. **Failure of formation**
   - Transverse arrest
   - Longitudinal arrest
II. **Failure of differentiation of parts**
   - Soft tissue
   - Osseous
III. **Duplication**
IV. **Overgrowth** (hyperplasia)
V. **Undergrowth** (hypoplasia)
VI. **Constriction band syndrome**
VII. **Generalized anomalies and syndromes**
   - Certain disorders may fit into multiple classes or may **not** fit perfectly into a specific class.
   - General congenital anomalies are not discussed in this chapter.
     - **Failure of formation:** Radial and ulnar ray deficiencies/dysplasias; central ray deficiencies (true cleft hand)
     - **Failure of differentiation:** Arthrogryposis (soft tissue, disseminated)
     - **Symbrachydactyly** (not easily classified)
     - **Generalized anomalies (chromosomal):** Madelung's deformity

SYNDACTYLY

CLASS
- Failure of differentiation (class II)

ETIOLOGIC FACTORS
- Unknown failure of the process of recession at web spaces

INCIDENCE
- 1:2000 live births
- Ten times more common in Caucasians than African Americans
- Twice as common in males than females
- No difference between bilateral and unilateral
- Long and ring finger most commonly affected (57%)[5]
- Thumb-index finger most rare (3%)[3]

FAMILY HISTORY
- Reported in 15%-40% of cases
- **Autosomal dominant inheritance with variable penetrance** when no other associated anomalies are present

ANATOMY
- Cleland's and Grayson's ligaments are thickened and coalesced
- Web space palmar fascia extensive and thick
- Joints may be stiff
- **Simple (cutaneous) form**
  - Ligaments usually normal
  - Duplicated sheaths, tendons, nerves, vessels
- **In complex and complicated forms**
  - Fusion levels vary
  - Fingernail synechia
  - Abnormal tendons (especially in acrocephalosyndactyly, Apert's syndrome)

CLINICAL PRESENTATION
- **Types**
  - **Simple (cutaneous):** No bony fusion
  - **Complex (osseous):** Presence of bony fusion
  - **Complicated:** Complicated by polydactyly
  - **Incomplete:** Web is recessed to a degree
  - **Complete:** No web present; syndactyly to fingertips
  - **Acrosyndactyly:** Associated with congenital band syndrome *(Streeter's syndrome)*
  - Usually isolated but may be associated with a multitude of syndromes and other congenital anomalies

IMAGING
- **Mandatory posteroanterior radiograph:** To evaluate bony involvement and transverse bars (bony segments) or more complicated proximal joint and bony abnormalities
- False positive and false negative results possible because of incomplete ossification, presence of delta phalanx, duplications, or bony synostosis

- **Arteriography**
  - May be helpful in complex cases (e.g., Apert's syndrome)

TREATMENT
- **Timing**
  - Up to 40 different surgical techniques available
  - **Early** operative intervention only warranted for **border digits** or when **complex** (e.g., Apert's with transverse bony components)
  - **Most commonly:** Assurance and waiting until hand is larger (18-24 months) is best treatment choice
- **Simple syndactyly**
  - Make use of dorsal skin and limit skin grafting.
  - Use dorsal skin to lay into future proximal web space.
  - **Avoid scars and incisions in web space.**
    - ► Incisions in web space can lead to "web creep" postoperatively.
  - Use interdigitated ulnar and radial-based mirror image Z-flaps (Fig. 51-1).
  - Use full-thickness skin grafts with precisely templated designs.
  - Make flaps large and simple.
  - Preserve paratenon.
  - Identify neurovascular bundles proximally and volarly first.
    - ► There may be a nonduplicated vascular supply.
    - ► Vascular bifurcation level is the limit of proximal separation.
    - ► Turn down tourniquet at least once to evaluate blood flow after separation of digits.
  - Bolster skin grafts with templated Xeroform® (Integrity Medical Devices, Hammonton, NJ), gauze, and Steri-Strips™ (3M, St. Paul, MN).
  - Long-arm cast placement that covers fingertips prevents operative failure resulting from infection and early mobility.
  - Tip reconstruction: Use Hentz "pulp-plasty" with composite graft or Buck-Gramcko "stiletto flap" to optimize tip fullness and contour[1] (Fig. 51-2)

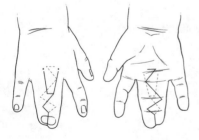

Fig. 51-1 Incision markings for correction of syndactyly. Note interdigitating mirror flaps. (From Carter P, Ezaki M. Disorders of the upper extremity. In Herring JA, Tachdjian MO, eds. Tachdjian's Pediatric Orthopedics From the Texas Scottish Rite Hospital for Children, vol 1, 3rd ed. Philadelphia: WB Saunders, 2001, p 438.)

Fig. 51-2 Hentz "pulp-plasty." Composite graft for radial or ulnar pulp defects after correction of syndactyly. (From Carter P, Ezaki M. Disorders of the upper extremity. In Herring JA, Tachdjian MO, eds. Tachdjian's Pediatric Orthopedics From the Texas Scottish Rite Hospital for Children, vol 1, 3rd ed. Philadelphia: WB Saunders, 2001, p 441.)

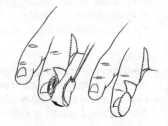

- **Complex syndactyly**
  - Use technique similar to that described previously.
  - Address bony elements with excision while preserving joints when possible.
  - Preserve extensor and flexor tendon slips to each separated digit.
  - Plan on case-by-case basis because presentation is quite variable.

CAMPTODACTYLY

CLASS
- Failure of differentiation; soft tissue (class II)
- Congenital constriction deformity of the proximal interphalangeal (PIP) joint
- **Classically defined as involving the little finger**

ETIOLOGIC FACTORS
- Unclear
- **Common theories**
  - Abnormal lumbrical insertions and morphology
  - Extra or abnormal flexor digitorum superficialis slips
  - Abnormal extensor or PIP capsular structures

INCIDENCE
- Approximately 1% of population
  - Likely an underestimate because of underreporting
- Up to 20% can present in adolescent females

CLINICAL PRESENTATION
- Abnormal flexion posture of PIP joint (commonly little finger) that may be reducible versus irreducible.
- If actively reducible while stabilizing metacarpophalangeal (MP) joint, problem is MP joint instability.

> TIP: Always note the exact degree of flexion contraction and passive/active correction possible.

- Pain on extension (passive) may imply abnormal musculature (lumbrical).
- If associated brachydactyly and very stiff PIP joint without flexion-extension creases, then consider *symphalangism* diagnosis.

IMAGING
- **True lateral radiograph of PIP joint is mandatory.**
  - Sometimes a bony synostosis is present.
- Dorsal ridge of proximal phalanx at PIP joint is often chiseled (flattened).
  - Flattened dorsal phalanx is often irreversible after correction.

TREATMENT[3]
- Very difficult problem with numerous approaches described
- Complete correction never achieved

- **Nonoperative treatment**
  - When contracture less than 30 degrees, surgery rarely indicated
  - Splinting (dynamic versus static)
    ▸ If correction achieved, splinting may be necessary in adolescence because of recurrence during growth spurts
  - Stretching exercises
- **Operative treatment**
  - Reserve operation for failure of conservative treatments.
  - Operation is usually required when **contracture is more than 30 degrees.**
  - If passive MP stability during examination allows active extension of PIP joint, consider a "lasso" procedure using FDS slip.
  - Severe contraction (more than 90 degrees) may require surgery because splint fitting is difficult.
  - **Technique**
    ▸ Examine FDS and lumbricals with zigzag incision.
    ▸ Release accessory collateral ligaments if necessary.

TIP: Similar to an open capsular contracture release, perform a minimalist stepwise release of tethering structures until satisfactory correction is achieved.

  ▸ After release, soft tissue defect can be covered with either a midlateral proximally based triangular rotation flap or a full-thickness skin graft.
  ▸ Maintain PIP joint in position by using K-wires.

CLINODACTYLY

CLASS
- Failure of differentiation (osseous; class II)

ETIOLOGIC FACTORS
- Unknown

FAMILY HISTORY
- Congenital ulnar angulation of small finger can be inherited in **autosomal dominant fashion with variable expression.**
- **May be associated with syndromes** such as Apert's (triphalangeal thumbs and symbrachydactyly).
- Phalanx may be trapezoidal, triangular, or "C-shaped" (bracketed) around one corner of phalangeal base.
- *Delta phalanx* is the name for the triangular shape of the bony wedge.
  - Bracket and abnormal shape prevents proper longitudinal growth.
- **Clinical presentation**
  - Digit (commonly little finger) is abnormally angled.
  - Pain should not be a prevalent feature.
  - Limited motion when delta or bracketed phalanx is present.
  - Most common site is **middle phalanx of small finger.**

IMAGING

- Plain radiographs in at least two views are necessary to evaluate growth plates and bony anomalies (e.g., presence of delta and bracketed phalanx).

TREATMENT

> TIP: Any skin deficiencies after correction may require Z-plasty.

- Should always use K-wires to hold corrections in place
- Bracket resection with preservation of growth plate and fat graft
  - Works well when true delta phalanx is resected
  - Can be performed when child is age 3-4 years
- Closing wedge osteotomy
  - Indicated when trapezoidal phalanx is present
  - Wait until skeletal maturity
- Opening wedge osteotomy
- Reverse wedge osteotomy

POLYDACTYLY

CLASS
- Duplication (class III)

INCIDENCE
- Unknown
- **Most common deformity of the hand**
- True incidence skewed by "amputation" of extra digits in newborn nurseries
- African Americans: 1:300 (ulnar polydactyly)
- Caucasians: 1:3000

ULNAR-SIDED POLYDACTYLY (POSTAXIAL)
Duplication of little finger
- More common in blacks
- Strong inheritance pattern of dominant gene with variable penetrance
- Rare to have other associated disorders
- **General classification** (used for ulnar-sided polydactyly)
  Type I: No skeletal tissue
  Type II: Skeletal attachment to enlarged or bifid phalanx or metacarpal
  Type III: Complete duplication including metacarpal bone
- **Treatment**
  - Ligate when narrow stalk is present with two ligation clips.
  - Allow autoamputation while in cast over several weeks.
  - Broad-based stalk requires operative separation with possible ligament reconstruction.

RADIAL POLYDACTYLY (PREAXIAL)

- More common in Caucasians
- May have dominant inheritance
- **Triphalangeal thumbs:** Historically linked to **thalidomide ingestion** by mothers
- Other abnormalities and disorders possibly present (e.g., visceral deformities)
- **Syndromal associations**
  - Can involve every organ system (thorough workup necessary)
  - Orofacial abnormalities
  - Bone dysplasias
  - Mental retardation
  - *Examples:* Blackfan-Diamond anemia, Carpenter's syndrome, Bloom's syndrome, trisomy 13, Holt-Oram syndrome (triphalangeal thumb; atrial and ventricular septal defects, PDA, anomalous vessels), Fanconi pancytopenia (triphalangeal thumb), TAR syndrome
- Genetic disorder in Hox gene may be responsible
- Increase folding of AER. "Ruffle" in the hand plate[1]
- **Variations:** Soft tissue narrow stalk or bony elements with remnants or whole tendons, ligaments, and neurovascular tissue
- Surgical reconstruction more complicated
  - Reconstruct/preserve ligaments, delineate and preserve neurovascular supply (may not be duplicated)
  - Tendon reconstruction/reposition (insertions frequently eccentric or split)
  - Correction of angular deformity (caused by wedge-shaped *delta phalanx*)
  - Ulnar thumb most often best one to preserve

IMAGING

- Radiographic evaluation probably not necessary in ulnar polydactyly but helpful and required in radial polydactyly and triphalangeal thumb workup
- Can be misleading because ossification not complete

WASSEL CLASSIFICATION OF THUMB DUPLICATION (Fig. 51-3)

Differentiation of types I-IV: Based on whether duplication is at or between joints
  Type I: Least common—2%[5]
  Type IV: Most common—43%[5]
  Type VII: Most complex and requires at least one triphalangeal thumb

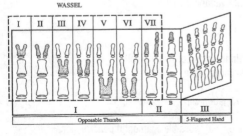

Fig. 51-3 Thumb polydactyly: Wassel classification as modified by McKusick and Temtamy. (From Carter P, Ezaki M. Disorders of the upper extremity. In Herring JA, Tachdjian MO, eds. Tachdjian's Pediatric Orthopedics From the Texas Scottish Rite Hospital for Children, vol 1, 3rd ed. Philadelphia: WB Saunders, 2001, p 422.)

TREATMENT
- **General guidelines**
  - Floating thumb with narrow stalk: Simple ligation
  - All others except floating thumb: Wait until 6-18 months
  - In general, **ulnar thumb preserved to save the ulnar collateral ligament (UCL),** which provides MP joint stability
    - ▶ Stabilizes power pinch
    - ▶ Preserve epiphyseal plates
- **Wassel types I and II**
  - If each duplication is symmetrical and of equal size, **Bilhaut-Cloquet procedure** may be used with or without modifications (Fig. 51-4).
  - Close nail plate and repair as meticulously as possible.
  - Preserve pulp margins.

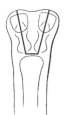 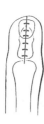

Fig. 51-4   Bilhaut-Cloquet operation. Good for symmetrical bifid thumb polydactyly. (From Carter P, Ezaki M. Disorders of the upper extremity. In Herring JA, Tachdjian MO, eds. Tachdjian's Pediatric Orthopedics From the Texas Scottish Rite Hospital for Children, vol 1, 3rd ed. Philadelphia: WB Saunders, 2001, p 426.)

- **Wassel type III**
  - If duplication is bifid, Bilhaut-Cloquet procedure can be performed; otherwise delete smaller thumb.
- **Wassel type IV**
  - Use racquet-shaped incision with proximal and distal extensions (as Zs if necessary).[1]
  - Preserve UCL and reduce radial metacarpal condyle (Fig. 51-5).
  - Reposition eccentric extensor and flexor tendons.
  - Identify and preserve abductor pollicis brevis.
  - Detach radial collateral ligament, trim metacarpal condyle, and reattach on preserved thumb.
  - Shell out radial thumb (the one usually excised) sharply.
  - Preserve growth plates.
  - Retrograde pin with K-wire(s).
- **Wassel type V and VI**
  - Reconstruct basal joint.

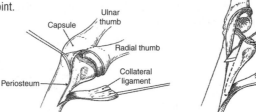

Fig. 51-5   Correction of thumb polydactyly. Trimming of radial facet of metacarpal head to prevent bony prominence after correction. Note preservation of radial collateral ligament. (From Carter P, Ezaki M. Disorders of the upper extremity. In Herring JA, Tachdjian MO, eds. Tachdjian's Pediatric Orthopedics From the Texas Scottish Rite Hospital for Children, vol 1, 3rd ed. Philadelphia: WB Saunders, 2001, p 430.)

MACRODACTYLY

CLASS:
- Overgrowth (class IV)

CLASSIFICATION
- Four types described by Upton[6]
  Type I: Macrodactyly with lipofibromatosis of nerve
  - Enlarged portion in specific nerve (median) distribution
  - Static subtype
    - Born with large digit(s), enlarge proportionately with age
  - **Progressive subtype**
    - Near-normal at birth; by age 3 enlarge disproportionately
    - Progressive growth until epiphyseal closure
  Type II: Associated with **neurofibromatosis** (von Recklinghausen's disease)
  Type III: Macrodactyly with hyperostosis: Very rare
  Type IV: Macrodactyly with hemihypertrophy

ETIOLOGIC FACTORS
- Largely unknown
- Most common theory: Nerve-stimulated pathology with abnormal neural control in sensory distribution of peripheral nerve (median)

CLINICAL PRESENTATION
Type I
- Index then middle finger most commonly involved
  - Multiple digits three times more likely to be involved
- Predilection of median nerve distribution
- 90% of cases unilateral
- Hyperextension (anterior growth > dorsal growth) and clinodactyly (deviates toward normal side)
Type II
- **Usual signs of neurofibromatosis**
  - Less fatty infiltration of nerve; more fibrous
  - Six or more café-au-lait spots, multiple nodular peripheral nerve tumors
  - Autosomal dominant
  - Skeletal abnormalities (30%): Scoliosis, bowing, tibial pseudarthrosis
  - Seizures, mental retardation possible
  - Often bilateral
- Enlarged metacarpal and phalangeal heads
Type III
- No enchondromas
- Abnormal nerves not typically present
  - No proliferation of fat or neural elements
- Not inherited
- Incision scars prone to hypertrophy
Type IV
- One extremity developing more than the other
- Forearm and arm also involved

- Not inherited
- Ipsilateral upper and lower extremity involved
- Typical ulnar drift and flexion contraction of MP joints
- Enlarged thenar and hypothenar eminences
  - ▸ Adduction contraction of thumb
- May have renal, adrenal, and brain involvement

IMAGING
- **Comparison plain radiographs** are required to document growth variation.
- **Arteriogram** or **MRA** may be required to rule out vascular malformations.

TREATMENTS

> TIP: Psychological consequences can be disastrous, and school-aged ridicule may be severe because this deformity is difficult to conceal. Social counseling and thorough family discussions are imperative.

- Repeat surgery is often necessary and involves different forms of debulking.
- Involved digit is **never normal.**
- **Treatment goals[1]:**
  - Control or reduce size
  - Maintain sensibility as much as feasible
  - Maintain useful motion, especially of thumb joints
- **Common procedures:**
  - Skin and subcutaneous resection
  - Extensive neurolysis, resection
  - Epiphysiodesis
  - Angulation, recession, and narrowing-type osteotomies
  - Arthrodesis
  - Amputation

> TIP: Amputation is a very reasonable option for a useless digit that is grotesque and a source of embarrassment. Most described procedures are unsatisfactory and ultimately continue to create deformities.

THUMB HYPOPLASIA

CLASS:
- Undergrowth (class V)
  - May go unnoticed by parents until fine motor skills begin and the thumb is noted to be less involved or smaller in comparison with the contralateral thumb

BACKGROUND FACTORS
- Involves radial half of upper limb
- May be associated with a hypoplastic or absent radius, and other radial dysplasias

- **Mandatory evaluation for other anomalies**
  - **Holt-Oram syndrome:** Autosomal dominant, septal defects, tetralogy of Fallot, mitral valve prolapse, PDA
  - **VACTERL:** *V*ertebral, *A*nal, *C*ardiac, *Tracheo*E*sophageal fistula, *R*enal, and *L*ower extremity abnormalities
  - **Blood dyscrasias**
    - ▸ **TAR:** *T*hrombocytopenia *A*bsent *R*adius syndrome
    - ▸ **Fanconi anemia:** Autosomal dominant, poor long-term prognosis

ANATOMY

- Small to absent intrinsic and extrinsic tendons/muscles, smaller bony anatomy, joint instability or absence
- *Caveat:* Look for ***pollex abductus,*** which is an abnormal insertion of the flexor pollicis longus into the extensor mechanism
  - Causes abduction on thumb flexion
  - May also be present in radial polydactyly

CLASSIFICATION

- Modified Blauth classification, by Manske[7,8]
  Type 1: Diminution of thenar muscle bulk, smaller thumb elements
  Type 2: Type 1, plus lessened thumb-index web space, MP joint instability from UCL, lack of thumb to palmar abduction motion
  Type 3A: Even less bony (metacarpal) element; stable carpometacarpal (CMC) joint
  Type 3B: Type 3, with unstable CMC joint
  Type 4: Floating thumb; *(pouce flottant)* small pedicle holding floating thumb with no bony elements
  Type 5: Completely absent thumb

IMAGING

- Multiview plain radiographs mandatory to assess the joints (especially CMC and MP joints)

TREATMENT

> TIP: The decision whether to perform a pollicization is based on CMC joint presence and integrity.

- Reconstruction of the thumb addressing all components
- **Types 1-3A**
  - Opponensplasty with ring-finger FDS in addition to UCL stabilization and thumb-index web space deepening with a four-flap Z-plasty (Fig. 51-6)[1,4]
  - Use of abductor digiti quinti transfer (Huber) to augment opponensplasty described but is very weak as a sole transfer and scars down easily
- **Types 3B, 4, and 5**
  - Formal pollicization with index finger
  - Need to assess mobility of index finger before decision to perform pollicization
    - ▸ Joint stiffness can ensue

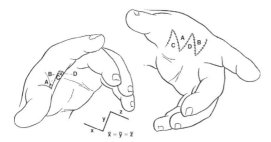

Fig. 51-6   Thumb-index web space deepening with four-flap reconstruction. (From Carter P, Ezaki M. Disorders of the upper extremity. In Herring JA, Tachdjian MO, eds. Tachdjian's Pediatric Orthopedics From the Texas Scottish Rite Hospital for Children, vol 1, 3rd ed. Philadelphia: WB Saunders, 2001, p 445.)

TIP: If the child does not bring the index finger into play or move it during the examination, he or she is not likely to move it as a new thumb after pollicization.

- **A normal-sized thumb with normal range of motion should never be expected or promised to the family.**
- More severe dysplasia or lack of elements will produce less pinch strength, thumb stability, and flexibility.

CONGENITAL BAND SYNDROME

CLASS
- Constriction band syndrome (class VI)
- Commonly known as **Streeter's syndrome**
- Unclear etiologic factors dating back to Hippocrates

CLASSIFICATION BY PATTERSON[9]
Type I: Simple constriction ring
Type II: Constriction ring with deformity of distal part
Type III: Constriction with variable fusion of distal parts (acrosyndactyly)
Type IV: Complete intrauterine disruption

ETIOLOGIC FACTORS
- **Two main theories: Internal theory** (intrinsic) and **amniotic band theory** (extrinsic)
  - **Intrinsic theory** (Streeter)
    ▸ Internal defect in embryo with possible genetic or sporadic etiologic factors
  - **Extrinsic theory:**
    ▸ Amniotic band may compress or encircle extremity or distal segment causing local compression that heals and results in cleft
    ▸ Carter and Ezaki[1] theorize that swallowing of amniotic band may explain associated cleft lips, palates
- **Clinical presentation**
  - **Check prenatal history**
    ▸ Oligohydramnios, premature contractions, ruptures
    ▸ Three-dimensional ultrasonography may improve intrauterine diagnosis

- Distal segment of extremity may present as **venous** and **edematous** (blue, purple, possibly weeping)
  - ▶ Initially observe most cases, even if edematous, as long as no vascular embarrassment distally. If necessary can do hemi–Z release (50% of constriction)
  - ▶ Early correction often suboptimal because Z-flaps are small and amount of correction is minimal with poor cosmetic result
- Often confused with symbrachydactyly (distal "nubbins")
- **Acrosyndactyly**
  - ▶ Seen with Apert's syndrome
  - ▶ May have fistulas and clefts or sinus tracts distal to web
    - ✦ Can evaluate with a small probe

IMAGING
- Plain radiographs help evaluate any underlying bony abnormality and depth of soft tissue involved

TREATMENT
- Impending amputations are rarely salvageable (dried necrotic segment in newborn).
- If there is neurologic compromise, earlier release is required.
- Puffy digits that show no circulatory compromise can be watched.
- **Reconstruction**
  - Best to wait until extremity is larger (2-3 years) so that larger, more effective flaps can be used.
  - Must excise full thickness of abnormal, scarred ring basin.
  - **Upton and Tan method**
    - ▶ Reverse (mirror) Z-flap of subcutaneous tissue from Z-flaps on skin layer and close as two layers
    - ▶ Not feasible for fingers
  - Staging not always necessary
  - **Procedures for acrosyndactyly**
    - ▶ Early but minimal surgery
    - ▶ Thumb web deepening (four-flap Z-plasty)
    - ▶ Release of small skin bridges
    - ▶ Amputations sometimes warranted
    - ▶ Delayed reconstruction

TRIGGER THUMB

BACKGROUND
- *Not a true congenital deformity; not in any classification scheme*
- Develops within the first 2 years of life
- Bilateral in 25% of cases
- Thickening of FPL tendon *(Notta's node)*, which catches on first anular pulley

CLINICAL PRESENTATION
- Thumb interphalangeal joint catches in flexion and rest of thumb normal
- *Notta's node* palpable as moving with tendon at MP joint level
- Often discovered by parents when thumb fixed in flexion

IMAGING
- Not necessary unless trauma suspected

TREATMENT
- Conservative splinting and steroid injections are not very useful (different from adult trigger fingers).
- Easiest and most effective treatment is complete release of A1 pulley of thumb in controlled operating room environment.
  - Preserve as much pulley as possible after ranging tendon excursion in operating room.
- Cast with thumb tip exposed and in abduction-extension for minimal time, and allow early motion to prevent tendinous adhesions.

KEY POINTS

✔ Need first to rule out associated syndromes and other health concerns that may be occult or not diagnosed by the referring physician.

✔ Timing of corrective surgery is critical and should be weighed against anaesthetic risk (greater risk if <6 months old), severity of deformity, and the goal of completing operative treatments by the time the child is school age, which is when peer ridicule begins.

✔ Certain conditions have many operative descriptions associated with them. This may be a clue that an optimal treatment is not yet available (e.g., macrodactyly).

✔ Always consider basic hand surgery tenets, such as adequate blood supply, sensation, preservation of function, and basic goal of achieving a functional prehensile hand (sensate thumb opposition, pinch, and grip ability).

✔ Do not interfere with skeletal growth (be wary of growth plates).

✔ Social rehabilitation and support is as important as any other form of treatment.

✔ Many of these children do very well if they are appropriately managed, and go on to lead happy, successful, independent lives.

REFERENCES

1. Carter P, Ezaki M. Disorders of the upper extremity. In Herring JA, Tachdjian MO, eds. Tachdjian's Pediatric Orthopedics From the Texas Scottish Rite Hospital for Children, vol 1, 3rd ed. Philadelphia: WB Saunders, 2001, pp 379-507.
2. McCarroll HR. Congenital anomalies: A 25-year overview. J Hand Surg Am 25:1007-1037, 2000.
3. Dr. Peter Carter. Personal communication.
4. Ezaki M, Kay SP, Light TR, et al. Congenital hand deformities. In Green DP, Hotchkiss RN, Pederson WC, eds. Operative Hand Surgery, vol 2, 4th ed. New York: Churchill Livingstone, 1994, pp 325-551.
5. Flatt AE. Care of Congenital Hand Anomalies, 2nd ed. St Louis: Quality Medical Publishing, 1994.
6. Upton J. Congenital anomalies of the hand and forearm. In McCarthy JG, ed. Plastic Surgery, vol 8, Philadelphia: WB Saunders, 1990.
7. Blauth W. Der hypoplastiche Daumen. Arch Orthop Unfallchir 62:225, 1967.
8. Manske PR, McCarroll HR Jr. Index finger pollicization for a congenitally absent or nonfunctioning thumb. J Hand Surg Am 10:606-613, 1985.
9. Patterson TJ. Congenital ring-constrictions. Br J Plast Surg 14:1-31, 1961.

52. Carpal Bone Fractures

Joshua A. Lemmon

Carpal bone fractures are significant wrist injuries that occur either in isolation or in association with more global carpal soft tissue injuries (see Chapter 53).[1]

SCAPHOID

FRACTURE INCIDENCE (Fig. 52-1)

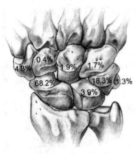

Fig. 52-1 Relative incidence of carpal bone fractures.

- The **scaphoid** is the **most frequently fractured carpal bone,** accounting for **70%** of all carpal bone fractures.[2]
- These fractures occur most commonly in young men (age 15-30 years).
- Scaphoid fractures are uncommon in children; the carpus is primarily cartilaginous and more resilient to injury.

ANATOMY
- The scaphoid (from Greek *skaphos*) has a unique shape, often described as "boat-shaped" or "peanut-shaped."
- The surface is **almost entirely articular** and covered with cartilage, except a thin strip across the dorsal waist. Nutrient foramina are in this nonarticular region, allowing for vascular supply.
- **Vascular supply**[3]
  - Two predominant vascular pedicles from the radial artery supply the scaphoid:
    - ▸ **Scaphoid tubercle:** Branch supplies the distal 20% of scaphoid
    - ▸ **Dorsal ridge vessels:** Small perforating branches coming off radial artery penetrate through several foramina to supply proximal 80% of scaphoid
  - No perforators supplying the scaphoid are found proximal to the waist, but a retrograde vascular supply is present.

TIP: The unusual retrograde vascular supply limits healing of proximal scaphoid fractures and is the reason for the increased risk of avascular necrosis, delayed union, and nonunion.

KINEMATICS

- Wrist kinematics are discussed in Chapter 53.
- The scaphoid and scapholunate interosseous ligament are important for the coordination of proximal and distal carpal row motion.
- Unstable scaphoid fractures allow the lunate and proximal scaphoid to extend while the distal scaphoid continues to flex. This creates a **dorsal intercalated segment instability (DISI).**
  - Creates an altered distribution of carpal loading and results in degenerative disease and progressive arthritic changes

MECHANISMS OF INJURY (Fig. 52-2)

- **Two mechanisms**
  1. **Hyperextension:** With forced hyperextension to 95-100 degrees, the proximal half of the scaphoid is stabilized while the distal pole is unsupported. Load applied to the scaphoid is then concentrated at the waist (junction of supported and unsupported zones), and fracture occurs.[4]
  2. **Axial load (punch):** With the wrist in neutral position, an axial load is transmitted from the second metacarpal through the trapezium and trapezoid to impart volar shear force on the distal pole of the scaphoid. Fracture occurs most frequently at waist.[5]

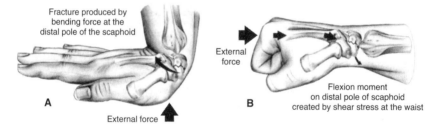

Fig. 52-2 Mechanism of scaphoid fracture. **A,** Hyperextension. **B,** Axial load. (From Wolfe SW. Fractures of the carpus: Scaphoid fractures. In Berger RA, Weiss A-PC, eds. Hand Surgery. Philadelpia: Lippincott, 2004, pp 351-408.)

EVALUATION

- **History**
  - Age
  - Sex
  - Handedness
  - Occupation
  - Mechanism of injury: Usually a fall on outstretched hand
  - Time of injury

- **Physical examination**
  - **Radial-sided wrist pain, edema, and ecchymosis:** Signs may be subtle
  - **Specific signs**
    - ▶ Tenderness in the anatomic snuffbox: Dorsal wrist between first and third dorsal compartments
    - ▶ Tenderness over the volar scaphoid tubercle
    - ▶ Tenderness with axial compression: Apply force axially through the first metacarpal

> TIP: The clinical signs of scaphoid fracture are often inaccurate. Diagnosis relies mostly on high-quality radiography.

RADIOGRAPHIC IMAGING
- **Five views of the wrist**[2]
  1. Posterior-anterior (PA)
  2. Lateral
  3. Oblique
  4. Fisted PA: Extends scaphoid and accentuates waist fracture
  5. Navicular view: Fisted, semipronated, ulnar deviation

> TIP: In a setting of high clinical suspicion, normal radiographs do not exclude a fracture. Place the patient in a thumb-spica splint and repeat the examination and radiographic images after 10-14 days.

- **Bone scan**
  - Performed when initial and repeated plain radiographs are normal, but the clinical suspicion for scaphoid fracture remains high.
  - Increased activity is seen in the fractured scaphoid.
- **CT scan**
  - Obtain when plain radiographs demonstrate a nondisplaced fracture
  - Allows for more detailed examination of the scaphoid; reliably demonstrates when a fracture is displaced[6]
- **MRI**
  - Can detect presence or absence of acute fracture
  - Expense often makes use impractical

TREATMENT
- **Nondisplaced fractures**
  - **Nearly all nondisplaced scaphoid fractures heal well with immobilization.**
  - Immobilize fractures in a long-arm thumb-spica cast for 6 weeks followed by 6 weeks in a short-arm thumb-spica cast.
    - ▶ Short-arm casts show a trend toward higher nonunion rates.[7]
  - Consider operative treatment with internal fixation (including percutaneous screw fixations) for high-demand patients who cannot tolerate 12 weeks of immobilization.
  - Internal fixation is also recommended for proximal pole fractures because of high rates of nonunion and avascular necrosis.[8]
- **Displaced fractures**
  - **All displaced scaphoid fractures require operative treatment.**

- Multiple operative techniques are used and continue to evolve.
  - ▸ **Percutaneous screw fixation:** Frequently used by modern surgeons
  - ▸ **Open reduction with screw fixation**
    - ✦ Solid (Herbert) or cannulated screws are placed across the fracture; these screws are designed to apply compression across the fracture site.
    - ✦ **Volar** approaches are often recommended to preserve vascular supply to the scaphoid.
    - ✦ **Dorsal** approaches permit better exposure of the proximal pole.

TIP: K-wires can be placed and used as "joysticks" to aid in reduction.

  - ▸ **Percutaneous screw fixation**[9]
    - ✦ This is the most recent innovation.
    - ✦ Cannulated screws are drilled over guidewires placed using fluoroscopy.
    - ✦ Arthroscopy is used to assist and evaluate reduction.
    - ✦ Early results are promising.

COMPLICATIONS

- **Malunion**
  - **Improper reduction can lead to healing with inadequate alignment.**
  - A *humpback deformity* is the most common malunion.
    - ▸ *The distal pole of the scaphoid is flexed while the proximal pole is extended*
    - ▸ Creates an angulated scaphoid in lateral radiographs
    - ▸ Can lead to chronic pain, poor mobility, reduced grip strength, and degenerative arthritis
    - ▸ Treatment options (controversial)
      - ✦ Reoperate early[10]
      - ✦ Employ a conservative, nonoperative approach[11]
- **Delayed union**
  - Occurs when symptoms persist and there is no radiographic evidence of union after 4 months of adequate immobilization.
  - Treatment is controversial: Most surgeons treat with additional immobilization and observation.
- **Nonunion**
  - Trabeculation fails across the fracture site, and the ends become sclerotic.
  - Nonunions progress to degenerative arthritis and **S**caphoid **N**onunion **A**dvanced **C**ollapse **(SNAC)** wrist deformities.
  - Treatment options are controversial: Vary according to anatomic location.
    - ▸ Most surgeons suggest screw fixation and bone grafting of waist and distal pole nonunions, and vascularized bone grafting and screw fixation of proximal pole nonunions.[12]

FRACTURES OF OTHER CARPAL BONES

TRIQUETRUM[13]

- Second most commonly fractured carpal bone
- **Two fracture types:**
  1. **Dorsal rim:** Avulsion fractures
     - ▸ Dorsal intercarpal ligament or lunotriquetral avulsions may pull small bony fragments off the dorsal rim.

▸ Close inspection is required to detect wrist instability patterns or dislocations (see Chapter 53).
▸ Hyperextension and ulnar deviation can force impaction with the ulnar styloid, and a small ulnar-sided fracture of the dorsal rim occurs.

2. **Body**
▸ Isolated body fractures can occur from direct impact at the ulnar body of the hand, involving the medial tuberosity.
▸ Other body fractures (sagittal, transverse, or comminuted) usually are secondary to crush injuries or part of a more complex global wrist injury.

- **Treatment**
  - Dorsal rim fractures usually heal with immobilization for 4 weeks in a short-arm cast.
  - Displaced body fractures require open reduction and internal fixation (ORIF) along with treatment of any associated ligamentous injuries or dislocations.

HAMATE

- **Two fracture types:**
  1. **Hamulus:** "Hook" of the hamate fractures
     ▸ These fractures occur most commonly by direct trauma to the hand while holding a racket, club, or bat (Fig. 52-3). Also may be caused by falls on an outstretched hand.
     ▸ Patients present with pain and tenderness over the hamate and with ulnar-sided hand edema.
     ▸ A careful ulnar nerve examination, especially of the deep (motor) branch, should be performed to exclude associated nerve injury.
     ▸ Specialized radiographs (lateral, oblique, and carpal tunnel views) are needed to view the fracture.
     ▸ CT scans are often required for adequate diagnosis.
     ▸ Presentation of small finger flexor tendon injuries can be delayed until pseudarthrosis and degenerative bony changes lead to attrition ruptures of the tendon.[14]
  2. **Hamate body**
     ▸ These fractures usually represent a more complex wrist injury with axial fracture-dislocation patterns (see Chapter 53).
     ▸ These fractures most commonly result from a closed fist injury with axial force transmitted through the fourth and fifth metacarpals.
       ⋆ The hamate is fractured in the coronal plane at the fourth or fifth carpal metacarpal (CMC); it dislocates dorsally.

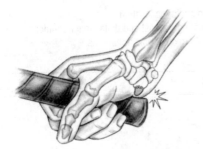

Fig. 52-3 Mechanism of injury in hook of the hamate fractures. (From Sennwald GR. Carpal bone fractures other than the scaphoid. In Berger RA, Weiss A, eds. Hand Surgery. Philadelphia: Lippincott, 2004, pp 409-423.)

■ **Treatment**
- Nondisplaced hamulus fractures usually are treated with cast immobilization, but recent data suggest that early surgical treatment yields the best results.[15]
- Treatment options for hamulus fractures include ORIF or excision of the fragment.
- Nondisplaced hamate body fractures should be treated with cast immobilization.
- Most hamate body fractures require ORIF because of other associated wrist injuries.

TRAPEZIUM
■ **Ridge fractures**
- **These are caused most commonly by avulsion of the transverse carpal ligament.**

> TIP: Carpal tunnel syndrome may occur in association with trapezium fractures and should be specifically excluded.

- Fractures are thought to occur with hyperextension and abduction force to the thumb.
- Treat with immobilization, although nonunions can result and should be treated with excision of bony fragment.

■ **Body fractures**
- These can occur when the wrist is forced into extension and radial deviation, crushing the trapezium into the radial styloid.
- Fractures also are found in association with first metacarpal-base fractures.
- Displaced body fractures should be treated with open reduction and rigid internal fixation.

CAPITATE
■ Half of these fractures are isolated, and half occur in association with other carpal injuries, e.g., greater-arc injuries (see Chapter 53).
■ Multiple mechanisms are described for these fractures including the **anvil mechanism,** when hyperextension crushes the capitate into the radius (Fig. 52-4).
  - In this situation, a transverse body fracture occurs with 180-degree rotation of the proximal fragment.
■ Dorsal articular fractures can occur in association with third metacarpal base fractures or third CMC dislocations.

■ **Treatment**
- Nondisplaced capitate fractures should be treated with cast immobilization, as long as ligamentous instability is excluded.
- Displaced fractures can be treated with closed reduction and percutaneous pin fixation or open reduction, ligament repair, and internal fixation.

> TIP: Avascular necrosis of the proximal fragment is a recognized long-term sequela; therefore patients should be followed closely.

LUNATE
■ Rare fractures that usually occur in association with ligamentous injuries of the wrist
- **Volar pole**
  ▶ These fractures often result from avulsion of the long and short radiolunate ligaments.
  ▶ Treat with anatomic reduction, giving attention to establishing normal ligamentous anatomy to support the midcarpal joint.

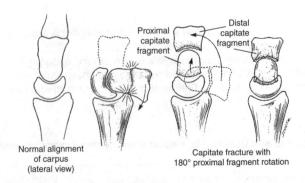

Normal alignment
of carpus
(lateral view)

Proximal
capitate
fragment

Distal
capitate
fragment

Capitate fracture with
180° proximal fragment rotation

Fig. 52-4   Anvil mechanism resulting in capitate body fracture. (From Shah MA, Viegas SF. Fractures of the carpal bones excluding the scaphoid. J Am Soc Surg Hand 2:129-139, 2002.)

- **Dorsal pole**
  - ▶ Avulsion of the scapholunate or lunotriquetral ligaments can cause fractures, although these ligaments usually avulse off the neighboring bones rather than the lunate itself.
  - ▶ Treatment should include repair of any associated ligamentous injuries.
- **Body**
  - ▶ These fractures result from axial compression between the capitate and the lunate fossa on the radius.
  - ▶ Careful evaluation with CT scan is needed to assess displacement.
  - ▶ Displaced fractures require open reduction and fixation.

CAUTION: All lunate fractures can progress to avascular necrosis (Kienbock's disease).

TIP: A meticulous carpal ligamentous exam is needed when evaluating lunate fractures because of the high rate of associated injuries.

TRAPEZOID

- This is the *least* **frequently fractured carpal bone.**
- The bone is **well-protected** by the surrounding osseous anatomy, trapezium, second metacarpal base, scaphoid, capitate, and strong carpal ligaments.
- Displaced fractures require anatomic reduction and fixation, and nondisplaced fractures should be treated with immobilization.[13]

PISIFORM

- This is a **sesamoid bone** rather than true carpal bone.
- It lies within sheath of flexor carpi ulnaris tendon.
- Fractures occur as a result of direct trauma.
- Plain radiographs frequently do not demonstrate these injuries, and CT scans may be necessary for diagnosis.
- The **ulnar nerve** is in close proximity, and therefore *careful nerve examination is imperative.*

■ **Treatment**
- **Acute fractures** should be treated with **splint immobilization.**
- **Chronic discomfort** and **nonunion** is best treated with **pisiform excision.**

KEY POINTS

✔ The scaphoid is the most commonly fractured carpal bone.

✔ The trapezoid is the least frequently fractured carpal bone.

✔ CT scans are necessary to accurately differentiate displaced and nondisplaced scaphoid fractures.

✔ Early operative treatment of nondisplaced scaphoid fractures can decrease the need for prolonged immobilization.

✔ Close follow-up is necessary for the treatment of scaphoid fractures to diagnose and treat delayed unions and nonunions.

✔ Whenever a carpal bone is fractured, median and ulnar nerve function should be carefully evaluated.

✔ Fractures of the triquetrum, hamate, lunate, and capitate often signal broader carpal injuries; precise imaging and a meticulous ligamentous examination are mandatory.

REFERENCES

1. Garcia-Elias M. Carpal bone fractures. In Watson HK, Weinzweig J, eds. The Wrist. Philadelphia: Lippincott, 2001, pp 173-186.
2. Wolfe SW. Fractures of the carpus: Scaphoid fractures. In Berger RA, Weiss A-PC, eds. Hand Surgery. Philadelphia: Lippincott, 2004, pp 381-408.
3. Gelberman RH, Panagis JS, Taleisnik J, et al. The arterial anatomy of the human carpus. Part I. The extraosseous vascularity. J Hand Surg Am 8:367-376, 1983.
4. Weber ER, Chao EY. An experimental approach to the mechanism of scaphoid waist fractures. J Hand Surg Am 3:142-148, 1978.
5. Horii E, Nakamura R, Watanabe K, et al. Scaphoid fracture as a puncher's fracture. J Orthop Trauma 8:107-110, 1994.
6. Nakamura R, Imaeda T, Horii E, et al. Analysis of scaphoid fracture displacement by three-dimensional computed tomography. J Hand Surg Am 16:485-492, 1991.
7. Gellman H, Caputo RJ, Carter V, et al. Comparison of short and long thumb-spica casts for non-displaced fractures of the carpal scaphoid. J Bone Joint Surg Am 71:354-357, 1989.
8. Krimmer H. Management of acute fractures and nonunions of the proximal pole of the scaphoid. J Hand Surg Br 27:245-248, 2002.
9. Slade JF III, Jaskwhich D. Percutaneous fixation of scaphoid fractures. Hand Clin 17:553-574, 2001.
10. Nakamura P, Imaeda T, Miura T, et al. Scaphoid malunion. J Bone Joint Surg Br 73:134-137, 1991.
11. Jiranek WA, Ruby LK, Millender LB, et al. Long-term results after Russe bone-grafting: The effect of malunion of the scaphoid. J Bone Joint Surg Am 74:1217-1228, 1992.
12. Merrell GA, Wolfe SW, Slade JF III, et al. Treatment of scaphoid non-unions: Quantitative meta-analysis of the literature. J Hand Surg Am 27:685-691, 2002.
13. Shah MA, Viegas SF. Fractures of the carpal bones excluding the scaphoid. J Am Soc Surg Hand 2:129-139, 2002.
14. Neviaser RJ. Fractures of the hook of the hamate. J Hand Surg Am 11:207-210, 1986.
15. Scheufler O, Andresen R, Radmer S, et al. Hook of hamate fractures: Critical evaluation of different therapeutic procedures. Plast Reconstr Surg 115:488-497, 2005.

53. Carpal Instability and Dislocations

Joshua A. Lemmon

WRIST ANATOMY AND KINEMATICS[1]

The wrist is a complex joint that connects the distal forearm and the hand.

EIGHT CARPAL BONES (Fig. 53-1)
- Arranged as a **distal** and **proximal** carpal row
- **Proximal row**
  - Scaphoid (proximal pole)
  - Lunate
  - Triquetrum
- **Distal row**
  - Trapezium
  - Trapezoid
  - Capitate
  - Hamate
- **Pisiform**
  - **Sesamoid bone:** Lies within flexor carpi ulnaris tendon

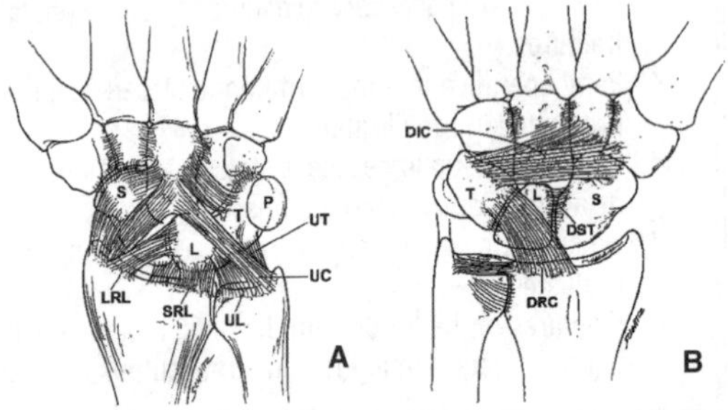

COMPLEX LIGAMENTOUS SUPPORT SYSTEM (see Fig. 53-1)
- **Extrinsic ligaments:** From radius and ulna to carpal bones
- **Intrinsic ligaments:** Interconnect carpal bones
- In general, **volar ligaments stronger** than dorsal ligaments

Fig. 53-1 The ligamentous anatomy of the volar (**A**) and dorsal (**B**) wrist. *DIC,* Dorsal intercarpal ligament; *DRC,* dorsal radiocapitate ligament; *DST,* dorsal scaphotriquetral ligament; *L,* lunate; *LRL,* long radiolunate ligament; *P,* pisiform; *S,* scaphoid; *SRL,* short radiolunate ligament; *T,* triquetrum; *UC,* ulnocapitate ligament; *UL,* ulnolunate ligament; *UT,* ulnotriquetral ligament. (From Butterfield WL, Joshi A, Lichtman D. Lunotriquetral injuries. J Am Soc Surg Hand 2:195-203, 2002.)

KINEMATICS AND INSTABILITY PATTERNS
- The proximal and distal carpal rows must move in a coordinated fashion to function as a stable joint.[2]
  - The proximal and distal rows move in synchrony with flexion and extension.
  - The movements are more complex during ulnar and radial deviation.
    - **Radial deviation:** The scaphoid flexes, the lunate and triquetrum follow passively into flexion with the scaphoid.
    - **Ulnar deviation:** The triquetrum is guided into extension by its articulation with the hamate, and the entire proximal row moves into extension with the triquetrum.
    - Coordinated carpal motion is possible because of the ligamentous support.
- When ligamentous support is absent, there is uncoordinated carpal motion (Fig. 53-2).
  - A scapholunate ligament disruption allows the lunate to extend when the scaphoid is flexed and creates a *dorsal intercalated segment instability* (DISI) deformity.
  - A lunotriquetral ligament injury permits lunate flexion with a normally aligned scaphoid and creates a volar (or palmar) intercalated segment instability (VISI) deformity.

Fig. 53-2   DISI and VISI deformities. *C*, Capitate; *L*, lunate; *R*, radius. (From Muzaffar AR, Hand V. Fractures and dislocations: The wrist: Congenital anomalies. Sel Read Plast Surg 9:36, 2003.)

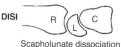

DISI

Scapholunate dissociation

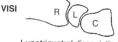

VISI

Lunotriquetral dissociation

LIGAMENTOUS INJURIES AND DISLOCATIONS

MECHANISM OF INJURY

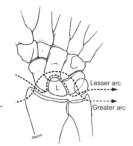

- **Mayfield** described the pathomechanics of progressive carpal injury.[3]
  - When loading occurs to the extended and ulnarly deviated wrist, the force dissipates through one of two arcs (Fig. 53-3).
    - ▶ **Greater arc:** Injury progresses through **carpal bones**
    - ▶ **Lesser arc:** Injury progresses only through **ligaments**

Fig. 53-3   Greater and lesser arcs of progressive carpal instability and injury. *L*, Lunate. (From Butterfield WL, Joshi A, Lichtman D. Lunotriquetral injuries. J Am Soc Surg Hand 2:195-203, 2002.)

TIP: Carpal dislocations and injuries usually result from extreme hyperextension, ulnar deviation, and intercarpal supination; they can be caused by motor vehicle collisions or falls from a height.

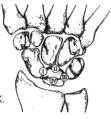

- In this model, ligamentous injuries occur in a **stepwise progression.**
  - Scapholunate
  - Midcarpal capsule (radioscaphocapitate ligament)
  - Lunotriquetral ligament
  - Dorsal radiocarpal ligament (Fig. 53-4)

Fig. 53-4   Stages of progressive perilunar instability. *I*, Scapholunate failure. *II*, Capitolunate failure. *III*, Triquetrolunate failure. *IV*, Dorsal radiocarpal ligament failure. (From Mayfield JK, Johnson RP, Kilcoyne RK. Carpal dislocation: Pathomechanics and progressive periulnar instability. J Hand Surg Am 5:226-241, 1980.)

LIGAMENTOUS INJURIES

- **Scapholunate (interosseous) ligament injuries**[4]
  - **Anatomy**
    - ▶ The scapholunate ligament is a C-shaped structure that connects the dorsal, proximal, and volar surfaces of the scaphoid and lunate (Fig. 53-5).
    - ▶ Several extrinsic volar ligaments lend additional support to the volar portion of this ligament.

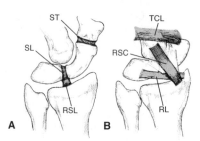

Fig. 53-5   A, Intrinsic ligaments. *RSL,* Radioscapholunate ligament; *SL,* scapholunate ligament; *ST,* scaphotrapezial ligament. **B,** Extrinsic ligaments. *RL,* radiolunate ligament; *RSC,* radioscaphocapitate ligament; *TCL,* transverse carpal ligament.

- **Mechanisms**
  - ▸ When an impact occurs to the hypothenar region, with the wrist in extension and ulnar deviation, the capitate is driven between the scaphoid and lunate. The lunate is pushed ulnarly and volarly; the scaphoid is pushed radially and dorsally.
    - ◆ The ligament will rupture given sufficient force, usually pulling away from the scaphoid and remaining attached to the lunate.
  - ▸ Abnormalities also can be congenital (usually bilateral) or degenerative (e.g., arthritis).
- **History**
  - ▸ Patients complain of **radial-sided wrist pain and weakness,** especially with loading activities.
  - ▸ Patients usually have a history of a fall or sudden load on the wrist.
- **Physical examination**
  - ▸ Radial-sided wrist edema
  - ▸ **Tenderness in radial snuffbox** or over the scapholunate interval just distal to Lister's tubercle
  - ▸ Discomfort at extremes of wrist extension and radial deviation
  - ▸ **Positive ballottement test:** Dorsal-volar stress of the scapholunate interval
  - ▸ **Positive Watson (scaphoid shift) test:** "Clunk" felt during dynamic wrist loading; scaphoid subluxates over dorsal rim of the radius when the wrist is moved from ulnar to radial deviation
- **Imaging**
  - ▸ Six views of the wrist: posteroanterior (PA), lateral, radial and ulnar deviation, flexion and extension
    - ◆ **Increased scapholunate gap (>3 mm):** Often called a *Terry Thomas sign,* referring to famous English comedian with large gap between his central incisors

---

TIP: The scapholunate gap always should be compared with the asymptomatic wrist because up to 5 mm is considered within normal limits.

  - ◆ *Cortical ring sign:* Represents hyperflexed scaphoid wherein the distal pole is seen on end and appears as a cortical ring within 7 mm of the proximal pole
  - ◆ Dorsiflexed lunate with a flexed scaphoid on lateral view: A DISI deformity
  - ◆ Increased scapholunate angle
  - ▸ **Cineradiography or stress radiographs:** Allow detection of dynamic injuries that are thought to occur with injury to only dorsal portion of the ligament
  - ▸ **Midcarpal or radiocarpal arthrography:** Used when standard radiographs are normal, as common in subacute injuries
    - ◆ Contrast defines complete injuries, partial injuries, and other wrist pathologies.
    - ◆ Contrast passing from the radiocarpal joint to the midcarpal joint indicates a perforation in the ligament.
  - ▸ **MRI**
    - ◆ Requires an experienced radiologist
    - ◆ Not well-supported in the literature[5]
  - ▸ **Arthroscopy**
    - ◆ **Gold standard for assessing the scapholunate ligament**
    - ◆ Aids staging the severity of the injury[6]
- **Treatment**
  - ▸ There is no consensus on the treatment of scapholunate ligament injuries.
  - ▸ Treatment options depend on the chronicity of the injury.
    - ◆ **Acute injuries:** Within **3 weeks** of injury

* **Subacute injuries:** Within **3-6 weeks** of injury
* **Chronic injuries:** Greater than **6 weeks** from injury
▶ Table 53-1 illustrates an algorithm for treatment.[4]

Table 53-1   *Surgical Treatment of Scapholunate Injuries*

Type	Radiographic Presentation	Treatment
Subacute	Dynamic deformity*	Conservative (splinting), arthroscopic pinning, capsulodesis
Acute	Static deformity	Open repair of SLIL
Late (chronic)	Static deformity	Open repair of SLIL and capsulodesis, capsulodesis alone, tenodesis alone, intercarpal fusion (STT or SC)

*Dynamic deformity is present during stress (motion radiographs); positive clinical stress testing, positive arthroscopy, but negative arthrogram and normal static radiographs.
SC, Scaphocapitate; *SLIL,* scapholunate interosseous ligament injury; *STT,* scaphotrapezial-trapezoid.
From Walsh JJ, Berger RA, Cooney WP, et al. Current status of scapholunate interosseous ligament injuries. J Am Acad Orthop Surg 10:32-42, 2002.

■ **Lunotriquetral ligament injuries**[7,8]
* **Anatomy**
  ▶ This is a C-shaped interosseous ligament spanning the proximal, volar, and dorsal surfaces of the lunate and triquetrum.
  ▶ The ligament allows coordinated motion between the triquetrum and lunate.
  ▶ Ligament injury results in the lunate flexing with the scaphoid and proximal migration of the triquetrum during ulnar deviation, showing a **VISI** pattern of instability.
* **Mechanism**
  ▶ Injury often occurs as part of progressive perilunate instability, mentioned previously (see Fig. 53-5).
    * Occurs as the event just before complete lunate dislocation
    * Results from forceful hyperextension and ulnar deviation
  ▶ Injury can also occur in isolation, showing a reverse perilunate instability pattern.[9]
    * Results from falling on outstretched hand in extension, with pronation and radial deviation
  ▶ Chronic degenerative conditions can also result in instability.[8]
    * Ulnar abutment syndrome
    * Inflammatory and crystalline arthropathies
* **History**
  ▶ Presentation is variable.
  ▶ Patients usually recall a specific inciting event, usually a fall on an outstretched hand.
  ▶ Symptoms may appear weeks to months following the injury.
  ▶ Patients complain of **ulnar-sided wrist pain and weakness,** exacerbated by heavy use of the hand.
  ▶ Patients may also describe a "clunk" or "clicking" when moving the wrist in radial-ulnar deviation.
* **Physical examination**
  ▶ Tenderness is found over the lunotriquetral joint, immediately deep to the extensor digiti minimi tendon.
  ▶ **Provocative tests**
    * **Positive ballottement test:** Increased anteroposterior laxity, with pain, in lunotriquetral interval
    * **Positive shear test:** Dorsal force directed on triquetrum while stabilizing the lunate demonstrates increased laxity and elicits pain

• **Positive lateral compression test:** Pressure placed on medial tubercle of the triquetrum between the flexor carpi ulnaris (FCU) and extensor carpi ulnaris (ECU) tendons elicits pain

> TIP: Always check positive provocative tests against the contralateral side.

• **Imaging**
  ▸ For patients with isolated lunotriquetral injuries, the radiographic appearance is often normal.
  ▸ **Obtain PA and lateral views of the wrist.**
    ◆ May not demonstrate any findings if injury stable (or dynamic)
    ◆ **Often a disruption in Gilula's arcs 1 and 2** (Fig. 53-6)
  ▸ The triquetrum moves proximally.
  ▸ Lunotriquetral overlap also can be present.
    ◆ Lateral view should be inspected for VISI deformity

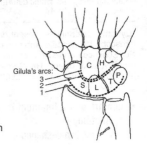

Fig. 53-6 Gilula's arcs: Smooth arcs that are formed by normal proximal and distal joint surfaces of the proximal carpal row (*1* and *2*) and the normal proximal joint surface of the capitate and hamate *(3)*. *C,* Capitate; *H,* hamate; *L,* lunate; *P,* pisiform; *S,* scaphoid; *T,* triquetrum. (From Butterfield WL, Joshi A, Lichtman D. Lunotriquetral injuries. J Am Soc Surg Hand 2:195-203, 2002.)

  ▸ **Cineradiography or stress radiographs (clenched fist, ulnar or radial deviation)** allow detection of dynamic injuries.
  ▸ **Midcarpal or radiocarpal arthrography**
    ◆ Rarely used
    ◆ Mostly replaced by arthroscopy
  ▸ **Arthroscopy[10]**
    ◆ **Gold standard for assessing lunotriquetral joint**
    ◆ Allows complete examination of wrist and triangular fibrocartilage complex
    ◆ Additionally, arthroscopic treatment can be performed for various soft tissue injuries
• **Treatment**
• **There is no consensus on the treatment of lunotriquetral injuries.**
• Treatment options depend on the **stability, chronicity,** and **severity** of the injury as well as the demands of the patient.
  ▸ **Nonsurgical management**
    ◆ Indicated for stable or degenerative conditions
    ◆ Immobilization using a molded cast with supporting pad under the pisiform or protective splint to prevent pronation
    ◆ Nonsteroidal antiinflammatory drugs or corticosteroid injections
    ◆ Consider arthroscopy if no improvement of symptoms within 6 weeks[7]
  ▸ **Surgical management**
    ◆ **Arthroscopic debridement**
      - Usually performed at same time as diagnostic arthroscopy
      - Debridement of synovial hyperplasia in the fibrocartilaginous portion for symptomatic relief[11]
    ◆ **Percutaneous pin fixation**
      - Only performed if no static VISI deformity
      - Arthroscopic guidance to examine the lunotriquetral alignment
      - Immobilization postoperatively for 8 weeks before pin removal and rehabilitation

* **Open repair**
  - Reserved for treating acute injuries
  - Dorsal or volar approaches
  - Ligament repaired directly with suture, bone tunnels, or suture anchors
  - Percutaneous pin fixation and immobilization also required
* **Ligament reconstruction**
  - Performed when treating chronic and severe injuries with attenuated ligament remnants
  - Slip of ECU passed through drill holes and looped around the lunate and triquetrum to reconstruct ligament
  - Also, osteoligamentous autografts may be used (from dorsal capitohamate joint or tarsal joints)
* **Lunotriquetral arthrodesis**
  - Consider for chronic dissociations
* **Salvage procedures**
  - Indicated for patients with long-term static VISI deformities
  - Options: Proximal row carpectomy, four-corner arthrodesis, or total wrist arthrodesis

PERILUNATE INJURIES AND PERILUNATE FRACTURE-DISLOCATIONS

- **Lesser-arc injuries (dorsal perilunate or lunate dislocations)**[3,12,13]
- **Anatomy**
  - ▸ The ligamentous anatomy of the wrist was reviewed earlier in this chapter.
  - ▸ **Space of Poirier**
    * Area on the volar wrist capsule devoid of substantial ligamentous stability
    * **Site of capsular weakness that tears during perilunate injury**
- **Mechanism**
  - ▸ As with scapholunate ligament injuries, these injuries result from forceful wrist hyperextension, ulnar deviation, and intercarpal supination.
  - ▸ **A progressive perilunate instability pattern ensues** (see Fig. 53-4).
    * Purely ligamentous injuries result from progressive injury along the **lesser arc** (see Fig. 53-3). **Stage I—Scapholunate dissociation:** Scaphoid is forced into extension while the lunate is restrained by extrinsic ligamentous support, and torque results in scapholunate ligament disruption.
    Stage II—Lunocapitate dislocation: Dorsal ligamentous attachments to lunate are disrupted, space of Poirier is torn volarly, and capitate is dislocated dorsally relative to lunate.
    Stage III—Lunotriquetral ligament disruption
    Stage IV—Lunate dislocation: External force pulls capitate proximally, which pushes lunate into volar dislocation after disruption of dorsal extrinsic ligamentous support.
    * Perilunate fracture-dislocations result from progression along the **greater arc** (see Fig. 53-3 and "Greater-Arc Injuries" later).
- **History**
  - ▸ Patients present with a painful and swollen wrist, after a high-energy hyperextension injury (usually a fall from a height or a motor vehicle collision).
- **Physical examination**
  - ▸ Wrist is acutely edematous.
  - ▸ Range of motion is very limited.
  - ▸ **Careful attention to sensation in the median nerve distribution is necessary.**

CAUTION: As the lunate dislocates, the median nerve can be compressed acutely. Carefully elicit signs and symptoms to facilitate early carpal tunnel release, if necessary.

- **Imaging**
  - ▸ Obtain PA and lateral views of the wrist.
    - ✦ **Gilula's arcs show multilevel disruption** with overlapping of bones across the midcarpal joint.
    - ✦ The lunate appears **triangular.**
    - ✦ The lateral view demonstrates the *spilled teapot sign* as the lunate tips volarly.
      - - Dorsal dislocation of the capitate (perilunate dislocation) or complete volar dislocation of the lunate (lunate dislocation) are seen with severe injuries.
  - ▸ Traction views, CT scans, or repeat radiographs (after reduction) are required to accurately diagnose any articular fractures obscured by a bony overlap.
- **Treatment**
  - ▸ **Closed reduction and immobilization**
    - ✦ *Closed reduction is the first step in all treatment methods.*

TIP: Closed reduction is performed most easily with a regional block and intravenous sedation. 10-15 minutes of uninterrupted traction should precede any attempt at reduction.

  - - **Tavernier's method** (Fig. 53-7)
    - ✦ Immobilization for 3 to 12 weeks is advocated by most surgeons.
  - ▸ Careful follow-up with serial radiographs is necessary because loss of reduction can occur.

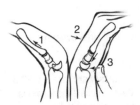

Fig. 53-7   Tavernier's method for reduction of perilunate dislocations. *1,* Apply manual traction on the slightly extended wrist. *2,* Stabilize the lunate volarly with a thumb and slowly flex the wrist without releasing traction until a snap occurs. This indicates that the proximal pole of the capitate has overcome the dorsal lip of the lunate. *3,* Traction is released and the wrist is brought back to neutral or slight flexion. Check reduction with a radiograph.

  - ▸ **Closed reduction and percutaneous pin fixation**
    - ✦ Careful reduction is obtained, and slight adjustments to carpal alignment are made intraoperatively.
    - ✦ Percutaneous pins are placed to hold reduction.
    - ✦ Immobilize with cast (initially) and then use a splint for 12 weeks.
  - ▸ **Open reduction, internal fixation, and ligament repair**
    - ✦ **Most surgeons consider this method the treatment of choice.**
    - ✦ This method allows for removal of intraarticular debris, more accurate reduction, and direct repair of ligamentous injuries (scapholunate ligament and volar capsule).
    - ✦ Dorsal or dorsal-volar combination approaches are used.

CARPAL FRACTURE-DISLOCATIONS

GREATER-ARC INJURIES[12,13]

- If force travels along the greater arc (see Fig. 53-3), **bony fractures** rather than ligament injuries are generated.
- Injuries are named as perilunate dislocations along with associated fractures.
  - **Transscaphoid perilunate dislocation:** Fracture of scaphoid

> TIP: Transscaphoid perilunate dislocation is the most common pattern of carpal dislocation.

  - **Transscaphoid, transcapitate perilunate dislocation:** Fracture of scaphoid and capitate

> TIP: The proximal pole of the capitate fractures and rotates 90 to 180 degrees, making closed reduction nearly impossible.

  - **Transscaphoid, transcapitate, transtriquetral perilunate dislocation:** Extremely rare
  - **Transtriquetral perilunate dislocation:** Fracture of triquetrum
- Treatment options are identical to those for lesser-arc injuries.
  - **Open reduction and internal fixation** is treatment of choice

AXIAL FRACTURE-DISLOCATIONS[14]

- These injuries usually result from a severe crush with dorsal-volar compression.
- The carpus divides longitudinally, with one portion remaining aligned with the radius and the other displacing to the radial or ulnar side; the metacarpals follow their carpal attachments.
- **Types** (Fig. 53-8)
  - **Axial-radial fracture-dislocations:** Radial column of carpus displaced distally and radially
    - ▶ Peritrapezoid
    - ▶ Peritrapezium
    - ▶ Transtrapezium
  - **Axial-ulnar fracture-dislocations:** Ulnar column displaced proximally and ulnarly
    - ▶ Transhamate peripisiform
    - ▶ Perihamate peripisiform
    - ▶ Perihamate transtriquetrum
- Associated soft tissue (vessel, nerve, and tendon) injuries are almost universal in these injury patterns.
- Dorsal approaches obtain fracture reduction and fixation.
- Volar approaches are necessary to repair associated soft tissue injuries.
- Outcomes are limited by associated tendon and nerve injuries.

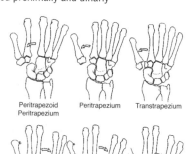

Peritrapezoid   Peritrapezium   Transtrapezium
Peritrapezium

Transhamate   Perihamate   Perihamate
peripisiform   peripisiform   transtriquetrum

Fig. 53-8   Axial fracture-dislocations of the carpus. (From Yaghoubian R, Goebel F, Musgrave DS, et al. Diagnosis and management of acute fracture-dislocation of the carpus. Orthop Clin North Am 32:295-305, 2001.)

ISOLATED CARPAL DISLOCATIONS[12]

- Isolated carpal bone dislocations, without the patterns described here, are extremely rare.
- These dislocations can occur when a localized force is concentrated over a single carpal bone.
- Treatment options include closed reduction, carpal bone excision, or open reduction and internal fixation.

KEY POINTS

✔ Carpal instability patterns are usually predictable.
✔ Lesser-arc injuries are ligamentous, and greater-arc injuries are bony.
✔ Scapholunate and lunotriquetral ligament injuries are best evaluated by wrist arthroscopy.
✔ Perilunate dislocations and fracture-dislocations should be treated with early open reduction, internal fixation, and ligament repair, when possible.

REFERENCES

1. Idler RS. Anatomy and biomechanics of the digital flexor tendons. Hand Clin 1:3-11, 1985.
2. Horii E, Garcia-Elias M, An KN, et al. A kinematic study of the lunotriquetral dissociations. J Hand Surg Am 23:425-431, 1998.
3. Mayfield J, Johnson RP, Kilcoyne RK, et al. Carpal dislocation: Pathomechanics and progressive perilunar instability. J Hand Surg Am 5:226-241, 1980.
4. Walsh JJ, Berger RA, Cooney WP, et al. Current status of scapholunate interosseous ligament injuries. J Am Acad Orthop Surg 10:32-42, 2002.
5. Cooney WP, Dobyns JH, Linscheid RL, et al. Arthroscopy of the wrist: Anatomy and classification of carpal instability. Arthroscopy 6:133-140, 1990.
6. Geissler WB, Freeland AE, Savoie FH, et al. Intracarpal soft-tissue lesions associated with an intra-articular fracture of the distal end of the radius. J Bone Joint Surg Am 78:357-365, 1996.
7. Butterfield WL, Joshi A, Lichtman D, et al. Lunotriquetral injuries. J Am Soc Surg Hand 2:195-203, 2002.
8. Berger RA. Lunotriquetral joint. In Berger RA, Weiss A-PC, eds. Hand Surgery. Philadelphia: Lippincott, 2004, pp 495-509.
9. Reagan DS, Linscheid RL, Dobyns JH, et al. Lunotriquetral sprains. J Hand Surg Am 9:502-514, 1984.
10. Osterman AL, Seidman G. The role of arthroscopy in the treatment of lunatotriquetral ligament injuries. Hand Clin 11:41-50, 1995.
11. Weiss AP, Sachar K, Glowack KA, et al. Arthroscopic debridement alone for intercarpal ligament tears. J Hand Surg Am 22:344-349, 1997.
12. Garcia-Elias M, Geissler WB. Carpal instability. In Green DP, Hotchkiss RN, Pederson WC, et al, eds. Green's Operative Hand Surgery, 5th ed. Philadelphia: Churchill Livingstone, 2005.
13. Garcia-Elias M. Perilunar injuries including fracture dislocations. In Berger RA, Weiss A-PC, eds. Hand Surgery. Philadelphia: Lippincott, 2004, pp 511-523.
14. Yaghoubian R, Goebel F, Musgrave DS, et al. Diagnosis and management of acute fracture-dislocation of the carpus. Orthop Clin North Am 32:295-305, 2001.

54. Metacarpal and Phalangeal Fractures

Danielle M. LeBlanc

DEMOGRAPHICS

- **Most common fractures of the upper extremity**
- **Outer rays** (thumb and fifth finger) most commonly injured
- Incidence peaks between ages 10 and 40 years

ANATOMY

- **Diaphysis:** Main shaft of bone
- **Metaphysis:** Flared end of bone
- **Physis:** Growth plate

FRACTURE TERMINOLOGY

- **Closed:** Intact skin over fracture and hematoma
- **Open:** Wound allowing interaction between fracture and environment
- **Simple:** Two bone fragments
- **Comminuted:** More than two bone fragments
- **Transverse:** Fracture perpendicular to long axis of bone
- **Oblique:** Fracture tangential to long axis of bone
- **Spiral:** Fracture plane oblique and rotated
- **Impaction:** End-on stress force causing compression without displacement
- **Longitudinal:** Parallel to long axis of bone
- **Pathologic:** Fracture in tumor-laden or osteoporotic bone
- **Stress:** Fracture in normal bone caused by cyclic loading
- **Greenstick:** Incomplete fracture involving only one cortex
- **Avulsion:** Bone chip caused by distraction forces on tendon or ligament
- **Intraarticular:** Through articular surface

SALTER-HARRIS FRACTURE CLASSIFICATION: PEDIATRIC FRACTURES (Fig. 54-1)

Salter-Harris I: Through growth plate only
Salter-Harris II: Through metaphysis and growth plate
Salter-Harris III: Through epiphysis and growth plate
Salter-Harris IV: Through epiphysis, growth plate, and metaphysis
Salter-Harris V: Crushed growth plate

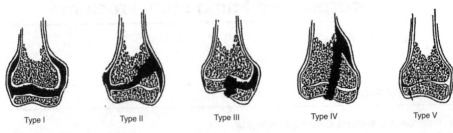

Type I   Type II   Type III   Type IV   Type V

Fig. 54-1   Salter-Harris fracture classifications. (From Crenshaw AH. Surgical approach. In Crenshaw AH, ed. Campbell's Operative Orthopedics, 7th ed. St Louis: Mosby, 1987.)

THREE PHASES OF FRACTURE HEALING

INFLAMMATION
- Starts immediately and lasts several days
- Formation of hematoma
- Infiltration of hematopoietic cells and osteogenic precursors

REPAIR
- Begins at less than 24 hours and peaks at 2-3 weeks
- Collagen deposition and cartilaginous callus formation over fracture site
- Endochondral ossification

REMODELING
- Lasts months to years depending on type of fracture
- Lamellar bone formation and repopulation of marrow
- Resorption of callus

TIP: External callus is not visible on plain radiographs until 3-6 weeks after formation. Clinical bony union averages 4-8 weeks; however, total bony healing time is approximately 5-7 months.[1]

DIAGNOSIS

- History and physical examination of the hand are covered in Chapter 50.
- Radiographic evaluation includes three views.
  - Anteroposterior
  - Lateral
  - Oblique

TREATMENT

A treatment plan depends on many factors:
- Patient age, occupation, health, and compliance

- Fracture location and geometry
- Clinical deformity
- Open or closed classification
- Associated soft tissue injury
- Stability

COMPLICATIONS

INFECTION
- Incidence 2.04%-11% in open fractures
- Usually results from contaminated wound or delay in treatment
- Antibiotics generally recommended for 24 hours for open fractures
- Management: Eradicate sepsis, obtain union of fracture, and regain function

MALUNION
- **Malrotation:** Functional impairment caused by digital overlap on flexion
- **Angulation:** Lateral or volar angle deformity
- **Shortening:** Prevents balance of extensor or flexor excursion
- All types of malunion: Usually corrected with osteotomy, with or without bone graft

NONUNION
Nonunion occurs when fracture site fails to heal.
- Usually results from unstable fracture reduction, contamination
- Treatment: Corrective osteotomy and possible bone graft

LOSS OF MOTION
- Tendon adhesions
- Capsular contracture
- Immobilization for more than 4 weeks
- Associated joint injury
- Multiple fractures per finger
- Crush injury

METACARPAL FRACTURES

METACARPAL HEAD FRACTURES
- Rare occurrence
- Result from axial loading, direct trauma, dislocation
- Usually intraarticular
- **Indications for treatment**[2]
  - **Nonoperative**
    - ► Closed fractures with articular congruency
    - ► Metacarpophalangeal (MP) joint stability by stress testing
    - ► Less than 20% articular surface involvement

- **Operative**
  - ▶ **Greater than 1 mm** articular step-off
  - ▶ Fixation technique depends on fragment size and number
- ■ **Treatment**[1]
  - **Simple fractures**
    - ▶ Surgically treated, open using dorsal approach with minicondylar plate or screws
    - ▶ K-wires also used, but may delay joint mobilization
  - **Comminuted fractures**
    - ▶ K-wire fixation or cerclage wire preferred because less risk of avascular necrosis
    - ▶ External fixator required if proximal phalanx also fractured or severe soft tissue loss
  - **Severe comminuted fractures**
    - ▶ May benefit from implant arthroplasty **except in index finger** (implant failure common because of shear stress), **extensive metacarpal bone loss**, or **extensive soft tissue loss**
    - ▶ MP arthrodesis only a salvage procedure

METACARPAL NECK FRACTURES

- ■ Common occurrence
- ■ Occur when axial load applied to clenched fist
- ■ **Apex dorsal angulation** because intrinsic muscles lie volar to axis of rotation of MP joint and maintain flexed head posture[1]
- ■ Nonunion rare, malunion common
- ■ *Boxer's fracture:* Small metacarpal neck fracture
- ■ **Indications for treatment**
  - **Angulation deformity**
    - ▶ Index and middle fingers: At least 10-15 degrees
    - ▶ Ring finger: At least 30-40 degrees
    - ▶ Small finger: At least 50-60 degrees
  - **Rotational deformity** or **"scissoring"**: Digital overlap in flexion
  - **Shortening:** Greater than 3 mm

TIP: Fracture angulation is better compensated by ring and small fingers because carpometacarpal (CMC) joints have 20-30 degrees of mobility in sagittal plane, whereas index and middle fingers are less mobile at CMC joint.

- ■ **Treatment**[1,2]
  - **Closed reduction**
    - ▶ Perform under local anaesthetic or hematoma block.
    - ▶ **Jahss maneuver:** Flexing the MP joint to 90 degrees relaxes the intrinsic muscles and tightens collateral ligaments, allowing proximal phalanx to place upward pressure on metacarpal (MC) head while placing downward pressure on metacarpal shaft.
    - ▶ Stable reduction is held by molded splint with wrist neutral, MP joint flexed 90 degrees, and proximal interphalangeal (PIP) joint in extension for 12-14 days.
    - ▶ Unstable reduction can be treated by crossed K-wires or transverse K-wires applied to intact adjacent metacarpal shaft.

TIP: Closed reduction is difficult if fracture is more than 5-7 days old.[3]

- **Open reduction**
  - ▸ Dorsal approach is through a longitudinal incision adjacent to extensor tendon overlying fractured metacarpal; juncturae tendinum can be divided and repaired with permanent suture.
  - ▸ Use K-wires or minicondylar plate.
  - ▸ Immobilize for 10 days in molded splint; confirm alignment using radiography, then protect active range of motion.

METACARPAL SHAFT FRACTURES

- **Transverse, oblique, or spiral fractures**
  - • **Transverse:** Produced by axial loading through metacarpal head or direct blow
  - • **Oblique** and **spiral:** Fractures from torsional forces
- **Apex dorsal angulation:** Caused by interosseous muscles
- **Indications for treatment:**
  - • **Dorsal angulation**
    - ▸ Index or middle fingers: At least 10 degrees
    - ▸ Ring finger: At least 20 degrees
    - ▸ Small finger: At least 30 degrees
  - • **Rotational deformity:** Digital overlap in flexion
  - • **Shortening in excess of 3 mm:** Alters length-tension relationship of intrinsic muscles causing weakness

---

TIP: 10 degrees of rotation equals 1.5 cm of digital overlap.[4]

- **Treatment**
  - • **Nonoperative reduction**
    - ▸ Plaster immobilization in cast with wrist in 30 degrees extension, MP joints flexed 80-90 degrees, and interphalangeal (IP) joints extended until fracture site not tender, then mobilized
  - • **Operative reduction**
    - ▸ Indicated for **unstable reductions, multiple fractures, or open fractures**
    - ▸ Fixation method dependent on fracture pattern
    - ▸ Exposure through longitudinal dorsal incision adjacent to extensor tendon that overlies fractured metacarpal; juncturae tendinum divided and repaired with permanent suture; reduction held with bone clamps
    - ▸ **K-wire fixation:** Two parallel wires set transverse into adjacent metacarpal shaft
    - ▸ **Lag screw fixation:** Prevents compression and torsional forces; two bicortical screws placed at minimum two-screw diameter from fracture line, one in plane of fracture and one in plane that bisects longitudinal axis
    - ▸ **Plate fixation:** Requires four cortex (2-screw) fixation proximal and distal to fracture; plates can interfere with tendon excursion

---

TIP: Use lag screw technique for oblique or spiral fracture, when the ratio of length of fracture plane to width of bone is 2:1 to 3:1 at the fracture site.

SEGMENTAL LOSS OF METACARPAL SHAFT

NOTE: Segmental loss almost always involves open injury with soft tissue loss; initial management requires debridement.

- **Treatment**
  - Provisional stabilization and maintenance of metacarpal length is achieved with external fixator, transfixion pins, or spacer wires.
  - Immediate or delayed corticocancellous or cancellous bone grafting is performed with or without fixation.
  - Timing depends on stability of soft tissue coverage.

METACARPAL BASE FRACTURES

- Rare occurrence
- Result from axial load on volar flexed wrist or partially flexed thumb
- Usually intraarticular
- ***Bennett fracture:*** Unstable intraarticular fracture; subluxation of thumb at the volar ulnar aspect of the metacarpal base; anterior oblique ligament holds the fragment in anatomic position while remainder of base rotates away radially and dorsally
- ***Reverse Bennett fracture:*** Unstable intraarticular fracture; dislocation of fifth metacarpal base causing proximal and dorsal subluxation of metacarpal; displacement accentuated by flexor carpi ulnaris, extensor carpi ulnaris, and abductor digiti minimi
- ***Rolando fracture:*** Any comminuted intraarticular fracture of thumb metacarpal base
- **Indications for treatment**
  - **Usually operative** because of unstable dislocation component
  - Open versus closed technique depends on fracture morphology

---

TIP: Open reduction is indicated in multiple CMC joint dislocations.

- **Treatment**
  - **Simple fractures:** Closed, reduced, and stabilized with K-wire fixation
  - **Closed Bennett reduction technique:** Longitudinal traction with pressure on metacarpal base and thumb pronation; K-wires placed through thumb metacarpal into trapezium and second metacarpal
  - **Open Bennett fracture technique:** Performed through radial border incision located between abductor pollicis and thenar muscles with screw or K-wire fixation

---

TIP: No pin is necessary with a Bennett fracture fragment.

- **Rolando fracture fixation:** Closed K-wire preferred because of comminuted fragments; if feasible, miniplate fixation on larger fragments
- **Severely comminuted fractures:** May require oblique traction pin or quadrilateral external fixator
- **Reverse Bennett fracture dislocations:** Treated with closed reduction and K-wire fixation to fourth metacarpal and hamate
- **Open Reverse Bennett reduction:** Performed through dorsal ulnar incision with protection of dorsal sensory branch of ulnar nerve; fixation held with multiple K-wires

PHALANGEAL FRACTURES

DISTAL PHALANX FRACTURES

- Distal phalanx fractures are the **most commonly encountered fracture of the hand.**
- **Thumb** and **middle finger** are most commonly injured.
- See Chapters 56 and 57 for fingertip and nailbed injuries.
- **Classification**
  - **Tuft fractures**
    - ▶ Occur secondary to crushing injury
    - ▶ Involve laceration of nail matrix and pulp
  - **Shaft fractures**
    - ▶ Transverse or longitudinal orientation
  - **Intraarticular fractures**
    - ▶ Avulsion fracture of insertion of extensor tendon called **mallet finger**
    - ▶ Dorsal base fracture with secondary mallet finger deformity caused by hyperextension of distal interphalangeal (DIP) joint
    - ▶ Epiphyseal separation from hyperflexion common in children; can result in foreshortened digit and decreased range of motion at DIP joint
    - ▶ Volar base fracture from forceful flexion and profundus tendon avulsion
- **Treatment**
  - **Nondisplaced** fractures stabilized by surrounding tissue
  - **Comminuted** fragments reduced by careful approximation of soft tissues
  - **Displaced** fractures stabilized with longitudinal K-wires
  - Immobilization with finger cast for less than 3 weeks, excluding PIP joint

---

TIP: Comminuted tuft fractures often fail to unite but are stabilized by fibrous union.[5]

- Symptomatic nonunion may be treated by crossed K-wires and bone graft using open volar midline approach.[6]
- **Mallet finger** treatment discussed in Chapter 59.

MIDDLE AND PROXIMAL PHALANX FRACTURES[7]

- **Classification**[1,8]
  - **Unicondylar fractures**
    - ▶ Classified by Weiss and Hastings[9]
    - ▶ Inherently unstable
  - **Bicondylar fractures**
    - ▶ Nearly always displaced and comminuted
    - ▶ Difficult to treat
  - **Neck fractures**
    - ▶ Subcapital fractures uncommon in adults but common in children
  - **Shaft fractures**
    - ▶ Transverse, spiral, or oblique

> TIP: Proximal phalanx shaft fractures angle apex-volar because of flexion of the proximal fragment by the interossei. Middle phalanx shaft fractures can angle apex-volar or apex-dorsal, depending on the location of the fracture in relation to the insertion of the flexor digitorum superficialis (FDS) tendon.[10]

- **Base fractures**
  - ▸ Typically involve impaction with **apex volar** angulation
  - ▸ Up to 25 degrees of angulation tolerated but may result in loss of motion
  - ▸ *Malunion:* **"Pseudoclawing"** possible when hyperextension of MP at fracture site and extensor lag at PIP joint
  - ▸ **Lateral volar base avulsions:** Result of detached collateral ligament
  - ▸ **Gamekeeper's thumb:** Proximal phalanx avulsion of ulnar collateral ligament at ulnar volar base
  - ▸ **Dorsal base avulsion fractures:** From detached central slip with PIP dislocation (see Chapter 55)
- **Pilon fractures**
  - ▸ Comminuted intraarticular fractures at base of middle phalanx
  - ▸ Caused by axial load
- **Treatment**
  - **Articular fractures (condylar)**
    - ▸ Require stabilization with K-wires, miniplates or lag screws, depending on fracture morphology
    - ▸ Displaced fractures require open reduction using dorsal approach through central slip and lateral band
  - **Neck fractures**
    - ▸ **Nondisplaced fractures:** Can be treated with closed reduction and splinting
    - ▸ **Displaced fractures:** Head fragment often rotated 90 degrees with articular surface facing dorsal and fracture surface volar
    - ▸ Open reduction from dorsal approach with displacement of interposed volar plate and stabilization with K-wires
  - **Shaft fractures**
    - ▸ **Stable, nondisplaced fractures:** Require splinting in "safe" position (James' position) with MP flexion at 70 degrees and IP joints in extension to prevent collateral ligament and volar plate contracture
    - ▸ **Unstable, displaced fractures:** May require closed fixation with K-wires, lag screws, interosseous wires, or miniplates
    - ▸ **Comminuted shaft fractures:** May require external fixator
  - **Base fractures**
    - ▸ Reduction or correction osteotomy: Required if **angulation is at least 25 degrees** to prevent loss of motion and pseudoclaw deformity (hyperextension of MP at fracture site with extensor lag)
    - ▸ **Gamekeeper's thumb:** Requires fixation of fragment displacement that is at least 2 mm; also requires thumb spica immobilization
    - ▸ Displaced collateral ligament avulsion fractures of all other digits: Require open reduction and repair if joint laterally unstable
  - **Pilon fractures**
    - ▸ Usually require open reduction and fixation combined with dynamic splinting to preserve articular surface

INDICATIONS FOR METACARPAL AND PHALANGEAL FRACTURE FIXATION

Irreducible fractures
Malrotation (spinal and short oblique)
Intraarticular fractures
Subcapital fractures (phalangeal)
Open fractures
Segmental bone loss
Polytrauma with hand fractures
Multiple hand or wrist fractures
Fractures with soft tissue injury (e.g., vessel, tendon, nerve, skin)
Reconstruction (e.g., osteotomy)

From Stern PJ. Fractures of the metacarpals and phalanges. In Green DP, Hotchkiss RN, Pederson WC, eds. Green's Operative Hand Surgery, 4th ed. Philadelphia: Churchill Livingstone, 1999, pp 711-771.

KEY POINTS

✔ The Salter-Harris classification is used only with pediatric fractures.

✔ In general, metacarpal and phalangeal fractures are addressed operatively if there is scissoring, rotation, or shortening.

✔ The Jahss maneuver may help with closed reduction of a fifth metacarpal neck fracture (boxer's fracture).

✔ It only takes a small amount of rotation to produce a significant amount of digital overlap.

✔ Lag screws are ideal for large oblique fractures and should be placed perpendicular to the fracture and the long axis of the bone. Both should be at least 2 screw-head diameters away from the fracture.

✔ Avoid opening comminuted fractures, if possible.

REFERENCES

1. Stern PJ. Fractures of the metacarpals and phalanges. In Green DP, Hotchkiss RN, Pederson WC, eds. Green's Operative Hand Surgery, 4th ed. Philadelphia: Churchill Livingstone, 1999, pp 711-771.
2. Weinstein LP, Hanel DP. Metacarpal fractures. J Hand Surg Am 2:168-180, 2002.
3. Opgrande JD, Westphal SA. Fractures of the hand. Orthop Clin North Am 14:779-792, 1983.
4. Freeland AE, Jabaley ME, Hughes JL. Stable Fixation of the Hand and Wrist. New York: Springer-Verlag, 1986, p 55.
5. Schneider LH. Fractures of the distal phalanx. Hand Clin 4:537-547, 1988.
6. Itoh Y, Uchinishi K, Oka Y. Treatment of pseudarthrosis of the distal phalanx with the palmar midline approach. J Hand Surg Am 8:80-84, 1983.
7. Freeland AE, Sud V. Unicondylar and bicondylar proximal phalangeal fractures. J Hand Surg Am 1:14-24, 2001.
8. London PS. Sprains and fractures involving the interphalangeal joints. Hand 3:155-158, 1971.
9. Weiss AP, Hastings H II. Distal unicondylar fractures of the proximal phalanx. J Hand Surg Am 18:594-599,1993.
10. McNealy RW, Lichtenstein ME. Fractures of the metacarpals and phalanges. West J Surg Obstet Gynecol 43:156-161, 1935.

55. Phalangeal Dislocations

Rohit K. Khosla

CLINICAL EVALUATION OF THE JOINT[1-3]

- Assess functional stability of the joint under digital or wrist block.
- **Active stability**
  - Evaluate active range of motion of the involved joint.
  - Full or near-complete range of motion indicates joint stability.
  - *Dislocation with motion indicates an unstable joint.*
- **Passive stability**
  - Lateral stress is applied to joint at full extension and at 30 degrees of flexion to assess integrity of collateral ligaments.
  - Dorsal stress and volar stress are applied to joint.
  - Compare joint laxity with an uninjured digit and contralateral digit to confirm injury from patient's normal joint laxity.
- Review routine plain radiographs, which must include at least two views of the hand or digit (antero-posterior, lateral).
- Joint may dislocate in **dorsal, lateral,** or **volar** direction.

NOTE: Dislocations are described according to the position of the distal bone relative to normal joint alignment.

GRADING OF COLLATERAL LIGAMENT SPRAIN

Grade I: Gross stability with microscopic tear
Grade II: A grossly intact ligament with some abnormal laxity when joint is stressed
Grade III: Complete tear of collateral ligament with gross instability

FINGER METACARPOPHALANGEAL JOINT

ANATOMY
- **Features of metacarpophalangeal (MP) joint ligament box complex that resist ligament injury and dislocation**
  - Protected position at base of finger
  - Intrinsic ligamentous structure
  - Surrounding support structures, which include flexor and extensor tendon systems, sagittal bands, and tendons of the intrinsic muscles
- **Volar plate**
  - Forms floor of joint
  - Supported laterally by deep transverse metacarpal (intervolar plate) ligament that links each ligament box complex to the adjacent joint (Fig. 55-1).

540

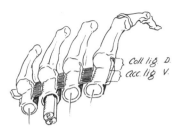

Fig. 55-1 The intervolar plate ligaments span in a transverse direction and link the ligament box complex of each MP joint, and provide increased stability to the volar plate. (From Eaton RG, Littler JW. Joint injuries and their sequelae. Clin Plast Surg 3:85-98, 1976.)

- **Cam effect**
  - A cam is a construct that translates rotary motion into linear motion.
  - The rotary flexion of the MP joint places linear stretch on the collateral ligaments.
  - The metacarpal head has a nonspherical shape and is wider on the volar side. Therefore the collateral ligaments become stretched taut in flexion relative to extension.
  - There is broader, more stable articulation between the metacarpal head and proximal phalanx with more than 70 degrees of flexion. **This produces increased lateral stability when the MP joint is in flexion and allows for some abduction-adduction when the joint is in extension.**

DORSAL MP JOINT DISLOCATION
- Usual mechanism of injury is **forced hyperextension of digit** (e.g., from a fall on an outstretched hand).
- These injuries are rare and are primarily seen in the **index finger** followed by the **small finger**.

TIP: Central digit MP dislocation is seen only with concomitant dislocation of a border digit.

CLASSIFICATION OF DORSAL MP JOINT DISLOCATION
- **Simple MP subluxation**
  - **Incomplete dislocation:** Proximal phalanx is locked in 60-80 degrees of hyperextension.
  - Reduce by flexing the wrist to relax flexor tendons. Then apply gentle distal and volar traction to the base of the proximal phalanx.
- **Complex MP subluxation**
  - **Complete and irreducible dislocation:** Metacarpal head protrudes volarly between the lumbrical and flexor tendons. Volar plate becomes impinged in the previous joint space.
  - Flexor tendon sheath remains attached to the volar plate and is held taut. Distal joints are held in flexion. This maintains a tight tendon-lumbrical encirclement and prevents reduction.
  - **Requires open reduction and release of the A1 pulley:** This relaxes the tension of the tendon-lumbrical mechanism.
  - Immobilize the MP joint postoperatively in 30 degrees of flexion for 2 weeks. Then allow active range of motion with 10-degree dorsal blocking splint for 2 weeks.

VOLAR MP JOINT DISLOCATION
- These injuries are extremely rare.
- **Mostly managed with closed reduction.** If unsuccessful, proceed with open reduction.

COLLATERAL LIGAMENT RUPTURE OF MP JOINT
- Isolated ulnar collateral ligament (UCL) rupture is extremely rare.
- Isolated radial collateral ligament (RCL) rupture is more common.

- Seen typically in athletes after forced ulnar deviation of digit with MP joints flexed.
- Typically seen in ulnar three digits.
- Typically presents late with persistent swelling and dysfunction of involved digit.
- Tenderness on radial aspect of joint. Pain with passive MP flexion. Instability of joint with ulnar deviation of proximal phalanx.
- **Treatment of RCL rupture**
  - Immobilize joint in 30 degrees of flexion for 3 weeks.
  - Reevaluate joint laxity at 3 weeks. Buddy-tape to adjacent digit for additional 2-3 weeks if joint instability persists.
  - Surgical repair indicated if instability or pain persists after more than 6 weeks of nonoperative treatment.

THUMB METACARPOPHALANGEAL JOINT

ANATOMY
- Range of motion of the thumb MP joint is the most variable in the body.
- Primary arc of motion is flexion-extension. Minor arcs of motion are abduction-adduction and pronation-supination.
- **Collateral ligaments** provide lateral stability.
  - **Proper collateral ligaments** arise from condyles of the metacarpal head and insert on the volar proximal phalanx.
  - **Accessory collateral ligaments** originate on the volar metacarpal head and insert on the sesamoid bones and volar plate.
  - Additional lateral stability is provided by thenar muscle secondary insertions via adductor and abductor aponeuroses.
- Volar support of the joint is provided by the volar plate and thenar intrinsic muscle insertions to sesamoid bones.

ACUTE UCL INJURY (SKIER'S THUMB)[4]
- **UCL** injuries are 10 times more common than **RCL** injuries in the thumb MP joint.
- Usually occur from forced radial deviation of the joint (e.g., falling on an outstretched hand with thumb abducted).

TIP: *Distal* tears of the UCL insertion are five times more common than *proximal* tears.

- **Avulsion fractures** of the proximal phalanx can occur with UCL tear.
  - Typically they are small fracture fragments that do not involve the articular surface. Manage with cast immobilization.
  - Large fracture fragments with more than 2 mm displacement require closed reduction percutaneous pinning (CRPP) or open reduction and internal fixation (ORIF).
- **Stener lesion**
  - Occurs only with complete UCL rupture.
  - Adductor aponeurosis sweeps the loose ligament away from its insertion on joint realignment.
  - **The UCL will not heal in this situation without surgical repair.**

- **Treatment of acute UCL ruptures**
  - **Partial UCL tears** are effectively treated with **cast immobilization** for 4 weeks. Follow with 2 weeks of splint immobilization with active range-of-motion exercises.
  - **Complete UCL** tears require **operative exploration and repair.**
    - ▸ Reattach ligament avulsions with a bone-anchoring technique.
    - ▸ Central ligament tears can be repaired with nonabsorbable braided sutures.
    - ▸ Immobilize postoperatively in thumb spica cast for 4 weeks. Follow with 2 weeks of splint immobilization and active range-of-motion exercises.

CHRONIC UCL INJURY (GAMEKEEPER'S THUMB)

- Seen in patients with untreated acute complete tear, unrecognized Stener lesion, or progressive attenuation of UCL.
- Patients present with chronic pain, swelling, and weakness of affected thumb.
  - *Chronic* is defined as symptoms **lasting longer than 6 weeks.**
- Need to rule out osteoarthritis of joint on plain radiographs before reconstruction.
- Surgical reconstruction of ligament best achieved with free tendon graft.
  - Must resect all scar and remnant of the UCL.
  - Options for tendon graft include palmaris longus, strip of flexor carpi radialis (FCR), abductor pollicus longus (APL), plantaris, or toe extensor.
  - Immobilize postoperatively in thumb spica cast for 6 weeks. Follow with 2 weeks of splint immobilization and active range-of-motion exercises.

RCL INJURY

- Occurs with forced adduction or torsion on a flexed MP joint
- No equivalent Stener-type lesion because abductor aponeurosis is much broader than adductor aponeurosis and prevents ligament interposition
- Can be torn on the proximal or distal end
- Treatment of acute RCL ruptures
  - **Manage partial tears nonoperatively,** similar to partial UCL injury.
  - Isolated complete tears can be managed nonoperatively, similar to partial tear.
  - **Operative repair** is indicated for **complete tears associated with volar subluxation of the proximal phalanx.** Repair with free tendon graft similar to complete UCL reconstruction.

DORSAL DISLOCATION OF THUMB MP JOINT

- Much more common than volar dislocations
- Seen with hyperextension injuries that cause complete rupture of volar plate with at least partial tear of collateral ligaments
- Most are easily reducible
  - Immobilize in 20 degrees of MP joint flexion for 2 weeks. Follow with active flexion in 20-degree dorsal blocking splint.
  - Immobilize for up to 4 weeks if there is a significant collateral ligament injury.

TIP: Irreducible dislocations are a result of entrapment of the volar plate, sesamoid bone, or flexor pollicis longus (FPL) and require open reduction.

PROXIMAL INTERPHALANGEAL JOINT

Dislocation of the proximal interphalangeal (PIP) joint is the most common ligament injury in the hand.

ANATOMY
- Normal 100- to 110-degree arc of rotation
- **Lateral collateral ligaments**
  - 2-3 mm thick
  - **Proper collateral ligament:** Inserts on volar base of middle phalanx
  - **Accessory collateral ligament:** Inserts on volar plate
  - Avulse proximally in 85% of injuries
- **Volar plate**
  - Forms floor of joint and is suspended laterally by collateral ligaments
  - Confluent with periosteum of proximal and middle phalanx
  - Prevents hyperextension and allows for full flexion
  - Secondary stabilizer against lateral deviation of joint when collateral ligaments are incompetent or torn
- **Ligament box complex** (Fig. 55-2)
  - Provides stability to PIP joint and strength that resists joint displacement
  - *Must be disrupted in at least two planes for dislocation to occur*

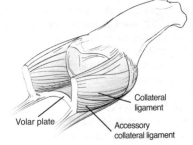

Collateral
ligament

Volar plate

Accessory
collateral ligament

Fig. 55-2   Ligament box complex provides joint stability.

DORSAL DISLOCATION OF THE PIP JOINT[5]
- These injuries are frequently seen with PIP joint hyperextension that includes longitudinal compression of digit.
- Avulsion of volar plate occurs distally in 80% of injuries.
- Proximal volar plate avulsion can produce a trapped osteochondral fragment between proximal and middle phalanx. This is irreducible and requires open reduction.

CLASSIFICATION OF DORSAL DISLOCATIONS
Type I (hyperextension): Partial or complete avulsion of volar plate. The middle phalanx locks in 70-80 degrees of hyperextension. Partial articulation of joint remains intact.

Type II (dorsal dislocation): Complete dorsal dislocation of middle phalanx. Avulsion of volar plate associated with major split of collateral ligaments. Base of middle phalanx rests on condyles of proximal phalanx without apposition of articular surface.

Type III (fracture-dislocation): Avulsion fracture of volar middle phalanx with volar plate.
- **Stable fracture-dislocation**
  - ▸ Small triangular fragment **less than 40% of volar articular surface** of middle phalanx
  - ▸ Dorsal portions of the collateral ligaments intact, which makes complex stable after reduction
- **Unstable fracture-dislocation**
  - ▸ **Disruption of more than 40% of volar articular surface** of middle phalanx
  - ▸ Most of collateral ligament-volar plate complex remains attached to fracture fragment
  - ▸ Difficult to maintain closed reduction

TREATMENT OF ACUTE PIP DISLOCATIONS[5,6]

Type I injury
- Closed reduction and immobilize in 20-30 degrees of flexion for 1 week
- Avoid prolonged immobilization.
- Edema and stiffness may persist for 6 months.

Type II injury
- Closed reduction and immobilize in 20-30 degrees of flexion for 2-3 weeks.

Stable type III injury
- Closed reduction and immobilize with dorsal blocking splint in 20-30 degrees of flexion for 3 weeks.
- Extension block splinting is effective. Must ensure adequate reduction before splinting. Start with dorsal blocking splint at degree of potential redisplacement. Reduce flexion of splint by 10-15 degrees each week.
- Follow with range-of-motion exercises after 3 weeks.

Unstable type III injury
- Dynamic skeletal traction techniques are effective for comminuted fracture patterns through base of middle phalanx.
- ORIF is effective when there is a large volar fracture fragment. Preserve the volar plate insertion to the fracture fragment. Stabilize with Kirschner wires or mini–lag screw.
- **Volar plate arthroplasty** is indicated when fracture-dislocation is not amenable to ORIF. Immobilize PIP joint for 3 weeks. Then allow unrestricted PIP flexion with dorsal blocking splint for 1-3 weeks. Then proceed with unrestricted active extension of joint. Best results are achieved if repair is made within 6 weeks of injury.

CHRONIC PIP SUBLUXATION (HYPEREXTENSION)

- Results from **untreated type I injury** resulting in **swan neck deformity**
- Pain as lateral bands that snap across the condyles of the proximal phalanx
- Must distinguish **volar plate injury** from **extensor mechanism imbalance**
  - Stabilize PIP joint in full extension and have patient actively extend distal interphalangeal (DIP) joint. Volar plate is damaged if DIP joint extends normally.
- Repaired with flexor digitorum superficialis (FDS) tenodesis ("sublimis sling")
  - The radial slip of the FDS tendon is passed through the proximal phalanx from the ulnar to the radial side.
  - Anchor tendon to the periosteum to hold PIP joint in 5 degrees of flexion.
  - Apply dorsal blocking splint and allow immediate active flexion.
  - Motion is unrestricted after 6 weeks.

LATERAL DISLOCATION OF PIP JOINT

- Seen with **rupture of collateral ligament** and at least **partial volar plate avulsion.**
- **Assess PIP stability after reduction of joint.** More than 20 degrees of deformity on lateral stress testing indicates complete collateral ligament disruption with injury to secondary stabilizer.
- Reduce and buddy-tape to adjacent uninjured digit.

TIP: Most lateral dislocations can be managed nonoperatively with early range of motion.

- Surgical repair is indicated for subacute or chronic injuries with persistent PIP instability and dysfunction.

VOLAR DISLOCATIONS OF PIP JOINT

- Rare injuries
- **Types of volar dislocations**
  - **Volar dislocation without rotation.** Tear through central slip of extensor mechanism.
  - **Volar rotatory subluxation** occurs when rotation occurs on one intact collateral ligament. The condyle of the proximal phalanx usually ruptures between the central slip of the extensor tendon and the ipsilateral lateral band as the middle phalanx displaces volarly.
  - Volar fracture-dislocation
- **Treatment**
  - Nonrotatory volar dislocations can be reduced easily. Splint in full extension for 4-6 weeks.

TIP: Most rotatory volar dislocations can be reduced and managed nonoperatively.

- ▶ Apply gentle traction with MP and PIP joints flexed to relax volarly displaced lateral band.
- ▶ Gentle rotatory motion disengages the intraarticular portion and allows for reduction.
- ▶ Test active range of motion of PIP joint after reduction.
- ▶ Immobilize in full extension for 6 weeks if unable to actively extend fully at PIP joint after closed reduction.
  - Volar fracture-dislocations should be managed with CRPP or ORIF with mini–lag screw. This depends on the size of the dorsal fracture fragment.

COLLATERAL LIGAMENT FIBROSIS

- This condition is a late inevitable consequence of PIP joint dislocation.
- Fibrosis evolves over **10-12 months** after injury.
- Minimize fibrosis with consistent rehabilitation as soon as joint is stable.
- Low-dose prednisone taper after 4 weeks of injury can reduce edema and enhance recovery of movement.
- **Collateral ligament excision for PIP contracture release**
  - Operative intervention indicated if range of motion is less than 60 degrees after compliant rehabilitation efforts and patient's quality of life is significantly impaired.
  - Both collateral ligaments usually must be excised. Lateral bands must be preserved.
  - Full passive range of motion must be achieved before testing active excursion.

DISTAL INTERPHALANGEAL JOINT AND THUMB INTERPHALANGEAL JOINT

ANATOMY

- Ligamentous anatomy of DIP joint and thumb IP joint is analogous to that of PIP joint.

DISLOCATIONS OF DIP AND THUMB IP JOINTS

- Much less frequent than PIP dislocations
- Enhanced stability of these joints provided by **adjacent insertions of flexor and extensor tendons**
- Usually dorsal or lateral
- **Can treat most with closed reduction;** joint immobilized with dorsal splint in slight flexion for 2-3 weeks

- Irreducible dislocations rare and usually caused by a trapped volar plate
  - Requires operative reduction

DORSAL FRACTURE-DISLOCATIONS OF DIP AND THUMB IP JOINTS
- Condition is a volar fracture fragment of distal phalanx.
- Stable closed reduction must be achieved if volar fracture fragment is not avulsed with FDP-FPL tendon.
- Operative intervention required if FDP-FPL is avulsed.
- Volar plate arthroplasty is indicated if there is an unstable fracture-dislocation.

KEY POINTS

- Dislocations are described as the position of the distal bone relative to normal joint alignment.
- The **Cam effect** describes the stretch of the digit MP joint collateral ligaments during flexion. This stabilizes the joint during flexion.
- Complete tears of the thumb MP ulnar collateral ligament are associated with **Stener lesions**. These require operative repair to prevent chronic joint instability.
- Dislocations of the PIP joint are the most common ligament injury in the hand.
- The ligament box complex must be disrupted in at least two planes for dislocation to occur.
- Unstable fractures-dislocations typically occur when more than 40% of the volar articular surface is disrupted.
- Volar plate arthroplasty is the most effective treatment for unstable type III injuries.
- Must distinguish volar plate injury from extensor tendon imbalance in patients with post-traumatic swan neck deformities before repair.
- Collateral ligament fibrosis will develop after PIP dislocations and will disrupt the function of the digit.
- Reduce the severity of collateral ligament fibrosis with early rehabilitation as soon as the joint is stable after injury.

REFERENCES

1. Glickel SZ, Barron OA, Catalano LW. Dislocations and ligament injuries in the digits. In Green DP, Hotchkiss RN, Pederson WC, et al, eds. Green's Operative Hand Surgery, 5th ed. Philadelphia: Churchill Livingstone, 2005, pp 343-388.
2. Jobe MT, Calandruccio JH. Fractures, dislocations and ligamentous injuries. In Canale ST, ed. Campbell's Operative Orthopaedics, 10th ed. New York: Elsevier, 2003, pp 3483-3526.
3. Eaton RG, Littler JW. Joint injuries and their sequelae. Clin Plast Surg 3:85-98, 1976.
4. Stener B. Skeletal injuries associated with rupture of the ulnar collateral ligament of the metacarpophalangeal joint of the thumb: A clinical and anatomic study. Acta Chir Scand 125:583-586, 1963.
5. Deitch MA, Kiefhaber TR, Comisar BR, et al. Dorsal fracture-dislocation in the proximal interphalangeal joint: Surgical complications and long-term results. J Hand Surg Am 24:914-923, 1994.
6. Eaton RG, Malerich MM. Volar plate arthroplasty of the proximal interphalangeal joint: A review of ten years' experience. J Hand Surg Am 5:260-268, 1980.

56. Fingertip Injuries

Joshua A. Lemmon

ANATOMY[1,2]

The **fingertip** is the portion of the digit **distal to the insertion of the profundus and extensor tendons** (Fig. 56-1).

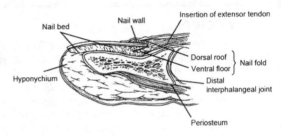

Fig. 56-1 Fingertip anatomy. (From Fassler PR. Fingertip injuries: Evaluation and treatment. J Am Acad Orthop Surg 4:84-92, 1996.)

PERIONYCHIUM
- Nail complex
- Constitutes dorsum of fingertip
- Begins approximately 1.2 mm distal to extensor tendon insertion
- See Chapter 57 for anatomic details
- Fingertip injuries: May involve nail plate, nail bed, hyponychium, eponychium, and paronychium

SKIN
- Glabrous
- Thick epidermis with deep papillary ridges that create fingerprints

PULP
- Fibrofatty tissue
- Rich vasculature
- Stabilized by fibrous septa extending from dermis to periosteum of distal phalanx
- Stabilized laterally to distal phalanx by extensions from Cleland's and Grayson's ligaments
- **Distal pulp:** Multipyramidal structure of fibroadipose tissue compartments
- **Proximal pulp:** Two layers of spherical tissue compartments
- Volar pulp: **56%** of fingertip volume[1]

INNERVATION
- Proper digital nerves split into **three branches (trifurcation)** just distal to the distal interphalangeal (DIP) joint.
- One branch innervates the nail bed, one the distal fingertip, and one the volar pulp.

VASCULAR SUPPLY
- The proper digital artery also divides into **three branches (trifurcation).**

- The three branches are interconnected distally by two anastomotic arches.
  - One arch is parallel to the lunula.
  - Second arch is parallel to the free edge of the nail.
- One branch continues laterally, and two dorsal branches arise from each artery.
  - One branch supplies nail fold.
  - The other branch arborizes at the level of the midnail and continues into the volar pulp.
- Venous drainage[3]
  - Dorsal veins are dominant.
  - Veins around the lateral nail wall and distal pulp form an arch over the distal phalanx, surrounding the nail fold proximally.
  - Midline, longitudinal veins connect to a middle venous arch over the middle phalanx.
  - Valves are present even in the most distal veins.

EVALUATION

HISTORY
- **Age:** Children are treated differently than adults, and older patients have limited treatment options.
- **Gender:** Aesthetic outcome is often more important to female patients.
- **Hand dominance:** Dominant-hand injuries are treated more aggressively.
- **Occupation:** A manual laborer might be treated differently than a musician.
- **Determine mechanism of injury.**
- **Tobacco use:** Random-pattern flaps are discouraged in smokers.
- **Comorbid medical illnesses:** Patients with rheumatoid arthritis or Dupuytren's disease may not be candidates for certain regional flaps because of contracture risk (e.g., thenar flap, cross-finger flap); patients with diabetes mellitus are prone to infection and wound healing difficulties.

PHYSICAL EXAMINATION
- Perform complete hand examination; do not neglect the rest of the hand.
- Give special attention to the injured digit.
  - Assess the flexor and extensor tendons.

TIP: Associated mallet injury is common.

  - Measure defect size (in cm^2).
  - Determine the composition of the missing or nonviable tissue (e.g., nail plate, nail bed, skin, pulp, bone).

TIP: This information may be best obtained after digital block anaesthesia and thorough irrigation.

  - Note the presence of exposed bone.
  - Evaluate the geometry of the injury to guide treatment (Fig. 56-2).

DIGIT-SPECIFIC RADIOGRAPHS
- Obtain anteroposterior (AP) and lateral films.
- Radiographs should include the amputated piece, if present.

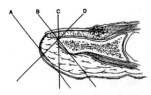

Fig. 56-2　Geometry of injury. *A*, Palmar oblique without exposed bone. *B*, Palmar oblique with exposed bone. *C*, Transverse. *D*, Dorsal oblique. (From Fassler PR. Fingertip injuries: Evaluation and treatment. J Am Acad Orthop Surg 4:84-92, 1996.)

TREATMENT PLANNING

The ideal treatment for a particular patient is either fingertip reconstruction or revision amputation. This decision should be made *along with the patient* by an experienced surgeon in a **patient-specific** and **digit-specific** fashion.

> TIP:　The size of the defect, the presence of exposed bone, and the geometry of the injury help guide reconstruction methods.

GOALS OF FINGERTIP RECONSTRUCTION
- Provide durable coverage.
- Preserve length.
- Preserve sensation.
- Minimize pain.
- Minimize donor site morbidity.
- Maintain joint function.
- Provide an aesthetically acceptable result.

RECONSTRUCTIVE OPTIONS: RECONSTRUCTIVE LADDER
- Healing by secondary intention
- Skin grafting
- Composite grafting
- Homodigital flaps
- Heterodigital flaps
- Regional flaps
- Microsurgical replantation or reconstruction

HOMODIGITAL FLAPS

- The source of donor tissue is the **injured digit.**
- These flaps provide immediate, near-normal sensibility.
- Donor tissue must be from outside the zone of injury.
- This method often requires a small amount of bone shortening to facilitate flap inset.

VOLAR V-Y ADVANCEMENT FLAP (ATASOY ET AL)[4]
- Useful for **dorsal oblique** and some **transverse** geometry injuries
- Uses tissue adjacent to wound
- Designed with wound edge as base of triangular flap

- Can only advance distal edge **1 cm** unless incision carried proximal to DIP flexion crease
- Can design flap more proximally to cross DIP flexion crease and include neurovascular pedicles for increased advancement (Fig. 56-3)

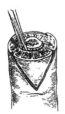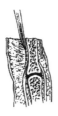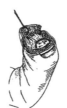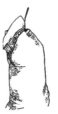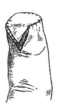

Fig. 56-3   Palmar V-Y advancement flap. (From Chao JD, Huang JM, Wiedrich TA. Local hand flaps. J Am Soc Surg Hand 1:28, 2002.)

Furlow's Modified Volar V-Y Advancement "Cup" Flap[5]
- Modification of classic V-Y volar advancement for volar oblique injuries
- Flap design extended across DIP and proximal interphalangeal (PIP) volar flexion creases
- Elevated just volar to flexor sheath, including neurovascular bundles laterally
- Flap advanced distally and lateral edges folded together and "cupped" over distal injury
- Use of digit possibly limited by postoperative fingertip and volar scars

Volar Advancement Flaps (Moberg)[6]
- Technique is used mostly for the **thumb** because of unique dorsal and volar blood supply.
- Radial and ulnar midaxial incisions are made dorsal to the neurovascular bundles, which are **included in the flap.**
- Flap elevation is in plane just volar to the tendon sheath.
- Advancement is limited to **1.0 cm** without additional modifications.
- A transverse incision at base increases advancement to **1.5 cm.**
- **Dellon's modification** of flap design into the web space increases advancement to **3.0 cm** (Fig. 56-4).

Fig. 56-4   Dellon's modification of palmar advancement flap to increase advancement. (From Rohrich RJ, Antrobus SD. Volar advancement flaps. In Blair WF, ed. Techniques in Hand Surgery. Baltimore: Williams & Wilkins, 1996, pp 39-47.)

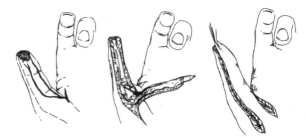

Bilateral Triangular V-Y Advancement Flaps (Kutler)[7]
- Described for **transverse amputations,** but perhaps most useful for **lateral oblique** injuries
- Triangular flaps designed along lateral aspects of distal tip
- Advanced distally and centrally to cover injury

Oblique Triangular Neurovascular Island Flap[8]

- Useful for **volar oblique** injuries up to 2 cm in size
- Unilateral triangular flap design
- Neurovascular pedicle dissection: Extend proximally to web space for increased advancement (Fig. 56-5)

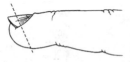 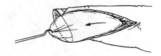 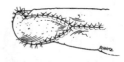

Fig. 56-5 Oblique triangular island flap. (From Chao JD, Huang JM, Wiedrich TA. Local hand flaps. J Am Soc Surg Hand 1:28, 2002.)

Other Homodigital Flaps

Surgeon familiarity and preference allows more frequent use of these techniques.

- Hueston's flap[9]
- Souquet's flap[10]
- Step-advancement flap[11]
- Reversed digital-artery flaps[12]

HETERODIGITAL FLAPS

- Can provide coverage for **larger areas than homodigital flaps**
- Violates a normal digit
- Often requires cortical relearning
- **Sensibility not as good as with homodigital flaps;** for example, protective sensation is preserved with cross-finger flaps but not tactile gnosis (0% tactile gnosis in 54 patients)[13]

Cross-Finger Flap[14] (Fig. 56-6)

- Useful for large **volar oblique** injuries
- Flap raised on dorsum of injured digit's adjacent middle phalanx and elevated just dorsal to paratenon
- Flap left pedicled to donor site along lateral margin adjacent to injured digit
- Injured finger flexed and flap inset over defect
- Flap division at 8 to 10 days
- Postoperative sensibility relatively poor (as previously described)
- Donor digit frequently bothered by cold intolerance and sensitivity
- Aesthetic deformity on dorsum of donor finger often troubling for women

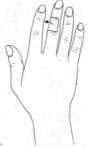 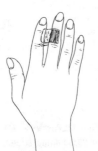 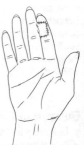

Fig. 56-6 Cross-finger flap.

Flap design　　Arc to adjacent digit　　Flap inset

HETERODIGITAL NEUROVASCULAR PEDICLE FLAPS (Fig. 56-7)[15]

- More commonly used for **ulnar thumb pulp defects**
- Can provide stable coverage for larger injuries than covered by homodigital flaps
- Donor site reconstructed with skin grafting
- Requires cortical relearning, which occurs in only 40% of cases[16]
- Involves dissection of middle or ring finger proper digital artery and nerve proximally to bifurcation of common digital source
- Larger volar access incisions necessary to tunnel pedicle and inset flap in defect

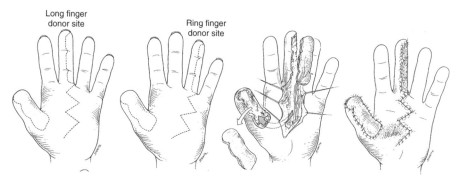

Fig. 56-7 Neurovascular pedicle flap. (From Green DP, Hotchkiss RN, Pederson WC, eds. Green's Operative Hand Surgery, 4th ed. Philadelphia: Churchill Livingstone, 1999.)

FIRST DORSAL METACARPAL ARTERY FLAP[17] (Fig. 56-8)

- Additional option for reconstructing volar thumb injuries
- Neurovascular pedicle flap based on dorsal first metacarpal artery
- Allows transfer of tissue from dorsum of index finger proximal phalanx
- Flap includes terminal branch of superficial radial nerve providing **protective sensation**
- Like other neurovascular pedicle flaps, requires cortical relearning and skin grafting of donor site

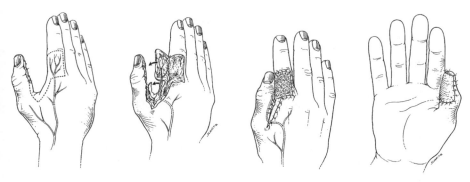

Fig. 56-8 First dorsal metacarpal artery flap. (From Green DP, Hotchkiss RN, Pederson WC, eds. Green's Operative Hand Surgery, 4th ed. Philadelphia: Churchill Livingstone, 1999.)

REGIONAL FLAPS

THENAR FLAP[18,19]

- Used for large **volar oblique** injuries of **index** and **middle** fingers
- Flap of skin and subcutaneous tissue elevated on thenar eminence
- Injured digit flexed and flap inset over injury
- Flap division at 10-14 days
- Often discouraged in patients older than 40 years for fear of joint contractures, but some report good results in older adults[20]
- **Contraindicated** in patients with rheumatoid arthritis, Dupuytren's disease, or other illnesses that preclude prolonged finger flexion

TREATMENT OF INJURY TYPES: AN ALGORITHMIC APPROACH

Treatment method selection follows focused injury evaluation with attention to **injury size** and **geometry,** as well as **patient-specific** and **digit-specific** factors.

SOFT TISSUE LOSS WITHOUT EXPOSED BONE (see Fig. 56-2, A)

- **Healing by secondary intention**
  - Digital tip injuries **less than 1.5 cm^2** heal with excellent results by secondary intention.[21]
  - **Procedure**
    - ▸ Local digital block with 1% lidocaine
    - ▸ Finger tourniquet not necessary, may hinder evaluation of viable tissue
    - ▸ Copious irrigation and cleansing with surgical scrub solution
    - ▸ Debridement of clearly nonviable tissue
    - ▸ Hemostasis obtained

TIP: Battery-operated cautery devices are helpful in the emergency department.

  - **Dressing options**
    - ▸ **Nonadherent gauze**
      - ◆ Permits home twice-daily dressing changes and wound treatment (e.g., sink hydrotherapy)
      - ◆ Best for heavily contaminated injuries
    - ▸ **Semiocclusive dressing** (e.g., Tegaderm™ [3M Corporation, St. Paul, MN], OpSite™ [Smith & Nephew Corporation, LaJolla, CA])
      - ◆ Can be changed each week by treating physician
      - ◆ Eliminates initial patient involvement in wound care
    - ▸ **Hyphecan cap** (Hainan Kangda Marine Biomedical Corp, Haikou, China)[22]
      - ◆ Chitin-derived biologic dressing left in place until healing is complete
  - **Postoperative care**
    - ▸ Average time for wound healing is **3-4 weeks,** but increased with larger wounds.
    - ▸ Desensitization and occupational therapy begins following soft tissue healing.
- **Skin grafting**
  - Full-thickness and split-thickness grafts are harvested from the **hypothenar eminence** and permit coverage with glabrous skin.

- Skin grafting does **not** provide consistently good results.[23]
  - ▶ Increased incidence of cold intolerance
  - ▶ Increased incidence of postoperative tenderness
  - ▶ Does not shorten period of unfitness for work
- For these reasons, skin grafting should be used only in instances where the wound is too large for healing by secondary intention and other techniques for reconstruction are not feasible or impractical (e.g., large volar skin avulsion without exposed tendon or bone).

SOFT TISSUE LOSS WITH EXPOSED BONE

- **Bone shortening**
  - In some circumstances, the bone can be minimally shortened to convert an injury with exposed bone to one without exposed bone, thus permitting healing by secondary intention.
  - This procedure is performed only for small wounds (<1.5 cm²) with a minimal area of exposed bone.
  - The distal phalanx serves as the support for the nail bed; therefore the **nail bed must be shortened 2 mm proximal to the distal extent of the distal phalanx** to prevent postoperative hook-nail deformity.[24]

TIP: The bone should never be shortened beyond the insertion of the flexor or extensor tendons.

- **Dorsal oblique injury**
  - Relative preservation of volar tip pulp and glabrous skin
  - Reconstruction with **volar V-Y advancement flap** (see Fig. 56-2, *D*)
  - **Procedure** (see Fig. 56-3)
    1. Digital block with 1% lidocaine
    2. Thorough irrigation and cleansing
    3. Debridement of nonviable tissue
    4. Finger exsanguination and digital tourniquet
    5. Sterile matrix removed 2 mm proximal to the end of distal phalanx
    6. Flap designed with wound edge as the base of a triangular flap
    7. Full-thickness elevation of volar flap under loupe magnification
    8. Fibrous septa that anchor pulp sharply released from distal phalanx
    9. Flap mobilized distally
    10. Limited bone shortening, as needed, to facilitate inset
    11. Inset into defect, secured to nail bed with 6-0 chromic gut suture
    12. Lateral edges contoured and secured with 5-0 nylon suture
    13. Donor site closed in V-Y fashion
    14. Bulky dressing or volar protective splint applied
    15. Desensitization and occupational therapy following soft tissue healing
- **Volar oblique injury** (see Fig. 56-2, *B*)
  - Technique preserves nail complex, but leaves deficiencies in volar skin and pulp.
  - Technique should be **digit-specific** to preserve most important aspects of each digit.
  - **Thumb**
    - ▶ Maintaining sensation is important for precision.
    - ▶ Sensation is best with homodigital flaps.
    - ▶ The **classic thumb tip procedure is the Moberg volar advancement flap**.[6]
    - ▶ Modifications may be required to increase advancement as described previously.

- ► Heterodigital flaps are required for large injuries (e.g., Littler neurovascular island flap, cross-finger flap, or first dorsal metacarpal artery flap).
- **Index finger**
  - ► Like the thumb, the index finger is involved with pinch grip and precision activity.
  - ► **Sensibility is of greatest importance.**
  - ► Use homodigital flap reconstruction when possible.
    - • **Furlow's modified volar V-Y advancement** can be used for large injuries (up to 1.5 cm^2).
    - • Larger injuries, up to 2 cm^2, can be reconstructed with **homodigital oblique triangular neurovascular island flap** (see Fig. 56-5).
  - ► **Thenar flaps** are preferred over cross-finger flaps for larger injuries; postoperative sensibility is better, whereas cross-finger flaps rarely achieve more than protective sensation.[13,25]

TIP: The thenar flap is the best option for large injuries of the index finger tip.

- ► A Moberg volar advancement flap is feasible for the index finger, but unlike the thumb the index finger has no dedicated dorsal arterial supply.
  - • Dorsal skin is supplied by perforating branches of the common digital arteries.
  - • Dorsal skin necrosis can occur unless these branches are preserved.
  - • To preserve these branches a vertical spreading technique is used during flap elevation, rather than sharp dissection.
  - • Excellent results are reported.
  - • Advancement is limited to 1.5 cm.

TIP: This is a difficult technique to use on the index finger, and should be done meticulously and only by an experienced surgeon.

- **Middle finger**
  - ► The middle or long finger is the central digit of the hand; its **length** is required for a normal aesthetic pattern of the hand.
  - ► **Sensibility is of secondary importance to length.**
  - ► Because most homodigital flaps require some bone shortening, the thenar flap should be used initially to limit any shortening.
- **Ring and small fingers**
  - ► The main role of the ulnar two digits is **power grip.**
  - ► Durable coverage, length, minimal pain, and adequate joint mobility are the most important considerations.
  - ► Sensibility is of limited importance.
  - ► Homodigital flaps may sacrifice length, as previously indicated.
  - ► Additionally, homodigital flaps can result in volar scars that extend across the contact surface of these fingers during power grip.
  - ► **A heterodigital, cross-finger flap is an appropriate reconstructive method.**
    - • Limited postoperative sensibility is attained, but length and durable coverage are preserved, volar scars are avoided, and metacarpophalangeal (MP) and PIP joint mobility are maintained.
  - ► **Procedure (for ring finger)**
    1. Best performed in operating room with regional anaesthesia
    2. Injury irrigation, cleansing, and debridement

3. Upper extremity exsanguination and tourniquet
4. Flap designed on dorsum of middle finger over middle phalanx
5. Flap elevated just dorsal to extensor paratenon; elevated from radial to ulnar direction
6. Full-thickness skin graft harvested from forearm and secured to radial border of the injury on ring finger
7. Ring finger flexed into position and flap inset over injury and skin graft secured over donor site
8. Volar protective splint applied
9. Flap divided in 8-10 days
10. Desensitization and occupational therapy started after soft tissue healed

- **Transverse injury** (see Fig. 56-2, *C*)

This type of injury results in equal deficiencies in the volar pulp and dorsal nail complex.

- Use techniques described for dorsal oblique and volar oblique injuries.
  - ▸ **Volar V-Y advancement flaps** are useful for relatively distal injuries, but require prohibitive bone shortening if the injury goes through the proximal half of the sterile matrix.
  - ▸ Other **homodigital, heterodigital,** or **regional flaps** are used as described for volar oblique injuries.

- **Lateral oblique injury**
  - Use with injury in the sagittal plane and with radial or ulnar-sided tissue loss.
  - Previously mentioned homodigital flaps can be used.
  - Additionally, a **lateral pulp flap** may be used.[26]
    - ▸ The remaining volar pulp is sharply elevated off the periosteum of the distal phalanx and advanced laterally into the defect; a raw surface remains on the lateral aspect.
    - ▸ The wound is allowed to reepithelialize with moist wound care.

COMPOSITE GRAFTING

- Nonmicrosurgical replantation of amputated fingertip
- Typically recommended only for children younger than age 2-6 years[27,28]
- **Not recommended for those older than 6 years**
- May use just a biologic dressing that allows for underlying healing by secondary intention
- Attempts have been made to improve graft take by using postoperative cooling and subcutaneous pocket placement
- Discouraged in severe crush injuries

REVISION AMPUTATION

INDICATIONS

- Patient preference
  - Manual laborers may request a well-performed termination rather than a reconstruction to speed recovery and return to work.
- Heavy contamination and human bites should be staged with initial debridement and delayed amputation.
- Injury **proximal to the lunula** is best treated with **nail ablation** and **revision amputation.**
- Perform if injury is proximal to the insertion of the flexor or extensor tendons.

TECHNICAL CONSIDERATIONS

- The remaining skeleton should be contoured to a smooth, tapered end.
- The distal phalanx should be completely removed, if injured.

- Digital nerves should be divided at least 1 cm proximal to the injury and placed away from contact surfaces.
- Digital arteries and dorsal veins should be ligated or cauterized to prevent hematomas.
- To prevent a *"quadrigia effect"* the profundus tendon should **not** be advanced distally. The quadrigia effect is a restriction in flexion of adjacent digits, resulting from a common muscular origin of the profundus tendons.
- The profundus tendon can be secured to the A4 pulley to prevent a **"lumbrical plus"** deformity; extension at the PIP with attempted flexion results from retracting flexor digitorum profundus (FDP) tendon and lumbrical origin, increasing lumbrical pull.
- Completely ablate the nail bed, including the dorsal roof, to prevent problematic remnants.

MICROSURGICAL REPLANTATION

- These techniques are practiced and reported mostly in Japan and other Asian countries, where cultural differences place greater importance on the presence of a normal fingertip.
- Replantation of fingertips occurs only at tertiary referral centers in the United States.
- Replantation should be considered in all children, young women, and musicians.

KEY POINTS

- ✔ Injuries without exposed bone that are less than 1.5 cm^2 are best managed with healing by secondary intention.
- ✔ Skin grafting should rarely be used.
- ✔ Injury geometry dictates reconstructive options.
- ✔ Homodigital flaps provide better postoperative sensibility than heterodigital flaps and are preferred for the thumb and index fingers.
- ✔ Shortening should be avoided, if at all possible, when treating middle fingertip injuries.
- ✔ Composite grafting should be performed only in children less than 6 years old.
- ✔ Revision amputation is a preferred treatment for many patients and should be discussed with every patient before pursuing fingertip reconstruction.

REFERENCES

1. Murai M, Lau HK, Pereira BP, et al. A cadaver study on volume and surface area of the fingertip. J Hand Surg Am 22:935-941, 1997.
2. Zook EG. Anatomy and physiology of the perionychium. Hand Clin 6:1-7, 1990.
3. Moss SH, Schwartz KS, von Drasek-Ascher G, et al. Digital venous anatomy. J Hand Surg Am 10:473-482, 1985.
4. Atasoy E, Ioakimidis E, Kasdan ML, et al. Reconstruction of the amputated finger tip with a triangular volar flap. A new surgical procedure. J Bone Joint Surg Am 52:921-926, 1970.
5. Furlow LT Jr. V-Y "cup" flap for volar oblique amputation of fingers. J Hand Surg Br 9:253-256, 1984.
6. Moberg E. Aspects of sensation in reconstructive surgery of the upper extremity. J Bone Joint Surg Am 46:817-825, 1964.
7. Kutler W. A new method for fingertip amputation. JAMA 133:29-30, 1947.

8. Venkataswami R, Subramanian N. Oblique triangular flap: A new method of repair for oblique amputations of the fingertip and thumb. Plast Reconstr Surg 66:296-300, 1980.
9. Hueston J. Local flap repair of fingertip injuries. Plast Reconstr Surg 37:349-350, 1966.
10. Souquet R. The asymmetric arterial advancement flap in distal pulp loss (modified Hueston's flap). Ann Chir Main 4:233-238, 1985.
11. Evans DM, Martin DL. Step-advancement flap for fingertip reconstruction. Br J Plast Surg 41:105-111, 1988.
12. Lai CS, Lin SD, Chou CK, et al. A versatile method for reconstruction of finger defects: Reverse digital artery flap. Br J Plast Surg 45:443-453, 1992.
13. Nishikawa H, Smith PJ. The recovery of sensation and function after cross-finger flaps for fingertip injury. J Hand Surg Br 17:102-107, 1992.
14. Gurdin M, Pangman WJ. The repair of surface defects of fingers by trans-digital flaps. Plast Reconstr Surg 5:368-371, 1950.
15. Littler JW. The neurovascular pedicle method of digital transposition for reconstruction of the thumb. Plast Reconstr Surg 12:303-319, 1953.
16. Oka Y. Sensory function of the neurovascular island flap in thumb reconstruction: Comparison of original and modified procedures. J Hand Surg Am 25:637-643, 2000.
17. Holevich J. A new method of restoring sensibility to the thumb. J Bone Joint Surg Br 45:496-502, 1963.
18. Gatewood MD. A plastic repair of finger defects without hospitalization. JAMA 87:1479, 1926.
19. Flatt AE. The thenar flap. J Bone Joint Surg Br 39:80-85, 1957.
20. Barbato BD, Guelmi K, Romano SJ, et al. Thenar flap rehabilitated: A review of 20 cases. Ann Plast Surg 37:135-139, 1996.
21. Mennen U, Weise A. Fingertip injuries management with semi-occlusive dressing. J Hand Surg Br 18:416-422, 1993.
22. Halim AS, Stone CA, Devaraj VS. The Hyphecan cap: A biological fingertip dressing. Injury 29:261-263, 1998.
23. Holm A, Zachariae L. Fingertip lesion: An evaluation of conservative treatment versus free skin grafting. Acta Orthop Scand 45:382-392, 1974.
24. Kumar VP, Satku K. Treatment and prevention of "hook nail" deformity with anatomic correlation. J Hand Surg Am 18:617-620, 1993.
25. Melone CP Jr, Beasley RW, Carstens JH Jr. The thenar flap: Analysis of its use in 150 cases. J Hand Surg Am 7:291-297, 1982.
26. Elliot D, Jigjinni VS. The lateral pulp flap. J Hand Surg Br 18:423-426, 1993.
27. Elsahy NI. When to replant a fingertip after its complete amputation. Plast Reconstr Surg 60:14-21, 1977.
28. Moiemen NS, Elliot D. Composite graft replacement of digital tips. A study in children. J Hand Surg Br 22:346-352, 1997.

57. Nail Bed Injuries

Joshua A. Lemmon

ANATOMY[1,2] (Fig. 57-1)

NAIL PLATE
- Composed of hard, keratinized, squamous cells attached to nail bed
- Loosely attached to germinal matrix, but densely adherent to sterile matrix

HYPONYCHIUM
- Junction of sterile matrix and fingertip skin beneath distal nail margin
- Subject to heavy contamination because material accumulates during process of scratching and interaction with environment
- Keratin plug acts as mechanical barrier
  - Large numbers of polymorphonuclear leukocytes and lymphocytes present, serve as immunologic barrier

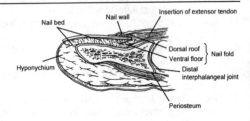

Fig. 57-1 Nail bed anatomy. (From Fassler PR. Fingertip injuries: Evaluation and treatment. J Am Acad Orthop Surg 4:84-92, 1996.)

TIP: Subungual infections are rare unless this barrier is compromised by prolonged immersion in alkaline fluids, soaps, or oils.

PARONYCHIUM
- Extends along lateral border of nail

EPONYCHIUM
- Distal portion of nail fold where it is attached to the surface of nail

NAIL FOLD
- Composed of the ventral floor and the dorsal roof
- **Ventral floor:** Site of the **germinal matrix**
- **Dorsal roof:** Hosts cells that impart **nail shine**

LUNULA
- White arc just distal to the eponychium
- Caused by **persistence of nail cell nuclei** in the germinal matrix
- Distal to this location, nuclei are absent and the nail is clear

GERMINAL MATRIX
- Lies on ventral floor proximal to distal border of lunula
- Immediately distal to the insertion of extensor tendon
- Responsible for **90%** of nail production

STERILE MATRIX
- Nail bed distal to lunula
- Tightly adherent to overlying nail plate and to periosteum of distal phalanx
- Secondary site of nail production

PHYSIOLOGY AND FUNCTION[1-3]

NAIL GROWTH OCCURS IN THREE LOCATIONS
1. **Germinal matrix**
   - Produces nail by **gradient parakeratosis**
     - Basilar cells, close to the distal phalanx periosteum, duplicate and enlarge (macrocytosis).
     - Newly formed cells are driven dorsally in a column toward the nail.
     - These cells flatten and elongate in response to the resistance of the nail, assimilate into the nail itself, and stream distally.
     - Cells initially retain nuclei, but slowly lose them as cells become nonviable.
     - When cells reach the distal lunula, so few nuclei remain that the nail becomes clear.
2. **Dorsal roof of nail fold**
   - Produces nail by same mechanism as germinal matrix, but these cells lose nuclei more rapidly
   - Imparts shine to nail plate
3. **Sterile matrix**
   - Amount of nail produced in this location varies by individual
   - Adds squamous cells, contributing to **nail strength** and **thickness**
   - Continued nail growth permits nail adherence; overlying nail plate is securely anchored by linear ridges in sterile matrix epithelium

VARIABLE NAIL GROWTH
- Nail growth rate generally **3-4 mm** per month
- **Growth more rapid in:**
  - Longer digits
  - Summer months
  - Young persons
    - Growth is twice as rapid in persons less than age 30 years as for those more than age 80 years; growth is in inverse proportion for intermediate ages.
  - Nail biters

TIP: It takes about 100 days to grow a complete nail.

NAIL FUNCTION
- The fingernail serves as a counterforce to the fingertip pad, increasing its sensitivity.
  - **Two-point discrimination drops when the fingernail is absent.**
- The fingernail is used almost exclusively for picking up fine objects (e.g., pins, needles).

FREQUENCY, MECHANISMS, AND CLASSIFICATION OF TRAUMATIC NAIL BED INJURIES

FREQUENCY
- The hand is the most frequently injured body part, and the **fingertip** is the most commonly injured part of the hand.[4,5]
- These injuries are most common in males, age 4-30 years.
- **Middle** and **ring fingers** are the most commonly injured.[6]
- Most injuries involve the **nail bed** and the **soft tissue of the fingertip.**

> TIP: Fifty percent of nail bed injuries are associated with distal phalangeal fractures, so make certain a radiograph is obtained.

ETIOLOGIC FACTORS AND MECHANISMS[3]
- The nail bed is positioned between two relatively unyielding structures, the **distal phalanx** and the **nail plate;** thus it is well protected.
- The required force must be great enough either to cause fracture of the distal phalanx or to deform the nail plate.
- Most injuries result from a crushing force, compressing the delicate nail bed between solid nail plate and solid bone.
- Other injuries result from penetration of the nail plate by foreign objects such as machinery or tools.

CLASSIFICATION
- **Injury type**[7]
    Type I: Small (<25%) subungual hematoma
    Type II: Larger (50%) subungual hematoma
    Type III: Nail bed laceration associated with distal phalangeal fracture
    Type IV: Nail bed fragmentation
    Type V: Nail bed avulsion
- **Laceration type** (in order of increasing severity)
    - Simple lacerations
    - Stellate lacerations
    - Severe crush
    - Nail bed avulsion

PROGNOSIS
- Determined by extent of injury
- Associated with poor aesthetic and functional outcomes
- Comminuted distal phalanx fracture
- Severe soft tissue loss
- Nail bed fragmentation or avulsion lacerations

EVALUATION

HISTORY
- Age
- Gender (aesthetic importance of nail greater in women)
- Handedness
- Occupation
- Mechanism of injury
- Time of injury

COMPLETE HAND EXAMINATION
- Special attention to injured digit
  - Extension tendon function: Mallet deformity possible
  - Flexor tendon function
  - Tip sensation

DIGIT-SPECIFIC RADIOGRAPHS
- Anterior-posterior (AP) and true lateral views

> TIP: A true lateral of a particular digit is obtained easily by asking for a lateral radiograph of that digit's fingernail.

DIGITAL BLOCK
- Often necessary to clean fingertip and completely assess injury

TREATMENT

UNDERLYING PHALANGEAL FRACTURES
- **Tuft fractures** are best managed with only **protective splinting.**
- More proximally significant or displaced fractures should be managed as described in Chapter 54.
- The nail bed injury is repaired following skeletal fixation.

SIMPLE SUBUNGUAL HEMATOMA (TYPE I, TYPE II INJURIES)
Historically, nail removal and nail bed inspection and repair were recommended if the hematoma stained more than 25% to 50% of the nail bed. More recent data suggest that **trephination alone** gives equivalent good results with all hematoma sizes.[8]
- **Nail trephination for subungual hematoma**
  - **Indications**
    - Nail margin and nail plate intact
    - No associated displaced distal phalanx fracture
    - Patient complains of pain; otherwise, observation alone sufficient
  - **Technique**
    - Use a digital block with 1% lidocaine without epinephrine.
    - No digital tourniquet is necessary.
    - Ophthalmic battery-powered cautery or heated paperclip is used to penetrate nail plate and evacuate underlying hematoma.

- ▸ Irrigate with isotonic saline.
- ▸ Cover with nonadherent and sterile gauze.
- ▸ Protective finger splint is applied for 1 week.
- ▸ Prescribe antibiotics for a tuft fracture.

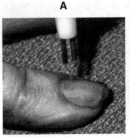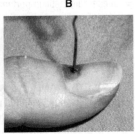

Fig. 57-2   Nail trephination with ophthalmic cautery **(A)** or heated paperclip **(B)**.

TIP: Sharp instruments injure the underlying nail bed.

SIMPLE AND STELLATE LACERATIONS (TYPE III INJURIES)[9]

- Nail plate is removed and the nail bed is explored when nail margin or nail plate is disrupted and when associated with a displaced fracture of distal phalanx.
- Nail bed lacerations are common in these situations.
- **Nail bed laceration primary repair:**
  - **Indications**
    - ▸ Simple or stellate nail bed lacerations
  - **Technique**
    - ▸ Use a digital block with 1% lidocaine without epinephrine.
    - ▸ Exsanguinate finger and create a tourniquet at base of finger using half-inch Penrose drain or small sterile glove.
    - ▸ Remove nail with Freer elevator, tenotomy scissors, or curved iris scissors.
      - ✦ *Careful technique is mandatory to prevent iatrogenic nail bed injury.*
    - ▸ If laceration involves germinal matrix, incisions should be made perpendicular to nail fold margin to allow elevation of the nail fold and improve exposure.
    - ▸ Examine laceration and perform minimal debridement; crushed and bruised nail beds often survive.
    - ▸ Running 6-0 or 7-0 chromic gut suture repairs simple lacerations.
    - ▸ Interrupted and running sutures are often necessary to accurately repair stellate lacerations.
    - ▸ If the nail plate is available, replace it in the nail fold.
      - ✦ This splints the repair and prevents formation of nail fold adhesions (synechiae), which lead to postinjury ridging.
      - ✦ Drainage is through a hole made in the nail plate.
    - ▸ When the nail plate is not available or excessively damaged, secure silicone sheeting or sterile foil (from suture package or nonadherent gauze package) over the repair and in the nail fold.
    - ▸ Hold nail plate or other material in place with 5-0 chromic or nylon half-buried horizontal mattress suture, secured proximal to the nail fold; suture is removed at first postoperative visit.
    - ▸ Place nonadherent, sterile gauze and a protective finger splint for dressing.

TIP: Always use loupe magnification.

NAIL BED AVULSIONS AND SEVERE CRUSH INJURIES (TYPE IV, TYPE V INJURIES)[10-13]

■ **Characteristics**
- Common in industrial workers, carpenters, and manual laborers who work with power machinery (e.g., saws, belts, drills, and presses)
- Large areas of nail bed tissue absent or irreparably damaged
- If left to heal by secondary intention, **uniformly poor** results with misshapen and nonadherent nail plates
- Replace like tissue with like tissue; avulsed nail bed or nail bed grafting used when possible

TIP: When nail bed grafting is not possible, split-thickness skin grafts can be placed over the defect, but nonadherent nail plates and poor aesthetic outcomes are common.

■ **Nail bed avulsion repair with retained segment**
- **Indications**
  ▶ Injury too complex for primary repair
  ▶ Large segment of nail bed tissue retained on avulsed portion of nail plate
- **Technique**
  ▶ Digital block and exposure as for type III injuries
  ▶ Avulsed segment of nail bed carefully removed from back of nail plate and used as free graft
    ◆ Removed segment placed directly on periosteum with good results
    ◆ Secured with 7-0 chromic gut suture under loupe magnification
  ▶ Dressing and nail plate replacement and postoperative treatment as for type III injuries
■ **Nail bed avulsion repair with lateral bipedicle advancement**
- **Indications**
  ▶ Narrow (<2 mm) germinal matrix avulsions
  ▶ Narrow (<2 mm) sterile matrix avulsions (less frequently described)
- **Technique**
  ▶ Digital block, finger tourniquet, and exposure as for type III injuries
  ▶ Nail bed undermining performed lateral to defect on either side
    ◆ Performed with Freer or Cottle periosteal elevator
    ◆ Usually requires extensive undermining to lateral nail fold
  ▶ Tissue advanced medially to cover defect
  ▶ Sutured with 6-0 or 7-0 chromic gut suture
    ◆ **Must be tension free** or suture will tear the tissue and create nail deformity
■ **Nail bed avulsion repair with split-thickness nail bed graft**[11-13]
- **Indications**
  ▶ Large area of avulsed or irreparably damaged sterile matrix
  ▶ Retained segment not available
- **Technique**
  ▶ Discuss potential donor sites (same digit, toe, etc.) with patient.
  ▶ Technique is best performed in operating room.
  ▶ Use digital or regional block with digital or upper extremity exsanguination and tourniquet.
  ▶ Expose nail bed as described previously.

▸ Template of defect is made using foil from suture package.
▸ If defect is less than 50% of nail bed, a split-thickness nail bed graft can be harvested from the same digit using the foil template.
▸ When defect is larger than 50% of nail bed, a split-thickness nail bed graft should be harvested from the great toe.[12]
▸ Harvest split-thickness nail graft with No. 15 scalpel.
  • View blade through nail bed at all times to ensure proper thickness (0.007-0.010 inch).
  • Harvesting is best done using an operating microscope.
▸ Sew graft in place with 7-0 chromic gut suture; proper longitudinal orientation is not necessary for injuries in the sterile matrix.
▸ The nail plate makes the best dressing when available; otherwise, fine mesh gauze or silicone sheeting can be used with excellent results.
▸ Dressings will be pushed forward and off by the new advancing nail.
▸ Protective splinting is performed as previously described.

■ **Nail bed avulsion repair with full-thickness nail bed graft**
  • **Indications**
    ▸ Germinal matrix avulsion injuries too wide (>2 mm) for repair with bipedicled advancement
  • **Technique**
    ▸ Procedure begins as with split-thickness technique.
    ▸ The lateral nail bed of the great toe is the best donor site.
    ▸ Remove toenail, elevate the nail fold, and excise the lateral nail bed (full-thickness) from distal margin to most proximal extent of germinal matrix.
    ▸ Close donor site by advancement of lateral nail fold and primary closure.
    ▸ Use template to design graft dimensions.
    ▸ Secure graft to defect with 7-0 chromic gut suture.
      • **MUST** maintain proper longitudinal orientation
    ▸ Use nail plate, fine mesh gauze, or silicone sheeting for dressing.

POSTOPERATIVE CARE

■ Protective digital splint and bulky dressing suffice for adults unless associated injury requires greater immobilization.
■ More bulky, usually plaster, immobilization is required to ensure compliance in children.
■ Antibiotics are recommended if there is an associated distal phalanx fracture.
■ Patients are seen in office, and dressings are removed after 5-7 days.
■ Protective splinting is continued for 2 weeks.
■ Desensitization protocols and occupational therapy should be started after soft tissue healing is adequate.
■ Follow up monthly for 3 months and then at 6 months and 1 year.
■ Three nail cycles (approximately 1 year) are required before final nail appearance can be assessed reliably.

MICROVASCULAR NAIL BED RECONSTRUCTION[14]

■ Reconstructions are most common in Asian countries, where the aesthetic importance of the hand is culturally more significant than in other parts of the world.

- Free-distal toe flap transfer to an injured digit creates foot donor-site defects and additional scars on the recipient digit.
- More recent techniques, including short-pedicle free-nail transfer, free-pulp flaps and use of bone grafts for distal phalanx reconstruction, limit recipient scarring and demonstrate improved aesthetic outcome.
- These techniques require advanced equipment and microsurgical skill.
- These techniques should be considered for children and young females and performed in specialized centers.

KEY POINTS

✔ Nail production occurs primarily in the germinal matrix.
✔ It takes 100 days to grow a fingernail.
✔ Nail trephination is the best treatment for simple subungual hematomas.
✔ Loupe magnification and fine, absorbable sutures are necessary for all nail bed repairs.
✔ The nail plate makes the best dressing for the nail bed.
✔ Split-thickness nail bed grafting is best for sterile matrix avulsion injuries.
✔ Full-thickness nail bed grafting is best for germinal matrix avulsion injuries.

REFERENCES

1. Zook EG. Anatomy and physiology of the perionychium. Hand Clin 18:553-559, 2002.
2. Zook EG. Anatomy and physiology of the perionychium. Hand Clin 6:1-7, 1990.
3. Guy RJ. The etiologies and mechanisms of nail bed injuries. Hand Clin 6:9-19, 1990.
4. Chau N, Gauchard GC, Siegfried C, et al. Relationships of job, age, and life condition with the causes and severity of occupational injuries in construction workers. Int Arch Occup Environ Health 77:60-66, 2004.
5. Sorock GS, Lombardi DA, Hauser RB, et al. Acute traumatic occupational hand injuries: Type, location, and severity. J Occup Environ Med 44:345-351, 2002.
6. Zook EG, Guy RJ, Russell RC. A study of nail bed injuries: Causes, treatment, and prognosis. J Hand Surg Am 9:247-252, 1984.
7. Van Beek AL, Kassan MA, Adson MH, et al. Management of acute fingernail injuries. Hand Clin 6:23-35, 1990.
8. Roser SE, Gellman H. Comparison of nail bed repair versus nail trephination for subungual hematomas in children. J Hand Surg Am 24:1166-1170, 1999.
9. Brown RE. Acute nail bed injuries. Hand Clin 18:561-575, 2002.
10. Shepard GH. Management of acute nail bed avulsions. Hand Clin 6:39-56, 1990.
11. Shepard GH. Perionychial grafts in trauma and reconstruction. Hand Clin 18:595-614, 2002.
12. Brown RE, Zook EG, Russell RC. Fingertip reconstruction with flaps and nail bed grafts. J Hand Surg Am 24:345-351, 1999.
13. Hsieh SC, Chen SL, Chen TM, et al. Thin split-thickness toenail bed grafts for avulsed nail bed defects. Ann Plast Surg 52:375-379, 2004.
14. Endo T, Nakayama Y. Microtransfers for nail and fingertip replacement. Hand Clin 18:615-622, 2002.

58. Flexor Tendon Injuries

Joshua A. Lemmon
Blake A. Morrison

ANATOMY[1-6]

MUSCLES AND TENDONS
- Flexion of the fingers and thumb is powered by the **flexor digitorum profundus** (FDP), **flexor digitorum superficialis** (FDS), and **flexor pollicis longus** (FPL) **muscles.**
  - Each FDS tendon divides into two equal halves at the level of the metacarpal head.
    - ▸ Each half rotates laterally and dorsally around the FDP tendon.
    - ▸ The slips rejoin deep to the FDP tendon at *Camper's chiasma* (Fig. 58-1).
    - ▸ The FDS then inserts on the volar aspect of the middle phalanx as two separate slips.

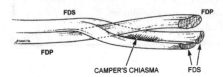

Fig. 58-1 Arrangement of flexor digitorum profundus *(FDP)* and flexor digitorum superficialis *(FDS)* tendons within the flexor tendon sheath. (From Idler RS. Anatomy and biomechanics of the digital flexor tendons. Hand Clin 1:4, 1985.)

- **FDS** tendons power flexion of the **proximal interphalangeal (PIP) joints.**
- **FDP** tendons power flexion of the **distal interphalangeal (DIP) joints.**
- Each FDP tendon inserts on the base of the distal phalanx.
- Tendons of these muscles each lie within a tendon sheath.
  - The sheath is a synovial-lined channel that allows smooth tendon gliding.
  - The synovial fluid environment provides tendon nutrition.
  - Each sheath is reinforced with thickened areas known as **pulleys.**

PULLEY SYSTEM
- Pulleys hold the tendons close to the phalanges, maximizing mechanical efficiency.
- There are **five annular** and **three cruciate** pulleys (Fig. 58-2).
- Transverse fibers of the **p**almar **a**poneurosis make up the **PA pulley**, also known as the **A1 pulley.**

> TIP: The A2 and A4 pulleys are the most important for proper flexor tendon function.

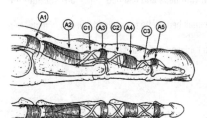

Fig. 58-2 Components of the flexor tendon sheath. A1-A5 are annular pulleys. C1-C3 are cruciate pulleys. (From Idler RS. Anatomy and biomechanics of the digital flexor tendons. Hand Clin 1:4, 1985.)

- The **pulley system of the thumb** reflects its unique anatomy, with one less tendon and one less intercalated joint than the fingers.

TENDON NUTRITION
- **Direct vascular supply**
  - **Musculotendinous junction:** Supplies short segment near the proximal end of the tendon
  - **Bony junction (Sharpey's fibers):** Supplies a short distal segment
  - **Vincula:** Fibrovascular structures that directly supply the tendons within the tendon sheath (Fig. 58-3)
- **Synovial diffusion:** Provides most of the tendon nutrition within the sheath

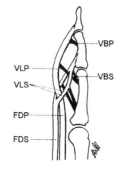

Fig. 58-3   Vincula of the flexor tendons. *FDP,* Flexor digitorum profundus; *FDS,* flexor digitorum superficialis; *VBP,* vinculum breve profundus; *VBS,* vinculum breve superficialis; *VLP,* vinculum longum profundus; *VLS,* vinculum longum superficialis. (From Kleinert HE, Lubahn JD. Current state of flexor tendon surgery. Ann Chir Main 3:10, 1984.)

FLEXOR TENDON ZONES
A universal nomenclature for flexor tendon injuries has been established. Recommended techniques and prognoses vary by zone.
- **Five zones for fingers** (Fig. 58-4)
  Zone I: Distal to insertion of the FDS
  Zone II: From A1 pulley to FDS insertion (within the sheath)
  Zone III: From distal end of the carpal tunnel to A1 pulley
  Zone IV: Within the carpal tunnel
  Zone V: Proximal to the carpal tunnel
- **Five zones for thumb**
  Zone T I: Distal to interphalangeal (IP) joint
  Zone T II: From A1 pulley to IP joint
  Zone T III: Over thenar eminence
  Zone T IV: Within the carpal tunnel
  Zone T V: Proximal to the carpal tunnel

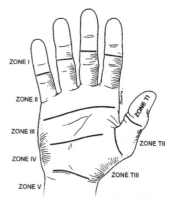

Fig. 58-4   Flexor tendon zones of the digits. (From Strickland JW. Flexor tendon repair. Hand Clin 1:56, 1985.)

HISTOLOGY[7]

TENDON COMPOSITION
- **Collagen:** Mostly type I
- **Ground substance:** Elastin and various mucopolysaccharides
- **Tenocytes:** Specialized fibroblasts

TENDON STRUCTURE
- **Endotenon:** Fascicular arrangement with bundles of tenocytes and collagen fibers held together by fine layer of connective tissue
- **Epitenon:** Septa of endotenon joined together externally to form fibrous outer layer
- **Paratenon:** Tendons covered by loose layer of adventitial tissue proximal to tendon sheath

PATIENT EVALUATION

HISTORY
- Age
- Handedness
- Occupation
- Mechanism of injury, including how hand was positioned during the injury
- Time of injury
- Previous treatment

PHYSICAL EXAMINATION
- Characterize and document open wounds.
- Evaluate arterial supply to the digit; handheld Doppler probes are useful.
- Evaluate for nerve injury.

> TIP: Sensation should be evaluated with static and moving two-point discrimination tests before using local anaesthetic.

- Test individual tendon function.
  - Each FDS and FDP must be assessed while blocking movement of adjacent digits.
- Recognize normal variants.
  - FDS tendon for small finger is absent in **15%** of the population.
  - **Linburg's syndrome:** Adhesions between FPL tendon and index finger FDP tendon within the carpal tunnel cause the index finger to flex with flexion of the thumb IP; found in **30%** of the population.

HAND RADIOGRAPHS
- Anteroposterior (AP), lateral, and oblique views

PREOPERATIVE CONSIDERATIONS, TIMING OF REPAIR, AND TREATMENT OPTIONS[8-12]

> TIP: Emergency flexor tendon repair is not required unless the digit is devascularized.

PRIMARY REPAIR (<24 HOURS)
- Preferred option when feasible
- **Contraindications**
  - Gross contamination or human bites

- Evidence of active infection (cellulitis, purulence)
- Lack of stable soft tissue coverage

DELAYED PRIMARY REPAIR (>24 HOURS BUT <2 WEEKS)
- Reasonable option for heavily contaminated wounds
- Functional results comparable to primary repair

SECONDARY REPAIR
- **Early (2-5 weeks)**
  - Performed before significant muscle contraction
  - Functional results similar to delayed primary repair
  - Increased risk of infection and prolonged edema with longer repair delay
- **Late (>5 weeks)**
  - Presence of tendon edema and softening
  - Repair without advancement and extensive deficit prohibited by significant muscular contraction
  - **Best treatments: Tendon graft or transfer**

TIP: The FDP tendon may be advanced up to, *but not more than,* 1 cm. Because the FDP tendons have a common muscle belly, excessive advancement creates a *quadrigia effect,* in which a flexion deformity appears in the repaired digit, and the adjacent digits are hyperextended.

TENDON GRAFTING
Segmental tendon loss or muscular contracture necessitates grafting for repair.
- **Single-stage**
  - Requires adequate tendon sheath and pulleys, soft tissue coverage, and supple joints
  - **Common donors**
    - ▶ Palmaris longus (13 cm)
    - ▶ Plantaris (31 cm)
    - ▶ Long-toe extensor (30 cm)
- **Two-stage: Used when tendon sheath is unusable**
  - **First stage**
    - ▶ Native tendon is excised.
    - ▶ Pulleys are reconstructed as necessary.
    - ▶ A silicone rod **(Hunter rod)** is sutured to distal tendon stump; rod induces formation of a **pseudosheath** within approximately 8 weeks.
  - **Second stage**
    - ▶ Tendon graft is sutured to the distal end of silicone rod and pulled through pseudosheath.
    - ▶ The **proximal** juncture is made with a **Pulvertaft weave.**
    - ▶ The **distal** juncture is made with a **pull-out suture** or **suture anchor** to bone.
    - ▶ Tension is adjusted so that the cascade of fingers is slightly tighter in the grafted digit.

TENDON TRANSFER
- Limited indications for flexor tendon repair
- Used when proximal muscle unusable because of denervation, direct injury, or contraction
- See Chapter 60 for more detailed information

OTHER OPTIONS

- For patients in whom normal active motion of DIP joint is not essential.
  - Arthrodesis
  - Capsulodesis
  - Tenodesis

OPERATIVE PRINCIPLES[12-15]

GENERAL TECHNICAL CONSIDERATIONS

- Flexor tendon repair should be performed in the operating room with loupe magnification.
- Incisions should be designed to **maintain viability of skin flaps, permit wide exposure,** and **prohibit formation of scar contractures:** Midlateral, volar zigzag, or combinations that incorporate traumatic laceration (Fig. 58-5).
- Minimal traumatic handling of the tendon surface limits subsequent adhesion formation.

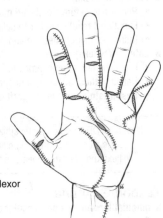

Fig. 58-5   Surgical exposure of the flexor tendon sheath.

REPAIR STRENGTH AND TECHNIQUE

- **Initial strength of the repair is proportional to the size and number of suture strands crossing the repair site.**
- Multiple methods exist for placing core sutures.
  - The most popular methods are shown in Fig. 58-6.
- **Pulvertaft weave**
  - Repair by weaving together the proximal and distal tendon ends.
  - As the strongest juncture, it is capable of immediate active motion.
  - Bulk prohibits use outside of zones III or V.
  - Technique is suitable only for **tendon grafts** or **transfers** because of additional length requirement.

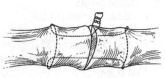

Modified Kessler

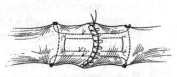

Indiana technique

Fig. 58-6   Popular core suture techniques for end-to-end tendon repair. (From Seiler JG. Flexor tendon repair. J Am Soc Surg Hand 1:177, 2001.)

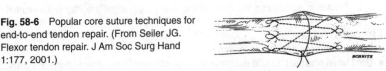

Six-Strand technique

PARTIAL TENDON LACERATIONS

- Technique is controversial.
- Oblique or beveled lacerations can catch on a pulley, so should be repaired with a few simple sutures.
- Most agree that tendon lacerations involving **more than 50% of tendon diameter** should be formally repaired with both core suture and epitendinous repair.
- Early mobilization is imperative.

ZONE I INJURIES

- **Sharp injuries: Lacerations**
  - Vincula: Usually holds proximal tendon end within injured digit
  - DIP volar plate examined and repaired if necessary
  - Distal FDP tendon with 5 mm stump required to place adequate core sutures
  - If sufficient distal length not available, reinsert with a **pull-out suture** tied over a dorsal button or use direct fixation to bone with **suture anchor(s)**

TIP: A monofilament pull-out suture is easier to remove and less susceptible to infection than braided suture material.

- **Avulsion injuries: "Jersey finger"**

These injuries are most common in **young men who participate in contact sports.** They occur because of forced extension during maximal profundus contraction.

  - **Types**

    Type I: FDP tendon retracts into palm with rupture of both vincula.
    - Requires repair within 1 week because tendon will degenerate without the nutrition of either the vincula or synovial diffusion.
    - Treat as for sharp injuries.

    Type II: FDP tendon avulses with small fragment of distal phalanx; the long vinculum remains intact, and the tendon retracts to the level of the PIP joint.
    - Repair can be delayed up to 6 weeks.
    - Pull-out suture or suture anchor is used as for sharp injuries.

    Type III: Large bony fragment is avulsed with the tendon and is prevented from retraction beyond the middle phalanx by the A4 pulley
    - Use open reduction and Kirschner-wire fixation if the fragment is large enough, otherwise use a pull-out suture secured over dorsal button.

    Type IV: Avulsion fracture of the distal phalanx combines with tendon avulsion from the fragment with tendon retraction.

- **Late treatment options and salvage procedures:** Secondary tendon grafts, tenodesis, and DIP capsulodesis or arthrodesis

ZONE II INJURIES

- **Historically associated with poor results,** acute repair used to be discouraged, given the name *"no man's land."*
  - Acute repair is now recommended because of improved techniques and results.
- Repair of both FDP and FDS is advocated by most, except in cases of massive injury (e.g., replantation) when repair of only FDP acceptable.

- Wide exposure is required.
- Neurovascular bundles are identified and protected.
- Transection of annular pulleys is avoided; instead windows can be made in tendon sheath by opening cruciate pulleys.
- **Tendon retrieval methods:**
  - Proximal to distal "milking" or use of reverse Esmarch's tourniquet
  - Skin hook passed retrograde into tendon sheath to grasp tendon end
  - Proximal (volar) incision made to expose proximal tendon end; small catheter used to pull tendon distally through pulley system to the repair site
- **Four to six core strands** of 3-0 or 4-0 braided or monofilament nonabsorbable suture are placed for repair.
- Strength and improved tendon gliding are added through use of **epitendinous suture** of running 5-0 or 6-0 monofilament polypropylene.

Zone III Injuries
- Repaired with same operative technique as for zone II
- **Prognosis better** than for zone II injuries
  - Repair bulk less important and postoperative adhesions less constricting
  - Functional results usually dictated by results of associated nerve repair

Zone IV Injuries
- Exacting technique must be used because tolerances within the carpal tunnel are similar to those for zone II.
- Operative technique is as for zone II.
- To prevent bowstringing, **transverse carpal ligament should be repaired** following tendon repair.

Zone V Injuries
- Repair with core sutures as described previously, but epitendinous suture is *not* necessary.
- Associated injuries in the median and ulnar nerves result in more disability than do tendon injuries themselves.

POSTOPERATIVE CARE AND REHABILITATION[16-18]

Extension Block-Splint
- Wrist at neutral to 30 degrees of flexion
- Metacarpophalangeal (MP) joints at 45-70 degrees of flexion
- Should maintain IP joints in near-full extension or slight flexion (15 degrees)
- Sutures removed after 2 weeks

Rehabilitation Protocols
- Early controlled mobilization protocols are now standard care, except for young children.
  - **Duran-Houser[19]:** Early passive range of motion
  - **Kleinert[20]:** Active extension, passive flexion
  - Multiple variations and modifications of these protocols described

COMPLICATIONS[19]

RUPTURES

- Occur in 5% of all repairs: slightly more common for FPL than for other finger tendons
- **Immediate exploration and re-repair recommended**
- Recurrent rupture best treated with secondary tendon reconstruction, tendon transfer, or arthrodesis

ADHESIONS

- Limited range of motion and function caused by postoperative and postinjury scars between tendon and surrounding structures
- **Increased likelihood of adhesions with prolonged immobilization and severe injury**
- **Consider tenolysis if:**
  - More than 3 months have elapsed since the tendon repair.
  - Tendon repair is intact, but there is a large discrepancy between total active range of motion (ROM) and total passive ROM.
  - Soft tissue is supple with normal or near-normal passive ROM.
  - There is no appreciable improvement in active ROM after 4-6 weeks of aggressive hand therapy.
- **Contractures**
  - Affect 17% of flexor tendon repairs[19]
  - Prevention and treatment primarily splinting
  - Open or closed capsulotomy reserved for severe and recalcitrant cases

---

KEY POINTS

- ✔ The best results are associated with early repair.
- ✔ Flexor tendon repair should be performed in the operating room, with a tourniquet and loupe magnification.
- ✔ The FDP tendon should not be advanced more than 1 cm.
- ✔ Proper splint placement and postoperative rehabilitation are as important as operative technique.

REFERENCES

1. Idler RS. Anatomy and biomechanics of the digital flexor tendons. Hand Clin 1:3-11, 1985.
2. Austin GJ, Leslie BM, Ruby LK, et al. Variations of the flexor digitorum superficialis of the small finger. J Hand Surg Am 14:262-267, 1989.
3. Doyle JR, Blythe WF. Macroscopic and functional anatomy of the flexor tendon sheath. J Bone Joint Surg Am 56:1094, 1974.
4. Doyle JR, Blythe WF. Anatomy of the flexor tendon sheath and pulleys of the thumb. J Hand Surg Am 2:149-151, 1977.
5. Doyle JR, Blythe WF. Anatomy of the flexor tendon sheath and pulley system: A current review. J Hand Surg Am 14:349-351, 1989.
6. Strickland JW. Development of flexor tendon surgery: Twenty-five years of progress. J Hand Surg Am 25:214-235, 2000.

7. Cohen MJ, Kaplan L. Histology and ultrastructure of the human flexor tendon sheath. J Hand Surg Am 12:25-29, 1987.

8. Strickland JW. Flexor tendon surgery. Part 1: Primary flexor tendon repair. J Hand Surg Br 14:261-272, 1989.

9. Steinberg DR. Acute flexor tendon injuries. Orthop Clin North Am 23:125-140, 1992.

10. Strickland JW. Flexor tendon injuries: I. Foundations of treatment. J Am Acad Orthop Surg 3:44-54, 1995.

11. Schneider LH, Bush DC. Primary care of flexor tendon injuries. Hand Clin 5:383-394, 1989.

12. Seiler JG. Flexor tendon repair. J Am Soc Surg of the Hand 1:177-191, 2001.

13. Strickland JW. Flexor tendon injuries: II. Operative technique. J Am Acad Orthop Surg 3:55-62, 1995.

14. Strickland JW. Flexor tendon injuries. Part 2. Flexor tendon repair. Orthop Rev 15:701-721, 1986.

15. Malerich M, Baird R, McMaster W, et al. Permissible limits of flexor digitorum profundus tendon advancement: An anatomic study. J Hand Surg Am 12:30-33, 1987.

16. Wang AW, Gupta A. Early motion after flexor tendon surgery. Hand Clin 12:43-55, 1996.

17. Bainbridge LC, Robertson C, Gillies D, et al. A comparison of post-operative mobilization of flexor tendon repairs with "passive flexion–active extension" and "controlled active motion" techniques. J Hand Surg Br 4:517-521, 1994.

18. Chow JA, Thomes LJ, Dovelle S, et al. Controlled motion rehabilitation after flexor tendon repair and grafting. A multi-centre study. J Bone Joint Surg Br 70:591-595, 1988.

19. Duran RJ, Houser RG. Controlled passive motion following flexor tendon repair in zones two and three. In American Association of Orthopaedic Surgeons Symposium on Tendon Surgery in the Hand. St Louis: CV Mosby, 1975, pp 105-111.

20. Kleinert HE, Kutz JE, Ashbell S. Primary repair of lacerated flexor tendons in "no man's land." J Bone Joint Surg Am 49:577, 1967.

21. Taras JS, Gray RM, Culp RW. Complications of flexor tendon injuries. Hand Clin 10:93-109, 1994.

59. Extensor Tendon Injuries

Bishr Hijazi
Blake A. Morrison

GENERAL CONSIDERATIONS[1]

- Concomitant neurovascular involvement is less common with extensor injuries.
  - Extensor tendons are relatively exposed, superficial structures.
  - The neurovascular bundles are guarded from dorsal injury by bone.
- Partial injuries are particularly common because of relatively flat extensor tendons in the digits.
- Penetrating injuries can easily involve underlying joints.

ANATOMY[2,3]

EXTRINSIC TENDONS
- Innervated by the **radial nerve**
- Cross the wrist under extensor retinaculum, which is divided into **six compartments** (Fig. 59-1)
  - **First compartment**
    - ▸ *Abductor pollicis longus* (APL)
      - ✦ Inserts into base of thumb metacarpal
      - ✦ Almost always multiple slips
    - ▸ *Extensor pollicis brevis* (EPB)
      - ✦ Inserts into base of thumb proximal phalanx
      - ✦ Rarely multiple slips
  - **Second compartment**
    - ▸ *Extensor carpi radialis longus* (ECRL)
      - ✦ Inserts into base of index finger metacarpal
    - ▸ *Extensor carpi radialis brevis* (ECRB)
      - ✦ Inserts into base of middle finger metacarpal
  - **Third compartment**
    - ▸ *Extensor pollicis longus* (EPL)
      - ✦ Inserts into base of thumb distal phalanx
      - ✦ Relative independence of action across all three joints because of multiple attachments to dorsal apparatus
  - **Fourth compartment**
    - ▸ *Extensor digitorum communis* (EDC)
      - ✦ Often has two slips to ring finger
      - ✦ Slip to small finger absent in up to **56%** of population

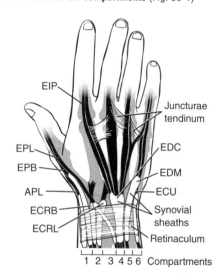

Fig. 59-1 Extensor compartments. *APL,* Abductor pollicis longus; *EDM,* extensor digiti minimi; *ECRB,* extensor carpi radialis brevis; *ECRL,* Extensor carpi radialis longus; *EDC,* Extensor digitorum communis; *ECU,* extensor carpi ulnaris; *EIP,* extensor indicis proprius; *EPB,* extensor pollicis brevis; *EPL,* extensor pollicis longus.

- ► *Extensor indicis proprius* (EIP)
  - ✦ Ulnar to EDC of index finger
  - ✦ **Most distal** musculotendinous junction
- **Fifth compartment**
  - ► *Extensor digiti minimi* (EDM) (also called *extensor digiti quinti* [EDQ])
    - ✦ Two slips in 80% of population
- **Sixth compartment**
  - ► *Extensor carpi ulnaris* (ECU)
    - ✦ **Only extensor tendon with a true sheath**
    - ✦ Tear of sheath: Leads to ulnar-sided wrist pain and popping sensation with subluxation of ECU

INTRINSICS

- **Dorsal interossei** (Fig. 59-2)
  - Innervated by **ulnar nerve**
  - Act to abduct fingers, flex metacarpophalangeals (MPs), and extend interphalangeals (IPs) (only with MP joints flexed)
- **Palmar (volar) interossei** (see Fig. 59-2)
  - Innervated by **ulnar nerve**
  - Act to adduct fingers, flex MPs, extend IPs (only with MP joints flexed)

TIP: The function of the interossei can be remembered by the mnemonics "DAB" (dorsal abduct) and "PAD" (palmar adduct)

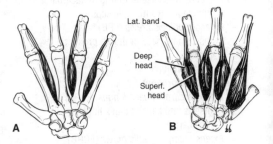

Fig. 59-2 Anatomy of the interosseous muscles.

- **Lumbricals** (Fig. 59-3)
  - **Ring** and **small** finger lumbricals innervated by **ulnar** nerve
  - **Index** and **middle** lumbricals innervated by **median** nerve
  - Prime extensors of IP joints, weak flexors of MP joints

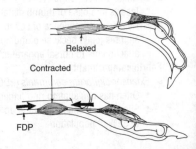

Fig. 59-3 The lumbrical muscle originates from the FDP tendon. When the lumbrical muscle is relaxed and the flexor profundus muscle contracts the IP joints flex. When the lumbrical contracts it extends the IP joints by relaxation of the profundus tendon distal to the lumbrical origin and by proximal pull on the lateral band and dorsal aponeurosis. (From Green DP, Hotchkiss RN, Pederson WC, et al, eds. Green's Operative Hand Surgery, 5th ed. Philadelphia: Churchill Livingstone, 2005, p 423.)

EXTENSOR MECHANISM
- Complex structures balance synergistic and antagonistic actions of extrinsics and intrinsics.
- Extensor tendon trifurcates into central slip and two lateral slips.
- Central slip inserts into base of middle phalanx, with fibers from lumbricals and interossei.
- Lateral slips join with lateral bands of intrinsics to form conjoined lateral bands.
- Conjoined lateral bands reunite over distal portion of middle phalanx to form terminal extensor tendon, which inserts into base of distal phalanx (Fig. 59-4).

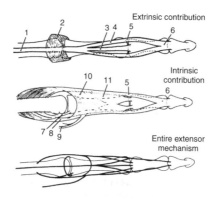

Fig. 59-4   Dorsal view of the extensor mechanism of the finger. Extrinsic and intrinsic contributions of the dorsal aponeurosis. *1,* Extensor tendon; *2,* sagittal band; *3,* central slip; *4,* lateral slip; *5,* conjoined lateral band; *6,* terminal tendon; *7,* superficial head and medial tendon of dorsal interosseous; *8,* deep head and lateral tendon of dorsal interosseous; *9,* lumbrical muscle and tendon; *10,* transverse fibers of dorsal aponeurosis; *11,* oblique fibers of dorsal aponeurosis. (From Green DP, Hotchkiss RN, Pederson WC, et al, eds. Green's Operative Hand Surgery, 5th ed. Philadelphia: Churchill Livingstone, 2005, p 422.)

JUNCTURAE
- Interconnect EDC tendons
- **Most variable anatomy of extensor system**
  - Consistency varies: Fascial, ligamentous, or tendinous
- Can provide some cross-tendon motion in cases of lacerated EDC tendons proximal to the juncturae, leading to misdiagnosis

SAGITTAL BANDS
- Originate from intermetacarpal plate on either side of metacarpal head
- Form dorsal expansion, or hood
- Maintain central slip of extensors over MP joints, preventing lateral subluxation
- Prevent MP joint hyperextension

EXTENSOR DIGITORUM BREVIS MANUS (EDBM)
- **Anomalous muscle** located on dorsal wrist, with tendons inserting into extensors of hand
- Approximately **3%** incidence
- Occasionally can produce pain and a mass effect when wrist is flexed
- **Often misdiagnosed as ganglion or other tumor**
- Treatment of choice is excision

PHYSIOLOGY OF TENDON HEALING

- See Chapter 58 for phases of tendon healing and tendon histology.

EXTENSOR TENDON HEALING: THREE SOURCES OF NUTRITION
- Endogenous circulation
- Synovial fluid diffusion (only under dorsal retinaculum)
- Exogenous circulation (from adhesions)

VASCULAR SUPPLY
- Like flexor tendons, there are multiple sources.
  - Musculotendinous junction
  - Bony insertion
  - Paratenon along length of tendon
  - Long mesotenon within synovial-lined dorsal retinaculum
- Unlike the flexor tendons, there are **no vincular vessels.**

ZONES OF INJURY[4]

- Universal, established nomenclature for extensor tendon injuries
- Recommended techniques and prognoses vary by zone
- **Nine zones:**
  Zone I: Over distal IP joint
  Zone II: Over middle phalanx
  Zone III: Over proximal IP joint
  Zone IV: Over proximal phalanx
  Zone V: Over MP joint
  Zone VI: Over dorsum of hand, distal to retinaculum
  Zone VII: Under dorsal retinaculum
  Zone VIII: Distal forearm
  Zone IX: Proximal forearm

TIP: The odd zones are over the joints; the even zones are in between.

RECOMMENDED REPAIR TECHNIQUE BY ZONE[5]

GENERAL CONSIDERATIONS
- Extensors are thin thus difficult to suture well.
- Kessler and Bunnell patterns are most popular for core sutures.
- Epitendinous sutures are usually 5-0 monofilament in a running cross-stitch, dorsal aspect only.
- Primary repair is preferred, except in cases of human bite or cellulitis.
- Injuries distal to the MP joints retract very little because the adjacent juncturae limit proximal migration.

TIP: Avoid large knots of monofilament suture outside the tendon, because they may be palpable under the thin dorsal soft tissue coverage. Braided core sutures are less conspicuous.

ZONE I (MALLET FINGER DEFORMITIES)

- Several **classification systems** have been proposed; the following was **described by Doyle.**[6]
    Type I: Closed injury with loss of tendon continuity, with or without small avulsion fracture
    Type II: Laceration at, or proximal to, DIP joint with loss of tendon continuity
    Type III: Deep abrasion with loss of skin, subcutaneous cover, and tendon substance
    Type IV A: Transepiphyseal plate fracture in children
    Type IV B: Fracture of 20%-50% of articular surface
    Type IV C: Fracture of more than 50% of articular surface, and volar subluxation of distal phalanx
- **Treatment by type**
    Type I
    - Immobilization of DIP joint only, in full extension
        * Dorsal or volar based aluminum foam splint, or plastic (Stack) splint
        * Requires at least 6 weeks of continuous extension followed with 2 weeks of splinting at night

---

TIP: Inform patients that *even one episode of flexion* "starts the clock over."

---

   * Careful observation of skin to avoid necrosis or maceration
   * Percutaneous pinning across DIP joint in full extension
     - May be warranted in certain occupations (e.g., surgeons)
     - Option for patients **incapable of compliance** (e.g., children)
    Type II
    - Running monofilament suture, incorporating skin and tendon
    - Remove suture after 10-14 days
    - Splint as for type I
    Type III
    - Typically requires flap reconstruction of soft tissue
    - Terminal extensor reconstructed secondarily with tendon graft
    Type IV
    - Closed reduction and percutaneous K-wire fixation when possible
    - Open reduction with transarticular K-wire and pull-out suture or K-wire fracture fragment fixation
    - Fixation protected with splint for 6 weeks, then K-wires removed and progressive motion begun
- **Mallet thumb**
    - Closed injuries treated by splinting, as with fingers
    - Open injuries treated with direct repair
        * EPL is substantial and holds suture well.
        * Repair is protected with splinting for 6 weeks.

ZONE II

- **Partial lacerations** *(less than 50% of surface)*
    - Repair is not required.
    - Debride frayed edges and provide closure or wound care.
    - Begin active motion after 7-10 days, or after wound is healed.

- **Lacerations greater than 50% of surface**
  - The tendon is often too thin for a core suture.
  - Repair with a running 4-0 suture, followed by 5-0 epitendinous cross-stitch.
  - Splint the DIP joint for 6 weeks, with DIP joint free.
- **Thumb**
  - The EPL can usually hold a core-type suture at this level.
  - Add an epitendinous suture.
  - Splint the IP joint for 6 weeks, with the MP joint free.
  - Some advocate short, forearm-based thumb spica cast with thumb in full extension.

ZONE III

- **Closed avulsion** *(boutonniere injury)*
  - Often misdiagnosed as a "jammed" or "sprained" finger
  - **Diagnosis**
    - ▸ Swelling and tenderness are observed at base of dorsal middle phalanx.
    - ▸ PIP joint extension exhibits weakness against resistance.
    - ▸ Extension function is preserved with only one lateral band intact.
    - ▸ MRI or ultrasound can confirm injury.
  - **Treatment**
    - ▸ Splint PIP in full extension for 6 weeks with MP and DIP joints free.
    - ▸ Follow with active PIP flexion and 2 weeks of splinting at night.
    - ▸ K-wire fixation of the PIP joint is an alternative.
    - ▸ Open reduction or reinsertion for avulsion fracture fragment is viewed using radiographs.
- **Open injury**
  - Use Kessler pattern 4-0 core suture, followed by 5-0 epitendinous cross-stitch (Fig. 59-5).
  - The PIP joint is violated easily; **irrigate thoroughly.**
  - Splint as for previously described closed injury.
  - Inadequate distal stump of tendon can be addressed by drilling a transverse hole through dorsal base of middle phalanx.
  - **Primary goal of treatment: Prevent development of boutonniere deformity** *(DIP hyperextension with flexion deformity of the PIP joint.)*
    - ▸ Deformity can take weeks to develop because **lateral bands slowly migrate volarly.**
    - ▸ Secondary reconstruction of chronic boutonnieres is difficult.
    - ▸ Prevention is much easier than treatment.

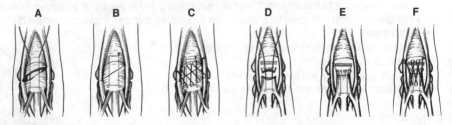

Fig. 59-5 Techniques for repair of zone III lacerations. **A-C,** Central slip laceration with sufficient tendon to repair with core suture and oversew with Silfverskiöld epitendinous stitch. **D-F,** The core stitch can be passed through a trough in the base of the middle phalanx when the tendon laceration is distal, leaving a small stump of central slip. (From Green DP, Hotchkiss RN, Pederson WC, et al, eds. Green's Operative Hand Surgery, 5th ed. Philadelphia: Churchill Livingstone, 2005, p 202.)

■ **Thumb**
- Injury to one or both of the extensors (EPL or EPB) is possible.
- Both tendons are large enough for core sutures.
- Splint with wrist in 30 degrees of extension; thumb IP and MP joints are in extension for 3 weeks.
- Establish progressive active motion over next 4 weeks.

ZONE IV

■ **Partial injuries** are common because the tendon is broad at this level.
■ Repair central tendon laceration with 4-0 core suture and 5-0 epitendinous cross-stitch.
■ Maintain exact length relationships.
■ Splint with wrist in 30-degree extension, MP joints in 45-70 degrees flexion, and IP joints in extension.
■ Begin passive extension after 1 week and gentle active extension at 4 weeks.
■ Isolated lateral band laceration can be repaired with a single 5-0 epitendinous cross-stitch.
■ Thumb is treated as previously described for zone III injury.

ZONE V

■ **Open tendon lacerations**

CAUTION: Beware of a wound from a closed-fist strike ("fight bite"). Victims of such altercations are notoriously evasive when interviewed.

- Review radiographs carefully.
- Debride wound edges and irrigate thoroughly.
- **Leave human bite wounds open.**
- Lacerations at this level are often partial.
- Repair large lacerations as for zone IV injuries.
- Postoperative management is as for zone IV injuries.

■ **Open sagittal band laceration**
- Must be repaired to prevent subluxation of the tendon.
- Use cross-stitch of 4-0 or 5-0 suture.
- Splint with MP joints in full extension for 3-5 days, then follow with gentle flexion and extension exercises.
- Avoid abduction or adduction by buddy-taping to the adjacent finger.

■ **Closed sagittal band injury**
- Injury occurs following blunt trauma, forceful extension, or flexion of digit.
- **Diagnosis**
  ▶ Tenderness, swelling, and inability to actively extend MP joint
  ▶ Subluxation of extensor tendon (usually ulnar) with flexion
  ▶ Patient capable of holding finger in extension once passively positioned
- **Treatment**
  ▶ **Acute injuries (within 2 weeks)**
    ✦ Flexion block-splint that holds MP joints in extension for 6 weeks
  ▶ **Late injuries (after 2 weeks)**
    ✦ Primary repair when possible, or one of many reconstructive procedures

- **Thumb**
  - APL or EPB can be lacerated.
  - **Look for concomitant injuries to the superficial radial nerve branches or the radial artery.**
  - Either tendon can be repaired as for zone III injury.

> TIP: An APL laceration near its insertion can be treated with reinsertion into the metacarpal base.

ZONE VI

- Tendons are substantial enough for core sutures.
- Prognosis tends to be very good in this zone, with adhesions uncommon.
- Use postoperative splint as for zone IV injury.

ZONE VII

- Tendons are substantial enough for core sutures.
- Treatment of retinacular rent is controversial.
  - **Traditional approach**
    - ▸ Excise portion of the retinaculum adjacent to the repair.
    - ▸ Preserve a distal or proximal portion of retinaculum to prevent bowstringing.
  - **Alternative approach**
    - ▸ Repair the retinacular rent and use dynamic splint early (after 10 days).
    - ▸ Use postoperative splint as for zone IV injury.

ZONE VIII

- **Associated neurovascular injuries are common;** document with a thorough examination.
- Lacerated tendons hold core sutures well.
- **Lacerations or avulsions at musculotendinous juncture**
  - Approximate tendon to the fibrous septa of the muscle belly.
  - Splint statically with wrist in 40-degree extension, MP joints in 20-degree flexion, and fingers free for 5 weeks.
  - **These repairs are tenuous;** use tendon transfers as salvage procedures.

ZONE IX

- Injuries at this level are usually from penetrating trauma and require thorough exploration.
- **Nerve injuries are common** and should be repaired primarily.
- Repair muscle bellies with **multiple figure-eight absorbable sutures.**
- Immobilize with wrist in extension, MP joints in 20 degrees of flexion, and fingers free for 4 weeks.
- Follow with 2 weeks of night splinting.
- Immobilize elbow at 90 degrees if repaired muscles originate at or above the elbow.
- Use tendon transfers as salvage procedures.

COMPLICATIONS

RUPTURE

- As with flexor tendons, **explore immediately and repeat repair.**

ADHESIONS
- Occurrence is less likely than with flexor repairs.
- Adhesions to the supple dorsal soft tissues can move and eventually break away with remodeling.
- When necessary, tenolysis can be performed with no need for pulley reconstruction.
- Preserve the sagittal bands.
- The dorsal retinaculum can be sacrificed when substantially involved.

SEQUENCE OF EXTENSOR IMBALANCE
- Swan neck deformity
- Boutonniere deformity
- Extrinsic tightness
- Intrinsic tightness
- Extensor tendon subluxation with ulnar drift

KEY POINTS
- Partial injuries are common with extensor tendons.
- All extrinsic extensors are innervated by the radial nerve.
- The interossei are innervated by the ulnar nerve.
- The index finger (IF) and middle finger (MF) lumbricals are innervated by the median nerve, and the ring finger (RF) and small finger (SF) are innervated by the ulnar nerve.
- There are **six** dorsal wrist compartments.
- Extensor tendon lacerations may be camouflaged by the cross-tendon action of the juncturae tendinum.
- There are **nine zones** of the extensor tendon versus five of the flexor tendon. Odd zones are over joints and even zones are over bones.
- A Bunnell suture technique frequently is the most useful because of the broad, flat nature of the extensor.
- Boutonniere and swan neck deformities can result from extensor tendon imbalance following subpunctural repair on neglected injuries.

REFERENCES

1. American Society for Surgery of the Hand. History and general examination. In The Hand: Examination and Diagnosis, 2nd ed. New York: Churchill Livingstone, 1983, pp 3-10.
2. Agur AMR, Lee MJ, eds. Grant's Atlas of Anatomy, 10th ed. Baltimore: Lippincott, 1999.
3. el-Badawi MG, Butt MM, al-Zuhair AG, et al. Extensor tendons of the fingers: Arrangement and variations— II. Clin Anat 8:391-398, 1995.
4. Blair WF, Steyers CM. Extensor tendon injuries. Orthop Clin North Am 23:141-148, 1992.
5. Green DP, Hotchkiss RN, Pederson WC, et al, eds. Green's Operative Hand Surgery, 5th ed. Philadelphia: Churchill Livingstone, 2005.
6. Doyle JR. Extensor tendons—Acute injuries. In Green DP, ed. Green's Operative Hand Surgery, 3rd ed. New York: Churchill Livingstone, 1993.

60. Tendon Transfers

Bishr Hijazi
Blake A. Morrison

GENERAL PRINCIPLES[1,2]

- **Basic concepts**
  - The power of a functioning muscle and tendon unit can be used to activate a nonfunctioning unit.
  - Tendon transfers are justified to restore **functional** motion in the hand, not just motion.
  - See Table 60-1 for a list of abbreviations used in this chapter.

Table 60-1 *Forearm and Hand Muscle Abbreviations*

PL: Palmaris longus	**FCU:** Flexor carpi ulnaris	**ECU:** Extensor carpi ulnaris	**APL:** Adductor pollicis longus
FDS: Flexor digitorum superficialis	**FCR:** Flexor carpi radialis	**EPL:** Extensor pollicis longus	**APB:** Adductor pollicis brevis
FPL: Flexor pollicis longus	**FPB:** Flexor pollicis brevis	**EPB:** Extensor pollicis brevis	**OP:** Opponens pollicis
PT: Pronator teres	**EDC:** Extensor digiti communis	**EIP:** Extensor indicis proprius	**FDM:** Flexor digiti minimi
PQ: Pronator quadratus	**ECRB:** Extensor carpi radialis brevis	**EDM:** Extensor digiti minimi	**ADM:** Abductor digiti minimi
FDP: Flexor digitorum profundus	**ECRL:** Extensor carpi radialis longus	**BR:** Brachioradialis	**ODM:** Opponens digiti minimi

- **One muscle, one function**
  - A tendon will move only the joint with the tightest attachment.
  - If a single tendon must be transferred to two or more tendons, ensure that the excursion of each is the same.
- **Similar force of contraction**
  - The chosen donor must have adequate strength for the new function.
  - Expect the transferred tendon **to lose one grade of strength.**
  - Overly powerful muscles can lead to joint deformity.
- **Adequate excursion**
  - Use the **3-5-7 rule** as a practical guide, based on the insertion of the various hand tendons.
    - **Wrist level** (e.g., wrist extensors, flexors): **3.3 cm long**
    - **Metacarpophalangeal (MP) joint level** (e.g., finger extensors): **5.0 cm long**
    - **Finger tips** (e.g., FDP, FDS): **7.0 cm long**
  - Tenodesis at the wrist increases excursion by **2.5 cm.**
  - Dissection of the muscle from surrounding fascial attachments (e.g., BR) can increase excursion substantially.

586

- *Need straightest line of action possible*
  - Parallel the line of action of the muscle being replaced.
  - Power is maximized.
- *Preservation of tenodesis action of the wrist (synergism)*
  - Muscles transferred within a synergistic group are easier to retrain than muscles from an antagonistic group.
  - **"Fist" group**
    - ▶ Wrist extensors (Make a tight fist and feel the tension of your ECRB and ECRL.)
    - ▶ Finger and thumb flexors
    - ▶ Digital adductors
    - ▶ Forearm pronators
  - **"Open hand" group**
    - ▶ Wrist flexors (Fully extend your hand, feel the FCU, FCR, and PL tendons' tension.)
    - ▶ Finger and thumb extensors
    - ▶ Digital abductors
    - ▶ Forearm supinators
- *Expendability of donors*
  - Avoid significant functional deficit from loss of the donor's original function.
  - For example, the PL is inadequate as a sole remaining wrist flexor.

ALTERNATIVES

- **Nerve repair**
  - Preferred treatment when possible
  - Possible for up to 87% of cases
- **Primary tendon repair or tendon graft**
  - Primary repair is preferred when ends of injured tendon are suitable.
  - No task reeducation is required.
  - Muscles used are already correct in power, amplitude, and direction of pull.
- **Tenodesis**
  - Consider when prognosis for tendon transfer is poor.
  - Providing a fixed origin for a tendon may position a joint for acceptable movement.
- **Arthrodesis**
  - May provide adequate stability for desired function
  - Typically reduces number of muscle and tendon motors needed
- **Nerve transfer**
  - Theoretical advantages in rehabilitation
    - ▶ No adhesions to tendon junctions
    - ▶ Power, amplitude, and direction of pull all correct
  - Technically very demanding
- **Amputation**
  - May be indicated in extreme cases
  - Tends to shorten rehabilitation time

INDICATIONS

- **Nerve injury**
  - This is the **most common indication.**
  - Smaller, more distal nerve branches are less likely to require transfer.
  - Transfers can be performed for **temporary function** while waiting for nerve recovery.
- **Muscle or tendon injury**
  - Trauma
  - Disease processes (e.g., poliomyelitis, rheumatoid arthritis)
- **Spastic disorders (e.g., cerebral palsy)**
  - Tendon transfers are far less predictable.
  - *Never perform a transfer to a limb with athetoid movements.*

CONTRAINDICATIONS

- **Advanced age**
  - Reeducation of movement is more difficult.
  - Need for power movements decreases.
- **Unmotivated patients**
  - Patients unconcerned with disability are unlikely to retrain transferred function.
  - Patients must be cognizant of loss of function.
- **Lack of a specific task deficit**
  - Transfers are planned to provide specific tasks (e.g., opening doors).
  - Transfers are not performed simply to replace lost motion.
- **Systemic disease**
  - If functional loss is because of systemic disease, it must be under medical control before attempting tendon transfer.

EVALUATION

- **Thorough history**
  - Determine duration of disability.
  - Have the patient list specific task deficits.
  - Evaluate status of any systemic diseases.
  - Ensure that patient's expectations are realistic.
  - Confirm patient's motivation to comply with rehabilitation.
- **Careful examination to determine functional deficit**
  - Which nerve injured, and at what level
  - Which muscles or tendons injured
  - Associated injuries (e.g., skeletal, sensory nerve)
  - Potential donor availability
- **Complex deficits planning chart**
  - List functional deficits, working motors, and available donor motors.
  - Match donors to needs to stage transfers.

TIMING

IMMEDIATE TENDON TRANSFERS

- Done when prognosis for nerve recovery **poor**
  - Destruction of large portion of muscle
  - Proximal destruction of nerve or large segmental loss
  - Advanced age
- For **temporary function** while waiting for nerve repair
  - PT to ECRB transfer (e.g., after radial nerve palsy)
  - Serves as **"internal splint"**
    - ▸ Obviates need for external splint
    - ▸ Supplements extension once recovery begins

DELAYED TENDON TRANSFERS

- Perform after **expected recovery period** of injured nerve.
  - Measure distance from point of injury to muscle in millimeters.
  - Distance in millimeters plus 30 provides the number of days for defining the expected recovery period.
- **Perform only after the following requirements have been met:**
  - Skeletal stability
  - Supple soft tissue coverage
  - Joint mobility
  - Adequate (i.e., at least protective) sensation
  - Correction of any contractures

TENDON TRANSFERS FOR SPECIFIC NERVE PALSIES

LOW RADIAL NERVE PALSY

- **Affected innervations**
  - ECRB (variably)
  - ECU
  - Finger and thumb extensors
  - Supinator
- **Functional deficits and recommended options**
  - **Finger extension, one of the following:**
    - ▸ FCR to EDC
    - ▸ FCU to EDC
    - ▸ FDS of ring or middle finger to EDC
  - **Thumb extension and radial abduction**
    - ▸ PL to EPL
    - ▸ FDS of ring or middle finger to EPL
    - ▸ FCR to APL; EPB and FDS to EPL

TIP: Avoid transferring the FCR and FCU in the same extremity. PL alone is inadequate for flexion of the wrist.

- **Radial deviation of wrist because of unopposed ERCL action**
  - ECRL to ECRB (side-to-side)

HIGH RADIAL NERVE PALSY

- **Affected innervations**
  - Same as for low radial nerve palsy, plus ECRL and BR
- **Functional deficits**
  - Same as for low palsy, plus wrist extension
- **Recommended options**
  - PT to ECRB for wrist extension
  - Other deficits treated as for low palsy

LOW MEDIAN NERVE PALSY (LEVEL OF WRIST)

- **Affected innervations**
  - Thenar eminence: APB, OP, and superficial head of FPB
  - Lumbricals to index and middle fingers
  - Sensory nerves to palm, thumb, index, middle, and radial ring fingers
- **Functional deficits and recommended options**
  - **Thumb opposition**
    - FDS of ring finger
    - EIP
    - PL *(Camitz procedure)*
    - ADM *(Huber procedure)*
  - All of these options insert into the APB, or split APB and EPL.

NOTE: All of these require construction of a pulley to redirect the direction of pull.

HIGH MEDIAN NERVE PALSY[2,3]

- **Affected innervations**
  - Same as for low median nerve palsy plus:
    - FPL, FDS, FDP to index and half of FDP to middle finger
    - PQ and PT (variably)
    - FCR
- **Functional deficits**
  - Same as for low palsy plus:
    - Flexion of thumb and index fingers
    - Weakness of flexion of middle finger
    - Weakness or loss of pronation
- **Recommended options**
  - **For thumb flexion**
    - BR to FPL
    - ECRL or ECRB to FPL
  - **For index and middle finger flexion**
    - Transfer side-to-side to intact ulnar FDPs
    - ECRL to FDPs
  - Reroute biceps if pronation too weak to overcome supination

NOTE: Loss of pronation is a significant disability.

- Opposition treated as for low median nerve palsy

LOW ULNAR NERVE PALSY[3,4]

- **Affected innervations**
  - Hypothenar eminence: ADM, ODM, and FDM
  - Lumbricals to ring and small fingers
  - Adductor pollicis
  - Deep head of FPB
  - Dorsal and palmar interossei
  - Sensory nerves to small and ulnar ring fingers
- **Functional deficits**
  - Clawing of ring and small fingers
  - Inadequate pinch between index finger and thumb
  - Persistent abduction of small finger *(Wartenberg's sign)*
  - Loss of power grip
- **Recommended options**
  - **Multiple procedures described for correction of clawing**
    - ▶ FDS to lateral bands
    - ▶ FDS to A1 pulley *(Zancolli lasso)*[5] or A2 pulley
    - ▶ ECRB or ECRL to lateral bands
  - **For key pinch**
    - ▶ BR to adductor pollicis tendon of thumb
    - ▶ ECRB to same
    - ▶ FDS of long or ring finger to same
    - ▶ EIP to same
    - ▶ MP or interphalangeal (IP) joint fusion in thumb
  - **For Wartenberg's sign**
    - ▶ Ulnar half of EDM to radial proximal phalanx of small finger or A2 pulley
  - **For power grip**
    - ▶ ECRL to lateral bands, proximal phalanx, or A2 pulleys
    - ▶ BR to same

HIGH ULNAR NERVE PALSY[3,4]

- **Affected innervations**
  - Same as for low ulnar nerve palsy plus:
    - ▶ FDP to ring and small finger
    - ▶ FCU
- **Functional deficits**
  - Inadequate pinch
  - Wartenberg's sign
  - Loss of power grip
  - No clawing because no longer an imbalance of extrinsics versus intrinsics
- **Recommended options**
  - See section on low ulnar nerve palsy.
  - Perform FCR to FCU transfer in rare cases of radial wrist deviation causing dysfunction.

TENDON TRANSFERS FOR DISEASE

RHEUMATOID ARTHRITIS[2]

- **Causes of ruptures**
  - **Tenosynovitis**—Attrition from tendon rubbing over bone damaged by chronic synovitis
  - **Flexor pollicis longus** *(Mannerfelt lesion)*
    - ▶ **Most common rupture in rheumatoid arthritis**
    - ▶ Secondary to attrition over scaphoid
    - ▶ Only apparent in patients with functional IP joint
    - ▶ **Treatment**
      - ✦ Resection of bony spicule causing rupture
      - ✦ Intercalated tendon graft
      - ✦ Tendon transfer with FDS from middle or ring finger
  - **Extensor pollicis longus rupture**
    - ▶ Secondary to tenosynovitis or attrition
    - ▶ **Treatment**
      - ✦ Tenosynovectomy
      - ✦ Excision of any bone spikes
      - ✦ EIP to EPL transfer
  - **Finger extensor rupture**
    - ▶ Secondary to tenosynovitis or attrition over ulnar head
    - ▶ Often starts at small finger, followed by ring finger, middle finger, etc., because intact tendons shift ulnarly
    - ▶ **Treatment**
      - ✦ **Single tendon:** Transfer to adjacent intact tendon.
      - ✦ **Two tendons:** Transfer to adjacent tendon, with or without EIP transfer to small finger.
      - ✦ **Multiple tendons:** Transfer as for two tendons, with or without FDS of ring finger.
      - ✦ **Multiple ruptures with MP joint disease:** Address MP joints by arthroplasty, as with first part of staged reconstruction.
      - ✦ Perform dorsal tenosynovectomy, with or without distal ulnar excision.

CEREBRAL PALSY

- **Many tendon transfers are used, typically to augment or balance wrist or digital extension.**
  - FCU to ECRB
  - ECU to ECRB
  - FCU to EDC
  - BR to ECRB

NOTE: Tendon transfers are less predictable for cerebral palsy patients.

- **Athetoid movement**
  - Involuntary movement that varies from spastic to flaccid
  - *Tendon transfers typically too unpredictable to be useful*

POLIOMYELITIS
- Muscles often regain function, particularly those affected early.
- **Delay tendon transfers** until no recovery of weakness is documented for at least 6 months.

LEPROSY (HANSEN'S DISEASE)
- Most common deficits requiring tendon transfer are clawing, loss of opposition, and key pinch.
- See sections on ulnar and median nerve palsies for details about procedures.
- **Disease must be under control before surgery.**

ROUTINE POSTOPERATIVE CARE

- **Immobilization**
  - Transfers are typically immobilized for the first 4 weeks.
  - Splint in a position that minimizes tension on the transfer.
  - Any joints that can be left free without placing tension on the transfer are mobilized passively.
- **Mobilization**
  - Begin protected mobilization at week 4.
  - Typically, no strengthening is allowed until week 6-8.
  - By late mobilization phase (week 6), patients are splinted only at night.
- **Strengthening**
  - Resistance exercises are added gradually, beginning at week 6-8.

COMPLICATIONS

- **Rupture**
  - **Low incidence with Pulvertaft weaves**
  - Immediate exploration and repair recommended
- **Adhesions**
  - Likelihood is reduced by routing the transferred tendon through scar-free subcutaneous tissue.

CAUTION: Do not orient incisions directly over the path of the transferred tendon.

- **Improper tension**
  - All tendon transfers tend to stretch with time.

TIP: Start with some initial overcorrection.

KEY POINTS

✔ Adherence to the general principles optimizes results.
✔ Nerve injury is the most common indication for tendon transfers.
✔ Never perform a tendon transfer to a limb with athetoid movements.
✔ For complex decisions, prepare a planning chart.
✔ Immediate tendon transfer can be performed when prognosis for nerve recovery is dismal and/or when seeking temporary function while waiting for nerve recovery (serves as an "internal splint").
✔ Tenosynovitis causes tendon rupture with rheumatoid arthritis because the tendon rubs over damaged bone.

REFERENCES

1. Beasley RW. Principles of tendon transfer. Orthop Clin North Am 1:433-438, 1970.
2. Phalen GS, Miller RC. The transfer of wrist extensor muscles to restore or reinforce flexion power of the fingers and opposition of the thumb. J Bone Joint Surg Am 29:993-997, 1947.
3. Brand PW. Tendon transfers for median and ulnar nerve paralysis. Orthop Clin North Am 1:447-454, 1970.
4. Mayer L. Operative reconstruction of the paralysed upper extremity. J Bone Joint Surg 21:377-383, 1939.
5. Zancolli EA, Cozzi EP. Atlas of Surgical Anatomy of the Hand. New York: Churchill Livingstone, 1992.

61. Amputations

David S. Chang

GENERAL CONSIDERATIONS

- **Trauma** is the most common cause of amputations.
- Are all digits necessary for patient's occupation?
- What is patient's attitude toward amputation?

INDICATIONS

- Multiple-level injury
- Complex, nonsalvageable, traumatic injuries
- Poor candidate for replantation (e.g., other life-threatening trauma, significant smoker)
- Medical comorbidities
- Significant vascular disorders
- Necrosis
- Infection
- Tumors

CONTRAINDICATIONS

- **There are no absolute contraindications to amputation.**
- Potentially amputated part is in good condition.
- Patient is a good candidate for replantation (see Chapter 62).

GOALS

- Preserve length
- Durable coverage
- Preserve useful sensibility
- Prevent symptomatic neuromas
- Prevent adjacent joint contractures
- Minimize morbidity
- Early prosthetic fitting
- Early return to work and recreation

LEVEL OF INJURY[1,2]

FINGER
- **Technique**
  1. Administer adequate anaesthesia.
  2. Administer preoperative antibiotics and tetanus prophylaxis.
  3. Remove gross wound contamination.
  4. After field is prepared and draped, irrigate wound thoroughly with saline under tourniquet control.
  5. Debride devitalized tissue.
  6. Assess soft tissue coverage and shorten bone, if necessary, to allow for primary closure.
  7. Use volar skin for distal stump coverage if possible, or use a fishmouth incision (Fig. 61-1).
  8. Cut back flexor and extensor tendons, depending on level of amputation. **Do not suture tendon ends to stump.**
  9. Identify digital nerves and transect proximal to amputation site to prevent symptomatic neuromas.
  10. Close the stump with interrupted nonabsorbable sutures (e.g., 4-0 nylon).
  11. Place a splint and begin range of motion exercises 3-5 days postoperatively.

> TIP: Most traumatic finger amputations can be managed in the emergency department with a digital block and finger tourniquet.

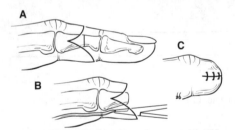

Fig. 61-1 Use of volar and dorsal skin flaps for stump coverage. Volar flaps are preferable for greater sensibility.

- **Outcomes**
  - Primary digital amputation can result in better function and quicker return to work than complex reconstruction or replantation.[3]
  - Symptomatic neuromas can be prevented by transecting nerve proximal to the stump to allow retraction into uninjured tissue.
  - Early return to work can prevent symptomatic neuromas.[4]
  - Cold intolerance and dysesthesia are common complications that usually resolve, but may last up to 2 years.[5]

SPECIFIC AMPUTATIONS
- **Digital tip** (see Chapter 56)
- **Through distal interphalangeal (DIP) or posterior interphalangeal (PIP) joint**
  - Use skeletal shortening and primary closure.
  - Use rongeur to contour shape of stump, and **remove articular cartilage** to prevent necrosis or infection.
  - Avoid lumbrical plus deformity.

▸ Transection of flexor digitorum profundus (FDP) tendon and retraction proximally pulls on lumbrical. As finger is flexed, lumbrical puts tension on lateral bands of extensor mechanism causing extension of PIP joint.

▸ Treat by sectioning lumbrical tendon (can be done later).

- **Through middle or proximal phalanx**
  • Use skeletal shortening and primary closure with dorsal and volar skin flaps (fishmouth incision).
- **Proximal to proximal phalanx:** Intrinsic muscles allow flexion up to 45 degrees unless amputation is at or near metacarpophalangeal (MP) joint; in which case preserving a very short proximal phalanx may **impair function;** *consider ray amputation.*

CAUTION: *Do not tether flexor tendons* because this can prevent excursion of flexors to remaining fingers (quadrigia effect).

TIP: If an injury to the middle phalanx is proximal to flexor digitorum superficialis (FDS) tendon, the need to preserve length is obviated because there will be no PIP joint motion without the FDS tendon.

- **Through thumb**
  • See Chapter 63 for algorithmic approach to thumb reconstruction.
  • Restoring sensibility is important for restoring function.
  • If no bone is exposed can allow to heal by secondary intention.
  • Coverage of exposed bone can be done with crossfinger flap or radially innervated sensory flap.
- **Multiple digits**
  • Preserve as much viable tissue as possible for later reconstruction.

HAND

- **Ray amputation**
  • Amputation at or near MP joint is best treated with partial metacarpal resection.
  • Power grip, key pinch, and supination strength will be reduced, which must be weighed against disability associated with the gap created by the missing finger.
  • Small objects can fall through the gap created by the missing digit, especially with the long and ring fingers.

TIP: Ray amputation can be performed electively and is rarely indicated at the time of initial trauma.

- **Technique**
  1. Make incision over dorsum of metacarpal.
  2. Divide extensor tendon.
  3. Dissect periosteum off metacarpal needing resection.
  4. Perform osteotomy at metacarpal base.
  5. Third-ray amputations can be managed with index metacarpal transposition[6] or suture of deep intervolar plate ligaments to close the space between the index and long fingers.[7]
  6. Fourth-ray amputations can be managed similar to third-ray amputations, with transposition of fifth metacarpal or suture of deep intervolar plate ligaments.

7. Fifth-ray amputations require preservation of metacarpal base because of insertions of flexor carpi ulnaris (FCU) and extensor carpi ulnaris (ECU) tendons.
8. Distract flexor tendons and transect.
9. Transect neurovascular bundles.
10. Trim skin flaps and close wound primarily.

- **Outcomes**
  - Ray amputations result in **15%-20% loss of grip strength**[8-10] and narrowing of the palm.
  - **Index-ray amputations** also result in **50% loss of pronation strength.**[8]
  - Border-ray translocation to a central position can improve cosmetic results.

WRIST

- **Through carpus**
  - Functional restoration results are worse than those for more distal amputations.
  - Initially preserve as much tissue as possible.
  - Preserve radiocarpal joint if possible, which may allow for a functional prosthesis.
- **Wrist disarticulation**
  - This method is preferable to long, below-elbow amputations.
  - Preservation of distal radioulnar and radial styloid allows for full supination and pronation, as well as better-fitting prosthesis.
  - Ligate radial and ulnar arteries and transect nerves proximal to end of stump.
  - Pull flexor and extensor tendons distally and transect; allow to retract proximally.
  - Use fishmouth incision with long volar flap and short dorsal flap.

FOREARM AND ABOVE

- **Below elbow**
  - Preserve as much length as possible to allow pronation and supination.
  - Make anterior and posterior flaps equal in length.
  - Shorten bone proximally.
  - Nerves should be ligated and buried under muscle, if possible.
  - Smooth bone with rasp.
  - Use circumferential dressing with elastic bandage to prevent postoperative edema.
  - Encourage elbow and shoulder motion to prevent contracture.
  - Fit with prosthesis at 6 weeks, when edema has subsided.
- **Elbow disarticulation**
  - This method is preferable to above-elbow amputation, when possible, because it allows transmission of humeral rotation to prosthesis.
  - If the patient is thin, use brachialis, biceps, or triceps muscle to cover the end of humerus.
- **Above elbow**
  - Additional bone resection to close wound is not indicated; use skin grafts, if necessary, to preserve length.
  - Amputations near the axillary fold are functionally equivalent to shoulder disarticulation.

TIP: Maintain as much length as possible.

KEY POINTS

✔ In traumatic amputations, address life-threatening injuries first (i.e., follow ABCs).
✔ Assess patient in emergency department for replantation.
✔ Prevent neuromas by cutting back ends of nerves and bury stump in soft tissue/muscle away from incision site.
✔ For digital amputations, do not suture flexor or extensor tendons to stump.
✔ Preserve length.

REFERENCES

1. Adamson GJ, Palmer RE. Amputations. In Achauer BM, Erikson E, Guyuron B, et al, eds. Plastic Surgery: Indications, Operations, and Outcomes. St Louis: Mosby, 2000, p 1831.
2. Louis DS, Jebson PJ, Graham T. Amputations. In Green DP, Hotchkiss RN, Pederson WC, eds. Green's Operative Hand Surgery, 4th ed. Philadelphia: Churchill Livingstone, 1999, pp 48-94.
3. Jones JM, Schenck RR, Chesney RB. Digital replantation and amputation: Comparison of function. J Hand Surg Am 7:183-189, 1982.
4. Fisher GT, Boswick JA Jr. Neuroma formation following digital amputations. J Trauma 23:136-142, 1983.
5. Backman C, Nystrom A, Backman C. Cold-induced arterial spasm after digital amputation. J Hand Surg Br 16:378-381, 1981.
6. Carroll RE. Transposition of the index finger to replace the middle finger. Clin Orthop 15:27-34, 1959.
7. Steichen JB, Idler RS. Results of central ray resection without bony transposition. J Hand Surg Am 11:466-474, 1986.
8. Murray JF, Carman W, MacKenzie JK. Transmetacarpal amputation of the index finger: A clinical assessment of hand strength and complications. J Hand Surg Am 2:471-481, 1977.
9. Garcia-Moral CA, Putman-Mullins J, Taylor PA, et al. Ray resection of the index finger. Orthop Trans 15:71, 1991.
10. Melikyan EY, Beg MS, Woodbridge S, et al. The functional results of ray amputation. Hand Surg 8:47-51, 2003.

62. Replantation

Ashkan Ghavami

INDICATIONS AND CONTRAINDICATIONS[1-3]

INDICATIONS
- Thumb
- Single digit distal to flexor digitorum superficialis (FDS) insertion (zone I)
- Multiple digits
- Hand amputation through palm
- Hand amputation (distal wrist)
- Any part in a child
- More proximal arm (sharp, clean injury pattern)

CONTRAINDICATIONS
- Single digits proximal to FDS insertion (zone II) (see next section)
- Severely crushed or mangled parts
- Multiple-level amputations
- Multiple traumas or severe medical problems (relative contraindication)

SPECIFIC CASES

SINGLE-DIGIT REPLANTATION
- **Distal to zone II** (distal to FDS tendon insertion)
  - Favorable outcomes
  - Fewer secondary operations
- **Within zone II**
  - Function after replantation even after secondary operations (e.g., extensive tenolysis) is usually poor.
- **Exceptions**
  - Musician or other person requiring all 10 digits
  - Children
  - Thumb amputations (see later)
  - Cultural reasons (e.g., in Japan a missing digit has criminal connotations)

FINGERTIP AMPUTATIONS DISTAL TO OR AT DISTAL INTERPHALANGEAL (DIP) JOINT
- Expert technical skills and experience needed
- Main difficulties are venous paucity and venous repair
- **Tamai's fingertip classification[4]**
  - **Zone 1**
    - Distal to lunula
    - Volar venous plexus used for venous repair

- ▸ Options when venous repair not possible: Arterial-venous (A-V) shunting, nail bed bleed or heparin therapy, leech therapy

Zone 2
- ▸ DIP joint to lunula
- ▸ Digital arteries and dorsal veins used

> TIP: Occupation should be considered in the decision-making process. Many laborers prefer revision amputations at this level to allow quick return to work with adequate functional results.

RING AVULSION INJURIES

- **Ring finger classifications**[5]
  - **Type I:** Soft tissue injury *without* vascular compromise
    - ▸ *Treatment:* Standard neurovascular approach
  - **Type II:** Soft tissue damage *with* arterial and/or venous compromise
    - ▸ *Treatment:* May require coverage of vascular repairs using local flap or flow-through venous flap harvested as skin and soft tissue attached to underlying vein graft from forearm
  - **Type III:** *Complete degloving* of soft tissues; most controversial; function poor even with successful skin envelope revascularization
    - ▸ *Treatment:* Primary-ray amputation[5]
- **Thumb:** Similar to any other type of thumb injury or amputation, warrants every attempt at replantation

CHILDREN

- **Every attempt should be made to replant, no matter what the type of amputation,** *except severe crushes or multiple-level injuries.*
- **Distal amputations**
  - Such amputations may require only percutaneous needle for osteosynthesis.
  - Nerve repair is not always required.
  - Direct neurotization may allow normal two-point discrimination.[6]
  - Amputated part may survive as a "composite graft" without the need for microanastomosis. Neoepithelialization is often present under eschar.
- Better functional results are seen overall, likely secondary to greater neuronal regenerative capacity in children.
- Parents should be informed that a replanted finger can grow slower than other digits.[6]

> TIP: Avoid a running microvascular suture technique, which may increase vessel stenosis rate as child grows.[6]

PREOPERATIVE WORKUP

BEFORE TRANSFER

- Stabilize patient.
- Wrap amputated part in moist gauze, place in ziplock bag or specimen container, and place on ice (4° C).
- Prevent warm ischemia.
  - Duration is preferably less than 6 hours.
  - More than 12 hours duration generally precludes digital replantation.

- Sensitivity to warm ischemia increases in proportion to the amount of muscle mass in the amputated part (e.g., forearm amputation tolerates markedly less ischemia [maximum 4-6 hours] than digital level amputation).
- Optimize cold ischemia.
  - Optimal cooling can allow up to 24 hours cold ischemia.
  - Up to 30-40 hours cold ischemia has been reported for digital replantation, with one report of 94 hours.[7]

NOTE: These are rare cases and *NOT recommended*.

  - More proximal injuries with more muscle mass tolerate 10-12 hours cold ischemia.
- Alert other surgeons from replant team.
- The OR should be called to prepare staff, check microscope availability, create slush and warming fluid, obtain ICU bed, etc.

ON ARRIVAL AT ER
- Obtain thorough history.
  - Type of force, mechanism, machine, etc., resulting in amputation
  - Exact time of injury (to calculate accurate ischemia duration)
- Perform preliminary examination of stump and amputated parts.
  - **Avoid:**
    - ▸ Repeated manipulation of extremity (may increase vasospasm)
    - ▸ Digital blocks (decreases vascular flow)
- Assure hemodynamic stability.
- Obtain radiographs of stump and amputated parts.
- Start IV broad-spectrum antibiotics.
- Start tetanus prophylaxis.
- Points for consent:
  - Potential replant failure
  - Need for further surgery (e.g., secondary procedures such as tenolysis and capsulotomy)
  - Prolonged rehabilitation course
    - ▸ Realistic prognosis (e.g., sensation, mobility, and function)

TIP: Always take into account age, occupation, mental stability of patient, and presence of severe systemic injuries during the preoperative consultation and decision-making process.

SURGICAL PRINCIPLES

ANAESTHESIA ADJUNCTS
- Brachial plexus blocks or axillary blocks may assist with vasodilation and postoperative patient comfort.

GENERAL PREPARATION
- Well-padded operating table
- Foley catheter
- Tourniquets on upper extremity and leg for possible nerve, vein, or skin grafts

MULTIPLE-DIGIT AMPUTATIONS
- Consider future function and replant position.
  - **Finger with highest chance of success is replanted first** (e.g., if index finger and middle finger are amputated and middle finger is not replantable, replant index finger in middle finger position to prevent a gap and help with grip).[8]

MAJOR LIMB OR PROXIMAL AMPUTATIONS
- **Reperfusion shunts** used for arterial inflow early in proximal level amputations
  - Fasciotomies
  - Nerve tunnel releases
  - Intrinsic compartment decompression
- High-volume blood transfusions
- Often several subsequent tissue (muscle) debridements required
- May require later free-functional muscle transfer for biceps function

HAND REPLANTATION
- Shunt for reperfusion to reduce ischemia duration
- Proximal and distal flexor and extensor tendons tagged before osteosynthesis
  - Flexor tendons need precise anatomic organization.
  - Repair as many tendons as possible.
- Wrist level approach
  - Bone shortening (proximal row carpectomy) may be required.

SURGICAL TECHNIQUE: DIGITAL REPLANTATION

OPERATIVE SEQUENCE

TIP: Optimize use of "spare parts" from nonsalvageable tissue. An example is harvesting a digital nerve from a nonreplantable digit to use for a nerve graft.

- **Two-team approach**
  - **First team**
    1. Brings amputated part(s) to OR as soon as possible (can precede patient's OR arrival)
    2. Examines part(s) thoroughly with loupes or under microscope; part(s) held on back table
    3. Obtains appropriate exposure (if possible, incorporating lacerations present) (Fig. 62-1)
       - Bilateral longitudinal, midaxial incisions, or
       - Volar Bruner (zigzag) and dorsal longitudinal incisions
    4. Identifies and tags all neurovascular structures
       - Nerves: 6-0 black nylon
       - Arteries and veins: 6-0 Prolene® (Ethicon, Inc., Somerville, NJ)
    5. For bony preparation, places two Kirschner wires in retrograde fashion
  - **Second team**
    1. Works concurrently
    2. Begins with meticulous exploration, debridement, and irrigation of proximal part

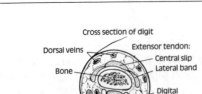
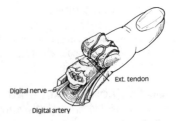

Fig. 62-1 Exposure of neurovascular structures to be labeled on an amputated part. (From Callico CG, Replantation and revascularization of the upper extremity. In May JW Jr, Littler JW, eds. McCarthy's Plastic Surgery, vol 7. The Hand. Philadelphia: WB Saunders, 1990.)

3. Identifies and tags all vital structures on proximal part
   * Nerves, arteries, and veins
   * Flexor and extensor tendons: May place core sutures before osteosynthesis to simplify later tendon coaptation
4. Performs bony shortening as necessary (no more than 5-10 mm for digits)
   * Fractures through joints often require fusion.

> TIP: Rigid fixation with low-profile plates, screws, or 90-90 intraosseous wiring allows for earlier motion protocols and lower nonunion rates.

- **Vessel damage evaluation**
  - **Normal vessel:** Pearly gray with no petechiae ("paprika")
  - **Ribbon sign ("corkscrew"):** Tortuous-appearing vessel from avulsion or traction injury
  - **Red-line sign:** Red streak along neurovascular bundle implying distal vessel damage

NOTE: Ribbon and red-line signs are poor prognostic indicators.

  - **Cobweb sign:** Multilaceration-like pattern on vessel wall (Fig. 62-2)
  - **Telescope sign:** Lumen telescopes away from outer vessel wall and past cut edge
  - **Terminal thrombus:** Presence indicates vessel wall disruption or damage
  - **Measles sign:** Pinpoint (petechial) bruising along vessel wall
    ► Result of high pressure from thrombus, usually after anastomosis complete
  - **Sausage sign:** Ballooning of vessel from thrombus

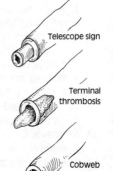

Telescope sign

Terminal thrombosis

Cobweb sign

Fig. 62-2 Signs of arterial damage should be appreciated, including the telescope, cobweb, and ribbon signs or terminal thrombosis, which require freshening of the vessel. (From Callico CG, Replantation and revascularization of the upper extremity. In May JW Jr, Littler JW, eds. McCarthy's Plastic Surgery, vol 7. The Hand. Philadelphia: WB Saunders, 1990.)

TIP: If signs of vessel damage are present, do not hesitate to cut back vessel as much as required. It is better to graft a vein than be concerned for vessel integrity with replant failure postoperatively.

- **Perform the following after tourniquet deflation:**
  - ▸ **Spurt test:** Vessel must have strong pressure head.
    - ✦ Inadequate pressure necessitates more vessel resection.
  - ▸ **Patency test:** Milking of vessel is used to check back-bleeding and inflow patency.

TIP: Performing all the previous sequences during one tourniquet run (2 hours) expedites the operation. Pooling of blood and clots can make later identification of vital structures, especially nerves, more challenging.

- **Vein graft harvest**
  - One surgeon (from either team, as soon as available) begins harvesting vein graft(s) from forearm or leg, if required.
  - Volar forearm veins are good size-matches for digital vessels.
  - **Common vein graft indications:**
    - ▸ **Thumb replants:** Often require vein interposition graft from ulnar digital artery (larger caliber than radial side) to radial artery in anatomic snuffbox
    - ▸ **Ring avulsions**
    - ▸ **Segmental tissue loss**
- **Osteosynthesis completed**
- **Extensor and flexor tendon repair**
  - Use standard 4-core suturing method of choice after edges are tidied up, e.g., modified Kessler-Tajima technique using 3-0 or 4-0 Ethibond® (Ethicon, Inc., Somerville, NJ).
  - Consider excision of FDS in zone II.
- **Primary digital nerve repair** (when possible)
  - Done under operative microscope
  - Epineurial suturing technique: 9-0 or 10-0 black nylon
  - Options if primary repair not feasible (see Chapter 68):
    - ▸ Autogenous nerve graft, polyglycolic acid conduit, vein graft (gap ≤2 cm)
    - ▸ Minimal joint repositioning
- **Microvascular artery repair**
  - A well-executed microsurgical technique is imperative.
  - Cut back artery to healthy intimal level.
  - One good artery is required.
  - Use 4% topical lidocaine (Xylocaine®) and/or papaverine solution for vasospasm.

TIP: Allow at least 10 minutes for vasospasm to clear before manipulating anastomosis.

- **Microvascular venous anastomosis**
  - **Use at least two veins** to avoid venous congestion.
    - ▸ Dorsal veins are larger and do not interfere with repair of volar structures.
    - ▸ Procedure can be done before arterial repair.

- **Without venous repair, approximately 80% of replants fail.**[4]
- **Closure**
  - Use skin closure, skin grafting, or local flaps, if needed.
  - Avoid any tension on the skin closure.
    - ▸ It is better to leave loose and allow healing by granulation (or skin graft).
- **Dressing**
  - Antibiotic ointment
  - Nonadherent gauze **(avoid circumferential wrapping),** fluffy or bulky dressing
  - Accessibility to fingertips needed for postoperative monitoring
  - Protective splinting

TIP:　Use Doppler before leaving OR and elevate extremity on foam pillow (e.g., Carter pillow).

- **Perioperative pharmacologic treatment**
  - 325 mg aspirin given per rectum before leaving OR
    - ▸ Aspirin inhibits platelet aggregation at the anastomosis at this dose level.
    - ▸ Heparin can be given during clamp removal of arterial anastomosis (1500-2500 units).

POSTOPERATIVE MANAGEMENT

ICU MONITORING
- 24-48 hours with frequent monitoring
- Clinical assessment
  - Capillary refill
  - Color
  - Turgor
  - Temperature
- Transcutaneous Doppler checks every hour
- Laser-Doppler flowmetry
- Transcutaneous oxygen monitors
- Temperature probes
- Warm ambient temperature and warm extremity; use warming blankets (e.g., Bair Hugger® [Arizant Healthcare, Eden Prairie, MN]) to keep digit warm
  - Marked temperature decrease possibly a result of arterial inflow problem
- Adequate IV hydration

PHARMACOLOGIC THERAPY
- **Antibiotics:** First-generation cephalosporin
- **Aspirin:** 325 mg (or 81 mg) by mouth every day for approximately 3 weeks postoperatively
- **Chlorpromazine:** 25 mg by mouth three times per day
  - Possesses antianxiety and vasodilation properties (for 3-5 days)
- **Other agents:** Calcium channel blockers and dipyridamole (Persantine®)
  - For vasodilation or as antivasospastic agent

- **Dextran-40**
  - **Test-dose** required with dextran
  - **Antiplatelet** and **antifibrin** function, in addition to volume expansion
  - Can be given during anastomosis (25 ml/hr) and then for 5 days postoperatively
- **Systemic heparinization**
  - **Not** commonly required
  - Used if anastomotic revision made or concern for thrombosis (severe crush injuries)
  - Used along with nail plate removal and heparin-soaked pledget if venous repair not done or tenuous
- **Leech therapy:** Valuable if signs of venous congestion not alleviated with other measures
  - *Hirudin,* an anticoagulant (thrombin inhibitor), is secreted by leeches during feeding; its use allows for continued bleeding from site.
  - Leeches usually fall off patient 10-15 minutes after feeding.
  - **Prophylaxis against *Aeromonas hydrophila* infection is required.**
    - ▸ Third-generation cephalosporin, quinolones (avoid in children), or trimethoprim plus sulfamethoxazole (TMP/Sulfa)
- **Smoking cessation:** At least 1 month postreplantation

REPLANT FAILURE AND SECONDARY PROCEDURES

Digits that undergo revision and "struggle to survive" show very poor eventual function.[3]

> TIP: If there is a problem in the OR, do not leave until it is corrected. If a postoperative problem is not remedied by conservative measures, go back to the OR as soon as possible for reexploration.

ARTERIAL INSUFFICIENCY
- Accounts for up to **60%** of failures[9]
- **Signs**
  - Pale color
  - Poor turgor
  - Cool finger with slow capillary refill
  - Little to no bleeding from needle prick test
- **Treatment**
  1. *If any doubts about patency, return to the OR immediately!*
  2. Warm finger.
  3. Loosen dressing.
  4. Use antivasospastic drugs.
  5. Improve pain control.
  6. Use bupivacaine (Marcaine®) block (vasodilation).
  7. Use heparin.

VENOUS INSUFFICIENCY
- Purple: Rapid capillary refill
- Congested, with dark bleeding from needle prick
- Increased tissue turgor

- **Treatment**
  1. Increase elevation of extremity.
  2. Loosen dressing and sutures.
  3. Use systemic heparin.
  4. Remove nail plate with heparin-soaked pledgets.
  5. Use leech therapy.
  6. Return to OR for reexploration.

OUTCOMES

OVERALL SUCCESS RATES
- Range from 54% to 82%[10]
- Success rates for guillotine-type injuries: 77% versus 49% for crush amputations[9]

FUNCTIONAL OUTCOMES
- Approximately 70% achieve two-point discrimination at less than 15 mm.[4]
  - **Factors affecting two-point discrimination**[10]
    - ▸ Patient age: **Best results with children**
    - ▸ Level and mechanism of injury (see previous sections)
    - ▸ Success of sensory reeducation
- Approximately 50% total active motion (TAM) and 50% grip strength for average replant result[11]
  - **Total active motion**[13]
    - ▸ Injury distal to FDS tendon insertion gives better results.
    - ▸ TAM, when subtracting minor contribution of metacarpophalangeal (MP) joint, is 85.5 degrees at middle phalanx level and 80 degrees for proximal phalanx.
    - ▸ Therefore range-of-motion is improved significantly with joint preservation, especially with the proximal interphalangeal (PIP) and MP joints.
- **Largest major limb replant review**[12]
  - 11 out of 24 had more than 50% TAM; 19 out of 24 had protective sensation; and 22 out of 24 were satisfied with function and appearance.
- **Flexor tenolysis**[11]
  - The average TAM improvement is 43%.
  - Thumb replants show less improvement.

COMPLICATIONS AND SECONDARY PROCEDURES
- **Secondary surgery**[1]
  - Required in **60%** of cases
  - More common among replants proximal to FDS insertion
  - **Incidence of procedures**
    - ▸ Extensor and flexor tenolysis or release of joint contractures: 67%
    - ▸ Open reduction and internal fixation (ORIF) correction of nonunions: 22%
    - ▸ Digital replants proximal to FDS insertion: 93% with secondary surgery
    - ▸ Thumb amputations: 11%
- Flexor or extensor tenolysis
- Neurolysis, with or without nerve grafting
- Nonunion, malunion
- Amputations

OTHER COMPLICATIONS

- Cold intolerance: Often improves postoperatively over 2 years[8]
- Chronic pain (chronic regional pain syndrome)

KEY POINTS

- ✔ Every attempt must be made for replantation in children.
- ✔ Prompt arrival at the replantation center and a two-team approach is essential to decrease ischemia duration and improve success.
- ✔ Signs of vessel injury must be recognized with resection of damaged vessel.
- ✔ All neurovascular structures and tendons must be delineated and tagged, preferably within one tourniquet run.
- ✔ When possible, rigid bony fixation should be performed to allow early motion-rehabilitation protocols.
- ✔ Close postoperative monitoring with multiple modalities and pharmacologic support (aspirin, vasodilation medications, analgesics, or anxiolytics) should be instituted.
- ✔ When conservative measures fail, return to the OR for reexploration as soon as possible.
- ✔ Usually secondary procedures are not required but can provide meaningful functional recovery when performed.

REFERENCES

1. Chao JJ, Castello JR, English JM, et al. Microsurgery: Free-tissue transfer and replantation. Sel Read Plast Surg 9(11), 2000.
2. Goldner RD, Urbaniak JR. Replantation. In Green DP, Hotchkiss RN, Pederson WC, eds. Green's Operative Hand Surgery, vol 2, 4th ed. Philadelphia: Churchill Livingstone, 1999, pp 1139-1157.
3. Pederson WC. Replantation. Plast Reconstr Surg 107:823-841, 2001.
4. Tamai S. Twenty years' experience of limb replantation: Review of 293 upper extremity replants. J Hand Surg 7:549-556, 1982.
5. Urbaniak JR, Evans JP, Bright DS. Microvascular management of ring avulsion injuries. J Hand Surg Am 6:25-30, 1981.
6. Merle M, Dautel G. Advances in digital replantation. Clin Plast Surg 24:87-105, 1997.
7. Wei FC, Chen HC, Chuang CC. Three successful digital replantations in a patient after 84, 86, and 94 hours cold ischemia time. Plast Reconstr Surg 82:346-350, 1988.
8. Buncke GM, Buncke HJ, Kind GM, et al. Replantation. In Russell RC, ed. Plastic Surgery: Indications, Operations, and Outcomes, vol 4. St Louis: Mosby, 2000, pp 2131-2147.
9. O'Brien BM. Replantation surgery. Clin Plast Surg 1:405-426, 1974.
10. Wilhelmi BJ, Lee WP, Pagensteert GI, et al. Replantation in the mutilated hand. Hand Clin 19:89-120, 2003.
11. Jupiter JB, Pess GM, Bour CJ, et al. Results of flexor tendon tenolysis after replantation of the hand. J Hand Surg Am 14:35-44, 1989.
12. Russell RC, O'Brien BM, Morrison WA, et al. The late functional results of upper limb revascularization and replantation. J Hand Surg Am 9:623-633, 1984.
13. Chiu HY, Shieh SJ. Multivariate analysis of factors influencing the functional recovery after finger replantation or revascularization. Microsurgery 16:713-717, 1995.

63. Thumb Reconstruction

David W. Mathes

Reconstruction of the thumb can be assessed by dividing the first ray into proximal, middle, and distal thirds. The middle third can be further subdivided into proximal and distal halves (Fig. 63-1).[1-3]

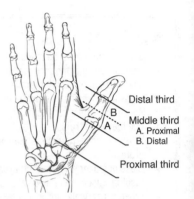

Distal third

Middle third
A. Proximal
B. Distal

Proximal third

Fig. 63-1 Areas of thumb loss: Distal third, middle third, and proximal third. The middle third is subdivided into proximal *(A)* and distal *(B)*.

AMPUTATION THROUGH THE DISTAL THIRD

- This is a *compensated amputation.*
  - **Minimal functional impairment**
- **Efforts should be directed at:**
  - Restoring skeletal stability
  - Providing well-padded soft tissue coverage
  - Ensuring satisfactory sensory perception
- Choice of procedure depends on the **amount** and **depth** of tissue loss.
- An attempt should be made to salvage all viable tissue.
- Injuries to the volar pad surface can be reconstructed by the same coverage techniques used on the fingers, but the approach is modified to preserve length.

> TIP: Completion amputation is the most common option for those seeking a rapid return to work.

Volar Advancement Flap (Moberg Flap)[4] (Fig. 63-2)
- **Indications**
  - Use for avulsions of **less than 50%** of the volar surface
  - Can resurface as much as **1.5 cm²**
  - Advantage of bringing **sensory-innervated skin** to resurface the pad of the thumb
  - Subcutaneous tissue and both neurovascular bundles included in volar flap
- **Technical tips**
  - Procedure is performed under thumb tourniquet.
  - Ragged bone is trimmed from the distal phalanx.
  - Midaxial incisions are made on the ulnar and radial side of the thumb and extended to the proximal thumb crease.
  - Do not disturb the underlying flexor tendon.

610

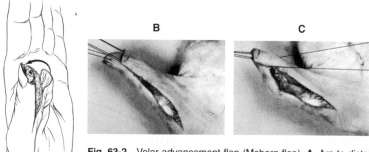

Fig. 63-2   Volar advancement flap (Moberg flap). **A,** Arc to distal phalanx of thumb. **B,** Elevation of flap. **C,** Coverage of distal phalanx of thumb.

- Flex the thumb at the metacarpophalangeal (MP) joint at 30 degrees and the interphalangeal (IP) joint at 45 degrees.
- Distal edge of the flap is sutured to remaining nail, nail bed, or terminal skin remnant.
- The addition of proximal releasing incision can increase coverage.
  - ▸ Full-thickness skin graft is needed to cover donor site.

CROSS-FINGER FLAP (Fig. 63-3)

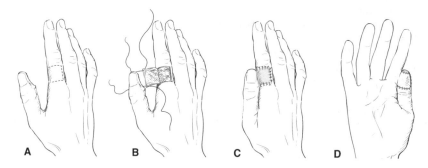

Fig. 63-3   Cross-finger flap from the index finger to the thumb. **A,** Large defect involving most of the distal pulp of the thumb; outline of the cross-finger flap on the proximal phalanx of the index finger. **B,** Placement of the flap on the thumb defect. **C** and **D,** Position of the thumb and cross-finger flap with a free graft covering the donor defect.

■ Indications
- Use to resurface entire volar surface of the distal phalanx.
- Use when skin grafting will not provide stable coverage.
- Design cross-finger flap from proximal phalanx of the index finger.
- Coverage and adequate sensory recovery are both provided.
■ Disadvantages
- Obvious dorsal donor site
- Occasional problems with digital joint stiffness or thumb web contracture

■ **Technical tips**
- Perform under tourniquet.
- Use a template of defect to design flap.
- Thumb is positioned against index finger to determine level.
- Slightly oblique configuration aids in positioning.
- During flap harvest, careful preservation of all small veins is essential.
- Flap can be divided at 3 weeks.

NEUROVASCULAR ISLAND PEDICLED FLAPS[5]

■ **Indications**
- Should be used when **one or both digital nerves have been lost,** as well as for a soft tissue loss, because failure to restore nerve continuity will lead to impairment of pinch and grasp.
- Amount of tissue harvested must match the defect.

■ **Disadvantages**
- Donor site morbidity
- Technically demanding

■ **Technical tips**
- Perform under tourniquet.
- Donor tissue is designed from the ulnar pad of the middle finger.
- If median nerve is lost, then donor is radial side of ring finger.

RADIAL SENSORY-INNERVATED CROSS-FINGER FLAP (FIRST DORSAL METACARPAL ARTERY FLAP)[6]

This flap provides a large cross-finger pedicle flap that brings with it a sensory branch of the radial nerve.

■ **Indications**
- **For use when the defect requires:**
  ▸ Substantial resurfacing (up to 4 cm)
  ▸ Need for innervated skin

■ **Technical tips**
- Defect of template is designed.
- Suitable flap is designed over the dorsum of the proximal phalanx of the index finger with the base just volar to the midlateral line.
- Flap design can be single, dual, or island flap

AMPUTATION THROUGH THE MIDDLE THIRD

■ The **middle third** can be divided into **distal** and **proximal** components.
■ **Functional deficits**
- Loss of **fine pinch** and **strong grasp**
- Acceptable carpometacarpal (CMC) joint rotation retained in most thumbs
- Variable preservation of adequate thumb-index cleft
■ **Functional requirements**
- Length
- Preservation of sensibility, mobility, and stability
- Pain-free thumb

■ **To achieve functional goals the procedures must:**
  • Create **relative ray lengthening** by deepening the first web space *(distal half of the middle third)*
  • **Add bone length** *(proximal half of the middle third)*

TIP: The best results for the proximal half are often obtained using free toe transfer techniques
       (great toe or second toe).

PROCEDURES THAT DEEPEN THE FIRST WEB SPACE
■ **Web space Z-plasty (two or four flap)** (Fig. 63-4)[7]
  • **Indications**
    ▸ The skin must be pliable.
    ▸ The first metacarpal must be mobile with no evidence of muscle contracture.

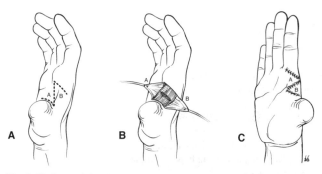

Fig. 63-4   Simple Z-plasty of the thumb web. **A,** Design of the Z-plasty. Preferred angles are approximately 60 degrees. **B,** Flaps reflected with partial recession of the web space musculature. **C,** Appearance of the flaps after reversal and suture. Corner sutures are preferred in the tips of the flaps.

  • **Advantages**
    ▸ Simple procedure with little morbidity
  • **Disadvantages**
    ▸ Does not provide much functional improvement
    ▸ Resulting cleft may look unnatural
  • **Technical tips**
    ▸ The longitudinal axis of the Z-plasty should be on the **distal ridge of the first web space.**
    ▸ Length gain is between 1.5 and 2 cm.
    ▸ Release of part of the first interosseous muscle and proximal transfer of the insertion of the adductor pollicis can be added for additional length.
■ **Dorsal rotation flap** (Fig. 63-5)[8]
  • **Indications**
    ▸ Injury with thumb loss and adjacent tissue injury through the first web space **with contracture of the first metacarpal**
    ▸ Need to restore the web space
  • **Advantage**
    ▸ Minimal morbidity

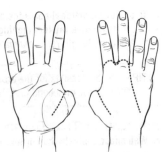

Fig. 63-5   Dorsal rotation flap. (From Canale
ST. Campbell's Operative Orthopedics, vol 4,
10th ed. St Louis: Mosby, 2003.)

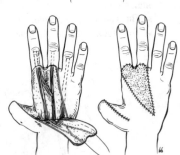

- **Disadvantages**
  - ▸ No direct improvement of thumb function
  - ▸ Need for skin graft to donor site
- **Technical tips**
  - ▸ Perform sequential division of all restraining skin, muscle, scar, and capsular adhesions.
  - ▸ Both the oblique and transverse heads of the adductor are divided.
  - ▸ Additional reconstructive procedures such as tendon transfer may be needed.

PROCEDURES THAT ADD BONE LENGTH

These procedures are often used for reconstruction of the proximal half because of the need for length. **The addition of 2 cm of length can significantly improve the function of the thumb.**

- ■ **Pollicization of an injured or normal digit**[9]
  - • **Indications**
    - ▸ Can be performed acutely or in delayed fashion when the thumb is not replantable
  - • **Advantages**
    - ▸ Minimal sacrifice of hand function
    - ▸ Excellent cosmetic and functional recovery
  - • **Disadvantage**
    - ▸ Narrows the palm
  - • **Technical tips**
    - ▸ Use the nonfunctional injured finger (classically the index finger) for reconstruction, if applicable.
    - ▸ **Ring finger** is best **normal** digit to harvest and use for thumb reconstruction.
- ■ **Metacarpal distraction osteogensis**[10]

This simple and reliable technique increases length without sacrificing another digit or toe.

- • **Indications**
  - ▸ The patient must have:
    - ✦ Two thirds of the first metacarpal
    - ✦ Adequate skin and subcutaneous coverage over the stump
  - ▸ Procedure can increase the length up to 3-3.5 cm
- • **Complications**
  - ▸ Nonunion
  - ▸ Tissue necrosis
  - ▸ Bone reabsorption

- **Technical tips**
  - ▸ Distract the metacarpal gradually over several weeks (1 mm/day over a period of 25-40 days).
  - ▸ Bone grafting is needed in those older than 25 years and in cases of a gap larger than 3 cm.
  - ▸ Most need a subsequent web space deepening procedure.
- **Osteoplastic reconstruction**
  - **Indications**
    - ▸ Partial or distal subtotal amputations.
    - ▸ Other fingers are either normal or too damaged to use.
    - ▸ Other lengthening procedures (such as toe transfer) are not an option.
  - **Advantage**
    - ▸ No digit is sacrificed
  - **Disadvantages**
    - ▸ Multistage procedure
    - ▸ Results may not be aesthetic
    - ▸ Additional neurovascular flap required for sensibility
  - **Technical tips**
    - ▸ Iliac bone best source for bone graft
    - ▸ Soft tissue coverage of bone shaft
      - ✦ Tubed abdominal or groin flap
      - ✦ Reverse radial forearm flap
      - ✦ Anterolateral thigh flap

AMPUTATION THROUGH THE PROXIMAL THIRD

- The entire thumb and at least the distal third of the first metacarpal are lost.
- Reconstruction must provide a **total thumb.**
- **Required length** will usually be **more than 5 cm.**

RECONSTRUCTION OPTIONS

- **Pollicization of an injured index finger** (see previous discussion)
  - Best acute option at the time of injury
  - Can be performed as long as the neurovascular status of the index digit is adequate
- **Free toe transfer**

TOE-TO-THUMB TRANSFER[11,12]

- Complete or partial toe transfer is an effective way to reconstruct an absent or deficient thumb.
- **There are three central questions to be addressed before embarking on a toe-to-thumb transfer.**
  1. **Is toe transfer the best surgical option?**
     - ▸ Patient considerations
       - ✦ Age
       - ✦ Motivation
       - ✦ Handedness
       - ✦ Functional requirements at work
       - ✦ Bilateral

▸ Better discriminative sensation and fine motor control with pollicization
▸ Better strength with toe transfer
▸ Possibility of local reconstructive options
▸ **Contraindications**
  ✦ Vascular abnormalities
  ✦ Significant comorbidity precluding extended anaesthesia time
  ✦ Cultural footwear preferences

2. **When should the procedure be done?**
▸ **Urgent** toe-to-thumb transfer
  ✦ Thumb salvage after soft tissue avulsion can be treated with an urgent wraparound flap.
▸ **Delayed** toe-to-thumb transfer
  ✦ Functional capability of a hand with a shortened or absent thumb is not immediately apparent.
  ✦ Patient may find new length more or less functional.
  ✦ Patient needs to understand donor site morbidity in foot.

3. **Which toe transplant procedure is indicated?**
▸ Can restore certain attributes of a functional thumb
  ✦ Excellent cosmetic appearance
  ✦ Strength
  ✦ Stability
  ✦ Movement (restore pinch and grasp)
  ✦ Sensation
  ✦ Growth (critical importance for children)
▸ **Advantages**
  ✦ Single operation
  ✦ Ideal length
  ✦ Good mobility (restores pinch and grasp)
  ✦ Good sensation
  ✦ Similar to thumb in appearance
  ✦ Glabrous skin and nail support
  ✦ Growth potential (of critical importance for children)
▸ **Disadvantages**
  ✦ Loss of toe
  ✦ Requires microvascular expertise
  ✦ Lengthy operation
  ✦ Donor site morbitity
▸ **Foot donor site anatomy**
  ✦ First dorsal metatarsal artery supplies the great and second toes and usually arises from the dorsalis pedis artery.
  ✦ Venous drainage is by the superficial dorsal veins to the greater saphenous vein.
  ✦ Volar digital nerves arise from the medial plantar nerve.
▸ **Whole great toe transfer** (Fig. 63-6)
  ✦ Great toe offers optimal mobility and excellent strength.
  ✦ Use the ipsilateral great toe.
  ✦ Appearance is somewhat compromised.
    - Great toe is **20% larger** than the thumb.
    - Great toenail is broader and shorter.
    - Donor site is not aesthetic.

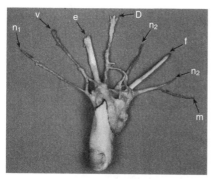

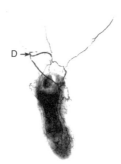

Dorsal surface of flap   Radiographic view

Fig. 63-6   Surgical anatomy of the great toe. *D,* First dorsal metatarsal artery (dominant pedicle); *e,* extensor pollicis longus; *f,* flexor pollicis longus; *m,* first plantar metatarsal artery (minor pedicle); *n₁,* dorsal digital nerve; *n₂,* plantar digital nerve; *v,* superficial vein.

- ✦ Neurovascular bundles of the toe are plantar to midaxial line
  - Lateral bundle is larger than the medial bundle.
  - Two levels of veins are available.
- ▶ **Second-toe transfer**
- ✦ Second toe is thinner, nail is shorter.
- ✦ **Advantages**
  - Second metatarsal and metatarsophalangeal joints can be harvested
  - Offers a good donor site and good sensation after transfer
- ✦ **Disadvantages**
  - Reconstructed thumb can be narrower than native thumb
  - Not as strong as great toe
  - Skin problems and need for skin grafts
- ▶ **Wraparound procedure**
- ✦ Soft tissue flap and nail from great toe transferred
- ✦ Osseous support provided by iliac bone graft
- ✦ **Advantages**
  - Good sensation
  - Adequate strength
  - Excellent aesthetic replacement for missing thumb
- ✦ **Disadvantages**
  - Poor mobility
  - Bone resorption
- ▶ **Trimmed toe technique**
- ✦ Smaller structure that is capable of movement
- ✦ Great toe trimmed to size of thumb
- ✦ **Advantages**
  - Good sensation, strength, and appearance
  - Excellent mobility

- **Disadvantages**
  - Complicated procedure
  - Cannot be used in children
- ▸ **Partial toe transfer (pulp, nail, or joint used)**
  - ✦ Second metatarsophalangeal joint
  - ✦ Skin of first web site
  - ✦ Pulp skin
  - ✦ Nail and dorsal skin

■ **Selection of toe transfer procedure**
- • **At or distal to interphalangeal joint**
  - ▸ No need for toe transplant
- • **Through proximal phalanx with intact MP joint**
  - ▸ Wraparound transfer provides better appearance than great toe.
  - ▸ No motion is possible at IP joint.

CAUTION: The wraparound procedure should not be used for children (because of growth restriction).

  - ▸ **Trimmed toe** is better with mobility intact.
  - ▸ **Second toe** may result in a mallet deformity.
  - ▸ **Great toe** provides best strength.
- • **Distal half of metacarpal**
  - ▸ **Great toe** is the best option.
  - ▸ Great toe must be harvested at metatarsophalangeal joint.
  - ▸ Thenar muscle should be reconstructed, or **opposition transfer** should be done.
  - ▸ If the great toe is too short, then the second toe can be harvested.
- • **Proximal half of metacarpal to MP joint.**
  - ▸ **Second toe** is best option.
  - ▸ Second toe is skin deficient and muscle must be covered by skin grafts.
  - ▸ An **opposition transfer** should be done.
- • **Proximal to the metacarpal**
  - ▸ Reconstruction is difficult because of lack of metacarpal bone.
  - ▸ **Pollicization of the index finger** is often the best option.
  - ▸ If other fingers are injured, then toe transfer is indicated.
  - ▸ Second toe, including the metatarsal, is harvested.
  - ▸ If index metacarpal is still intact, it can be pollicized before the toe transfer, improving the functional outcome.
- • **Partial thumb loss**
  - ▸ Missing portion can be replaced with part from toe (vascularized spare part).
  - ▸ Largest of the partial toe transfers is the wraparound flap.

KEY POINTS

✔ A useful algorithm for evaluating thumb defects is to divide the thumb into thirds.
✔ The choice of the correct procedure depends on *defect, location, size,* and *requirements for sensibility and durability.*
✔ The goals of reconstruction are *primary stable wound healing* and *early active use.*
✔ The toe wraparound procedure should not be used in children because of growth restriction.

REFERENCES

1. Kleinman W, Strickland JW. Thumb reconstruction. In Green DP, Hotchkiss RN, Pederson WC, eds. Green's Operative Hand Surgery, vol 2, 4th ed. Philadelphia: Churchill Livingstone, 1999.
2. Eaton CJ. Thumb reconstruction. In Aston SJ, Beasley RW, Thorne CHM, eds. Grabb and Smith's Plastic Surgery, 5th ed. Philadelphia: Lippincott-Raven, 1991.
3. Lister G. The choice of procedure following thumb amputation. Clin Orthop Relat Res 195:45-51, 1985.
4. Keim HA, Grantham SA. Volar-flap advancement for thumb and finger-tip injuries. Clin Orthop Relat Res 66:109-112, 1969.
5. Foucher G, Khouri RK. Digital reconstruction with island flaps [review]. Clin Plast Surg 24:1-32, 1997.
6. El-Khatib HA. Clinical experiences with the extended first dorsal metacarpal artery island flap for thumb reconstruction. J Hand Surg Am 23:647-652, 1998.
7. Eaton CJ, Lister GD. Treatment of skin and soft-tissue loss of the thumb. Hand Clin 8:71-97, 1992.
8. Emerson ET, Krizek TJ, Greenwald DP. Anatomy, physiology, and functional restoration of the thumb [review]. Ann Plast Surg 36:180-191, 1996.
9. Foucher G, Rostane S, Chammas M, et al. Transfer of a severely damaged digit to reconstruct an amputated thumb. J Bone Joint Surg Am 78:1889-1896, 1996.
10. Moy OJ, Clayton PA, Sherwin DS. Reconstruction of traumatic or congenital amputation of the thumb by distraction-lengthening [review]. Hand Clin 81:57-62, 1992.
11. Morrison WA. Thumb reconstruction: A review and philosophy of management. J Hand Surg Br 17:383-390, 1992.
12. Lister GD, Kalisman M, Tsai TM. Reconstruction of the hand with free microneurovascular toe-to-hand transfer: Experience with 54 toe transfers. Plast Reconstr Surg 71:372-386, 1983.

64. Soft Tissue Coverage of the Hand and Upper Extremity

Ashkan Ghavami

PRINCIPLES

- Wound control
  - Eradication of infection
  - Establishment of stable, reliable wound
- When possible, replace important tactile surfaces with similar tissue that can be reinnervated.
  - Example: Neurovascular axial flap to the radial volar thumb tip
- Begin with simple options and move to more complex choices, if required, while minimizing donor and patient morbidity.
- Consider patient's overall medical condition, occupation, hobbies, and priorities during surgical planning.

NOTE: Fingertip flaps are covered in Chapter 56.

SKIN GRAFTS

INDICATIONS
- Clean wound
- Well-vascularized wound bed
- Tissue bulk or specific type of tissue not required
- Over tendons and fingers
  - Need paratenon intact (confirm with presence of "fat stippling")

ADVANTAGES
- Thin
- Conforms well to concave and convex surfaces of the hand
- Can provide for good cosmesis
- Minimal donor site morbidity

DISADVANTAGES
- Does not provide tissue bulk
- Poor reinnervation potential
- Wound contracture

TIP: Whenever possible, use full-thickness skin grafts (FTSG). Bring glabrous tissue with less secondary contracture, improved sensibility, and improved aesthetics rather than split-thickness skin grafts (STSG).

Ask patients where they prefer to have the graft taken from after all options have been discussed. This places some responsibilty on patients and helps to include them in the decision-making process.

FULL-THICKNESS SKIN GRAFT

TIP: When possible, take grafts from sites adjacent to previous scars.

- **Hypothenar region** (at glabrous/nonglabrous junction)
  - May have hyperesthesia at donor site
- **Groin**
  - Donor site scar hidden in skin crease
  - May have increased rate of infection
- **Medial upper arm–medial epicondyle region**
  - Hyperesthesia/dysesthesia

TIP: Avoid the lateral upper arm as a donor site. There is an increased risk of hyperesthesia/dysesthesia and hypertrophic scarring.

POSTOPERATIVE CARE
- Nonadherent dressing (e.g., Xeroform®, OpSite™, Adaptic®) with tie-over bolster or vacuum-type dressing (e.g., VAC®)
  - Do not remove until day 5 (3-4 days for VAC)
- Splint immobilization of joints under or near skin graft
  - Decreases shearing
- "Piecrust" or trephinate if concern for fluid or hematoma
  - *Caveat:* With good hemostasis and bolster, usually not necessary

NOTE: Scars from trephination holes can be permanent.

LOCAL FLAPS[1-3]

TRANSPOSITION FLAPS
- **Z-plasty**
  - **Indications**
    - Web space deepening
    - Volar skin contractures
    - Hypertrophic scars

- **Contraindications**
  - ▸ Infection
  - ▸ Questionable skin flap vascularity
  - ▸ Poor soft tissue mobility or pliablity
- **Technical tips**
  - ▸ **Standard 60-degree Z-plasty** (75% increase in length along the long axis) with central limb over scar
    - ✦ Limbs should be equal length.
    - ✦ Central limbs should lay within joint flexion creases.
  - ▸ **Four-flap Z-plasty:** Increase in length of 150%
    - ✦ Four 60-degree equilateral triangles
  - ▸ **"Jumping man flap"** (five-flap Z-plasty)
    - ✦ Better for web space deepening than lengthening
- ■ **Limberg/rhomboid flap**
  - • Allows defect-closing tension to be distributed over larger surface area
  - • **Indications**
    - ▸ Small defects over dorsum of hand and digits
  - • **Contraindications**
    - ▸ Same as for Z-plasty
    - ▸ Large defects
  - • **Technical tips**
    - ▸ Pivot point: Base at a point farthest from defect (with or without back cuts)

TIP: Multiple Limberg flaps can be used when less tissue mobility is present (e.g., at the wrist).

ADVANCEMENT FLAPS
- ■ Allow direct advancement by using triangle-shaped back cuts (e.g., V-Y advancement flaps [see Chapter 56])
  - • **Atasoy-Kleinert:** Central volar fingertip advancement flap
  - • **Kutler flaps:** Bilateral triangular advancement flaps
  - • **Moberg flap:** Advancement flap for the thumb
- ■ May have axial and random blood supply patterns

AXIAL PATTERN FLAPS
- ■ Based on midlateral area of digit and incorporates a digital artery

CAUTION: A digital Allen's test must be done before the flap is elevated.

- ■ **Indications**
  - • Vary depending on flap capabilities; generally used for moderate-sized defects of dorsal and volar fingers
- ■ **Contraindications**
  - • Abnormal digital Allen's test
  - • Vascular disease
  - • Diabetes: Relative contraindication; use more conservative procedure

- **Technical tips**
  - Usually up to 1-2 cm wide and can extend along entire finger length
  - Requires contralateral digital artery patency
  - Branches to overlying skin paddle should not be disrupted
- **First dorsal metacarpal artery (FDMA) flap**

Axial flap including skin; subcutaneous tissue over dorsal proximal index finger
  - **Indication:** Optimal for thumb defects
  - **Technical tips**
    - ▸ Blood supply from first dorsal metacarpal artery off radial artery
    - ▸ Skin flap can be up to 3 cm by 3 cm
    - ▸ Can incorporate neural branches

TIP: Incorporate a strip of fascia over the first dorsal interosseous muscle into the pedicle for improved safe pedicle dissection.

- **Neurovascular island flaps**
  - Homodigital and heterodigital island flaps *(Littler type)*
- **C-ring flap cross-finger flap (Turkisk flap)**
  - **Indication**
    - ▸ Larger volar or dorsal defects, degloved finger stumps
  - **Contraindication**
    - ▸ Abnormal digital Allen's test
  - **Technical tips**
    - ▸ Based on digital artery, proximally or distally
    - ▸ Plane is superficial to paratenon
    - ▸ Small skin bridge to protect bundle but can be raised as an island

REGIONAL FLAPS

CROSS-FINGER FLAPS

- **Indication**
  - More than one third of the volar tissue of fingertip; exposed bone, tendon, and/or joint
- **Contraindications**
  - Coexisting disease with limited joint mobility
  - Elderly patient
  - Diabetes: Relative contraindication
- **Technical tips**
  - **Donor sites:** Middle finger used for thumb, index finger, or ring finger. Ring finger used to cover middle finger or small finger
  - Flap designed larger than defect (allows for contracture)
  - Raised on a hinge and inset; donor site covered with FTSG
  - Divided at 2 weeks

TIP: Hinge positions can be tested for optimal results by making a pattern of the defect and adjusting for optimal finger position.

Release Cleland's ligament to prevent flap kinking.

Use minimal sutures and avoid tension.

Use splint and/or K-wire to maintain joint positions.

CROSS-FINGER FLAP VARIATION
- **Innervated cross-finger flap**
  - **Indication:** Innervated tissue required (sensation critical)
  - **Technical tips**
    - Dorsal branch of proper digital nerve on donor divided proximally during flap elevation
    - Coapted to digital nerve of injured finger during flap inset
- **Reverse cross-finger flap**
  - **Indication:** Dorsal defects of the fingers
  - **Technical tips**
    - Adipodermal turnover flap
    - Skin graft after inset
    - Epidermis and papillary dermis skin lifted off with hinge contralateral to flap hinge
    - Skin placed back down on donor site after transposition
- **Cross-thumb flap**
  - **Indication:** Presence of defect on radial aspect of index finger
  - **Technical tips**
    - Based proximally overlying dorsal aspect of thumb proximal phalanx
    - Raised and inset similar to cross-finger flap

FILLET FLAP
- **Indications**
  - When "spare parts" are available from concomitant injury
    - Soft tissue preserved on another injured, nonsalvageable finger
  - Large volar or dorsal wounds
- **Contraindications**
  - Infection or unstable wound(s)
  - Severe crush or maceration of spare part(s)
- **Technical tips**
  - Longitudinal incision
  - Flap based on one or both digital vessels
  - After circumferential incision is made 5 mm proximal to nail fold, skin–subcutaneous flap elevated off of digit
  - Pulp tissue often excised
  - All dorsal veins ligated except one or two at side of hinge
  - Flap folded proximally, without tension, onto and into defect

TIP: When transposing to the digit, the flap can be made into an island. Use Bruner-type incisions to the palm for dissection. Rather than discarding excess, consider deepithelialization and filling of the wound third spaces.[3]

RADIAL FOREARM FLAP

- **Indications**
  - Small and large defects almost anywhere on the hand
    - ▶ Volar aspect
    - ▶ Dorsal aspect
    - ▶ First web space
  - When thin, pliable, reliable tissue is needed (can be bulky, especially in overweight patients)
- **Contraindications**
  - Abnormal wrist Allen's test, anomalous radial vessels
    - ▶ Up to **15%** of patients do **not** have a complete palmar arch
  - Forearm donor scar can be cosmetically unacceptable
  - Vasculopathy
    - ▶ Can produce cold intolerance of the hand, even in nonvasculopathic patients
- **Flap Variations**
  - Free tissue transfer
  - Fascia-only flap
  - Fasciocutaneous
  - Reverse radial pedicled
  - Neurosensory flap
- **Anatomy** (Fig. 64-1)
  - Dissection plane: Superficial to flexor digitorum superficialis and between flexor carpi radialis and brachioradialis muscles
  - Radial artery becomes very superficial distally in forearm with bifurcation just proximal to the wrist
  - Perforating vessels in forearm exist in fascial mesentery to supply skin and subcutaneous tissues (9-13 vessels; most are distal)
  - Venous drainage of flap
    - ▶ Venae comitantes
    - ▶ Can incorporate cephalic vein

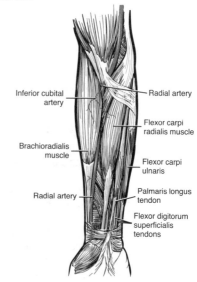

Inferior cubital artery
Radial artery
Flexor carpi radialis muscle
Brachioradialis muscle
Flexor carpi ulnaris
Radial artery
Palmaris longus tendon
Flexor digitorum superficialis tendons

Fig. 64-1   Local anatomy of the forearm.

TIP: Radial artery can be reconstituted (ideally with a nearby cephalic vein interposition vein graft) if hand perfusion becomes a concern.

REVERSE RADIAL ARTERY FOREARM FLAP (FASCIOCUTANEOUS)

- **Technical tips**
  - Design skin paddle.
    - ▶ Skin paddle can be up to 15 by 24 cm (entire volar forearm skin).
    - ▶ The more distal the defect, the more proximal the skin paddle.

> **TIP:** Use a template, and test pivot and flap reach by using nonelastic material (silk suture or lap pad) to simulate flap rotation arc and reach.

- Dissect from ulnar side to approach pedicle.
  - ▶ Raise flap from proximal to distal.
- Incise and elevate antebrachial fascia with skin paddle.

> **TIP:** It is helpful to suture the fascia to the skin edges to avoid fascial injury.

- Continue subfascial elevation to delineate radial vascular bundle and venae comitantes (in intermuscular septum), and ligate muscular perforators.
- Divide radial artery at proximal flap margin.

> **TIP:** The artery can be temporarily clamped first to test flap viablility.

- Rotate into defect.

> **TIP:** Avoid pedicle kinking. The best location for the pivot point is 2-3 cm proximal to the wrist. Tunnel or extend the incision. Avoid injury to the radial nerve dorsal sensory branches.

- Close donor defect partially and use skin for graft remaining portion.
  - ▶ FTSG may have better cosmesis.
  - ▶ Defects smaller than 5-6 cm wide are closed primarily.

POSTERIOR INTEROSSEOUS FLAP[4] (Fig. 64-2)
- Retrograde flap based on posterior interosseous artery (PIA)
- **Indications**
  - Defects at first web space, thumb, dorsal hand to level of proximal interphalangeal joint, palm, and wrist
  - When a thin, pliable flap needed
  - Radial forearm or other flaps contraindicated
- **Contraindications**
  - Do **not** attempt if significant wrist or forearm injury is present. Increased risk of PIA thrombosis.
- **Technical tips**
  - Make a line marking septocutaneous axis of flap from lateral epicondyle to ulnar styloid with 90-degree elbow flexion.
    - ▶ Skin paddle up to 6-7 cm wide
  - PIA is at junction of proximal and middle third of the line.
    - ▶ 7-14 fasciocutaneous perforators
  - PIA arises dorsally from the interosseous membrane, 6 cm distal to the lateral epicondyle.

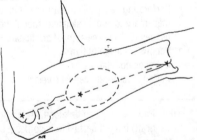

Fig. 64-2 Bony landmarks and location of skin paddle for the posterior interosseous artery flap. (From Gilbert A. Pedicle flaps of the upper limb. Philadelphia: Lippincott, 1992.)

- Center of flap is distal to most proximal perforators (proximal-middle third point).
- Pivot point is 2 cm proximal to ulnar styloid.
- PIA flap is raised radial to vessels.
- Dissect from proximal to distal, ligating muscular perforators.
- Ulnar border is raised (avoid injury to main perforator).
- Clamp and then ligate PIA proximal to main perforator.
- Can close donor site primarily if defect is smaller than 4 cm.

REVERSE ULNAR ARTERY FOREARM FLAP

- **Indications**
  - Defects of elbow (based proximally)
  - Dorsal or volar hand defects (based distally in retrograde fashion)
- **Advantages**
  - Less hair-bearing skin than reverse radial artery forearm flap
  - Better donor cosmesis than radial forearm flap
  - Excellent for elderly patients with thin skin and large dorsal defects (skin cancer or chemotherapy/chemical burns)
- **Disadvantages**
  - Ulnar artery is often the dominant blood supply to the hand.
  - Dissection is more difficult.
  - Adjacent ulnar nerve is at risk for injury.
- **Technical tips**
  - Similar principles to reverse radial artery forearm flap
  - Pedicle: Between flexor carpi ulnaris and FDS; ulnar nerve is deep to artery
  - Pivot point 2-4 cm proximal to pisiform

DISTANT FLAPS: PEDICLED

> TIP: Except for the epigastric and abdominal flaps (true random flaps), all can be used as free tissue transfers.

PEDICLED EPIGASTRIC/ABDOMINAL FLAPS

- **Indications**
  - Large or circumferential thumb defects
  - Large dorsal hand defects
  - Excellent for blast injuries with multiple amputated digits
- **Contraindications**
  - Elderly and disabled patients
    - ▸ Require joint positioning and prolonged immobilization
  - Diabetes: Relative contraindication
- **Technical tips**
  - Defect pattern is made and transposed to abdomen or chest.
  - Hand is brought to site to test position.
  - Flap is raised thick.
  - Avoid any tension on flap, or hinge kinking; use minimal sutures.

- Small donor defects can be closed primarily.
- Splint and bulky dressings are often required.
- Divide and inset at 2-3 weeks.
- As with most flaps, undermine minimally and stage debulking and revisions.
  ▸ Undermining less than 50% of flap is usually safe.

TIP: Skin graft donor defect if it is large, and there will be much less to close, if any at all, at division and inset. Flaps may also be tubed.

Secure the splint and dressing before the patient wakes up from anaesthesia.

GROIN FLAP

- Can be used as a random pattern flap, axial flap, or free flap
- **Indications**
  - Similar to abdominal/epigastric flap
- **Advantages**
  - When donor scar needs to be hidden (groin crease).
  - Can provide more tissue than epigastric/abdominal flaps.
  - Better vascularity. Can be made into an axial pattern flap.
- **Disadvantages**
  - More dependent positioning than previously discussed random pedicled flaps
  - Increased stiffness
- **Contraindications**
  - Chronic groin infection (e.g., intertrigo)
  - Lower extremity or upper extremity edema: Relative contraindication
- **Anatomy** (Fig. 64-3)
  - Flap based on **superficial circumflex iliac artery (SCIA)**
  - Pedicle parallel and 1 inch inferior to inguinal ligament
  - Commonly originates from femoral artery
- **Technical tips**
  - Pattern defect and decide on positioning of flap onto defect.

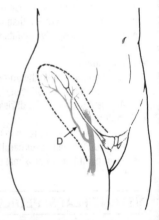

Fig. 64-3   Groin flap. The dominant pedicle is the superficial circumflex iliac artery (D).

TIP: Overall skin design can be elliptical for easier/more aesthetic primary closure.

- Using Doppler, mark artery to branch points where flap becomes random (at anterior superior iliac spine level).
- Incise deep fascia at level of inferior incision to find lateral border of sartorius.
- SCIA may be seen in deep subcutaneous tissue.
- Preserve the *lateral femoral cutaneous nerve;* as flap is raised from lateral to medial.

CAUTION: If the nerve is injured, the patient can have prolonged pain and dysesthesia.

TIP: Consider tubing the flap, unless all distal and lateral margins are needed to fit defect.

- Immobilize extremity with splint or cast; bulky dressing.
- Divide and complete inset at 2-3 weeks.
- Perform revisions and debulking as needed.

DISTANT FLAPS: FREE TISSUE TRANSFER[5,6]

LATERAL ARM FLAP

- **Indications**
  - Large dorsal or volar hand defects
  - Proximal multidigit defects
  - When radial forearm flaps are contraindicated
- **Contraindications**
  - Overweight patients: Flap can be excessively bulky
  - Epicondylitis or other inflammatory elbow disease
- **Advantages**
  - Pedicle can be extended.
  - Bone can be taken with flap.
  - Flap is ipsilateral to defect.
- **Disadvantages**
  - Can have poor appearance and hypersensitivity of donor site, elbow pain, numbness in the forearm, and excessive flap bulk
- **Technical tips**
  - **Blood supply:** Posterior radial collateral artery
  - **Nerve supply:** Posterior cutaneous nerve
  - Can be fasciocutaneous or a composite of fascia, muscle, tendon, and/or bone

SCAPULAR AND PARASCAPULAR FLAPS

- **Indications**
  - Large defects of arm and hand that do not require sensation
  - When bone is needed
    - ▶ Lateral border of scapula can be harvested for bony reconstruction.
- **Contraindications**
  - Similar to lateral arm flap
  - Bulky and commonly require secondary defatting and debulking
- **Technical tips**
  - **Blood supply:** Branch of circumflex scapular artery
  - **Scapular** flap based on **transverse branch** of circumflex scapular artery
  - **Parascapular** flap based on **descending branch**
    - ▶ Parascapular flap: Larger skin paddle and less conspicuous scar
  - Scapular osteocutaneous flap and latissimus dorsi flap can be combined on common vascular leash

LATISSIMUS DORSI MUSCLE FLAP

- **Anatomy**
  - **Blood supply:** Thoracodorsal artery and vein
  - Consistent long pedicle (up to 15 cm)

- **Indications**
  - Optimal for small to very large upper extremity wounds
  - Excellent for free functional tissue transfer
- **Advantages**
  - Large, broad flap
  - Can take segmental area of flap
  - Can be used as a free functional muscle transfer for large volar forearm injuries when hand reinnervation and wrist powering are required
- **Technical tips**
  - Details described in Chapter 43

SERRATUS ANTERIOR MUSCLE FLAP

- **Anatomy**
  - Arises from first nine ribs medial to axillary line and inserts into medial scapula
    - ▸ Segmental slips can be used
    - ▸ Can be taken as *fascia-only flap*
  - **Dual vascular supply** is *branch from thoracodorsal artery* (lower 3 slips) and *lateral thoracic artery* (upper 6 slips)
  - Can minimize motor deformity ("winging of scapula") by preserving motor and neurovascular segments
- **Indications**
  - Similar to previously mentioned free tissue flaps
- **Contraindications**
  - Previous latissimus flap harvest
  - Previous axillary dissection—*controversial.* Usually does not pose any problem if meticulous dissection performed
- **Advantages**
  - Can use different slips for multiple-finger soft tissue coverage
  - Reliable muscle
  - Easy dissection
  - Donor site morbidity very low

TEMPOROPARIETAL FASCIA FLAP

- **Anatomy**
  - **Blood supply:** Superficial temporal artery and vein
  - Based on fasciocutaneous perforators
    - ▸ Superior extension of SMAS
  - Maximal dimensions are 13 cm long by 9 cm wide
  - Auriculotemporal nerve divided during dissection
  - Can close donor defect primarily
- **Indications**
  - Good for small dorsal defects of the hand and wrist, especially in thin-skinned individuals
  - Wrapping of exposed, contracted tendons
    - ▸ Areolar surface provides good tissue for tendon gliding
  - Small three-dimensional defects in hand (e.g., after first web space release)
- **Contraindications**
  - Previous facial surgery

- **Advantages**
  - Very thin and extremely vascular tissue
  - Donor incision well hidden
- **Disadvantages**
  - Risk of palsy of frontal branch of facial nerve
  - Many hand surgeons not familiar with dissection
  - Risk of permanent alopecia

FIRST WEB SPACE FLAP[7]

- **Anatomy**
  - **Blood supply:** First dorsal metatarsal artery
    - ▸ Branch off of dorsalis pedis artery
    - ▸ Preoperative angiogram often required
  - **Nerve Supply:** Deep peroneal nerve and medial plantar nerve
  - Lateral region of great toe taken with combination of specific portion of pulp (according to defect), with all or partial nail
- **Indication**
  - Gold standard: A neurosensory flap to critical sensory areas of hand (pulp)
- **Advantages**
  - Allows thin glabrous skin with numerous sensory receptors
  - Excellent two-point discrimination
- **Contraindication**
  - Risk of toe devascularization
- **Disadvantage**
  - Difficult dissection

DORSALIS PEDIS FLAP[8]

- **Anatomy**
  - **Blood supply:** Dorsalis pedis artery
- **Advantages**
  - When thin, pliable skin over foot dorsum
  - Can be taken with underlying extensor tendon and can be innervated with superficial peroneal nerve
- **Disadvantage**
  - Healing problems at donor site

OTHER FREE TISSUE TRANSFER OPTIONS

RECTUS ABDOMINIS MUSCLE FLAP

- Very large, donor site morbidity
- Low in algorithm for upper extremity defects

ANTEROLATERAL THIGH FLAP

- Similar to radial forearm free flap in terms of bulk and pliability, but with a less-morbid donor site.

Gracilis Muscle Flap

- Long, minimal donor site morbidity
- Good for very lengthy or large arm defects and for limb salvage
- First choice for free functional tissue transfer to hand and arm (e.g., after Volkmann's contracture)

Key Points

- ✔ Properly control wound conditions (eradication of infection with culture-directed antimicrobial therapy, serial debridements, VAC therapy).
- ✔ Achieve absolute skeletal stability.
- ✔ Consider composite flaps of soft tissue, bone, tendon, and nerves when indicated.
- ✔ Prioritize reconstruction based on patient lifestyle and most critical functional deficits.
- ✔ Pedicled random and axial flaps are still simple and reliable options and can be workhorses for coverage of variety of hand defects.
- ✔ Institute rehabilitation protocols early on in reconstruction process.
- ✔ Do not hesitate to move to free tissue transfer when indicated. Complex wounds often require complex operations.

References

1. Jones NF, Lister GD. Free skin and composite flaps. In Green DP, Hotchkiss RN, Pederson WC, eds. Green's Operative Hand Surgery, vol 2, 4th ed. Philadelphia: Churchill Livingstone, 1999, pp 1159-1200.
2. Lister GD, Pederson CP. Skin flaps. In Green DP, Hotchkiss RN, Pederson WC, eds. Green's Operative Hand Surgery, vol 2, 4th ed. Philadelphia: Churchill Livingstone, 1999, pp 1783-1850.
3. Masson JA. Fingernails, infections, tumors and soft tissue reconstructions. Sel Read Plast Surg 9:19-27, 2002.
4. Zancolli EA, Angrigiani C. Posterior interosseous island forearm flap. J Hand Surg Br 13:130-135, 1988.
5. Strauch B, Yu HL, Chen ZW, et al. Atlas of Microvascular Surgery, Anatomy and Operative Approaches. New York: Thieme Medical Publishers, 1992, pp 44-68.
6. Upton J, Havlik RJ, Khouri RK. Refinements in hand coverage with microvascular free flaps. Clin Plast Surg 19:841-857, 1992.
7. May JW Jr, Chait LA, Cohen BE, et al. Free neurovascular flap from the first web space of the foot in hand reconstruction. J Hand Surg 2:387-393, 1977.
8. Zuker RM, Mantkelow RT. The dorsalis pedis free flap: Technique for elevation, foot closure, and flap application. Plast Reconstr Surg 77:93-104, 1986.

65. Compartment Syndrome

George Broughton II*

DEFINITION

- **Compartment syndrome** is a **limb-threatening** and **life-threatening** condition that occurs when perfusion pressure falls below tissue pressure in a closed anatomic space.
- Untreated compartment syndrome leads to tissue necrosis, permanent functional impairment, and, if severe, renal failure and death.

DEMOGRAPHICS

- Compartment syndrome has been found wherever a compartment is present: Hand, forearm, upper arm, abdomen, buttock, and entire lower extremity.
- Almost any injury can cause this syndrome, including injury from vigorous exercise.

INCIDENCE[1-4]

- **Anterior distal lower extremity** (secondary to its frequency of injury) is most common.
- Ranges of 2%-12% have been published.
- 30% of limbs develop compartment syndrome following vascular injury; however, this is not well documented and is most likely an estimate.
- McQueen and Court-Brown[3] retrospectively studied 164 patients diagnosed with compartment syndrome; 69% were associated with a fracture, one half of those being the tibia.

SEX

- Affects males more than females, which likely represents selection bias, because men are more often patients with traumatic injuries

PATHOPHYSIOLOGY[1,2,5-7]

- Compartment syndrome follows the path of ischemic injury.
  - "Container" pressure rises as more fluid is introduced into a fixed volume, and various fascial compartments have relatively fixed volumes.
  - Excess fluid or extraneous constriction increases pressure and decreases tissue perfusion until no oxygen is available for cellular metabolism.
  - Elevated perfusion pressure is the physiologic response to rising intracompartmental pressure.
  - As intracompartmental pressure rises, compensatory mechanisms are overwhelmed, and a cascade of injury develops.

---

*The opinions or assertions contained herein are the private views of the author and are not to be construed as official or as reflecting the views of the Department of the Army or the Department of Defense.

- **Tissue perfusion** is determined by measuring **capillary perfusion pressure (CPP) minus the interstitial fluid pressure.**
- Normal cellular metabolism requires **5-7 mm Hg** oxygen tension.
  - This tension is easily maintained when the CPP averages 25 mm Hg and the interstitial pressure averages 4-6 mm Hg.
  - In compartment syndrome, rising interstitial pressure overwhelms perfusion pressure.
- As intracompartmental pressure rises, venous pressure rises, and when venous pressure is higher than CPP, capillaries collapse.
  - The pressure at which collapse occurs is debated; however, **intracompartmental pressures greater than 30 mm Hg require intervention.** At this pressure, blood flow through the capillaries stops.
- Hypoxia causes tissues to undergo anaerobic metabolism.
  - Lactic acid accumulates, and with continued hypoxia, energy requirements are not met.
  - The ATP-dependent Na^+/K^+ pump fails, and the cellular membrane is unable to maintain the osmolar gradient.
  - The resulting edema causes more ischemia as pressure rises, and a self-perpetuating cycle leads to compartment syndrome.
  - Continued compression of nutrient capillaries exacerbates anoxia, which induces lipid peroxidation of the cell membrane, stimulates the inflammatory cascade, activates neutrophils, and generates hypoxanthine (a product of ATP breakdown—it forms the oxygen free radical superoxide).
  - The process eventually results in permanent damage, and the "no-reflow" phenomenon develops. (Reversal and correction of existing metabolic and structural deficits are not possible even if flow is reestablished.)
- Reperfusion of an ischemic compartment brings an abundant supply of oxygen that reacts with hypoxanthine to produce superoxide.
  - Iron from red blood cells reacts with hydrogen peroxide to form the highly toxic hydroxyl radical and other free radicals that potentiate the insult to the already damaged cell membranes.
  - These radicals also promote platelet aggregation and microvascular clotting, resulting in renewed ischemia.

DIAGNOSIS[1-3,8,9]

HISTORY
- Suspect compartment syndrome whenever significant pain occurs in an extremity after injury, especially if the extremity is tense.
- Compartment syndrome can be caused by increasing interstitial volume or decreasing size of the compartment.
- **The following mechanisms cause increased interstitial fluid production:**
  - Intensive muscle use (e.g., tetany, vigorous exercise, seizures)
  - Everyday exercise activities (e.g., stationary bicycle use, horseback riding)
  - Burns
  - Intraarterial injection (frequently iatrogenic)
  - Envenomation
  - Decreased serum osmolarity (e.g., nephrotic syndrome)
  - Infiltration injury
  - Hemorrhage (particularly from a large-vessel injury)
- **The following mechanisms can cause decreased compartment size:**
  - Military antishock trousers (MAST)

- Burns
- Casts
- Lying on a limb
  - ▶ Intracompartmental pressures have been measured in various positions common in drug overdoses[5]
    - ✦ 48 mm Hg with the head resting on forearm
    - ✦ 178 mm Hg when forearm under ribcage
    - ✦ 72 mm Hg when one leg folded under the other
- Usually the patient complains of severe pain out of proportion to examination and a burning sensation or tightness.
- The traditional five Ps of ischemia (i.e., pain, paresthesia, pallor, poikilothermia, and pulselessness) are not diagnostic of compartment syndrome. With the exception of pain and paresthesia, these traditional signs are unreliable, and the presence or absence of them should not affect injury management.

Pitfalls

- Obtunded patients and patients with spinal cord injuries
- Young children and infants

Maintain Suspicion

- High-velocity injuries
- Long bone fractures
- High-energy trauma
- Penetrating injuries (e.g., gunshot wounds, stabbings): Often cause arterial injury that can quickly lead to compartment syndrome
- Venous injuries: May cause compartment syndrome, but do not be misled by palpable pulses
- Crush injuries
- Anticoagulation therapy: Compartment syndrome requiring fasciotomy has been observed after simple venipuncture in patients undergoing anticoagulation therapy
- Intense physical activity: Compartment syndrome has been found in soldiers and athletes without trauma
  - Can be acute or chronic and have compartment pressures as high as those found in severe trauma

Physical Examination

- Follow-up physical examinations are important to determine whether any progression of symptoms exists.
- **Always compare the affected limb with the unaffected limb.**
- Severe pain at rest or with any movement should raise suspicion. **Pain during passive stretching** is one of the earliest clinical indicators of compartment syndrome.

TIP: Pain during passive stretching is one of the earliest indications of compartment syndrome and perhaps the most sensitive.

- Paresthesias: Sensory nerves are affected first, followed by motor nerves.
- Paralysis
- Weakness
- Tense limb

> **TIP:** Always compare the affected limb with the unaffected limb. A tense compartment is a sensitive sign.

CAUTION: Pulselessness is a *late* sign. (Too late!)

> **TIP:** The muscles most commonly affected are the flexor digitorum profundus in the forearm and the flexor hallucis longus in the leg because they lie against the bone.

LABORATORY STUDIES
- Blood chemistries: **Potassium** and **creatinine** levels important
- Complete blood count (CBC) with differential
- Creatine phosphokinase (CPK) and urine myoglobin
- Serum myoglobin
- Urine toxicology screen: May help define etiologic factors but rarely helpful for patient treatment
- Initial urinalysis: May be positive for blood but negative for RBC on microscopic analysis, which may indicate myoglobin in the urine (rhabdomyolysis)
- Prothrombin time (PT) and activated partial thromboplastin time (aPTT)

IMAGING STUDIES
- **Plain radiographs** of the affected extremity (looking for a fracture)
- **Ultrasonography** for evaluating arterial flow or revealing deep venous thrombosis (DVT)

NOTE: Ultrasonography is not helpful for diagnosis of compartment syndrome; however, it aids in the elimination of differential diagnoses.

COMPARTMENT PRESSURE MEASUREMENT
- Perform this test as soon as the diagnosis of compartment syndrome is considered.
- Various products are commercially available for direct pressure measurements through ACE Medical Equipment Inc. (Clearwater, FL) and Stryker (Kalamazoo, MI).

TREATMENT[1,2,6]

Many cases of compartment syndrome result from trauma. Follow advanced trauma life support (ATLS) guidelines to stabilize patient before attempting to address compartment syndrome.

PRINCIPLES
- **Early intervention is tremendously important.** Irreversible tissue injury starts approximately **6 hours** after onset of compartment syndrome.
- **Fasciotomy** remains the definitive therapy for compartment syndrome because of its well-documented, limb-saving results (Figs. 65-1 through 65-8).
- **IV hydration is essential.** A urine output goal should be 1-2 ml/kg/hour to prevent accumulation of myoglobin and subsequent renal dysfunction.

■ Positioning has little effect on intracompartmental pressure but affects mean arterial pressure to the affected limb.
• Keeping extremities level with the body decreases limb mean arterial pressure without changing intracompartmental pressure.
• Elevating the limb 35 cm in one study decreased the mean arterial perfusion pressure 23 mm Hg but did not change intracompartmental pressure.[7]

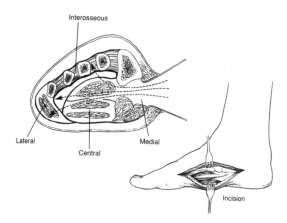

Fig. 65-1   Foot fasciotomy by medial incision. To decompress the four compartments of the foot using a medial approach, an incision is made along the plantar border of the first metatarsal allowing access to all four compartments. The incision can be extended proximally if the posterior tibial neurovascular bundle requires decompression as well. (From Aston SJ, Beasley RW, Thorne CHM, eds. Grabb and Smith's Plastic Surgery, 5th ed. Philadelphia: Lippincott-Raven, 1997, pp 1071.)

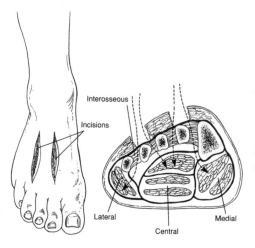

Fig. 65-2   Foot fasciotomy by dorsal incision. The dorsal approach to compartment decompression is performed along the second and fourth interspaces. All four compartments can then be released. (From Aston SJ, Beasley RW, Thorne CHM, eds. Grabb and Smith's Plastic Surgery, 5th ed. Philadelphia: Lippincott-Raven, 1997, pp 1071.)

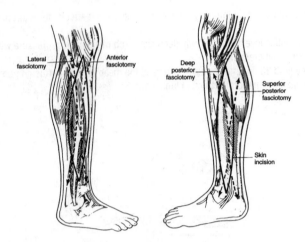

Fig. 65-3   Leg fasciotomy. Lateral and medial leg incisions for a four-compartment fasciotomy. The lateral and anterior compartments are decompressed through a lateral incision and the superficial and deep posterior compartments through a medial incision. (From Velmahos GC, Toutouzas KG. Vascular trauma and compartment syndromes. Surg Clin North Am 82:125, 2002.)

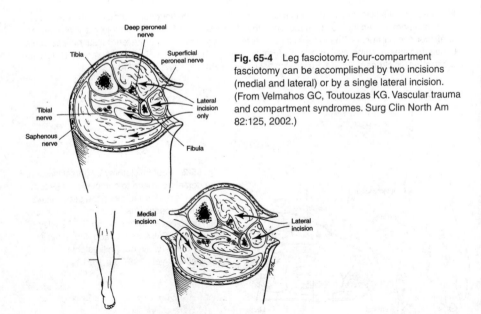

Fig. 65-4   Leg fasciotomy. Four-compartment fasciotomy can be accomplished by two incisions (medial and lateral) or by a single lateral incision. (From Velmahos GC, Toutouzas KG. Vascular trauma and compartment syndromes. Surg Clin North Am 82:125, 2002.)

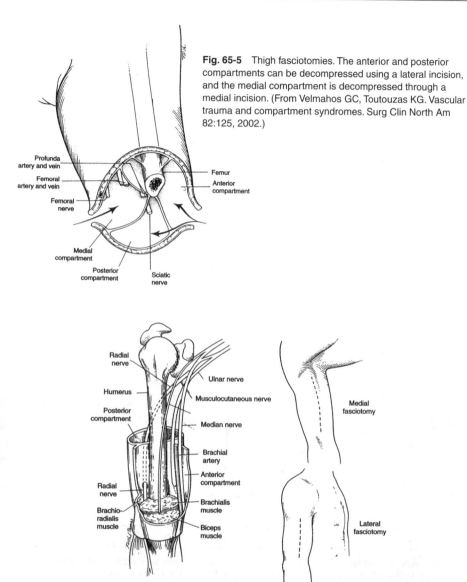

Fig. 65-5   Thigh fasciotomies. The anterior and posterior compartments can be decompressed using a lateral incision, and the medial compartment is decompressed through a medial incision. (From Velmahos GC, Toutouzas KG. Vascular trauma and compartment syndromes. Surg Clin North Am 82:125, 2002.)

Fig. 65-6   Arm fasciotomies. The anterior compartment is decompressed using a medial incision, and the posterior compartment is decompressed through a lateral incision. Notice that the ulnar and radial nerves travel in both compartments; therefore increased pressure in either produces symptoms along the distribution of both nerves. (From Velmahos GC, Toutouzas KG. Vascular trauma and compartment syndromes. Surg Clin North Am 82:125, 2002.)

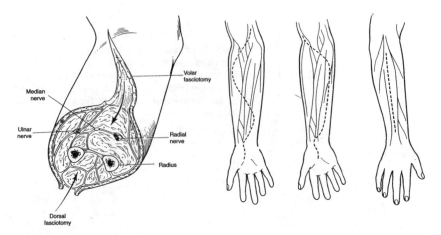

Fig. 65-7   Forearm fasciotomies. Volar (S-type or straight) and dorsal (straight) incisions are used for forearm fasciotomies. (From Velmahos GC, Toutouzas KG. Vascular trauma and compartment syndromes. Surg Clin North Am 82:125, 2002.)

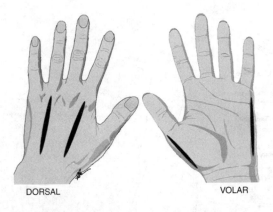

DORSAL   VOLAR

Fig. 65-8   Hand fasciotomy; volar and dorsal incisions for hand compartment releases.

CONTROVERSY

Debate exists regarding the threshold for fasciotomy. A number of researchers recommend 30 mm Hg, whereas others cite 45 mm Hg. Still others urge prophylactic fasciotomy at normal pressures to prevent compartment syndrome with high-risk injuries.

Convincing evidence indicates that debate should center on **delta-p** (Δp). Delta-p is a measure of **perfusion pressure** *(diastolic blood pressure minus intracompartmental pressure)*. Delta-p measurements of less than 30 mm Hg were used by McQueen and Court-Brown[3] for fasciotomy. Several patients with intracompartmental pressures of 40 mm Hg or greater were observed because the delta-p was greater than 30 mm Hg. Criteria were used in 116 patients without sequelae. The converse also is true, because patients with intracompartmental pressures less than 30 mm Hg but with low delta-p values have developed compartment syndrome (e.g., if the diastolic pressure is 40 mm Hg and the compartment pressure is 25 mm Hg; the delta-p is 15 mm Hg).

ENVENOMATIONS

- Studies have confirmed previously postulated theories that myonecrosis associated with compartment syndrome after envenomation is multifactorial and that fasciotomy may **not** prevent myonecrosis.[10]
- Myonecrosis is thought to result from a direct toxic effect of the venom and the inflammatory response. Therefore, these patients should be aggressively treated with antivenom if available, because this has been shown to decrease limb hypoperfusion.

POTENTIAL FUTURE TREATMENTS

MANNITOL

- Some authors have advocated the use of mannitol for compartment syndrome.[10,11] Although its use for rhabdomyolysis is well documented, its use for acute compartment syndrome is new.
- Daniels et al[11] treated with mannitol an Israeli soldier who developed compartment syndrome. After resolution, he was discharged without fasciotomy. Unfortunately, intracompartmental pressures were not measured, because the diagnosis was based on limb circumference and nerve conduction studies. Further investigation is warranted in this area.

HYPERBARIC OXYGEN (HBO)

- HBO therapy is a logical choice for compartment syndrome because it addresses the primary concern of ischemic injury.
- **HBO has many beneficial effects.**
  - It reduces edema through oxygen-induced vasoconstriction while maintaining oxygen perfusion.
  - It supports tissue healing in a similar mechanism by allowing oxygen delivery when perfusion pressure is low.
  - Reperfusion injury following compartment syndrome is an argument against HBO; however, HBO actually protects against reperfusion injury.
- Bouachour et al[12] performed a well-controlled randomized study with 31 patients following crush injury and demonstrated significant increase in complete healing ($p < 0.01$).
- Although HBO currently is only adjunctive therapy because of its limited availability, it should not be ignored.
- HBO may extend treatment duration, and it may not reverse etiologic factors, but it has been shown to be beneficial.

COMPLICATIONS[13]

- Permanent nerve damage
- Infection
- Loss of limb
- Cosmetic deformity from fasciotomy
- Death

OUTCOMES

- Outcome depends on both the **diagnosis** and the **time from injury to intervention.**
  - Rorabeck and Macnab[6] reported almost complete recovery of limb function if fasciotomy was performed **within 6 hours.**
  - Matsen et al[5] found necrosis **after 6 hours** of ischemia, which currently is the accepted upper limit of viability.
- The prognosis is excellent to poor, depending on **how quickly compartment syndrome is treated** and whether complications develop.
- Fitzgerald et al[14] reported the results of a retrospective study over an 8-year period of patients requiring fasciotomies of either upper or lower limbs.
  - Results for long-term morbidity are as follows:
    - Pain (10%)
    - Altered sensation within margins of the wound (77%)
    - Dry scaly skin (40%)
    - Pruritus (33%)
    - Discolored wounds (30%)
    - Swollen limbs (25%)
    - Tethered scars (26%)
    - Recurrent ulceration (13%)
    - Muscle herniation (13%)
    - Tethered tendon (7%)

KEY POINTS

- ✔ The prognosis for limb function is best if fasciotomy is performed within 6 hours of injury.
- ✔ Pain and paresthesia are the most diagnostic symptoms for compartment syndrome.
- ✔ Positioning has little effect on intracompartmental pressure but affects mean arterial pressure to the affected limb.
- ✔ Tissue perfusion is determined by CPP minus interstitial fluid pressure.

REFERENCES

1. Velmahos GC, Toutouzas KG. Vascular trauma and compartment syndromes. Surg Clin North Am 82:125-141, xxi, 2002.
2. McQueen MM, Gaston P, Court-Brown CM. Acute compartment syndrome. Who is at risk? J Bone Joint Surg Br 82:200-203, 2000.
3. McQueen MM, Court-Brown CM. Compartment monitoring in tibial fractures. The pressure threshold for decompression. J Bone Joint Surg Br 78:99-104, 1996.
4. Styf J, Wiger P. Abnormally increased intramuscular pressure in human legs: Comparison of two experimental models. J Trauma 45:133-139, 1998.
5. Matsen FA III, Winquist RA, Krugmire RB Jr. Diagnosis and management of compartmental syndromes. J Bone Joint Surg Am 62:286-291, 1980.
6. Rorabeck CH, Macnab I. The pathophysiology of the anterior tibial compartmental syndrome. Clin Orthop 113:52-57, 1975.

7. Seiler JG III, Casey PJ, Binford SH. Compartment syndromes of the upper extremity. J South Orthop Assoc 9:233-247, 2000.

8. Owen CA, Mubarak SJ, Hargens AR, et al. Intramuscular pressures with limb compression clarification of the pathogenesis of the drug-induced muscle-compartment syndrome. N Engl J Med 300:1169-1172, 1979.

9. Tanen DA, Danish DC, Grice GA, et al. Fasciotomy worsens the amount of myonecrosis in a porcine model of crotaline envenomation. Ann Emerg Med 44:99-104, 2004.

10. Better OS, Zinman C, Reis DN, et al. Hypertonic mannitol ameliorates intracompartmental tamponade in model compartment syndrome in the dog. Nephron 58:344-346, 1991.

11. Daniels M, Reichman J, Brezis M. Mannitol treatment for acute compartment syndrome. Nephron 79:492-493, 1998.

12. Bouachour G, Cronier P, Gouello JP, et al. Hyperbaric oxygen therapy in the management of crush injuries: A randomized double-blind placebo-controlled clinical trial. J Trauma 41:333-339, 1996.

13. Aston SJ, Beasley RW, Thorne CHM, eds. Grabb and Smith's Plastic Surgery, 5th ed. Philadelphia: Lippincott-Raven, 1997, pp 1071.

14. Fitzgerald AM, Gaston P, Wilson Y, et al. Long-term sequelae of fasciotomy wounds. Br J Plast Surg 53:690-693, 2000.

66. Upper Extremity Compression Syndromes

Edward M. Reece
Joshua A. Lemmon

ANATOMY[1-6]

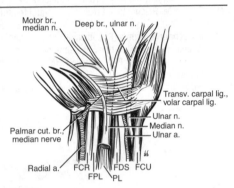

Fig. 66-1 Anatomy of the carpal tunnel. (*FCR*, Flexor carpi radialis; *FCU*, flexor carpi ulnaris; *FDS*, flexor digitorum superficialis; *FPL*, flexor pollicis longus; *PL*, palmaris longus.)

MEDIAN NERVE (C5-C7)

- Formed from **medial** and **lateral** cords of brachial plexus
- Courses between the brachialis muscle and intermuscular septum
  - Medial to the brachial artery
- Passes under ligament of Struthers at the supracondylar rim
  - Ligament associated with humeral head of the pronator teres muscle
- Crosses the antecubital fossa under the bicipital aponeurosis (lacertus fibrosis)
- Separates from artery to pass between heads of the pronator teres muscle
  - Anterior interosseous nerve descends on interosseous membrane
- Continues between the flexor digitorum profundus (FDP) and the flexor pollicis longus (FPL) muscle and behind pronator quadratus
- Median trunk continues deep to tendinous flexor digitorum superficialis (FDS) arch
- Travels distally under the palmaris longus (PL) tendon to enter the carpal tunnel
- Palmar cutaneous branch of the median nerve begins up to **5 cm** before tunnel
  - Provides sensory innervation to the thenar eminence
- **Carpal tunnel**[5]
  - **Floor:** Carpal bones
  - **Ulnar:** Hamate hook, triquetrum, pisiform
  - **Radial:** Scaphoid, trapezium, fascial septum
  - **Roof:** Transverse carpal ligament from scaphoid tuberosity/trapezium to pisiform and hamate hook
  - Nine tendons and the median nerve
  - **Variant branches of the median recurrent motor nerve:** Beyond the transverse carpal ligament, below the ligament, or through the ligament[6] (Fig. 66-1)
  - **Anterior interosseous nerve:** Reliably innervates pronator quadratus muscle and radiocarpal, radioulnar, and carpometacarpal (CMC) joints
  - **Median nerve:** Reliably innervates thenar hand musculature

RADIAL NERVE (C5-C7)

- Terminal branch **posterior cord**
- Bifurcates from axillary nerve running posterior to axillary/brachial artery
- Travels posterior to brachial artery, anterior to triceps/subscapularis muscle
- Proceeds posterior to profunda brachii artery between lateral/medial heads of triceps
- Transects lateral intermuscular septum with the radial collateral artery
  - 10 cm proximal to distal humerus
  - Between brachialis and brachioradialis muscle
  - Further distally enters between the brachialis and extensor carpi radialis longus (ECRL) muscle
- Traverses radial tunnel as soon as it is overlying tunnel floor
  - **Floor:** Radiocapitellar joint bursa
  - **Roof:** Brachioradialis tendon
  - **Lateral:** ECRL and extensor carpi radialis brevis (ECRB) tendons
  - **Medial:** Biceps tendon
  - End of tunnel is distal border of supinator muscle
- 1 cm lateral to the biceps tendon at the cubital fossa
- Splits at elbow, traverses the supinator medial and lateral heads
  - Deep branch **(posterior interosseous nerve [PIN])** passes under the arcade of Frohse and is distally adjacent to the extensor digitorum communis tendon
  - Branch enters the fourth compartment of the dorsal forearm
  - **Four areas of radial nerve compression** cross the elbow[3] (Fig. 66-2)
    1. Proximal to the radial tunnel (fibrous bands)
    2. Leash of Henry (radial recurrent artery)
    3. Extensor carpi radialis brevis originating tendon
    4. Arcade of Frohse (between the medial and lateral heads of the supinator)
  - **PIN reliably supplies** extensor indicis proprius muscle and extensor pollicis longus muscle

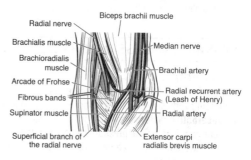

Fig. 66-2 Sites of compressions of the radial nerve at the radial tunnel.

Biceps brachii muscle
Radial nerve
Brachialis muscle
Median nerve
Brachioradialis muscle
Brachial artery
Arcade of Frohse
Fibrous bands
Radial recurrent artery (Leash of Henry)
Supinator muscle
Radial artery
Superficial branch of the radial nerve
Extensor carpi radialis brevis muscle

ULNAR NERVE (C8-T1)

- **Medial cord** terminal branch medial and posterior to brachial artery
- Transects medial intermuscular septum in middle arm to enter posterior arm
- Covered by arcade of Struthers **8 cm** proximal to medial epicondyle
- Passes dorsal to medial epicondyle
- **Cubital tunnel**
  - Nerve is covered by the flexor carpi ulnaris (FCU) tendon/arcuate ligament of Osborne for 4 mm.
  - Tunnel floor is composed of the capsule/median collateral ligaments.
  - Joint capsule/bursa of elbow is innervated by ulnar nerve.
- Innervates the FCU heads, passing between them

- Distally lies between the FDP/FDS muscle bellies
- Nerve tracks radial to FCU tendon and hook of hamate to enter **Guyon's canal** (Fig. 66-3)
  - Canal begins at proximal volar carpal ligament, ending with fibrous hypothenar origin ulnar to pisiform bone.

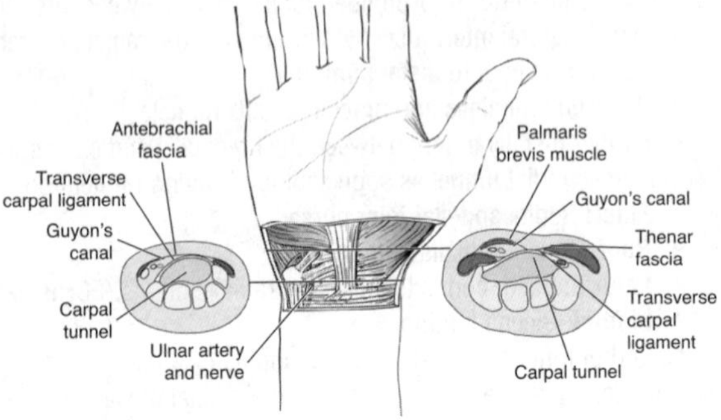

Fig. 66-3   Relationships of the ulnar nerve at the wrist.

- **Roof** is formed by FDP and transverse carpal ligament.
- **Ulnar border** is the pisiform/FCU.
- **Radial border** is the volar carpal ligament/hamate.
- Neurovascular bundle and fatty tissue run below abductor and flexor digiti minimi within the canal, separated by the transverse carpal ligament.
- Neurovascular motor bundle runs midvolarly after leaving canal (61%).
- Canal exit is bound by fascial arcade.
- **Reliably innervates** second/third dorsal interossei muscles
  - **Ulnar nerve palsy** is demonstrated by inability to deviate the extended middle finger ulnarly or radially while the hand is on a flat surface

NERVE COMPRESSION PHYSIOLOGY[4]

BACKGROUND
- Compression of **20 mm Hg or greater** interferes with nerve vasculature and has adverse effects on protein synthesis, axonal transport, saltatory conduction, and myelin sheath integrity.
- **Exacerbating factors** are vibration, prolonged stress loading, and prolonged nonneutral tendon excursion. Extraneural pressure can accelerate nerve damage additively.
- Motor system manifestations occur first as weakness, followed by numbness and tingling, and finally muscle atrophy.[5]
- **Associated comorbidities** are thyroid disorders, collagen vascular disease, and diabetes.

DIAGNOSIS[6]
- **History**
  - Determine patterns of paresthesia, pain, and weakness
  - Nocturnal disturbance
  - Presence or absence of neck pain
  - Work environment
  - Hand-arm vibratory syndrome (i.e., cold intolerance and weak, difficult pinch-grip) is secondary to environment and is not surgically correctible[7]

- **Physical examination**
  - Vibratory sense testing with tuning fork
  - Decreased vibratory perception in carpal tunnel syndrome and cubital tunnel syndrome
  - Semmes-Weinstein monofilament testing
  - Provocative examination (e.g., Phalen's sign, Tinel's sign)
  - Electrodiagnostic testing
  - Nerve conduction velocities/latencies provide objective measurement of neuropathy
  - Imaging
    - ▶ Plain radiographs
    - ▶ Magnetic resonance imaging
      - ✦ Indicated for soft tissue etiologic factors of neuropathy or suspected bone fracture

MEDIAN NERVE COMPRESSION

CARPAL TUNNEL SYNDROME (CTS)[7-11]

- Pain (worse at night) and numbness over the palmar hand with dose-dependent aggravation from repetitive movements
- **Diagnosis**
  - Nerve conduction studies show **motor latencies are usually greater than 4.5 msec** and **sensory latency is greater than 3.5 msec.**
  - **Pediatric CTS** commonly presents with **thenar atrophy** and is **often bilateral**—it is treated with the same algorithm as adult CTS.
  - Lumbrical musculature can occasionally violate the carpal tunnel, increasing the resting pressure.
- **Treatment**
  - **Nonsurgical**
    - ▶ Approximately 20% of patients are symptom free 1 year after steroid injection.
    - ▶ Patients with minimal symptoms have the most robust response.
  - **Surgical**
    - ▶ Neurolysis/epineurotomy *not* indicated in open release
    - ▶ Symptomatic improvement of sensation within 2 weeks
    - ▶ Nerve conduction improves by 3 months
    - ▶ Strength improves by 6 months
    - ▶ Reexploration indicated if postoperative symptoms persist
    - ▶ **Sensitive palmar scar** most common complication (62%)
    - ▶ **Open carpal tunnel release**
      - ✦ **Advantages**
        - Critical structures/anatomic variance made directly visible
        - Complete transverse carpal ligament release
        - Concomitant Guyon's canal decompression
      - ✦ **Disadvantages**
        - Bowstringing of tendons
        - Enlarged scar
        - Longer time to return to work
        - Traction neuritis

TIP: 93% of patients improve after nerve dissection and decompression.

- ▶ **Endoscopic carpal tunnel release**
  - ✦ **Advantages**
    - Decreased time to return to work
    - Smaller scar
  - ✦ **Disadvantages**
    - Higher rates of neuropraxia
    - Higher incidence of recurrent CTS, most often caused by incomplete transverse carpal ligament release; also adhesions and flexor tendon synovitis
    - Inability to view anatomic variants
      - Median recurrent motor nerve branches 50%-90% of the time beyond the transverse carpal ligament, 30% below the ligament, and approximately 23% through the ligament[2] (Fig. 66-4)

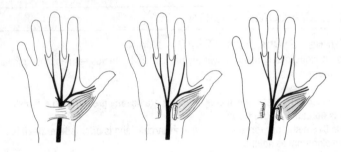

Fig. 66-4   Normal variation of the recurrent motor branch of the median nerve. (From Lanz U. Anatomical variations of the median nerve in the carpal tunnel. J Hand Surg 2:44, 1977.)

PRONATOR SYNDROME[12]

Forearm pain, paresthesia, and hypoesthesia occur over pronator teres distal to thumb and index finger. There is often no median nerve distribution weakness.

- ■ **Causes**
  - • **Median nerve adherence/compression at:**
    - ▶ Lacertus fibrosus
    - ▶ Pronator teres
    - ▶ Flexor digitorum superficialis
  - • Anomalies or vascular branches in the distal forearm
  - • Entrapment beneath Struthers' ligament at the distal humerus
- ■ **Diagnosis**
  - • **Tingling**
    - ▶ Tapping over the pronator teres
    - ▶ Elbow flexion
    - ▶ Forearm pronation
    - ▶ Active resistance to finger flexion
  - • Neuromuscular studies of limited benefit for diagnosis
- ■ **Treatment**
  - • Surgical release indicated with excellent results
  - • Release of Struthers' ligament, bicipital aponeurosis, and tendinous arch of the flexor digitorum superficialis

ANTERIOR INTEROSSEOUS SYNDROME[1,3,13]

Loss of function of the flexor pollicis longus, flexor digitorum profundus, and pronator quadratus

- **Sensation unaffected**
- **Causes**
  - Entrapment of median nerve in pronator teres muscle
- **Diagnosis**
  - Characteristic finding during examination is index finger extension at distal joint and increased flexion at proximal joint, generating a **pinch deformity**
  - Neuromuscular studies useful in diagnosis
- **Treatment**
  - Anterior approach to the median nerve at the antecubital fossa with neurolysis using intraoperative magnification is highly effective in treatment

RADIAL NERVE COMPRESSION

RADIAL TUNNEL SYNDROME (POSTERIOR INTEROSSEOUS NERVE)

Pain during movement at the elbow (tennis elbow) radiating distally to the dorsal hand accompanied with tingling of the hand and weakness of grip[3,7]

- **Causes**
  - Repetitive elbow extension/rotation (weakness is a result of pain)
- **Diagnosis**
  - Radial nerve block is diagnostic and prognostic for surgical repair
  - **Middle finger test:** Pain over ECRB during forceful extension of the middle finger and elbow
  - Electrodiagnostic studies not indicated
- **Treatment**
  - Radial nerve release using the brachioradialis approach
  - Results only marginally beneficial

TIP: Nonoperative management of radial tunnel syndrome always should be pursued initially with NSAIDs, resting splints, and avoidance of inciting activity.

POSTERIOR INTEROSSEOUS NERVE SYNDROME

Weakness and pain during finger/wrist extension without sensory involvement

- **Causes**
  - Trauma
  - Acute bleeding from arteriovenous malformation
  - Rheumatoid arthritis inflammation at the elbow or radial head involvement
  - Soft tissue growing mass (e.g., lipoma)
  - Traction neuropraxia
- **Diagnosis**
  - Elbow plain films to assure no radial head displacement
  - Electrodiagnostic testing
  - Ultrasound evaluation of soft tissue masses
  - MRI: Operative planning if PIN etiologic factors involve soft tissue masses

- **Index finger extension failure with paresthesias (a classic physical finding)**
  - ▸ Tendinous compression of the nerve at the arcade of Frohse results in hand paresthesias at the wrist and loss of distal hand extension
- ■ **Treatment**
  - • **Nonoperative treatment**
    - ▸ Considered with new, sudden onset of symptoms
    - ▸ Up to 3-month trial resting splint
    - ▸ Steroid injections for patients with rheumatoid arthritis (RA)
  - • **Operative treatment**
    - ▸ **Anatomic sites**
      - ◆ Radiocapitellar joint fascia
      - ◆ Leash of Henry (radial recurrent vessel bundle)
      - ◆ ECRB lateral edge
      - ◆ Arcade of Frohse (supinator edge)
    - ▸ Anterior approach to expose the radial tunnel inlet
    - ▸ Posterior approach to the arcade of Frohse

ULNAR NERVE COMPRESSION

CUBITAL TUNNEL SYNDROME[3]
Ulnar-side forearm tingling and pain extending to the ring and small fingers that may involve weakness and atrophy
- ■ **Causes**
  - • Aponeurotic compression
  - • Tumor
  - • Trauma
  - • Anatomic variation
- ■ **Diagnosis**
  - • Provocative testing includes percussion over the cubital tunnel.
  - • Neuromuscular conductivity testing is of limited use for diagnosis.
  - • Plain films of elbow determine whether subluxation is present.
- ■ **Treatment**
  - • Posterior approach: Decompression of the cubital tunnel, avoiding damage to the medial cutaneous nerves of the arm
  - • Persistent ulnar neuropathy after decompression
  - • Submuscular ulnar nerve transposition indicated[14,15]

ULNAR TUNNEL SYNDROME (GUYON'S CANAL)[1,3]
Wrist pain with numbness, tingling, and burning in the small and ring fingers
- ■ **Three zones** (Fig. 66-5)

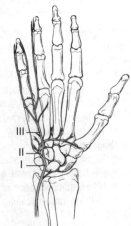

Fig. 66-5 Zones of ulnar nerve compression within Guyon's canal.

Zone 1 is proximal to the ulnar nerve bifurcation.
Zone 2 surrounds the ulnar nerve deep motor branch as it passes the hamate hook.
Zone 3 surrounds the superficial sensory ulnar nerve sensory branch.
- **Causes**
  - Carpal ganglion cyst
  - Occupational trauma
  - Vascular thrombosis/aneurysm
  - Synovial inflammation
- **Diagnosis**
  - Symptoms correlate with location of compression
    - ▸ Proximally, motor and sensory deficits occur (zone 1).
    - ▸ Distal to the canal, motor deficits frequently occur (zone 2).
    - ▸ Rarely isolated sensory deficits occur, which are distal (zone 3).
  - Semmes-Weinstein monofilament test
  - Two-point discrimination
  - Bedside intrinsic muscle motor testing
  - Plain films of the wrist and hand
  - CT scan of the wrist and hand if fracture suspected
  - Electrodiagnostic examination to help determine zone of injury
- **Treatment**
  - **Nonoperative**
    - ▸ NSAID medical therapy
    - ▸ Resting splint immobilization
    - ▸ Reduction of repetitive hand motion
  - **Operative**
    - ▸ Indicated with identifiable lesions
    - ▸ Release of the nerve requires both release of Guyon's canal and fascial arcade at the deep distal hiatus[16]
    - ▸ Complete release of the nerve from Guyon's canal

TIP: Pursue immediate ulnar nerve decompression after any wrist fracture with ulnar neuropathy or after ulnar neuropathy that persists longer than 24 hours.

TRACTION NEURITIS

Development of chronic pain following open carpal ligament release or transposition of the ulnar nerve
- **Causes**
  - Neuroma
  - Devascularization of nerve
  - Incomplete release during decompression or transposition
  - Adhesive median neuritis
- **Diagnosis**
  - Pain worsens during increased pressure over the site[17]
  - Often postoperative

■ **Treatment**
- Reexploration with external and internal neurolysis
- Cubital tunnel decompression, treating persistent pain with submuscular transposition or medial epicondylectomy
- Small percentage of patients do not improve after reexploration
- Usually secondary to scar formation; may progressively worsen
- End-stage traction neuritis
  ▶ External and internal neurolysis, epineurectomy, wrapped with local or free flap coverage

---

KEY POINTS

✔ History of the work environment is critical to compression neuropathy treatment.

✔ Operative intervention in carpal tunnel syndrome is indicated with **median nerve sensory latencies greater than 3.5 msec** and **median nerve motor latencies greater than 4.5 msec.**

✔ Nonoperative treatment of carpal tunnel syndrome has an **80%** rate of recurrent symptoms.

✔ Carpal tunnel syndrome release procedures must avoid injury to the median recurrent nerve.

✔ Testing the sensory distribution of the thenar eminence determines median nerve compression proximal or distal to the carpal tunnel.

✔ Inability to extend index finger with paresthesia is indicative of PIN syndrome.

✔ Ulnar nerve transposition is required if symptoms persist after cubital tunnel release.

✔ Traction neuritis mandates operative reexploration.

REFERENCES

1. Eversmann WW Jr. Entrapment and compression neuropathies. In Green DP, Hotchkiss RN, Pederson WC, eds. Green's Operative Hand Surgery, 4th ed. Philadelphia: Churchill Livingstone, 1998, pp 1404-1443.
2. Lanz U. Anatomical variations of the median nerve in the carpal tunnel. J Hand Surg 2:44, 1977.
3. Eversmann WW Jr. Compression and entrapment neuropathies of the upper extremity. J Hand Surg 8:759, 1983.
4. Rempel D, Dahlin L, Lundborg G. Pathophysiology of nerve compression syndromes: Response of peripheral nerves to loading. J Bone Joint Surg Am 81:1600, 1999.
5. Spinner M, Spencer PS. Nerve compression lesions of the upper extremity: A clinical and experimental review. Clin Orthop 104:46, 1974.
6. Dellon AL. Patient evaluation and management considerations in nerve compression. Hand Clin 8:229, 1992.
7. Stromberg T, Dahlin LB, Lundborg G. Vibrotactile sense in the hand-arm vibration syndrome. Scand J Work Environ Health 24:495, 1998.
8. Mackinnon SE, McCabe S, Murray JF, et al. Internal neurolysis fails to improve the results of primary carpal tunnel decompression. J Hand Surg Am 16:211, 1991.
9. Singh I, Khoo KMA, Krishnamoorthy S. The carpal tunnel syndrome: Clinical evaluation and results of surgical decompression. Ann Acad Med Singapore 23:94, 1994.
10. Shurr DG, Blair WF, Bassett G. Electromyographic changes after carpal tunnel release. J Hand Surg Am 11:876, 1986.
11. Botte MJ, von Schroeder HP, Abrams RA, et al. Recurrent carpal tunnel syndrome. Hand Clin 12:731, 1996.

12. Olehnik WK, Manske PR, Szerzinski J. Median nerve compression in the proximal forearm. J Hand Surg Am 19:121, 1994.
13. Hill NA, Howard FM, Huffer B. The incomplete anterior interosseous nerve syndrome. J Hand Surg Am 10:4, 1985.
14. Learmonth JR. A technique for transplanting the ulnar nerve. Surg Gynecol Obstet 75:792, 1942.
15. Amadio PC, Beckenbaugh RD. Entrapment of the ulnar nerve by the deep flexor-pronator aponeurosis. J Hand Surg Am 11:83, 1986.
16. Konig PS, Hage JJ, Bloem JJ, et al. Variations of the ulnar nerve and ulnar artery in Guyon's canal: A cadaveric study. J Hand Surg Am 19:617, 1994.
17. Jones NF, Shaw WW, Katz RG. Circumferential wrapping of a flap around a scarred peripheral nerve for salvage of end-stage traction neuritis. J Hand Surg Am 22:527, 1997.

67. Brachial Plexus

Ashkan Ghavami

ANATOMY (Fig. 67-1)

- **Roots:** Between anterior and middle scalene muscles to C5-T1
- **Trunks:** In posterior cervical triangle; upper, middle, and lower
- **Divisions:** Under clavicle and pectoralis minor; anterior and posterior
- **Cords:** Named for position **relative to axillary artery;** lateral, posterior, and median
- **Peripheral nerves:** From *terminal cord branches*
- Classified into **supraclavicular** or **infraclavicular** to assist in treatment planning
  - **Supraclavicular**
    - ▶ **Prognostic implications:** Carries poorer prognosis than infraclavicular
    - ▶ **Incidence:** 75% of patients[1]
    - ▶ Involves cervical roots, trunks, and divisions

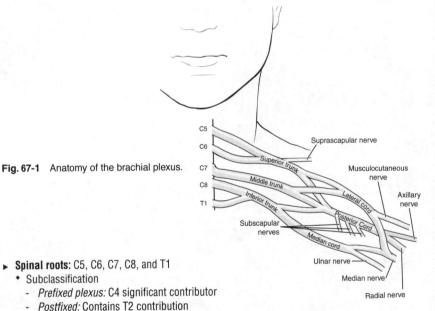

Fig. 67-1 Anatomy of the brachial plexus.

- ▶ **Spinal roots:** C5, C6, C7, C8, and T1
  - ✦ Subclassification
    - Prefixed plexus: C4 significant contributor
    - Postfixed: Contains T2 contribution
- **Infraclavicular**
  - ▶ Shoulder dislocations: Fractures often present
  - ▶ **Three cords** can be affected
    - ✦ *Lateral:* C5-C7 roots through anterior divisions of upper and middle trunks
    - ✦ *Medial:* C8 and T1 through anterior division of lateral trunk
    - ✦ *Posterior:* All roots contribute

ROOT AVULSIONS (PREGANGLIONIC OR SUPRAGANGLIONIC)

- Occur **proximal** to intraforaminal dorsal root ganglion (DRG)
- **No Wallerian degeneration** because axons continuous with DRG cell bodies
- Sensory action potentials present
- **Cannot be repaired with primary repair or nerve grafting** (often requires *neurotization* [nerve transfer])
- Denervation of paracervical muscles
- **Horner's syndrome:** C8 or T1 level injury
  - Ptosis
  - Miosis
  - Enophthalmos
  - Anhidrosis
- **Erb's point:** Convergence of C5 and C6 roots as they form upper trunk
  - Helps localize injury to upper roots
- Evaluate infraspinatus muscle
  - Provides external rotation of humerus
  - If intact, then lesion is at or distal to Erb's point

POSTGANGLIONIC OR INFRAGANGLIONIC

- Injury **distal** to DRG
- Paracervical muscles intact
- Rami communicans to sympathetic ganglion intact
- **Wallerian degeneration** in peripheral nerve fibers
- No action potentials recordable
- **Surgical repair with nerve grafts or primary repair possible** because proximal root intact and present, unlike preganglionic lesion

EPIDEMIOLOGY

OBSTETRIC INJURY[2]

- **Incidence:** 1.5 per 1000 term births
- **Risk factors**
  - Shoulder dystocia
  - Gestational diabetes
  - Forceps delivery
  - Vacuum extraction
  - Breech delivery
  - Macrosomia
  - Multiparity
- **Clinical presentation**[2]
  - Most patients (73%) present with upper root cervical injury **(Erb-Duchenne palsy)**
    - ▸ 4%-5% are bilateral
  - Usually mild traction injuries from large infant with shoulder dystocia or small infants presenting breech
  - **Indications for surgical exploration**
    - ▸ Absent biceps or deltoid function by 3 months *elsewhere Say 6 months*

- ▶ Absent elbow flexion and extension, wrist extension, or thumb/finger extension at 9 months of age
- ▶ Most explored before 9 months, but spontaneous recovery common

NONOBSTETRIC INJURY

- **Much more common** than obstetric injuries
- Mostly young male patients (up to 90% of cases), often from motor vehicle crashes (MVCs) or motorcycle crashes (MCCs)
- Frequently requires surgical intervention
  - Best results less than 6 months postinsult, no benefit after 2 years

NOTE: Many surgeons do not attempt reconstruction more than 1 year after injury because of irreversible muscle changes and neuronal cell body changes.

MECHANISM OF INJURY

TRACTION

- Downward direction (e.g., MCCs, skiing) from **forceful neck flexion** to contralateral side causes upper root or trunk injury.
- Upward (cephalad) direction with shoulder abduction greater than 90 degrees causes damage in lower plexus.
- Iatrogenic from surgical retraction or positioning causes extreme shoulder abduction, which is **most common.**

CRUSH

- In costoclavicular region between first rib and clavicle
- Often from direct trauma (MVCs), occupational injury (heavy object falling on shoulder), or football injury

COMPRESSION

- Adjacent tissues (bony fragments)
- Hematoma or pseudoaneurysm
- Cervical rib(s)
- Fibrous bands
- Prominent transverse process(es)
- Iatrogenic from positioning

DIRECT LACERATION

- Gunshot wounds (GSWs)
- Knife wounds

TIP: For GSWs, treat vascular injury acutely, tag nerve(s) for definitive exploration, and repair in 3 months.

INJURY PATTERN

OPEN

- Less common than closed traction-type injury patterns
- Concomitant vascular injury can increase injury severity
- Sharp injury
  - **Primary repair:** Along with repair of vascular or limb-threatening injury
  - **Delayed repair:** When zone of injury may be unclear
    - Explore and tag nerves out to length and reexplore in approximately 3-4 weeks with better wound conditions and when patient stable

---

TIP: In blast, crush, or stretch injuries, allow injury to mature for several weeks. This may help to identify scarred lesions later.

- **GSWs**
  - Rule out vascular injury
  - Often **mixed injury pattern** with neurapraxic component (Mackinnon sixth degree stage)
  - Observe for approximately 3 months
  - Explore by 3 months if no neural recovery seen

CLOSED TRACTION

- More common than open injury
- Young male patients (approximately 90%-95% of cases)
- **High-velocity** causes
  - MVCs
  - MCCs more than 80% of cases, with greater traction forces
  - Root avulsions more common
  - Reevaluate with examination and electrodiagnostics after 3 months observation
  - If evidence of recovery, then periodic reevaluation every 6-12 weeks
- **Low-velocity** causes
  - Sports injuries, bicycling, skiing, or falling from a height
  - Require same reevaluation and electrodiagnostic protocol as high-velocity injuries if no evidence of recovery

PATIENT EVALUATION

PRINCIPLES

- **Time interval from injury most important determinant of outcome**
  - Exact time threshold for evaluation and treatment is debatable, but less than 6 months is optimal, and no later than 12-18 months.
    - Less chance of end-organ denervation, muscle atrophy, and cell loss if treated in less than 6 months from initial injury.
- **Age vital to functional outcome**
  - **20 years old or younger:** Significantly better outcomes than older patients (see Chapter 68)
  - Older than 40 years: Prognosis worsens

- **Details of initial injury:** Help direct examination and diagnosis of injury pattern
  - **MVC**
    - ▶ Speed
    - ▶ Seat belt
    - ▶ Helmet
    - ▶ Airbag
    - ▶ Distance thrown
  - **Occupational**
    - ▶ Type of machine
    - ▶ Force and direction of pull
    - ▶ Falling object (i.e., weight of impact, location of impact, and head and neck position at time of impact)
    - ▶ Height of fall

PHYSICAL EXAMINATION

- **Motor**
  - Examine all muscle groups in upper extremity and shoulder
  - Document
    - ▶ Muscle grades
    - ▶ Atrophy
    - ▶ Joint mobility
    - ▶ Passive or active function
  - **Compare with contralateral side**
  - **Muscle/innervation**
    - ▶ Serratus muscle/long thoracic nerve (C5-C7 roots)
    - ▶ Supraspinatus and infraspinatus muscles/suprascapular nerve (C5-C6 roots)
    - ▶ Pectoralis major muscle/lateral and medial pectoral nerves (medial and lateral cords)
    - ▶ Latissimus by thoracodorsal nerve (posterior cord)
- **Vascular**
  - Peripheral pulses, including Allen's test and Doppler testing

---

TIP: Vascular injury can suggest severe nerve injury.

- **Sensory**
  - Touch, pain, two-point discrimination, and vibratory tests
  - **Tinel's sign:** Positive if paresthesias produced from percussion over most distal point of viable nerve fibers
    - ▶ Suggests most distal point of nerve regeneration
    - ▶ *Does not provide status of motor component*
    - ▶ Absence in supraclavicular region suggests total plexus avulsion with grave prognosis[3]

TIP: Estimate level of injury by conducting a detailed motor examination and by charting motor and sensory deficit patterns.

ELECTRODIAGNOSTIC TESTS

- **Electromyography (EMG)**
  - Delay 3-6 weeks to view fibrillations that have developed from denervated muscles
  - **Serial EMGs** for presence of reinnervation
    - ▸ Decreased fibrillations
    - ▸ Increased voluntary motor unit potentials (MUP)
    - ▸ Positive polyphasic low-amplitude potentials: Not indicative of injury level
- **Nerve conduction velocity**
  - Combined presence of sensory nerve action potential (SNAP), normal sensory conduction velocity in peripheral nerve, and paralyzed muscle
    - ▸ Indicates root avulsion with preservation of DRG
    - ▸ Not exact because absence of SNAP and sensory conduction could be present with double lesion (nerve rupture and root avulsion)[3,4]

TIP: In general, it is best to explore when the presence of root avulsion is suggested by denervation of posterior cervical muscles with paracervical fibrillations, intact sensory conduction velocities, and anaesthetic sensory dermatome.

IMAGING

- **Plain radiographs:** Indicated in acute setting
  - Cervical spine
  - Shoulder
  - Clavicle
  - Chest
  - Possible correlations
    - ▸ **Transverse process of cervical spine fracture:** *Root lesion*
    - ▸ **Hemidiaphragm elevation:** *Preganglionic, phrenic nerve* involved (phrenic and ipsilateral intercostal nerves as donor nerves contraindicated)
    - ▸ **Rib fractures:** *Intercostal nerves not usable as donors*
    - ▸ **Scapula and clavicle fractures:** *Compression, high-energy injury,* and *supraclavicular injury*
- **Cervical myelogram**[3]
  - Helps diagnose **pseudomeningoceles** and **root deviations,** which suggest presence of root avulsions
  - Excellent for C8 and T1 roots
    - ▸ False positive or negative in 9%
  - Perform at least 1 month after injury to allow pseudomeningocele formation
- **CT/myelography**
  - Excellent sensitivity (95%) and specificity (98%)[5]
- **MRI**
  - Noninvasive
  - No need to wait 4 weeks
  - Equivalent to CT/myelogram for root avulsions; less efficacious for lower root injury
- **Angiography**
  - Indicated in acute setting if vascular injury suspected
  - Can acutely explore open injuries without angiogram

PREOPERATIVE MANAGEMENT[4,6,7]

PHYSICAL THERAPY
- Maintain passive joint motion and appropriate splinting both preoperatively and postoperatively
- Motor reeducation and strengthening exercises if nerve transfers undertaken
- Electrical stimulation of nonfunctioning muscles used by some

PAIN MANAGEMENT
- Severe with total plexus avulsion
- Trial of gabapentin (Neurontin®) and referral to pain specialist for multipharmaceutical therapy
- Neurosurgical referral last resort for *intraspinal dorsal root coagulation*

TREATMENT PRINCIPLES

GENERAL PRINCIPLES
- Initially managed conservatively unless exact injury level known
- Lower trunk (C8 and T1) not reconstructed
- Evaluate whether nerve in continuity (indication for neurolysis) or nonviable/discontinuous (excision and nerve grafting) in other trunks

GOALS OF RECONSTRUCTION
- **Reconstitute elbow flexion:** First priority is to allow hand-to-mouth function.
- **Stabilize shoulder** to prevent subluxation and to support power across elbow.
- **Perform later reconstruction of wrist extension and finger flexion** through muscle/tendon unit transfers.
- **Reestablish sensation** through neurotization of median and ulnar nerves.

ACUTE BRACHIAL PLEXUS RECONSTRUCTION OR REPAIR DURING EXPLORATION[6]
- Allows primary nerve repair or use of shorter grafts because less nerve retraction
  - More scarring present during secondary operations
- If arm ischemia or vascular compromise with open injury:
  - Explore plexus at time of repair.
  - Define injury level.
  - Decompress lesions (e.g., evacuation of hematoma and bony reduction)

DELAYED REPAIR
- 4-6 weeks
- Lesion more accurately identified because of Wallerian degeneration and neuroma formation
- Noncontaminated wound
- Allows time for skeletal stability

NERVE GRAFTS AND TRANSFERS

NERVE GRAFTS

- Identify neuromas and lesions
- Resect all injured nerve to healthy fascicles
- Reconstruct with nerve graft
- Donors
  - Sural nerve (most common)
  - Medial antebrachial cutaneous (MABC)

TIP: Perform *intraoperative nerve stimulation* for nerve action potential (NAP) to determine whether large-diameter motor axons are continuous.

NERVE TRANSFERS

- **Indications**
  - Nonreconstructible injury (e.g., preganglionic root avulsions)
  - Very proximal postganglionic injury
- **Motor nerve transfers**
  - Same principles as tendon transfers
  - Preferably synergistic donor or recipient muscles
  - Maximal motor axon numbers
  - Donor nerves in close proximity to end-organ target
- **Sensory nerve transfers**
  - Hand sensation in critical areas (e.g., thumb and index fingers)
  - Timing not as important as for motor end targets

SPECIFIC PROCEDURES

ELBOW FLEXION

- *First priority*
- Reinnervation of **biceps** and **brachialis** muscles
- **Donors**[7]
  - **Oberlin transfer**
    - ▸ Redundant FCU fascicles of ulnar nerve used as donor for biceps reinnervation
  - **Intraplexus donors**
    - ▸ Medial pectoral branches and thoracodorsal nerve donors to musculocutaneous nerve recipient
  - **Extraplexal donor**
    - ▸ Distal spinal accessory nerve (after trapezial branch take-off, needs graft)
    - ▸ Phrenic nerve (contraindicated by respiratory compromise)
    - ▸ Intercostal nerves (third through fifth) require negative history of rib fracture, chest tube, and thoracotomy
    - ▸ Contralateral C7 root with or without vascularized ulnar nerve graft[3,4]

SHOULDER ABDUCTION

- Transfer to **suprascapular** and **axillary** nerves (infraspinatus/supraspinatus and deltoid, respectively)
- **Donors**
  - Distal spinal accessory nerve to suprascapular nerve (very synergistic)
  - Medial pectoral nerve to axillary nerve

TIP: When injury is severe and there is scarce donor availability, do not hesitate to perform shoulder fusion.

HAND SENSATION[7]

- **Donor nerves for transfer**
  - Intercostobrachial nerve
  - Intercostal sensory nerve
  - Supraclavicular nerve branches
- **Recipient nerves**
  - Ulnar nerve in upper arm
  - Lateral cord contribution to median nerve for thumb and radial digits
  - Transfer of fourth web space sensory nerve to first web space[7]

PALLIATIVE PROCEDURES/ADJUNCTIVE PROCEDURES

TIP: Consider palliative and adjunctive procedures if injury is older than 6-12 months and no recovery is seen.

TENDON TRANSFER

- Commonly indicated for **older patients** (>40 years)
- **Restoration of elbow flexion most common indication**
- **Operations**
  - Steindler flexorplasty using flexor pronator muscle
  - Pectoralis major
  - Latissimus dorsi
  - Triceps
- Restoration of hand intrinsic function and thumb opposition regardless of time from injury

FUNCTIONAL FREE-MUSCLE TRANSFER

- Usually indicated for elbow flexion
- Tendon transfers often preferred unless total plexus avulsion present requiring extraplexus neurotization (nerve transfers)[8]
- **Donor muscles:** Gracilis, rectus, or contralateral latissimus dorsi

ARTHRODESIS

- Shoulder fusion
- Small joint arthrodesis and tendon transfers to improve hand prehensile function, wrist fusion, and thumb fusion

POSTOPERATIVE CARE

- Limited immobilization to keep joint stiffness and scars or adhesions to a minimum
- Prefabricated splint for immobilization based on specific surgery
  - Timing varies from 10 to 14 days (nerve grafts equal less tension)
  - 14-21 days with direct nerve repair
  - Protective splinting for 6-8 weeks, then sling used for 1 more month
- Progressive therapy program based on surgery to increase passive range of motion (PROM) followed by increasing active range of motion (AROM) protocols

OUTCOMES

- Better results seen with more distal lesions (closer to target muscle)
- Motor nerve transfers commonly superior to nerve grafts, especially proximal lesions, with muscle grades ranging from 4 to 4+/5 on the Medical Research Council (MRC) scale for biceps flexion[9]
- Better outcome for postganglionic lesions over avulsion injuries[3,4,10] (outcomes for injuries involving upper roots even better[1,3,7,10])
- Higher postoperative muscle strength in younger patients (<20 years)
- 78% of patients compared with 90% of general population content with quality of life after reconstruction, although a negative impact was felt by some patients in the workplace[7]
- Job satisfaction rated as moderate to high with 75% of this group

TIP: Good functional recovery can result from a motivated patient; an expert surgical team that performs properly indicated, timely, and well-executed procedures; and implementation of appropriate postoperative rehabilitation.

KEY POINTS

- Most causes of brachial plexus are nonobstetric, closed injuries from MVCs or MCCs in young adult males.
- Nerve injury principles apply; therefore timely diagnosis of injury level and early intervention are required for optimal results.
- An initial observation period of 3 months for closed injuries is acceptable. If positive recovery is observed, then continue periodic reevaluation with physical examination and electrodiagnostic testing.
- Patients must be carefully selected (i.e., highly motivated, compliant, and cognitively aware of lengthy rehabilitation protocol and limitations of functional outcomes).
- Primary functional goal should be elbow flexion, followed by shoulder abduction.
- Tendon transfers, functional free-tissue transfers, and small and large joint arthrodesis (shoulder and wrist) play significant roles in treatment when functional recovery is poor.

REFERENCES

1. Alnot J. Traumatic brachial plexus lesions in the adult: Indications and results. Hand Clin 11:623-631, 1995.
2. Brunelli GA, Brunelli GR. Preoperative assessment of the adult plexus patient. Microsurgery 16:17-21, 1995.
3. Chuang DC. Neurotization procedures for brachial plexus injuries. Hand Clin 11:633-645, 1995.
4. Merrell GA, Barrie KA, Katz DL, et al. Results of nerve transfer techniques for restoration of shoulder and elbow function in the context of a meta-analysis of the English literature. J Hand Surg Am 26:303-314, 2001.
5. Roger B, Travers V, Laval-Jeantet M. Imaging of posttraumatic brachial plexus injury. Clin Orthop 237:57-61, 1988.
6. Shenaq SM, Kim JYS, Armenta AH, et al. The surgical treatment of obstetric brachial plexus palsy. Plast Reconstr Surg 113:54E-67E, 2004.
7. Terzis JK, Vekris MD, Soucacos PN. Brachial plexus. In Achauer BH, Eriksson E, Guyuron B, et al, eds. Plastic Surgery: Indications, Operations, and Outcomes, vol 4. St Louis: Mosby, 2000, pp 2075-2101.
8. Terzis JK, Papakonstantinou KC. The surgical treatment of brachial plexus injuries in adults. Plast Reconstr Surg 106:1097-1122, 2000.
9. Tomaino MM. Nonobstetrical brachial plexus injuries. J Am Soc Surg Hand 1:135-153, 2001.
10. Tung TH, Mackinnon SE. Brachial plexus injuries. Clin Plast Surg 30:269-287, 2003.

68. Nerve Injuries

Ashkan Ghavami

ANATOMY AND PHYSIOLOGY (Fig. 68-1)

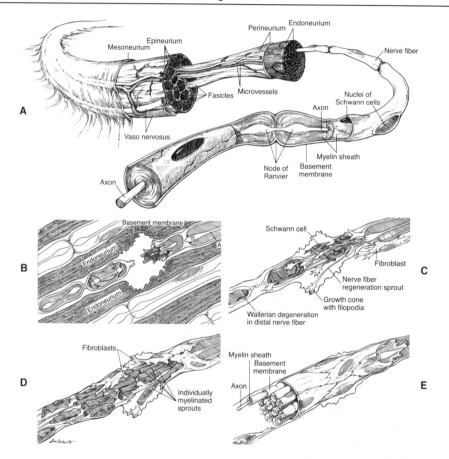

Fig. 68-1 Nerve anatomy and regeneration. **A,** The normal nerve consists of myelinated and unmyelinated axons. **B,** When a myelinated axon is injured, degeneration occurs distally and for a variable distance proximally. **C,** Multiple regenerating fibers sprout from the proximal axon forming a regenerating unit. A growth cone at the tip of each regenerating fiber samples the environment and advances the growth process distally. **D,** Schwann cells eventually myelinate the regenerating fibers. **E,** Because it is from a single nerve fiber, a regenerating unit that contains several fibers is formed, and each fiber is capable of functional connections. (From Brandt KE, Mackinnon SE. Microsurgical repair of peripheral nerves and nerve grafts. In Aston JS, Beasley RW, Throne CM, eds. Grabb and Smith's Plastic Surgery, 5th ed. New York: Lippincott-Raven, 1997.)

AXONS
- Peripheral nerve axons are surrounded by **endoneurium;** loose gelatinous collagen matrix, minimal tensile strength

SCHWANN CELL
- Surrounds individual **myelinated** axons (produces myelin), or surrounds several unmyelinated axons

NODE OF RANVIER
Gap at junction between Schwann cells
- Allows **rapid nerve conduction** as action potential depolarization jumps from one node of Ranvier to the next (3 to 150 m/sec versus 2 to 2.5 m/sec for unmyelinated axons)

FASCICLES
Grouped arrangement of axons with surrounding endoneurium
- Invested by internal (inner) epineurium
- Interconnect and branch proximally[1]
  - Makes matching fascicles more difficult proximally but fibers can be adjacent in a fascicular group

PERINEURIUM
Connective tissue encircling each fascicle
- Selective permeability
- Encircled by internal (inner) epineurium
  - Sutured in *fascicular repair*

OUTER EPINEURIUM
Outer sheath of peripheral nerve
- Sutured in *epineurial repair*
- Contains collagen and elastin fibers
- Surrounded by loose areolar tissue (mesoneurium)

MESONEURIUM
Outer adventitial layer of nerve
- Incorporated in epineurial repair
- Critical for nerve excursion and gliding

BLOOD SUPPLY
- **Arteriae nervosum (vaso nervosus)**
  - Enter nerve segmentally
  - Divide into longitudinal superficial branches in epineurium
  - Help guide proper orientation of nerve ends during repair
- **Extrinsic vessels** supply intrinsic longitudinal vessels in epineurium, which communicate with capillary plexus in perineurium
- **Capillary plexus**
  - Enters the endoneurium obliquely
  - Becomes occluded if endoneurial pressure rises because of injury (crush, edema)

MARTIN-GRUBER ANASTOMOSIS

- **Motor connections between ulnar and median nerves in forearm,** or distally between anterior interosseous nerve and ulnar branches
- Can be present in up to **17%** of the population
- **May mask the actual site of nerve injury** (e.g., a median nerve injury at elbow level with loss of all intrinsic muscle function, even though ulnar nerve intact)

RICHE-CANNIEU ANASTOMOSIS

- **Motor connections between median and ulnar nerves in *palm***
- Present in up to **70%** of the population
- **Also can mask injury pattern**

PATHOPHYSIOLOGY[2]

WALLERIAN DEGENERATION

- Nerve stump undergoes degeneration **distal** to axonotomy.
- Schwann cells proliferate and myelin breaks down.
- Schwann cells and macrophages replace neural tube and organize into **"bands of Bunger,"** providing a scaffold for regenerating axons.

CHROMATOLYSIS

- Mechanism of **proximal** neuronal cell body damage
- Axonal degeneration of axons in proximal stump
- **Growth cone** formed by individual axons creating numerous axonal sprouts (5-24 hours after injury)

GROWTH CONE

- Filopodia in cone explore neural tube and find correct distal stump by contact guidance and neurotropic factors.
- If incorrect distal stump and target organ are reached, sprouts are denied factors necessary for maturation.
- Approximately **50%** of axonal sprouts make incorrect connections.

NEUROTROPISM

- Chemotactic gradient toward proper distal stump that attracts regenerating axon toward correct end target

NEUROTROPHISM

- Trophic (nutritional) support provided to axons connecting with correct distal stump: Nerve growth factor (NGF), epidermal growth factor (EGF), insulin-like growth factor (IGF) I and II, etc.

MUSCLE DENERVATION

- Results in atrophy and interstitial fibrosis that is complete by 2-3 years after injury
- **Best reinnervation within 3 months of injury**
- Functional reinnervation possible up to **1 year after injury**
- **No reinnervation possible 2-3 years after injury**
- Outcome worse with **advanced age** (>40 years old) and **disuse**

SENSORY END ORGANS
- Best results seen in patients **less than 20 years old,** as with all nerve injuries
- **Mechanism**
  - Native nerve regeneration not required
  - Axonal collateral sprouting from adjacent axons present, allowing increased chance of successful reinnervation
- Delayed repairs (after more than 1 year): Only protective sensation achieved
- **Sunderland and Seddon classifications** (Table 68-1)

Table 68-1 *Two Classification Systems of Nerve Injuries*

Seddon	Sunderland	Disrupted Structure	Prognosis
Neuropraxia	1st degree	Axon (minimal)	Complete return in days or months
Axonotmesis	2nd degree	Axon (total, Wallerian degeneration)	Complete return in months
Neurotmesis	3rd degree	Axon, endoneurium	Mild/moderate reduction in function
Neurotmesis	4th degree	Axon, endoneurium, perineurium	Moderate reduction in function
Neurotmesis	5th degree	All structures	Marked reduction in functional return

From Gutowski KA. Hand II: Peripheral nerves and tendon transfers. Sel Read Plast Surg 9(33):1-19, 2003.

DIAGNOSIS

Diagnosing nerve injuries requires taking a complete history of the injury, performing accurate testing, and recording sensory and motor deficits.

TINEL'S SIGN
- Tapping over distal area of injury produces paresthesias.
- Axonal regeneration is suggested.

TWO-POINT DISCRIMINATION (2PD)
- **Static 2PD:** Up to 6 mm is normal for volar fingertip.
- **Moving 2PD:** 2-3 mm is normal when testing perpendicular to digit, moving longitudinally (proximal to distal).
- Must stay on ulnar and radial sides *without crossing over,* otherwise false results may occur from contralateral side of digit.

VIBRATION THRESHOLDS
- Very sensitive test

SEMMES-WEINSTEIN MONOFILAMENT
- Measures pressure thresholds
- Expensive and time-consuming, but very sensitive
- Can be performed early

PICK-UP TEST
- Performed during sensation reeducation

DAILY-LIVING TASK PERFORMANCE
- Used in rehabilitation protocols

ELECTRODIAGNOSTIC STUDIES
- Electromyogram (EMG) and/or nerve conduction velocity (NCV)
  - When unable to arrive at accurate diagnosis

SURGICAL PRINCIPLES[3]

OPEN INJURY REPAIR
- **Primary**
  - Within first 24 hours
  - Best for sharp lacerations, clean wounds, minimal to no crush component, no significant soft tissue damage
- **Delayed primary**
  - Within 1 week
  - Initial exploration to reveal previously listed contraindications for primary repair
  - Zone of injury allowed sufficient time to declare itself
- **Secondary**
  - Delay of more than 1 week
  - Unstable skeletal extremity
  - Significant vascular compromise
  - Associated life-threatening injuries

CLOSED OR BLUNT INJURY
- **Unexplored, closed injuries**
  - Waiting period of more than 6 weeks before electrodiagnostics employed
  - Reevaluation at 12 weeks with repeat of tests and expectation of regeneration occurring at approximately 1 mm/day; if recovery still incomplete, tests repeated
- **Operative exploration**
  - Indicated at 3 months when no clinical or electrical signs of reinnervation present (e.g., motor unit potentials)

NERVE REPAIR: TECHNICAL CONSIDERATIONS

PRINCIPLES OF NERVE REPAIR[4]
- Quantitative preoperative and postoperative assessment of sensory and motor function
- Microsurgical technique
- Primary repair when possible
- Tension-free repair
- Interpositional nerve grafts (when necessary)
- Avoidance of excessive postural movement

- Secondary repair if zone of injury indeterminate
- Sensory and motor reeducation

MICROSURGICAL PRINCIPLES

- Adequate magnification is required.
  - An operative microscope is preferred over surgical loupes (loupes ≥ 4× magnification).
  - Use 8-0, 9-0, or 10-0 interrupted monofilament nylon sutures.
- Cut back nerve ends to healthy tissue with a No. 15 or No. 11 blade against a rigid background (sterile tongue-blade works well).
- For soft end-to-end fascicle contact, trim fascicles that protrude outward.
- When motor-sensory topography is unclear:
  - Can use electrical stimulation tests intraoperatively if injury is acute
  - Immunohistochemical staining: Rarely clinically feasible—time-consuming and expensive
- Proximal and distal nerve can be safely mobilized for 1-2 cm (4%-25% of nerve length) to allow increased length and decreased tension on repair.[1,2]
  - Less mobilization is feasible in digits.
- Avoid excessive postural maneuvering to release tension.
  - Do not hesitate to use other options (e.g., grafting, vein graft, conduit) as indicated.

NERVE REPAIR OPTIONS (Fig. 68-2)

PERINEURIAL (FASCICULAR) REPAIR

NOTE: The superiority of perineurial repair over epineurial repair is not established.[1,5] However, it is more appropriate for nerves with fewer than five fascicles and for nerve grafting.

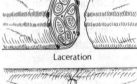

Laceration

- **Advantages**
  - More nerve stump myelination potential
  - Better perineurial tube alignment, more regenerating axons enter distal nerve, greater sensory and motor end-organ recovery[1]

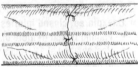

Epineurial Suture

- **Disadvantages**
  - Longer operative times
  - Increased fibrosis at repair
  - Potential vascular compromise
  - Suture crowding
  - Potential for fascicular mismatch

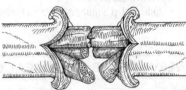

Group Fascicular Suture

Fig. 68-2 Nerve suturing techniques. (From Brushart T. Nerve repair and grafting. In Green DP, Hotchkiss RN, Pederson WC, eds. Green's Operative Hand Surgery, vol 2, 4th ed. Philadelphia: Churchill Livingstone, 1998.)

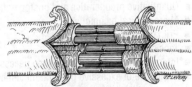

Individual Fascicular Suture

GROUP FASCICULAR REPAIR

- Indicated when nerve transection is at level where well-formed sensory and motor branches are easily identified
- Examples:[1]
  - **Median nerve:** 5 cm above wrist crease to end point in palm and several centimeters below elbow
  - **Ulnar nerve:** 7-8 cm proximal to wrist crease

EPINEURIAL REPAIR

- Best for digital nerves
- Outcomes similar to other types of nerve repair[5]
- Advantages
  - Short operative time
  - Technically simple
  - Less magnification requirements
  - Intraneural tissue not violated; less scarring
  - Good for primary and secondary repairs
- Disadvantages
  - May compromise specific fascicular alignment
  - Tension from retraction of cut nerve ends
  - Multiple sutures may be needed

> TIP: In general, no differences in outcomes have been seen when comparing epineurial repair with other types of repair.

NERVE GAP OPTIONS[6]

OPTIONS WITHOUT GRAFTING[7]

- **Neurotization (of distal end)**
  Direct implantation closer to target muscle by nerve transfer or direct implantation
- **Mobilization**
  - 4%-25% of nerve length safe[7,8]; general rule of 1-2 cm for most nerves
- **Transposition**
  - Ulnar nerve at elbow
- **Bone shortening**
  - Acceptable for digit and humeral shortening with multiple nerve involvement and comminution
  - Can have poor results because of alterations in biomechanics

NERVE GRAFTING

- **Autografts**
  - *Gold standard*
  - **Indication**
    - ▶ When end-to-end coaptation is under tension
  - **Ideal donor nerve**
    - ▶ Produces noncritical sensory deficit
    - ▶ Contains long, unbranched segments

- ► Easily accessible
- ► Overall, small diameter with large fascicles and few interfascicular connections
- • **Common donor nerves**
  - ► **Sural nerve** (30-40 cm)
    - ✦ **Most commonly used purely sensory nerve**
  - ► **Lateral antebrachial cutaneous nerve** (5-8 cm)
    - ✦ Preferred over medial antebrachial branch
  - ► Anterior branch of **medial antebrachial cutaneous nerve** (10-20 cm)
    - ✦ Good for digital nerve gaps longer than 1 cm
    - ✦ Can have hypersensitivity, dysesthesia of donor site
  - ► **Posterior interosseous nerve** (distal segment, terminal filament purely sensory)
    - ✦ Easily accessible on same extremity

VASCULARIZED NERVE GRAFTS[9]

- ■ Best for **extensive recipient bed scarring** and devascularity (e.g., radiation injury)
- ■ Very large donor nerve needed
- • Examples: Nonfunctional ulnar nerve sensory branch in proximal forearm or deep peroneal nerve

AUTOGENOUS INTERPOSITIONAL VEIN GRAFT

- ■ Less 2PD than with direct repair or nerve autograft
- ■ **Common indication:** Small gaps of **less than 3 cm** in nonessential peripheral sensory nerves
  - • Good for zone II injuries
- ■ Can collapse in center, leading to mechanical obstruction of regenerating nerve fibers

MUSCLE GRAFT

- ■ Muscle fascicles used directly as interposition graft
- ■ Not commonly used
- ■ Good results for sensory nerves in acute settings[7]

ALLOGRAFTS

- ■ Require appropriate pretreatment, preservation, and host immunosuppression
- ■ When neural regeneration complete, elements within allograft are entirely of host origin, therefore immunosuppression needed only temporarily

NERVE CONDUITS

- ■ Short distances (<3 cm)
- ■ Noncritical sensory areas
- ■ Patients who decline autogenous harvest[8]
- ■ Preliminary results good

NERVE TRANSFERS

- ■ Noncritical motor or sensory unit used to reconstruct important missing function
- ■ Indications[8,10,11]
  - • Brachial plexus injuries with no proximal nerve for grafting
  - • Proximal nerve injuries requiring long distance for regeneration
  - • Scarred bed in area with critical neurovascular structures

- Major limb trauma with loss of nerve segment
- Older injury and/or older patient
- Common nerve transfers: See Chapter 67

END-TO-SIDE REPAIR
- For sensory nerve injury having distal end without proximal neuronal source
- Worse outcomes than for primary repair and autograft
- Not indicated for motor nerves

POSTOPERATIVE CARE

- To protect the repair, the splint is placed in the OR without excessive postural positioning.
- Wounds should be examined within 1 week.
- Immobilization is continued for 2-4 weeks; then the splint is readjusted for protection, with joint position as close to optimal as possible.

REHABILITATION
- **Early (2-4 weeks)**
  - Mobilization proceeds with active, active-assisted, then passive range of motion exercises to avoid joint stiffness.
- **Late**
  - Seek sensory and motor reeducation.
  - Begin as soon as patient is able to perceive any type of sensory stimulus.
- **Sensory reeducation stages**
  1. Desensitization
  2. Early phase discrimination and localization
  3. Late phase discrimination and tactic gnosis

SECONDARY PROCEDURES[10]

- Internal neurolysis
- Recoaptation of the nerve
- Bypass nerve grafting
- Neuroma excision[9,10]
  - Usually at 3-4 months
  - Electrodiagnostic studies and clinical examination: Can include **nonprogressing Tinel's sign,** lack of functional recovery
  - Exploration indicated with or without intraoperative stimulation testing
  - Painful neuromas: If critical sensory region and distal nerve available, consider nerve autograft rather than excision and intramuscular or intraosseous transposition
    - ▶ Transposition (into bone, muscle) away from contact surface preferred with complete transections
  - Neuroma-in-continuity[7,12]
    - ▶ Lateral neuromas: Consider partial resection and perineurial repair of involved fascicles
    - ▶ Spindle-shaped neuromas: If fascicles-in-continuity, internal neurolysis required; if complete transection, resection and coaptation warranted

OUTCOMES

EVALUATION OF MOTOR AND SENSORY FUNCTION

- British Medical Research Council (MRC) grading system very useful

HIGHET'S METHOD OF END-RESULT EVALUATION AS MODIFIED BY DELLON ET AL

Motor Recovery

M0	No contraction
M1	Return of perceptible contraction on both proximal muscles
M2	Return of perceptible contraction in both proximal and distal muscles
M3	Return of function in both proximal and distal muscles to degree that all important muscles are sufficiently powerful to act against gravity
M4	Return of function as with stage M3; in addition, all synergistic and independent movements possible
M5	Complete recovery

Sensory Recovery

S0	Absence of sensory recovery
S1	Recovery of deep cutaneous pain sensibility within autonomous area of nerve
S2	Return of some degree of superficial cutaneous pain and tactile sensibility within autonomous area of nerve
S3	Return of superficial cutaneous pain and tactile sensibility throughout autonomous area, with disappearance of any previous overresponse
S3+	Return of sensibility as with stage S3; in addition, discrimination within autonomous area (7-15 mm)
S4	Complete recovery (2-point discrimination, 2-6 mm)

In the hand, proximal muscles are defined as extrinsic and distal muscles are intrinsic.
From Brushart T. Nerve repair and grafting. In Green DP, Hotchkiss RN, Pederson WC, eds. Green's Operative Hand Surgery, vol 2, 4th ed. Philadelphia: Churchill Livingstone, 1998.

SPECIFIC NERVES

- **Median:** Good to excellent results of motor component and sensation at wrist level; good to excellent results seen in more than one third of forearm-level repairs
  - Grafting: Fair to good results
- **Ulnar:** Less favorable, especially the motor component because need accurate reinnervation of distal intrinsics
  - Sensory recovery better than motor function recovery
- **Radial:** Poor results, with motor function poorer than sensation
  - M4 recovery in 20%-40% of patients[10]
- **Digital:** 2PD variable
  - Up to 95% of patients are S3+ or better with autogenous nerve grafting[10]

KEY POINTS

✔ Presence of Martin-Gruber and/or Riche-Cannieu connections can mask injury and confuse diagnosis. Explore laceration or wound when in doubt.

✔ Epineurial repair provides equivalent results in most situations, compared with other types of repair.

✔ Avoid tension on repair and be prepared to perform nerve autograft (or other type of graft, if appropriate) when gap exceeds 1-3 cm.

✔ Criteria for optimal results:
 Age, less than 20 years old
 Early repair, less than 3 months best
 Proximal injury

✔ Immobilization for 2-3 weeks, followed by a consistent rehabilitation program is key for successful treatment.

✔ Sensory recovery is often better than motor recovery.

✔ Follow results with clinical and electrophysiologic testing.

✔ If motor recovery is poor by 6 months to 1 year, consider appropriate tendon transfer(s).

REFERENCES

1. Jabaley ME. Current concepts of nerve repair. Clin Plast Surg 8:33-44, 1981.
2. Maggi SP, Lowe JB III, Mackinnon SE. Pathophysiology of nerve injury. Clin Plast Surg 30:109-126, 2003.
3. Novak CB. Evaluation of the nerve-injured patient. Clin Plast Surg 30:127-138, 2003.
4. Watchmaker GP, Mackinnon SE. Advances in peripheral nerve repair. Clin Plast Surg 24:63-73, 1997.
5. Young L, Wray RC, Weeks PM. A randomized prospective comparison of fascicular and epineural digital nerve repairs. Plast Reconstr Surg 68:89-93, 1981.
6. Millesi H. The nerve gap: Theory and clinical practice. Hand Clin 2:651-663, 1986.
7. Gutowski KA. Hand II: Peripheral nerve and tendon transfers. Sel Read Plast Surg 9(33), 2003.
8. Dvali L, Mackinnon SE. Nerve repair, grafting, and nerve transfers. Clin Plast Surg 30:203-221, 2003.
9. Taylor GI, Ham FJ. The free vascularized nerve graft. A further experimental and clinical application of microvascular techniques. Plast Reconstr Surg 57:413-426, 1976.
10. Mackinnon SE, Dellon AL. Surgery of the Peripheral Nerve. New York: Thieme, 1988.
11. Maser BM, Vedder N. Nerve repair and nerve grafting. In Achauer BM, Eriksson E, Guyuron B, et al, eds. Plastic Surgery: Indications, Operations, and Outcomes, vol 4. St Louis: Mosby, 2000, pp 2103-2113.
12. Vernadakis AJ, Koch H, Mackinnon SE. Management of neuromas. Clin Plast Surg 30:247-268, 2003.

69. Hand Infections

Bishr Hijazi
Blake A. Morrison

MICROBIOLOGY

- *Staphylococcus aureus* is the most common pathogen.
- *Streptococcus* spp are the next most common pathogens.
- **Immunocompromised hosts** are more likely to culture gram-negative anaerobes or unusual organisms.
- **Obtain cultures** before initiating antibiotic treatment using careful antiseptic techniques.
- **Methicillin-resistant** *S. aureus* **(MRSA)** is emerging as a common community-acquired organism in many areas. If resistance is common in your area, **treat for MRSA until cultures are identified.**

TIP: Many strains of MRSA are susceptible to trimethoprim/sulfamethoxazole, clindamycin, doxycycline, rifampin, tetracycline, and erythromycin, among others.

MEDICAL CONDITIONS WITH INCREASED RISK

- **Diabetes mellitus**
  - Hyperglycemia impairs polymorphonuclear (PMN) cell function.
  - Peripheral neuropathy may delay presentation.
- **Immunosuppressive conditions**
  - AIDS
  - Major debilitating medical conditions (e.g., liver disease, hematologic disease, or neoplasms)
  - Transplant patients
  - Patients with autoimmune disorders
- **Alcohol and drug abuse**
- **Malnutrition**
- **Renal failure**
- **Occupational or other behavioral factors increasing risk**
  - Dentists, dental hygienists, or others exposed to oral secretions: **Herpetic whitlow**
  - Dishwashers: **Chronic paronychia**
  - Nail biting: **Paronychia**

EVALUATION

HISTORY
- There is almost always a history of minor trauma, such as a splinter.
- Look for a history of systemic disease such as diabetes.
- Determine tetanus status.

676

- Expose and examine the entire upper extremity.
  - Notice any discoloration, edema, discharge, or lymphatic streaking; feel for any swelling, lymph node enlargement, or temperature change.
  - Compare results with opposite extremity, using it as a control.

RADIOLOGY
- Review for possible foreign bodies.
- Review for signs of osteomyelitis.
- Review for gas in the soft tissues.

SPECIFIC INFECTIONS[1-3]

CELLULITIS
Acute inflammation of the skin and subcutaneous tissues
- **Etiologic factors**
  - Usually caused by minor trauma, such as a scratch or splinter
  - Group A *Streptococcus* spp most common pathogens, followed by *Staphylococcus aureus*
- **Diagnosis:** Pain, swelling, and erythema, without abscess formation
- **Treatment**
  - Administer first-generation cephalosporin or penicillin as a first-line treatment.
  - Consider IV antibiotics for diabetics or when complicated by lymphangitis.
    - Monitor antibiotic treatment by encircling the visible cellulitic area using a pen; the erythema should retreat from the line centrally.
    - Consider changing antibiotic therapy to a more aggressive second line if no response.
    - Check your obtained culture by injecting 3 ml of saline solution at the cellulitic edge and aspirating back.
    - Consider the possibility of deep-seated abscess and the need for surgical drainage if antibiotic therapy is unsuccessful.
  - Adjust coverage for MRSA when prevalent.
  - Warm soaks, splinting, and elevation are important adjuncts.

PARONYCHIA[4,5]
An infection, including abscess, of the soft tissues surrounding the nail; occurs in acute and chronic forms
- **Acute infection**
  - **Etiologic factors**
    - **Most common infection type of the hand**
    - Associated with nail biting, poor manicure technique, or minor trauma
    - Usually *S. aureus,* occasionally anaerobes
  - **Diagnosis**
    - Patients present with pain, redness, and swelling around the nail.
    - Patients occasionally report drainage of pus.
  - **Treatment**
    - Elevate the nail fold with a No. 11 blade, pointing the tip away from the nail bed.
    - Culture and place a small wick of gauze under the nail fold.
    - Remove gauze after 48 hours and start sink hydrotherapy.
    - Prescribe oral antibiotics for 5-7 days.

▸ For pus collections under the nail plate, elevate the involved portion of the plate and remove just this portion of the nail.

- **Chronic infections**
  - **Etiologic factors**
    ▸ **Usually fungal** *(Candida albicans),* occasionally *Pseudomonas* spp, or atypical mycobacteria
    ▸ Associated with diabetes and chronic exposure to moisture (dishwashers, cafeteria workers)
  - **Diagnosis**
    ▸ Indurated, erythematous eponychium
    ▸ May have intermittent drainage, often a cheesy consistency
  - **Medical treatment**
    ▸ Topical antifungals tried first
    ▸ Eponychial marsupialization when conservative treatment fails
  - **Surgical treatment** (Fig. 69-1)
    ▸ A crescent-shaped portion of skin, proximal to eponychial fold, is excised.
    ▸ Any granulated tissue is removed.
    ▸ Wound is allowed to close by secondary intention.

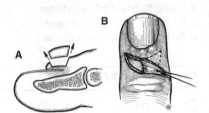

Fig. 69-1 Eponychial marsupialization for chronic paronychia. **A,** Lateral view showing the area of wedge-shaped excision; undisturbed matrix is stippled. **B,** Dorsal view of the crescent-shaped area of excision extending to the margins of the nail folds on each side. (From Green DP, Hotchkiss RN, Pederson WC, et al, eds. Green's Operative Hand Surgery, 5th ed. Philadelphia: Churchill Livingstone, 2005.)

FELON[4,5]

An abscess of the pulp of the thumb or fingertip

- **Etiologic factors**
  - Typically, a felon occurs after a puncture wound.
  - *S. aureus* is the most common pathogen.
  - Gram-negative microbes are possible, particularly in immunocompromised patients.
- **Diagnosis**
  - Patients have a **red, swollen, fluctuant fingertip,** which is exquisitely tender.
  - Patients often complain of throbbing pain that keeps them up at night.
- **Surgical treatment**
  - For an obvious pointing abscess, **open longitudinally over the point of maximum fluctuance.**
  - Otherwise use a **lateral incision over the midaxial line:** Ulnar for the index, middle, and ring fingers, but radial for the small finger and thumb.

TIP: Divide enough septa for thorough drainage, and stay dorsal to the neurovascular bundles.

- Pack loosely with gauze.
- Start sink hydrotherapy and daily dressing changes after 24-48 hours.
- Adjust antibiotics to culture results, when obtained.

HERPETIC WHITLOW[6]

A herpes simplex infection of the hand

- **Etiologic factors**
  - Herpes simplex virus types 1 and 2
- **Diagnosis**
  - Patients present with a **red, swollen, painful digit.**

- The pulp is not as tense as with a felon.
- **Clear vesicles** form, which may coalesce or become turbid.

NOTE: A whitlow tends to mimic a felon.

TIP: Whitlows and felons can usually be differentiated from the patient's history. Whitlows have a prodromal phase of 24-72 hours of burning pain before developing any skin changes.

■ **Treatment**
- **Do not incise** unless the whitlow is complicated by a secondary bacterial infection.
- Unroofing a vesicle is acceptable to obtain viral cultures or a Tzanck smear, if the diagnosis is in doubt.
- The process is generally **self-limiting.**
- **Acyclovir** may be used in severe cases, or for immunocompromised patients at risk for a life-threatening viremia.
- **Advise patients that about 20% will experience recurrences,** but these are typically less severe than the primary attack.

PALMAR SPACE ABSCESSES
Abscess formation within one of the potential spaces of the hand
■ **Etiologic factors**
- These abscesses typically occur after a puncture wound or other penetrating injury.
- *S. aureus* is the most common pathogen.
■ **Diagnosis**
- Presentation with pain, redness, and swelling over affected area
- **Web space abscess:** *Abducted posture of adjacent fingers*
- **Thenar abscess:** *Pain exacerbated by flexion or opposition of the thumb*
- **Midpalmar (subtendinous) space abscess:** *Pain on flexion of ulnar three fingers*
■ **Treatment**
- Perform incision and drainage in the operating room with tourniquet control.
- Multiple surgical approaches have been described.
- Avoid subsequent scar contractures in the web spaces.
- Avoid the motor branch of the median nerve to the thenar muscles.
- Start dressing changes in 24-48 hours.
- Use elevation, splinting, and IV antibiotics.

FLEXOR TENOSYNOVITIS[7]
An abscess within the flexor tendon sheath
■ **Etiologic factors**
- *S. aureus* the most common pathogen
- Usually a history of penetrating trauma; may occur as extension of a felon
- Rarely caused by hematogenous spread (suspect gonococci)
■ **Diagnosis: *Kanavel's four cardinal signs***
1. Pain on passive extension of the finger (earliest and most reliable sign of the four)
2. Fusiform swelling of digit
3. Tenderness over flexor tendon sheath
4. Partially flexed posture of digit

■ **Treatment**
- Very early cases *(less than 48 hours of symptoms)*
  - ► Splinting
  - ► Elevation
  - ► IV antibiotics

CAUTION: Patients must be reassessed after 24 hours and operated on emergently if they fail to improve.

- **Emergency incision and drainage** in the operating room required for most cases
  - ► **Surgical principles**
    - ✦ Perform with tourniquet control. If pus in the sheath is thin enough to be flushable, make limited incisions at the proximal and distal ends of the sheath, irrigate copiously with saline, and leave a catheter in place for 24-48 hours of irrigation postoperatively (Fig. 69-2).
    - ✦ **If the pus is thick,** open widely with a midlateral or Bruner incision, debride while preserving the pulleys, and pack with gauze. The wounds can be closed loosely after the infection subsides, usually after 5-7 days of dressing changes.

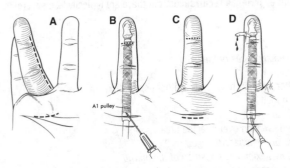

Fig. 69-2 Drainage of tendon sheath infections. **A,** Open drainage incisions through mid-axial approach. **B,** Sheath irrigation with distal opening of the sheath and proximal syringe irrigation. **C,** Incisions for intermittent through-and-through irrigation. **D,** Closed tendon sheath irrigation technique. (From Green DP, Hotchkiss RN, Pederson WC, et al, eds. Green's Operative Hand Surgery, 5th ed. Philadelphia: Churchill Livingstone, 2005.)

- **Treatment for all cases**
  - ► Rest in a splint
  - ► Heat and pain control
  - ► IV antibiotics
  - ► **Aggressive hand therapy as soon as feasible**

BITES
Classified according to source: Human or animal

■ **Human**
- **Etiologic factors**
  - ► **Bites are most common over the ring and small finger metacarpal head** *(fight bite).*
  - ► Organisms include the relatively virulent flora of the human mouth.
    - ✦ *Streptococcus viridans*
    - ✦ *S. aureus, Bacteroides* spp
    - ✦ *Eikenella corrodens*
- **Diagnosis**
  - ► Maintain a high index of suspicion for what may be a very unimpressive external wound.

TIP: Patients involved in fights are notoriously evasive during initial questioning.

▸ **The hand must be examined with the fingers fully flexed** to reproduce the orientation of skin, tendons, and joints at the time of impact.

▸ **Radiographs are mandatory.** Look for a tooth fragment, metacarpal head fracture, or air in the joint.

- **Treatment**
  1. **Explore in the operating room.**
  2. Irrigate the joint and debride wound edges.
  3. Allow to close by secondary intention or after 7 days of dressing changes.
  4. Use IV antibiotics, splinting, and elevation.
  5. Start hand therapy after 48-72 hours.

■ **Animal** (dog and cat bites)
- **Etiologic factors**
  ▸ *Dog bites are the most common.*
  ▸ *Cat bites are more likely to cause an abscess,* because their long, thin teeth are more likely to cause puncture wounds.
  ▸ Both bite types require coverage for *Pasteurella multocida,* as well as *Staphylococcus* spp, *Streptococcus* spp, and anaerobes.
- **Diagnosis**
  ▸ Determine tetanus status and investigate the possibility of rabies.
  ▸ Cat bites may cause **cat-scratch fever.**
    ✦ The patient presents with a small pustule at the wound site and painful lymphadenopathy proximally.
    ✦ The process is self-limiting and is treated with nonsteroidal antiinflammatory drugs (NSAIDs).
- **Treatment**
  ▸ All wounds should be irrigated thoroughly.
  ▸ Explore joints, when indicated, as for human bites.
  ▸ For dog bites, loosely approximate and sharply debride the skin edges.
  ▸ Substantial bite injuries may benefit from splinting and hand therapy.
  ▸ Cat bites rarely require closure.
  ▸ Administer antibiotics with coverage as described previously.

SEPTIC ARTHRITIS
Infection within a joint space
■ **Etiologic factors**
- These infections are typically secondary to a penetrating trauma; *S. aureus* is the most common pathogen.
- The infection may occur from hematogenous seeding.
  ▸ In **children,** search for an infectious source elsewhere in the body. *Streptococcus* spp, *Staphylococcus* spp, and *Haemophilus influenzae* are the most common pathogens.
  ▸ In **adults,** suspect gonococci.
■ **Diagnosis**
- A septic joint appears hot, swollen, erythematous, and tender, with marked pain during passive movement.

NOTE: Crystalline arthropathies can mimic septic arthritis or occur simultaneously.

- In the absence of a clear history of traumatic penetration, the joint should be aspirated to confirm the diagnosis. Be sure to send the aspirate for a Gram stain, culture, antibiotic sensitivity, and the presence of crystals.

- **Treatment**
  - All septic joints must be explored in the operating room.
  - The joint space is irrigated copiously and gently debrided.
  - The wound is packed open, with daily dressing changes until the wound closes by secondary intention.
  - Alternatively, the joint can be closed over an irrigation catheter and drain. The joint is then irrigated for 48-72 hours.
  - Use IV antibiotics, splinting, and elevation.
  - Begin hand therapy as soon as tolerated (after the drain is removed, if used).

NECROTIZING FASCIITIS[8]

Life- and limb-threatening, rapidly progressive infection of the subcutaneous tissue and fascia
- **Etiologic factors**
  - Commonly follows major or minor trauma
  - **Patients most at risk**
    - ▸ Diabetics
    - ▸ Elderly
    - ▸ Immunocompromised
  - Classically attributed to group A *Streptococcus* spp, but polymicrobial infections of aerobes and anaerobes in most cases
  - Closely related to gas gangrene caused by *Clostridia* spp
    - ▸ Demonstrates **crepitus** during physical examination and air in fascial planes on radiographs
- **Diagnosis**
  - Presents initially as a low-grade cellulitis; rapidly followed by cyanosis or bullae in the skin.
  - Patients typically appear diaphoretic, obtunded, and pale, with tachycardia (i.e., toxic/septic shock).
  - An area of cutaneous anaesthesia often follows the spread of the underlying infection.
  - **Foul-smelling, "dishwater" pus is evident.**
- **Treatment**
  - **Perform emergency, aggressive debridement of all nonviable tissue.**
  - Leave wounds open.

TIP: Silver sulfadiazine (Silvadene) cream is an excellent local antibiotic and helps prevent tendons and other critical structures from desiccating.

  - **Monitor in the ICU.** Sepsis associated with necrotizing fasciitis can cause significant hemodynamic instability.
  - **Repeat debridement** every 24 hours until the infection is under control. Some patients may require life-saving amputations.
  - **High-dose, broad-spectrum IV antibiotics** are administered, but surgical debridement is the cornerstone of treatment.
  - Consider **hyperbaric** treatment, particularly for **clostridial infections.**
  - Most patients will need secondary reconstruction of defects.

OSTEOMYELITIS[9]

A destructive infection of bones
- **Etiologic factors**
  - Osteomyelitis usually develops as a local extension of an adjacent felon, septic arthritis, flexor tenosynovitis, or after an open fracture.

- Occasionally, hematogenous spread is the cause.
- *Staphylococcus* spp and *Streptococcus* spp are the most common pathogens.
  ▸ Gram-negative, anaerobic, and polymicrobial infections can occur, particularly in immunocompromised patients.
- **Diagnosis**
- Patients have pain, swelling, and erythema over the affected bone, and may have a **chronically draining sinus.**
- It may be difficult, in early radiographs, to distinguish demineralization from the periosteal reaction of the overlying wound infection without bone involvement.
- A **bone scan or MRI** supports the diagnosis, when in doubt.
- **Treatment**
- Prescribe **antibiotics for a minimum of 4-6 weeks,** continuing as long as symptoms persist.
- **Antibiotic choice must be based on a bone biopsy and microbial culture.**
- Nonviable bone must be curetted back to bleeding, viable bone stock.
- Bone loss may require bone grafting and/or fracture fixation.
- Amputation rates as high as **39%** have been reported.

FUNGAL INFECTIONS

Common fungal infections of the upper extremity include **onychomycosis** (fungal infection of the nail) and **sporotrichosis** (granulomatous fungal infection of the subcutaneous tissue).
- **Onychomycosis *(tinea unguium)***
- **Etiologic factors**
  ▸ *Trichophyton rubrum* is the most common cause in the United States.
  ▸ *Candida albicans* is common in diabetics.
- **Diagnosis**
  ▸ Thickened, discolored nail
  ▸ Occasionally, flaky nail plates may separate from nail bed.
  ▸ Fungal cultures are obtained before initiating therapy, because different antifungal agents are used for each organism.
- **Treatment**
  ▸ *T. rubrum:* Oral terbinafine
  ▸ *C. albicans*
    ✦ **Topical:** Nystatin, miconazole, or econazole
    ✦ **Oral:** Ketoconazole, itraconazole, or griseofulvin
  ▸ **Removal of a thickened nail plate** can reduce the duration of oral therapy by 50%.
- **Sporotrichosis**
- **Etiologic factors**
  ▸ *Sporothrix schenckii* is the most common fungus on rose thorns, moss, and other plants.
  ▸ Typically, this infection develops after a puncture wound occurs while handling plants or soil.
- **Diagnosis**
  ▸ Patients present with a nodule at a puncture site, which later ulcerates.
  ▸ This is followed by **nodule formation** along lymphatic channels, which also ulcerate.
  ▸ A definitive diagnosis is made by **fungal culture** of a nodule aspirate.
- **Treatment**
  ▸ The classic treatment is the use of a **saturated solution of potassium iodide.**
  ▸ **Currently, potassium iodide is supplanted by itraconazole or fluconazole.**
  ▸ All oral antifungal regimens require **long-term treatment** for 3-6 months (at least 4 weeks after resolution of symptoms).

ATYPICAL MYCOBACTERIAL INFECTIONS
Relatively rare infections caused by nontubercular Mycobacterium *spp*
- **Etiologic factors**
  - Most cases in the hand are caused by *Mycobacterium marinum, M. kansasii,* and *M. terrae.*
  - *M. marinum* is indigenous to fresh and salt water.
  - Patients with any break in the skin can become infected after contact with fish, contaminated water, or other sources of the organism.
- **Diagnosis**
  - Suspect mycobacteria when a chronic skin lesion, draining sinus tract, or other infection fails to heal as expected.
  - A biopsy will show granulomas with negative fungal staining.
  - Culture in **Lowenstein-Jensen medium** at 31° C for up to 8 weeks.
- **Treatment**
  1. Surgical debridement of lesions
  2. Long-term antibiotics (2-6 months) specific for the organism

---

KEY POINTS
- ✔ Patient comorbidities can predispose to hand or finger infections.
- ✔ *Staphylococcus* spp and *Streptococcus* spp are usually the most common pathogens.
- ✔ MRSA is becoming more prevalent as a community-acquired pathogen.
- ✔ Paronychia (acute) is the most common hand infection.
- ✔ Chronic paronychia is a common fungal infection.
- ✔ Plan your incisions carefully, in general, to avoid exposing underlying vital structures while still allowing for adequate drainage.
- ✔ Whitlows resemble felons, although they can be differentiated by the patient's history and the presence of clear vesicles.
- ✔ Watch for Kanavel's four signs to diagnose flexor tenosynovitis.
- ✔ Include antibiotic coverage for *Eikenella* infections originating from human bites.
- ✔ Include antibiotic coverage for *Pasteurella* infections originating from cat and dog bites.
- ✔ Suspect necrotizing fasciitis if you see "dishwater" drainage and rapidly progressing cellulitis.

REFERENCES

1. Leddy J. Infections of the upper extremity. J Hand Surg Am 11:294-297, 1986.
2. Mann R, Peacock J. Hand infections in patients with diabetes mellitus. J Trauma 17:376-380, 1977.
3. Milford LW. The Hand, 2nd ed. St Louis: Mosby, 1982.
4. Canales F, Newmeyer W, Kilgore EJ. The treatment of felons and paronychias. Hand Clin 5:515-523, 1989.
5. Jebson P. Infections of the fingertip: Paronychias and felons. Hand Clin 5:547-555, 1998.
6. Carter SJ. Herpetic whitlow: Herpetic infections of the digits. J Hand Surg Am 4:93-94, 1979.
7. Neviaser RJ, Gunther SF. Tenosynovial infections in the hand: Diagnosis and management: I. Acute pyogenic tenosynovitis of the hand. In AAOS Instructional Course Lectures. St Louis: Mosby, 1980, pp 108-117.
8. Giuliano A, Lewis F Jr, Hadley K, et al. Bacteriology of necrotizing fasciitis. Am J Surg 134:52-57, 1977.
9. Reilly KE, Linz JC, Stern PJ, et al. Osteomyelitis of the tubular bones of the hand. J Hand Surg Am 22:644-649, 1997.

70. Benign and Malignant Masses of the Hand

Melissa A. Crosby

BENIGN SOFT TISSUE TUMORS[1-5]

GANGLION CYSTS

- **Demographics**
  - *Most frequent benign mass in the hand* (33%-69% of all hand tumors)
  - Two to three times more common in women, second to fourth decades
- **Pathologic conditions and etiologic factors**
  - Mucoid degeneration of fibrous connective tissue in joint capsules or tendon sheaths.
  - 10% of cases present after a specific, traumatic, antecedent event.
  - Repeated minor trauma may be an etiologic factor in development.
- **Diagnosis**
  - May present with or without pain
  - Most on dorsum (scapholunate ligament)
  - Mobile, **transilluminate,** may move with tendon
  - Radiographs **not** helpful to diagnose a ganglion cyst but may help rule out other conditions if diagnosis unclear
  - Histology
    - ▸ Compressed collagen
    - ▸ No synovial or epithelial cells
  - Cysts contain glucosamine, albumin, globulin, and hyaluronic acid
- **Types**
  - **Dorsal wrist ganglion**
    - ▸ Overlies scapholunate ligament
    - ▸ **70%** of all ganglia
    - ▸ Often occurs between third and fourth extensor compartments
  - **Volar wrist**
    - ▸ **Most frequent site in children** less than 10 years old and in 15%-20% of adult cases
    - ▸ Originates from flexor carpi radialis (FCR) tendon sheath, radiocarpal, or scaphotrapezial joints
    - ▸ **Adjacent to radial artery**
  - **Flexor tendon sheath ganglion (volar retinacular)**
    - ▸ Often at **A1 pulley** (or between A1 and A2 pulleys), base of digit
    - ▸ 3-8 mm diameter
    - ▸ Attached to tendon and **does not move with tendon**
    - ▸ Result of direct damage to fibrous sheath
    - ▸ Possibly delay or obviate need for surgery by using needle aspiration, steroid injection, and massage until rupture
  - **Mucous cysts**
    - ▸ **Dorsal aspect of P3** (digital phalanx) is associated with extensor tendon, joint, or joint capsule.
    - ▸ Longitudinal grooving of the nail is possible.

685

DIFFERENTIAL DIAGNOSIS OF SOFT TISSUE MASSES OF THE HAND

I. Wrist Ganglions

Neoplasms or Cysts

Xanthoma	Lymphangioma
Lipoma	Osteochondroma
Fibroma	Synovial sarcoma
Epidermoid inclusion cyst	Histiocytoma
Hemangioma	Chondrosarcoma

Infections

Tuberculosis	Secondary syphilis
Fungi	

Inflammation

Gout	Rheumatoid extensor tenosynovitis
Rheumatoid nodule	Bursitis

Posttraumatic

Scar	Foreign body granuloma

Other

Radial artery aneurysm	Anomalous muscle

II. Volar Retinacular Ganglions

Trigger finger	Inclusion cysts
Giant cell tumor	

III. Distal Interphalangeal Joint Ganglions

Giant cell tumor	Heberden's node
Inclusion cyst	

From Young L, Bartell T, Logan SE. Ganglions of the hand and wrist. South Med J 81:751-760, 1988.

- ▸ These cysts are found mostly in older women, associated with degenerative changes in the distal interphalangeal (DIP) joint.
- ▸ Radiographs show narrow space and osteophytes.
- ▸ The skin is thin and may rupture.
- ▸ **Always remove osteophytes at the time of excision, and look for occult cysts on the contralateral side.**
- • **Carpal bosses**
  - ▸ Painful masses on dorsal II or III metacarpal bases
  - ▸ Associated with arthritis
  - ▸ More common in the right hands of women in the third or fourth decades
  - ▸ Ganglia present 30% of the time
- ■ **Medical management**
  - • **Children:** Rosson and Walker,[6] 22 of 29 cases resolved with conservative treatment
  - • **Adult regression:** Approximately 38%-58% incidence
  - • **Treatment**
    - ▸ Aspiration
    - ▸ Injection of enzymes, sclerosing agents, or cortisone

- **Surgical management**
  - Surgery for pain, deformity, or limitation of function
  - Resection must include entire cyst wall, stalk, and joint surface
  - Do **not** need to close joint capsule
  - No splint postoperatively, if uncomplicated
  - Most return to work in a few days
- **Recurrence**
  - Treatment associated with 1%-50% recurrence **(mean 24%)**

GIANT CELL TUMORS

- **Demographics**
  - *Second most common hand tumor*
  - Generally in fourth to sixth decades
  - Also called *pigmented villonodular synovitis*
  - Occurs most commonly in radial three digits
- **Pathologic conditions and etiologic factors**
  - Probably reaction to injury
  - Growth interferes with functioning of hand
  - Often confused with ganglion, but giant cell tumors fixed to deeper tissues and may erode bone
- **Diagnosis**
  - Yellow subcutaneous mass usually evident
  - Fine needle aspiration (FNA) may help in difficult cases
  - Histology: Cells of fibrous xanthoma, spindle cells, foam cells
  - **May erode into bone,** infiltrate dermis
- **Treatment**
  - Marginal excision
- **Recurrence**
  - Common (5%-50%) because of incomplete excision or satellite lesions
  - Reexcise; may need arthrodesis; amputation rare

EPIDERMAL INCLUSION CYST

- **Demographics**
  - *Third most common tumor in the hand*
  - Most on palm and fingertips of people with occupations that predispose them to penetrating injuries
  - Evolution may take months to years
- **Pathologic conditions and etiologic factors**
  - Penetrating injury causes implantation of epidermal cells in the dermis.
- **Diagnosis**
  - Firm, spherical, nontender mass
  - Cyst material: Protein, cholesterol, and fat
  - May cause bone erosion
- **Treatment**
  - Must excise completely to avoid recurrence
- **Recurrence:** Low recurrence rate if excised completely

GLOMUS TUMOR
- **Demographics**
  - 1%-2% of all hand tumors
- **Pathologic conditions and etiologic factors**
  - Benign hamartoma of glomus apparatus (arterial-venous anastomosis involved in regulation of cutaneous circulation)
- **Diagnosis**
  - **Triad of symptoms**
    1. **Pain**
    2. **Pinpoint tenderness**
    3. **Cold sensitivity**
  - **Subungual** most common site
  - Multiple tumors in 25% of cases
  - **Nail-ridging** and red to bluish discoloration
  - Tumor less than 1 cm in diameter
  - Ultrasound with high frequency transducer detects lesion
  - Magnetic resonance imaging (MRI): High-signal intensity on transverse relaxation time (T2) weighted images
- **Treatment**
  - Local complete excision through sterile matrix
- **Recurrence:** Low incidence of recurrence if completely excised

ULNAR ARTERY ANEURYSM
- **Demographics**
  - Commonly seen in **carpenters** using hammers or in other laborers
  - Mostly in **men**
- **Pathologic conditions and etiologic factors**
  - Posttraumatic repetitive motion **(hypothenar hammer syndrome)** near ulnar artery
- **Diagnosis**
  - Pulsatile mass
  - Digital ischemic changes
  - Emboli
  - *Tinel's sign* of ulnar nerve often present
    - ▶ Allen's test to determine patency
  - Arteriogram results
- **Treatment**
  - Resection and ligation
  - Interposition, if collateral circulation inadequate
  - Consider lysis for emboli
- **Recurrence:** Rare

PERIPHERAL NERVE TUMORS
- **Demographics**
  - 1%-5% of all hand tumors
- **Pathologic conditions and etiologic factors**
  - Originate from Schwann cells
- **Diagnosis**
  - Evaluation with CT scan and MRI

- **Five types of peripheral nerve tumors**
  1. **Neurilemmoma (also called schwannoma)**
     - *Most common nerve tumor*
     - Prevalent in middle age
     - Asymptomatic nodular swellings extrinsic to nerve
     - Treatment: Enucleate
     - Recurrence: Rare
  2. **Neurofibroma**
     - Can proliferate within fiber
     - Functional abnormality possible, including paresthesias
     - Lesions seen before age 10 years
     - Can cause gigantism in affected part
     - Histology demonstrates mast cells
     - Treatment: Consider resection if primary repair possible
  3. **Neurofibromatosis (von Recklinghausen's disease)**
     - Autosomal dominant
     - Acoustic neuromas
     - Optic gliomas
     - Meningiomas
     - Gigantism of limb
     - More than 6 café au lait spots
     - Plexiform pattern
     - Sarcomatous degeneration in 10%-15% of cases
  4. **Neurofibrosarcoma**
     - 2%-3% of malignant hand tumors
     - Associated with von Recklinghausen's disease
     - Local extension or metastasis common
     - 90% mortality
     - Treatment: Wide excision if possible; if not, amputation recommended
  5. **Intraneural nonneural tumors:** Lipoma, hemangioma, lipofibromatosis hamartoma
     - **Recurrence:** Rare with complete excision

MALIGNANT SOFT TISSUE TUMORS[2-4,7]

SQUAMOUS CELL CANCER

- **Demographics**
  - *Most common malignant cutaneous tumor of hand*
  - *Most common malignancy of nail bed*
  - 11% of all squamous cell tumors
  - **Dorsum of hand** most common location
  - Elderly patients
  - Mostly in men
- **Pathologic conditions and etiologic factors**
  - Originate from spindle cell layer of epithelium
  - Originate in areas of premalignant conditions
    - Sun damage (solar radiation) main factor
    - Actinic keratosis

- ▶ Leukoplakia
- ▶ Radiation keratosis
- ▶ Scars
- ▶ Chronic ulcers
- ▶ Sinuses
- **Diagnosis**
  - Diagnosis assisted by biopsy
  - Appearance
    - ▶ Smooth
    - ▶ Verrucous
    - ▶ Papillomatous
    - ▶ Ulcerative
  - Aggressive metastatic rate more common in hand than any other part of body, especially if digital web space involved
- **Treatment**
  - Wide local surgical excision or Mohs' excision are mainstay of treatment
  - Destruction by electrodesiccation and curettage; cryosurgery limited to very superficial lesions
  - Medical interventions
    - ▶ Radiation treatment
    - ▶ Topical 5-fluorouracil for premalignant lesions
    - ▶ Systemic chemotherapy
- **Recurrence**
  - Depends on degree of cellular differentiation, depth of tumor invasion, and perineural invasion
  - 7% for well-differentiated tumors versus 28% for poorly-differentiated tumors

BASAL CELL CANCER

- **Demographics**
  - *Second most common cutaneous malignancy of hand*
  - 2%-3% of all basal cell cancers
  - Occur in middle-aged and elderly light-skinned individuals
- **Pathologic conditions and etiologic factors**
  - Does not arise from malignant changes in preexisting structures
  - Occur most often at sites with greatest concentration of pilosebaceous follicles
  - Up to 26 histologic variants described
  - Palmar variants associated with *Gorlin's syndrome,* also subungual
- **Diagnosis**
  - Diagnosis assisted by biopsy
  - Slow-growing tumors with skin atrophy, pink to red discoloration, telangiectasias, and ulceration in pearly lesions
  - Metastases uncommon, locally aggressive
- **Treatment**
  - Primary excision or Mohs' excision best treatment
  - Electrodesiccation and curettage, cryosurgery, and laser phototherapy for superficial lesions or poor surgical risk patients
  - Medical treatment may include:
    - ▶ Intralesional interferon injection
    - ▶ Chemotherapy
    - ▶ Radiation

- **Recurrence**
  - Increases with larger lesions
  - Increased rate with infiltrative nodular variants that have poorly-defined borders, sclerosing, and morpheaform variants

MELANOMA
- **Demographics**
  - 10%-20% of all melanomas found in the hand
  - Palmar or subungual locations common
- **Pathologic conditions and etiologic factors**
  - Sun exposure important etiologic factor
  - Consider dysplastic nevus syndrome
  - **Types**
    - ▸ Superficial spreading
    - ▸ Nodular
    - ▸ Acral-lentiginous
    - ▸ Lentigo maligna
- **Diagnosis**
  - Biopsy important to diagnosis: **Complete excisional biopsy preferred**
  - **Tumor thickness** only prognostic indicator
- **Treatment**
  - Wide local excision (WLE) or amputation; level not definitively determined, but **most agree with joint proximal to lesion**
  - Regional lymphadenectomy and sentinel lymph node dissection controversial; most often for intermediate-depth tumor
- Recurrence more common with increased tumor thickness

SARCOMA
- **Demographics**
  - Uncommon in hand
  - 15% in upper extremity
  - Young patients
- **Pathologic conditions and etiologic factors**
  - Share common mesodermal origin
  - Increased risk with previous exposure to radiation and herbicides
  - Increased risk in patients with neurofibromatosis and Li-Fraumeni syndrome
- **Diagnosis**
  - Painless mass with recent growth
  - Innocuous at presentation
  - Plain radiographs may demonstrate:
    - ▸ Soft tissue calcification
    - ▸ Fat density
    - ▸ Bony involvement
  - MRI helpful for defining pathologic anatomy and local extent of disease, and for preoperative planning
  - **Biopsy important**
    - ▸ Plan in line with limb salvage or amputation procedure.
  - Prone to local recurrence
  - High incidence of lymphatic spread and regional lymph node metastases

- **Seven types of sarcoma**
  1. **Epithelioid sarcoma**
     - *Most common subtype*
     - Possibly posttraumatic
     - Insidious
     - Originates on palm or volar surface of digits
     - Local recurrence common
     - Distant metastases common
  2. **Malignant fibrous histiocytoma**
     - Variable lesions
       - Superficial
       - Deep
       - Single
       - Multinodular
     - Extend along tissue planes
     - Metastasis through lymphatics or bloodstream
  3. **Alveolar rhabdomyosarcoma**
     - Thenar or hypothenar musculature
     - Highly malignant and devastating tumor
     - Rapidly growing deep mass when in palm of children
     - Prognosis poor even with multimodality therapy
  4. **Synovial sarcoma**
     - Originates in juxtaarticular soft tissues (tendon, tendon sheath, bursa)
     - Grow slowly over years on palmar surface of hand
     - Poor prognosis
     - High incidence of metastases
     - **Treatment**
       - Surgery
       - Radiotherapy
       - Chemotherapy
  5. **Fibrosarcoma**
     - **Origin**
       - Deep subcutaneous space
       - Facial septa
       - Muscle
     - Insidious
     - Hematogenous spread
  6. **Clear cell sarcoma**
     - Uncommon
     - Slow-growing
     - Deep mass attached to tendons and aponeuroses or fascia
     - Poor prognosis
     - Local recurrence high
     - **Treatment**
       - Surgery with node dissection
       - Radiation
       - Chemotherapy

7. Kaposi's sarcoma
- ▸ Prevalent in fourth or fifth decade
- ▸ Male/female ratio of 10:1
- ▸ Associated with **AIDS**
- ▸ Dark-blue to violaceous macules replaced by infiltrative plaques
- ▸ Diameter of 0.5-3 cm
- ▸ Treatment includes: Radiotherapy and chemotherapy
- ▸ Fulminating lesions, 6-12 months life expectancy
- ▸ If slower growing, up to 20-year life expectancy

BONY TUMORS OF THE HAND

Benign (G0)	Low-Grade Sarcomas (G1)	High-Grade Sarcomas (G2)
Bone	Giant cell tumor	Osteosarcoma
Enchondroma	Desmoplastic fibroma	Ewing's sarcoma
Osteochondroma	Chondrosarcoma (LG)	Lymphoma
Fibrous dysplasia	Parosteal osteosarcoma	Chondrosarcoma
Osteoid osteoma	Desmoid	Angiosarcoma
Bone cysts	Liposarcoma (LG)	Myeloma
Hemangioma	Fibrosarcoma (LG)	Synovioma
Osteoblastoma	Kaposi's sarcoma	Malignant fibrous histiocytoma
Soft tissue		Liposarcoma (HG)
Ganglion		Rhabdomyosarcoma
Giant cell tumor (tendon sheath)		Epithelioid sarcoma
Lipoma		Clear cell sarcoma
Neurilemmoma		Angiosarcoma
Chondromatosis		Hemangiopericytoma
Glomus tumor		Malignant schwannoma

From Mankin HJ. Principles of diagnosis and management of tumors of the hand. Hand Clin 3:185-195, 1987.

- ■ **Treatment principles for sarcoma**
  - • Wide surgical excision including 2-3 cm of normal tissue, with or without adjunctive radiotherapy and/or chemotherapy
  - • Prognosis poor
- ■ **Recurrence:** Rare if excised completely with adequate margins
- ■ **Metastatic factors**
  - • Very uncommon
  - • Kidney and lung involvement
  - • Distal phalanges common site
  - • With palliative treatment, survival is generally only 5 months

BENIGN BONE TUMORS[8,9]

CHONDROMA
- ■ **Demographics**
  - • *Most common benign cartilaginous tumors of the hand*
- ■ **Pathologic conditions and etiologic factors**
  - • Most result from aberrant focus of cartilage

- **Diagnosis**
  - Plain radiography often helpful
  - CT scan and MRI also useful
  - May be asymptomatic or present with pain from pathologic fracture or remodeling
- **Three types of chondromas**
  1. **Enchondromas**
     - ▶ Favor the **tubular bones** of the hand
     - ▶ Middle or proximal phalanges
     - ▶ Well-demarcated round or oval swellings
     - ▶ **Pathologic fracture may occur**
     - ▶ Radiolucent, expansile, diametaphyseal lesion that does not involve epiphyses
     - ▶ **Treatment:**
       - ◆ Curettage with or without cancellous bone grafting
       - ◆ If fracture present, allow to heal before curettage
  2. **Multiple enchondromas**
     - ▶ Rare
     - ▶ Known as *Ollier's disease*
     - ▶ *Maffucci's syndrome,* if associated with hemangiomas
     - ▶ 20% degenerate into chondrosarcoma
     - ▶ **Treatment:** Wide excision
  3. **Osteochondroma**
     - ▶ *Most common cartilaginous neoplasm overall*
     - ▶ Young patients
     - ▶ 1% risk of malignant transformation
     - ▶ Bony protuberances extending beyond metaphyseal cortex on narrow stalk seen in diagnostic radiographs
     - ▶ **Treatment:** Wide excision
- **Recurrence:** Rare with complete excision

ANEURYSMAL BONE CYST

- **Demographics**
  - 5% of all benign bone tumors
  - Equal sex distribution
  - Most common in second decade of life before closure of epiphyseal plate
- **Pathologic conditions and etiologic factors**
  - Unknown
- **Diagnosis**
  - Eccentric in metaphysis or diaphysis
  - Expansile
  - Lucent lesion on radiographs
- **Treatment**
  - Excision or curettage with bone grafting
- **Recurrence**
  - Up to 60% following curettage and bone grafting

OSTEOID OSTEOMA
- **Demographics**
  - Uncommon osteoblastic tumor in hand: 10% of all benign bone tumors
  - Two to three times more prevalent in males than females
  - Most prevalent in first and third decades
- **Pathologic conditions and etiologic factors**
  - Nidus of abnormal bone less than 1.5 cm in diameter
- **Diagnosis**
  - Distal phalanx most commonly affected
  - Painful, localized area over tubular bone
  - **Pain worse at night**
  - Relief of pain with nonsteroidal antiinflammatory drugs (NSAIDs)
  - Central area of lucency surrounded by zone of sclerotic bone seen in radiographs
  - Bone scintigraphy and CT scan useful
- **Treatment**
  - Complete excision with cancellous bone grafting
- **Recurrence**
  - 0%-25% after complete nidus excised

OSTEOBLASTOMA
- **Demographics**
  - Rare in hand
  - Prevalent in second to third decades
  - No sex predilection
- **Pathologic conditions and etiologic factors**
  - Poorly mineralized immature bars of neoplastic osteoid
- **Diagnosis**
  - Localized to carpus, especially scaphoid and tubular bones such as metacarpal
  - Larger than 1.5-2 cm
  - Localized swelling and pain
- **Treatment**
  - Complete resection of involved bone required
  - Radiotherapy helpful for tumor control
- **Recurrence**
  - Recurrence rare with wide en bloc excision

GIANT CELL TUMOR OF BONE
- **Demographics**
  - 2%-5% occur in hand
  - Prevalent in third to fifth decades
  - Incidence greater in females than in males
- **Pathologic conditions and etiologic factors**
  - Benign lesions based on histology, but behave in locally aggressive fashion, metastasize, and ultimately result in death
- **Diagnosis**
  - Solitary lesion
  - Dull constant pain, involves soft tissues

- Epiphyseal end of bone affected with extension into metaphysis
- Translucent with thin cortex in radiographs
- **Treatment**
  - Wide resection with autograft or allograft
  - Sarcomatous degeneration in 10% of cases
- **Recurrence:** High, at 75%

MALIGNANT BONE TUMORS

EWING'S SARCOMA
- **Demographics**
  - Rare in hand, 10% of all primary malignant bone tumors
  - Metacarpus most common site of involvement
  - Male/female incidence is 2:1
  - Young patients
- **Pathologic conditions and etiologic factors**
  - Neural cell origin
- **Diagnosis**
  - Focal, permeating, soft tissue mass with sclerotic reaction on radiographs
- **Treatment**
  - Poor prognosis, although the hand subset can have excellent local control with multimodal therapy, including adjuvant chemotherapy followed by surgical excision.
- **Recurrence:** Rare with complete excision and multimodal therapy

CHONDROSARCOMA
- **Demographics**
  - *Most common primary malignant bone tumor that occurs in the hand*
  - Most prevalent in sixth to eighth decades
- **Pathologic conditions and etiologic factors**
  - Occasionally associated with osteochondromas and multiple enchondromatosis
- **Diagnosis**
  - Epiphyseal area of proximal phalanx or metacarpal
  - Clinical course slow
  - Metastases late
  - Painful large mass near metacarpophalangeal joint
- **Treatment**
  - Amputation or ray resection
- **Recurrence**
  - Common because metastases may become apparent several years later

OSTEOSARCOMA
- **Demographics**
  - Rare tumor of hand: 0.18% incidence
  - Peak incidence in fourth to seventh decades, when hand involved
  - Male/female incidence is 2:1
- **Pathologic conditions and etiologic factors**
  - Mesenchymal origin: Immature, neoplastic osteoid directly produced by proliferating cellular stroma

- More frequent in irradiated bone, Paget's disease, fibrous dysplasia, giant cell tumors, solitary enchondroma, multiple enchondromas, and multiple osteochondromas
- **Diagnosis**
  - Persistent, increasing pain from rapidly growing mass
  - Sunburst pattern seen in plain radiographs
  - Further imaging may be needed for staging
  - Histology: Spindle-shaped cell
- **Treatment**
  - Wide local excision with adjuvant chemotherapy
  - Five-year survival rate 70% if no metastasis, 10%-20% with metastasis
- **Recurrence**
  - Rare with complete excision and no metastasis
- **Metastatic factors**
  - Very uncommon
  - Kidney and lung involvement
  - Distal phalanges common site
  - With palliative treatment, survival is generally only 5 months

---

KEY POINTS

- ✔ The most common tumor of the hand is an enchondroma (benign).
- ✔ The difference between Ollier's disease and Maffucci's syndrome is that Maffucci's syndrome is associated with soft tissue hemangiomas and lymphangiomas; both involve multiple enchondromas.
- ✔ Osteoid osteoma (benign) symptoms are relieved by NSAIDs.
- ✔ Despite excision, giant cell tumors have a high recurrence rate of 9%-30%.
- ✔ Pathologic fractures often are seen with enchondromas.
- ✔ The glomus tumor triad of symptoms includes pain, pinpoint tenderness, and cold sensitivity in the subungual location.

REFERENCES

1. Athanasian EA. Bone and soft tissue tumors. In Green DP, Hotchkiss RN, Pederson WC, eds. Green's Operative Hand Surgery, 4th ed. Philadelphia: Churchill Livingstone, 1998, pp 2223-2253.
2. Fleegler, EJ. Skin tumors. In Green DP, Hotchkiss RN, Pederson WC, eds. Green's Operative Hand Surgery, 4th ed. Philadelphia: Churchill Livingstone, 1998, pp 2184-2205.
3. Mankin HJ. Principles of diagnosis and management of tumors of the hand. Hand Clin 3:185-195, 1987.
4. Masson JA. Hand I: Fingernails, infections, tumors and soft-tissue reconstruction. Sel Read Plast Surg 8(32), 1999.
5. Nahra ME, Bucchieri JS. Ganglion cysts and other tumor related conditions of the hand and wrist. Hand Clin 20:249-260, 2004.
6. Rosson JW. The natural history of ganglia in children. J Bone Joint Surg Br 71:707-708, 1989.
7. TerKonda SP, Perdikis G. Non-melanotic skin tumors of the upper extremity. Hand Clin 20:293-301, 2004.
8. Feldman F. Primary bone tumors of the hand and carpus. Hand Clin 3:269-289, 1987.
9. Young L, Bartell T, Logan SE. Ganglions of the hand and wrist. South Med J 81:751-760, 1988.

71. Dupuytren's Disease

Bishr Hijazi
Blake A. Morrison

DEFINITION

Dupuytren's disease (DD) is a benign proliferative disorder that occurs in the fascia of the palm and digits resulting in nodules, cords, and disabling contractures of the fingers and the palm. Guillaume Dupuytren, a French surgeon, clarified the nature of this disease in 1831. His classic dissections and teachings led to the adoption of his name to identify the condition.

DEMOGRAPHICS

- The highest incidence is in Caucasian males of northern European ancestry.
- There is a greater prevalence in men until the age of 70, when it becomes equal.
- The Japanese population tends to contract a mild form of the disease characterized by nodule formation without cords or contractures.
- Both familial and sporadic forms exist.
- Proposed mode of inheritance is **autosomal dominant with variable penetrance.**
- Bilateral in **50%** of patients; when unilateral it usually involves the dominant hand.
- The **ulnar rays** of the hand are most commonly affected (ring > small > middle).
- **Dupuytren's diathesis** is an aggressive variant of the disease with earlier presentation and more rapid progression.
  - Knuckle pads over the dorsum of the proximal interphalangeal joints **(Garrod's pads)**
  - Penile fibromatosis **(Peyronie's disease)**
  - Plantar fibromatosis **(Ledderhose disease)**

ETIOLOGIC FACTORS AND PATHOPHYSIOLOGY

No single causative factor has been described. Many associated conditions have been implicated, but the data are still conflicting.
- **Alcohol**
  - **DD occurs more often in alcoholics,** with a possible liver-related mechanism, although this connection is controversial
- **Manual labor**
  - **No clear correlation,** with a possible microtrauma mechanism leading to myofibroblast contracture
- **Smoking**
  - Smoking has a **significant role in causation and progression of DD.**
  - Association with drinking may explain high prevalence in alcoholics.
  - Nicotine markedly decreases the blood flow to the hand; microvascular occlusion has been discovered in diseased tissue specimens from smokers.

- **Diabetes**
  - **More than twice as prevalent in diabetics**
  - More common in diabetics with retinopathy, suggesting a microangiopathic or ischemic mechanism (as in smoking)
- **Epilepsy**
  - No clear mechanism
  - Possible relation to anticonvulsants

ANATOMY/HISTOLOGY/PATHOLOGY[1,2]

- Dupuytren's fascia has a much higher percentage of **type III collagen** than normal fascia (40% compared with 5%).
- Collagen bands are normal structures of the digital and palmar fascias.
- **Affected structures:**
  - Spiral bands
  - Lateral digital sheets
  - Natatory ligaments
  - Pretendinous bands
  - Grayson's ligaments
- **Cleland's ligaments** (dorsal to the neurovascular bundle) do **not** become involved.
- **A self-perpetuating cycle has been proposed.**
  1. Local tissue ischemia leads to increased oxygen free radical production.
  2. The free radicals induce fibroblast production.
  3. Increased fibroblasts increase cell density.
  4. This leads to tissue contracture and further ischemia.
- For every band that becomes diseased, there is a corresponding cord of diseased tissue.
  - **Metacarpophalangeal (MP) joint:** *Pretendinous cord*
  - **Proximal interphalangeal (PIP) joint:** *Central, spiral,* and *lateral* cords
    - ▶ **Spiral cord:** Made up of pretendinous band, spiral band, lateral sheet, and Grayson's ligament
    - ▶ **Central cord:** Continuation of the pretendinous fibers in the palm to the digit
    - ▶ **Lateral cord:** Runs from natatory ligament to the lateral digital sheet
  - **Natatory cord:** Causes web-space contracture from diseased natatory ligament

NOTE: The cords are not random—they develop in a specific relationship to the organization of the digital and palmar fascia.

- Tissue factors that increase in DD are collagen type III, platelet-derived growth factor (PDGF), fibroblast growth factor (FGF), and transforming growth factor beta (TGF-β).

INDICATIONS FOR SURGERY AND PATIENT SELECTION

- **Surgery will not cure the disease.** Patients with unrealistic expectations should be approached with caution.
- In general, operate only for contractures leading to loss of function or difficulty with hygiene; encourage patients to relate specific tasks that DD limits them in performing.
- **MP joint** contracture can be recovered after essentially any duration, thus significant contractures can be tolerated before operative intervention is considered.

- **MP joint contracture greater than 30 degrees** is often cited as the threshold for surgery, but patients must be evaluated individually.
- **PIP joints** are more difficult to fully correct. Earlier intervention may be advisable. *Thus any degree of PIP contracture is considered an indication for surgery.*
- **Rapidly progressive** cases warrant **earlier operative treatment** than slowly progressive forms.
- **Increased sensitivity to the disease is suggested by:**
  - Young age
  - Strongly positive family history
  - Involvement of the radial side of the hand
  - Ectopic site involvement (diathesis)
  - Rapid rate of progression

> TIP: Hueston's tabletop test can indicate need for surgical intervention. The test is considered positive if the patient is unable to place all fingers in a flat position on a flat tabletop simultaneously.

NOTE: No staging system is currently in use for Dupuytren's disease.

CONTRAINDICATIONS TO SURGERY

RELATIVE
- Early MP joint contracture without functional consequence
- Nodules or cords of largely cosmetic concern
- Unrealistic patient expectations

ABSOLUTE
- Patients with a general medical condition that places them at an unreasonable risk for surgery

PREOPERATIVE WORKUP

Dupuytren's disease is a clinical diagnosis. No confirmatory lab work or studies are indicated.

HISTORY
- Progression of the disease
- Specific tasks that are compromised by contractures
- Family history of DD
- General medical history

PHYSICAL EXAMINATION
- Extent of the diseased tissue
- Involvement of the skin
- Presence and severity of joint contractures (Do not guess—measure!)
- Allen's test
- Involvement of the ectopic sites

TREATMENT[3,4]

NONSURGICAL OPTIONS

- Many modalities have been tried without consistent success (radiotherapy, ultrasound, colchicine, interferon).
- **Steroid injections** may be helpful for **isolated, painful palmar nodules,** but will not change the natural history of the disease.
- Collagenase injections show promise, but its role is not yet clear.
- Patients without functional limitations should be observed.

SURGICAL OPTIONS

- **Subcutaneous fasciotomy**
  Division of the fascia only with no resection through very limited incisions
  - **Least** effective option
  - Use only in **very sick or debilitated patients** who cannot tolerate more extensive surgery
- **Limited or partial fasciectomy**
  Grossly involved fascia is removed, often along with one or more rays, leaving most of the fascia behind
  - **Most commonly used technique**
- **Radical fasciectomy**
  Extensive resection of the palmar and digital fascia
  - **Highest complication rate,** particularly hematoma
- **Dermatofasciectomy** (McCash's open palm technique)
  Removal of the fascia and the overlying skin
  - Used most often for extensive skin involvement, severe PIP joint contractures, or recurrent cases
  - **Typically requires a skin graft closure,** occasionally a dorsal rotational flap closure.

INCISIONS

- **Longitudinal incisions** over the cords, closed with multiple Z-plasties
  - Most common technique
  - Allows some lengthening without substantial ischemic complications
- **Transverse incisions**
  - Commonly used in the palm
  - May leave portions open to close by secondary intention, reducing the risk of hematoma
- **Limited exposure** when multiple transverse incisions are used in the digits
- **Bruner incisions**
  - Limited lengthening by closing with V-Y flaps in each limb
  - May be more ischemic than longitudinal incisions, particularly at the flap tips (Fig. 71-1)

GOALS OF SURGERY

- The entire fascia is potentially at risk and should not be removed, because this is essentially impossible.
- The tension line should be altered, shielding residual Dupuytren's tissue from reuniting tensile strength (firebreak concept).
- The PIP joint contractures are addressed surgically if the contracture remains after fasciotomy.
  - Checkrein ligament release
  - Volar capsulotomy
  - Collateral ligament release

Fig. 71-1   A, Longitudinal incisions.
1, T-shaped; *2,* Lazy S (NOT recommended); *3,* Bruner incisions;
4, Multiple V-Y with Z-plasties on
either end; *5,* Midline longitudinal
incision. **B,** Transverse incisions.
1, Most commonly used; *2,* Multiple
short transverse incisions. **C,** Minimal exposure. *1,* Moerman's short
curved incisions; *2,* Fasciotomy
incisions; *3,* Limited fasciotomy
incisions.

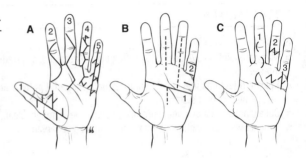

ROUTINE POSTOPERATIVE CARE

DRESSING
- Postoperative dressings or splint should be removed at 2-4 days to check wounds.
- Splinting can be omitted if the PIP joint is not involved.
- Sutures are removed at 2-3 weeks.
- Daily dressing changes are initiated for wounds left open.

SPLINTING
- Use an orthoplast splint in digital extension (some prefer position of function), fabricated at the first postoperative visit.
- **Static splinting at night** may continue for up to **3 months** depending on the severity of the contracture.
- **Serial splinting** may be required for cases in which vascular compromise does not allow full opera-tive extension.

MOBILIZATION
- **Begin mobilization at the first postoperative visit.**
- Patient is to perform range-of-motion exercises daily.

COMPLICATIONS

HEMATOMA
- Risk is reduced when the incision is left open (McCash technique).
- Remove the tourniquet before closing, and establish meticulous hemostasis.

DIGITAL NERVE OR ARTERY INJURIES

CAUTION: The neurovascular bundle typically will be displaced superficially toward the midline if the spiral cords are involved.

TIP: Dissection should start at the palm and proceed distally. Alternatively the bundles can be identified distal to the involved area and the dissection is directed proximally.

A tight piece of the diseased fascia can look like a nerve and vice versa; proceed cautiously.

FLAP NECROSIS
- Reduce risk with careful choice of incisions.
- Consider dermatofasciectomy for extensive skin involvement.

DUPUYTREN'S FLARE RESPONSE
- A form of **complex regional pain syndrome** (CRPS) or **reflex sympathetic dystrophy** (RSD)
- Institute early aggressive hand therapy
- Consider methylprednisolone (Medrol) dose pack, or other pharmacologic treatment
- Sympathetic blockade advocated by some

FAILURE TO CORRECT THE CONTRACTURE
- **Inadequate resection of the involved fascia**
- Failure to address PIP joint contracture
- Failure to recognize attenuation of central slip of the extensor tendon
- Poor compliance with hand therapy

TIP: Recurrence is not a complication; it is the natural history of the disease.

- **Consider:**
  - Arthrodesis
  - Repeat fasciectomy
  - Closing wedge osteotomy of the distal part of the proximal phalanx

OUTCOMES

- Restoration of motion after extended follow-up is good.
- Durability of PIP joint contracture correction is marginal.
- **Recurrence is common.**
  - Occurs in 50% of patients after 5 years
  - Occurs in 100% of patients after 10 years
- Decreased sensation is common following revision surgery.
  - 68% had decreased sensation.
  - 11% had anaesthetic digits.

KEY POINTS

✔ Dupuytren's disease most commonly affects older males of northern European descent.
✔ The palm, ring, and small fingers are the most commonly affected.
✔ DD is associated with alcoholism, diabetes, epilepsy, and HIV infection; it is inherited in an autosomal dominant fashion with variable penetrance.
✔ Dupuytren's diathesis is an aggressive form of the disease characterized by knuckle pads, foot, and penis involvement.
✔ Cleland's ligament is **not** affected by DD.
✔ Watch out for the neurovascular bundle when a spiral cord is present, because it is displaced more volarly, proximally, and midline than normal.
✔ Operate if there is a functionally restricting MP contracture or any PIP joint contracture, or if there are maceration and/or hygiene issues.

REFERENCES

1. McFarlane RM. Patterns of the diseased fascia in the fingers in Dupuytren's contracture. Plast Reconstr Surg 54:31-44, 1974.
2. McFarlane RM. On the origin and spread of Dupuytren's disease [review]. J Hand Surg Am 27:385-390, 2002.
3. Rives K, Gelberman R, Smith B, et al. Severe contractures of the proximal interphalangeal joint in Dupuytren's disease: Results of a prospective trial of operative correction and dynamic extension splinting. J Hand Surg Am 17:1153-1159, 1992.
4. Weinzweig N, Culver JE, Fleegler EJ. Severe contractures of the proximal interphalangeal joint in Dupuytren's disease: Combined fasciectomy with capsuloligamentous release versus fasciectomy alone. Plast Reconstr Surg 97:560-566, 1996.

72. Rheumatoid Arthritis

Ashkan Ghavami

Rheumatoid arthritis (RA) is a chronically progressive, autoimmune inflammatory disease process affecting synovial tissues.

CHARACTERISTICS[1,2]

- Invasion by *pannus* (inflammatory tissue)
  - Invades articular cartilage, joint spaces, ligamentous support, and flexor and extensor tendons
- Profound pain, **often worse in morning**
- Female/male ratio: 3:1

DIAGNOSIS

CLINICAL FINDINGS
- **Skin**
  - **Rheumatoid nodules**
    - ▸ Occur in 25% of patients
    - ▸ Subcutaneous inflammatory masses (at ulna near elbow)
    - ▸ Correlates with worse prognosis
- **Joints**
  - **"Z deformities"** from loss of joint tissue support (e.g., ulnar deviation of metacarpophalangeal [MP] joints caused by radial deviation of metacarpals)
  - **Arthritis mutilans:** Osteolysis with profound destruction of joint cartilage and bony surfaces
- **Tendons**
  - Tenosynovitis (50% incidence in RA overall)
  - Wrist tendon ruptures
    - ▸ Most common extensor ruptures are, in order of frequency:
      1. Extensor digiti minimi [EDM]
      2. Extensor digitorum communis [EDC] 5
      3. EDC 4
      4. Extensor pollicis longus [EPL]
      5. EDC 3
  - Flexor tendon triggering (trigger finger) sometimes leads to rupture; **flexor pollicis longus (FPL)** is most common flexor tendon rupture
  - Swan neck and boutonniere deformities
- **Muscles**
  - Intrinsic muscle atrophy from disuse
  - Inflammation
  - Cervical myopathy or nerve compression (particularly median and posterior interosseous nerves [PIN])

- **Nerves**
  - Inflammatory tenosynovitis involving carpal, cubital, and/or radial tunnels
  - Example: PIN compression and/or paralysis from radiohumeral joint synovitis
- **Vessels**
  - Vasculitis
  - Raynaud's phenomenon
- **Extraarticular involvement**
  - **Respiratory**
    - ► Nodules
    - ► Pleuritis
  - **Cardiac**
    - ► Valvular
    - ► Pericarditis
    - ► Myocarditis
  - **Hematologic:** Anemia
    - ► *Felty's syndrome;* also splenomegaly and lymphadenopathy
  - **Ocular**
    - ► Uveitis
    - ► Iritis
  - **Neurologic**
    - ► Polyneuropathy
  - **Multisystem**
    - ► Sjögren's syndrome

DIFFERENTIAL DIAGNOSIS

- Osteoarthritis (OA)
- Psoriatic arthritis
- Gout and pseudogout
- Systemic lupus erythematosus (SLE)
- Ankylosing spondylitis
- Scleroderma
- Reiter's syndrome
- Sjögren's syndrome

LABORATORY TESTS

- **Positive rheumatoid factor**
  - IgM or IgG rheumatoid factors present in **70%-80%** of RA patients (seropositivity indicates less favorable prognosis)
- Increased erythrocyte sedimentation rate (ESR) and C-reactive protein, decreased hemoglobin

IMAGING

- **Radiographs**
  - Periarticular osteoporosis and soft tissue swelling
  - Joint space narrowing
  - Marginal erosions
  - Symmetric bilateral involvement
  - Carpal ankylosis (bones appear fused)

Fig. 72-1 Characteristic ulnar deviation of metacarpophalangeal joints. Note the severe joint destruction, particularly at the metacarpophalangeal joints. Patient has had previous thumb metacarpophalangeal joint arthrodesis with tendon band technique. (Courtesy Denton Watumull, MD.)

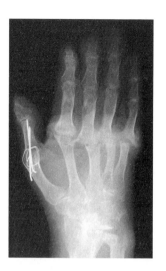

- Characteristic translation deformities (e.g., ulnar translation of carpus and ulnar deviation at MP joints) (Fig. 72-1)

DISEASE STAGING
- **Lister's three stages of RA**[3]
  - **Proliferative:** Synovial swelling causes pain, limited motion, and potential nerve compression.
  - **Destructive:** Synovial erosion results in tendon rupture, bone erosion, and capsular/ligament weakness.
  - **Reparative:** Extensive fibrosis causes tendon adherence and joint contractures.

RHEUMATOID VARIANTS AND AUTOIMMUNE DISEASES AFFECTING HANDS[4]

JUVENILE RHEUMATOID ARTHRITIS
- 80% of children are affected: Seronegative disease process.
- **Z deformities are reversed:** Ulnar deviation of metacarpals and radial deviation of digits.
- Swan neck and boutonniere deformities, tendon ruptures, and nerve compression are rare.

PSORIATIC ARTHRITIS
- Seronegative spondyloarthropathy
- Can have arthritis mutilans, similar to RA
- **Unlike RA**
  - Distal interphalangeal **(DIP)** joints involved
  - Fusiform digital swelling
  - Characteristic scaly extensor surface skin plaques
    - ▸ Often precedes joint involvement

SYSTEMIC LUPUS ERYTHEMATOSUS
- **Multisystem disease** in young women
  - Renal
  - Cardiac (pericarditis)
  - Respiratory, integument "butterfly" (malar) rash
- Commonly involves multiple joints, including hands
- **Hand findings**
  - Joints involved, but **no cartilage destruction** with **normal joint spaces**
  - **Hallmark:** Ligamentous and volar plate laxity; tendon subluxation

- **Mainstay treatment**
  - ▸ Pharmacologic
  - ▸ Splinting
  - ▸ Exercise

SCLERODERMA
- ■ **Can involve:**
  - • Skin
  - • Gastrointestinal tract
  - • Kidneys
  - • Lungs
  - • Heart
  - • Hands
- ■ Small vessel vasculitis

RAYNAUD'S PHENOMENON
- ■ Intermittent vasospasm: Decreased digital circulation, then skin ulcerations
- ■ Can progress to gangrene requiring digital amputation
- ■ Web-space contractures (first web space)
- ■ **CREST syndrome:** *Systemic sclerosis*
  - • **C**alcinosis
  - • **R**aynaud's phenomenon
  - • **E**sophageal dysfunction
  - • **S**clerodactyly
  - • **T**elangiectasias
- ■ **Hand deformities**
  - • Similar to RA
  - • Decreased circulation may cause wound-healing problems postoperatively

NONSURGICAL THERAPY

PHARMACOTHERAPY
- ■ *Mainstay of RA treatment*
- ■ **Medications**
  - • **NSAIDs:** First-line agents
    - ▸ Aspirin
    - ▸ Naproxen
    - ▸ Indomethacin
  - • **Corticosteroids**
    - ▸ Helpful as local injection
    - ▸ Systemic use for severe flare-ups
  - • **Immunomodulators:** Less commonly used
    - ▸ Azathioprine (Imuran®)
    - ▸ Methotrexate
    - ▸ Hydroquinones
    - ▸ Cyclosporine (Restasis®)

- **Antimonoclonal antibody compounds:** Have changed disease management and lessened severity of RA in developed countries
  - ▸ Etanercept (Enbrel®)
  - ▸ Infliximab (Remicade®)

INTRAARTICULAR STEROID INJECTIONS
- Indicated for severe joint pain
- Provides transient benefit
- Limited by multiple joint involvement

JOINT PROTECTION AND SPLINTING
- Decreases excess wear of joints and tendons; counteracts deforming forces
- Decreases deformity severity and can simplify surgical plan
- Does not prevent disease progression
- Must include non–weight-bearing exercise program

SURGICAL PRINCIPLES[3]

MULTIDISCIPLINARY APPROACH
- Rheumatologist
  - Maximize preoperative medical treatment
  - Ensure proper postoperative care
- Occupational therapists

GENERAL PRINCIPLES
- **Indications for surgery**
  - Progressive deformities that are **functionally limiting** or **painful** and have become **unresponsive to conservative therapy**

NOTE: The presence of a deformity is <u>not</u> by itself an indication for surgical treatment.

TIP: Timing and type of surgical treatment is critical and probably best reserved for hand surgeons specializing in RA surgery.

- **Surgical goals** (in order of decreasing importance)[4]
  - Operate on painful joints before other joints
  - Restore function; provide stability and mobility
  - Prevent further progression
    - ▸ Prophylactic tenosynovectomy
    - ▸ Carpal tunnel release with flexor tenosynovectomy
  - Cosmesis
    - ▸ More important for younger patients
- **Early tenosynovectomy**
  - Indicated if medical therapy fails within 6 months

NOTE: Tenosynovectomy is the most commonly indicated operation for RA.

- **Operative goal:** Decrease tendon rupture risk, decrease flexor tendon triggering, and decompress median nerve
- **Rheumatoid thumb:** 50% of hand function
- **Any** disability should be treated.
- **Silastic MP joint arthroplasty:** Decreases pain, increases function (MP joint arthroplasties are more effective than PIP joint arthroplasties)

TIP: Evaluate cervical spine preoperatively for subluxation. Takes precedence over upper extremity operations.

TENDONS

EXTENSOR TENDONS[5,6]
- **Dorsal tenosynovitis** (early finding)
- **Rupture**
  - **Mechanism:** Direct invasion versus weakening from pannus or mechanical attrition caused by dorsal osteophytes and prominent bony surfaces
  - Tenodesis mechanism (finger extension during passive wrist flexion) not present *(diagnostic)*
  - Rule out:
    - Tendon ulnar subluxation at MP joints
    - MP joint dislocation
    - Extensor paralysis (e.g., PIN paralysis: Positive tenodesis extension but no passive extension maintained)
  - **Vaughan-Jackson lesion:** Prominent ulnar head (styloid) causing EDC rupture and EDM rupture from attrition
- **Treatment and surgical principles**
  1. Use sharp dissection tenosynovectomy.
     - Can be prophylactic if tenosynovitis has lasted more than 6 months with medical therapy
  2. Preserve proximal extensor retinaculum and frayed (intact) tendons.
  3. Use retinacular flaps to stabilize tendons (e.g., extensor carpi ulnaris [ECU]) in position.
  4. Address ruptures when present.
     - **Tendon rupture repair**
       - **Single ruptures:** Suture distal stump to EDC
       - **Double ruptures:** Suture distal stumps to EDC; extensor indicis proprius (EIP) transfer
       - **Isolated EPL rupture:** EIP transfer
       - **Multiple ruptures:** Flexor digitorum superficialis (FDS) transfers

---

TIP: If rupture is caused by caput ulnae syndrome or other fixed joint abnormality, then correct the joint deformity (arthroplasty or arthrodesis) at the same time as or before tendon repair.

FLEXOR TENDONS
- **Treatment**
  - **Tenosynovectomy:** Similar to extensors
    - Indicated before any tendon operation and when simultaneous carpal tunnel or trigger finger release performed

NOTE: A1 pulley is not released for RA.

- **FPL rupture** *(Mannerfelt lesion)*
  - ▸ Commonly occurs from attrition by scaphoid bone osteophytes
  - ▸ Treatment
    - ✦ Tenosynovectomy
    - ✦ Osteophyte excision
    - ✦ FDS transfer (from index finger) or tendon graft
    - ✦ Interphalangeal joint arthrodesis
- **Flexor digitorum profundus (FDP) and FDS ruptures**
  - ▸ Caused by direct pannus invasion
  - ▸ Treatment
    - ✦ Tenosynovectomy
    - ✦ FDS slip excision
    - ✦ Adjacent FDP transfers for FDP rupture
    - ✦ Tendon grafting
    - ✦ DIP arthrodesis

SPECIFIC DEFORMITIES

SWAN NECK DEFORMITIES
- **Mechanism** (Fig. 72-2)
  - Intrinsic tightness
  - Hyperextension at PIP joint and lax volar plate
  - Eventual DIP/MP joint hyperflexion, PIP joint hyperextension
- **Treatment**
  - **Early stages:** Intrinsic release, flexor synovectomy, and lateral band transfer
    - ▸ Correct any subluxations of MP joint that are present.
    - ▸ If PIP joint is passively mobile at various MP angles, then splint PIP, fuse DIP, or reconstruct retinacular system.
  - **Late stage:** Joint destruction present
    - ▸ Use arthroplasty instead of arthrodesis

BOUTONNIERE DEFORMITIES
- **Mechanism** (see Fig. 72-2)
  - PIP joint synovitis causes extensor stretch (central slip attenuation).
  - Lateral bands move volarly and become fixed with tight oblique retinacular ligament of Landsmeer (ORL).
  - Hyperextension of DIP joint ensues.

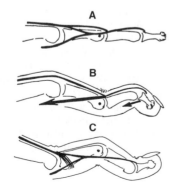

Fig. 72-2 Characteristic swan neck and boutonniere deformities. **A,** Normal. **B,** Swan neck. **C,** Boutonniere deformity. (From Lister G. Rheumatoid arthritis, its variants, and osteoarthritis. In Smith P. Lister's the Hand, 4th ed. London: Churchill Livingstone, 2002, pp 331-397.)

- **Treatment**
  - Use early synovectomy and dynamic splinting.
  - If PIP flexion is affected (but not fixed/frozen), then consider central slip shortening procedures, extensor tenotomy, or lateral band repositioning.
  - If deformity is severe (e.g., frozen PIP joint), consider arthroplasty over fusion.

ELBOW JOINTS

EXTRAARTICULAR DISEASE

- Synovitis, antecubital cysts, and bony spurs can cause PIN compression
- **Treatment:** Prompt nerve decompression

INTRAARTICULAR DISEASE

- **Treatment**
  - **Synovectomy and radial head excision**
    - ▶ 90% pain relief
  - **Elbow arthroplasty (controversial)**
    - ▶ Limited studies
    - ▶ Significant complication rates

SUBCUTANEOUS NODULES

- **Treatment**
  - Steroid injections can cause regression of nodule with possible ulceration.
  - If pain is significant, then excise.
    - ▶ Recurrence is common with nodules in any location.

WRIST JOINTS

TIP: Do not perform wrist operations before more distal surgery.

- **Synovectomy**
  - May help early for minimal deformity, slow disease, and painful, swollen wrists
- **Repositioning ECU and extensor carpi radialis longus (ECRL)**
  - Rebalances force vectors early in disease process
- **Wrist arthrodesis:** Total or limited
  - Predictable pain relief; best for low-demand patients or advanced disease
  - Radiolunate fusion: When midcarpal joints are normal
- **Wrist arthroplasty:** For higher-demand patients
  - **Biaxial total wrist devices:** Metal on plastic, cemented, or noncemented
    - ▶ **Complications:** Loosening, dislocation, soft tissue imbalance, infection
  - **Silicone (Swanson) total wrist implants**
    - ▶ For very-low-demand patients with little bone stock

▶ Must be willing to trade improvement in pain with minimal mobility
  ✦ *High complication rate:* Up to **65%** implant fracture rate,[1] subsidence, resorption around implant, particulate synovitis, high reoperation rate
■ **Distal radioulnar joint (DRUJ)**
  • Most stability is from ligamentous support.
  • Extensive synovitis and loss of triangular fibrocartilage complex (TFCC) support is common.
■ **Caput ulnae syndrome**
  • Dorsal ulnar head prominence
  • Carpal supination
  • ECU volar subluxation from DRUJ synovitis and capsular stretch
  • May have positive *piano key sign*
  • **Treatment**
    ▶ **Tenosynovectomy:** Never perform as isolated procedure
    ▶ **Darrach's procedure**
      ✦ Resection of distal 2 cm of ulnar head
      ✦ Stabilization of remaining stump
      ✦ **Indications**
        - Tendon impingement
        - Intractable pain at DRUJ
        - Deformity of DRUJ
        - Extensor tendon rupture from ulnar subluxation
    ▶ **Sauve-Kapandji (SK) procedure**
      ✦ Limited ulnar head osteotomy
      ✦ Arthrodesis from ulnar head to sigmoid notch
      ✦ Preserve an attached bony and soft tissue shelf to resist ulnar subluxation and DRUJ pain

NOTE: Newer variations of the Darrach and SK procedures involve interposition of soft tissue (e.g., pronator teres).

METACARPAL AND INTERPHALANGEAL JOINTS

■ **Mechanism:** MP joint ulnar collateral ligament and capsule attenuated to volar plate and stretched
  • Ulnar drift
  • Volar subluxation
  • Extensor tendon subluxation into intermetacarpal valleys
■ **Treatment**
  • Joint synovitis managed medically when problem isolated
  • Synovectomy
  • Ligament reconstruction
  • Intrinsic muscle release or transfer if ulnar drift is more than 30 degrees[1]
  • Joint reconstruction (arthroplasty or arthrodesis) if bone or cartilage erosion is significant
    ▶ **Arthroplasty**
      ✦ **Swanson implant:** Excellent functional results for MP joint; acts as a spacer
        - **Complications:** Fractures (although not an indication for removal) and synovitis
      ✦ **Pyrolytic carbon implant arthroplasty:** Good for PIP and MP joints

> **Arthrodesis**
  - Reserved for **IP joints** (especially DIP joint)
  - **PIP:** 40 degrees of flexion for the index finger, adding 5 degrees for each digit moving ulnarly to restore cascade
  - **DIP:** Up to 20 degrees of flexion
  - Index finger, metacarpal fusion: 5-10 degrees of supination to aid pinch mechanism

RHEUMATOID THUMB

BOUTONNIERE DEFORMITY

- **Etiologic factors**
  - Attenuation of extensor pollicis brevis (EPB)
  - Extensor hood laxity
  - Ulnar and volar subluxation of EPL caused by MP synovitis
  - Subluxation of proximal phalanx on the metacarpal head
  - Hyperextension of IP joint, flexion of MP joint
- **Treatment**
  - **Mild deformity:** MP joint synovectomy, EPL rerouting
  - **Moderate:** MP joint arthrodesis
    > MP joint arthroplasty if there is carpometacarpal (CMC) or IP level destruction
  - **Severe (fixed deformity):** MP arthroplasty or arthrodesis

SWAN NECK DEFORMITY

- **Etiologic factors**
  - CMC disease causing dorsoradial subluxation of thumb ray during opposition and grasp functions
- **Treatment**
  - CMC implant hemiarthroplasty for mild to moderate cases
  - MP joint fusion with resection arthroplasty of CMC and partial release of adductor and dorsal interosseous attachments

INTERPHALANGEAL JOINT

- **If unstable or destroyed**
  - Arthrodesis: procedure of choice to provide stable pinch with no functional loss; proximal joints must have adequate ROM

TIP: Determine arthrodesis angle by positioning thumb against tip of index finger.

METACARPOPHALANGEAL JOINT

- Synovectomy
- Arthrodesis: When articular bony or cartilaginous joint destruction present
  - Angles: 15 degrees of flexion, 5-10 degrees of abduction, and 20 degrees of pronation
- **Gamekeeper's thumb:** Reconstruction of ulnar collateral ligament (UCL) may be required using volar portion of abductor pollicis longus (APL) or free flexor carpi radialis (FCR) tendon graft

CARPOMETACARPAL JOINT
- Resection arthroplasty, ligament reconstruction, and soft tissue interposition
- Similar to thumb CMC osteoarthritis

OUTCOMES

TENOSYNOVECTOMY
- Does **not** alter course of joint disease progression
- Often performed with wrist arthrodesis or MP arthroplasty
- Good outcomes for pain and grip strength
- Poor ROM improvement

TENDON RUPTURE
- Variable reports
- Difficult to study because of different rupture combinations with varied stages of joint disease
- Less favorable outcomes when multiple ruptures

MP ARTHROPLASTY
- Short-term: Strength improved
- Long-term: Strength not maintained, but pain generally does not recur
- Correction of ulnar drift improves the gripping and pinching mechanism
- Total ROM not as improved as arc of motion
- Short-term daily hand function improvements good (few long-term studies)
- Late fractures often seen on radiographs, but not significant

WRIST ARTHROPLASTY
- Very limited indications for Swanson implants
  - Up to 90% have no pain or mild pain[1]
  - High complication rate (see previous discussion), but helps preserve daily activity mobility better than arthrodesis
- Biaxial metal implants possibly superior; are becoming more popular

WRIST ARTHRODESIS
- Treatment of choice for severe wrist disease and high-demand patients
- Up to 100% pain relief[1]

DRUJ
- SK procedure good for young patients
  - Improves cosmesis and wrist stability
  - Better wrist ROM and forearm rotation postoperatively than with Darrach's procedure
- Darrach's procedure with synovectomy and TFCC reconstruction: Procedure of choice for caput ulnae syndrome[2]

KEY POINTS
✔ Rheumatoid arthritis is always treated by a rheumatologist in conjunction with medical management.
✔ Limit surgical intervention to progressive deformities that become functionally limiting or painful and are unresponsive to conservative therapy.
✔ Tenosynovectomy is the most commonly indicated operation and can be beneficial as a prophylaxis if medical treatment fails for more than 6 months.
✔ Always evaluate cervical spine for subluxation preoperatively.
✔ When joints are destroyed or fixed, consider arthrodesis over arthroplasty. Continue to perform any indicated tendon procedures.
✔ MP joint arthroplasty provides high patient satisfaction.

REFERENCES

1. Brown FE, Collins ED, Harmatz AS. Rheumatoid arthritis of the hand and wrist. In Achauer BM, Elof E, Guyuron B. Plastic Surgery: Indications, Operations, and Outcomes, vol 4. St Louis: Mosby, 2000, pp 2249-2274.
2. Feldon P, Terrono AL, Nalebuff EA. Rheumatoid arthritis in the hand and wrist. In Green DP, Hotchkiss RN, Pederson WC, eds. Operative Hand Surgery, vol 2, 4th ed. Philadelphia: Churchill Livingstone, 1998, pp 1651-1739.
3. Lister G. Rheumatoid arthritis, its variants, and osteoarthritis. In Smith P. Lister's the Hand, 4th ed. London: Churchill Livingstone, 2002, pp 331-397.
4. O'Brien ET. Surgical principles and planning for the rheumatoid hand and wrist. Clin Plast Surg 23:407-419, 1996.
5. Masson JA. Hand IV: Extensor tendons, Dupuytren's disease, and rheumatoid arthritis. Sel Read Plast Surg 35:23-34, 2003.
6. Richards RA, Wilson RL. Management of extensor tendons and the distal radioulnar joint in rheumatoid arthritis. J Am Soc Surg Hand 3:132-144, 2003.

73. Osteoarthritis

Ashkan Ghavami

INCIDENCE AND ETIOLOGIC FACTORS[1]

- Up to **40%** of adults are affected.
  - 10% of those affected seek medical attention.
- The incidence for **women is much greater than for men** and usually occurs at ages greater than 40 years.
- Multiple genetic factors are likely.
- Commonly, osteoarthritis (OA) results from:
  - Aging
  - Major trauma
  - Daily, repetitive microtrauma to joint(s)

DIAGNOSIS

CLINICAL ASSESSMENT

- **Joints involved** (in order of decreasing occurrence)
  - Distal interphalangeal (DIP) joints
  - Carpometacarpal (CMC) joints
  - Proximal interphalangeal (PIP) joints
  - Scaphotrapeziotrapezoidal (STT) joints
- **Pain during stressed movements**
  - In contrast to those with rheumatoid arthritis (RA), OA patients have **less pain in the morning** and **more pain during the day.**
  - OA often interferes with sleep.
- **RA and its variants** (see Chapter 72) **must be ruled out** with a detailed history and appropriate lab tests.

PHYSICAL EXAMINATION

- Locate the point of maximum tenderness.
- Perform stressed maneuvers to elicit characteristic pain.
  - **Grind test** (e.g., for thumb CMC osteoarthritis, axially directed thumb grinding performed on trapeziometacarpal joint)
- Identify lax ligaments.

IMAGING

- **Radiographic findings**
  - Narrowed joint space (late disease)
  - Subchondral sclerosis (eburnation) or cyst formation
  - Bony exostosis and osteophyte production
- **Specific views:** Robert's view for CMC osteoarthritis and stress views for ligament laxity

NONOPERATIVE TREATMENT

- Nonsteroidal antiinflammatory drugs (NSAIDs)
  - Provide pain relief and slow the inflammatory process
- Splinting and exercise
- Steroid injections
  - Injections can provide good long-term relief in early disease.[2]
  - Example: With a treatment of one injection for thumb CMC arthritis, 80% of patients with stage I disease sustained pain relief beyond 18 months.[2]
  - Excess injections can further weaken ligamentous support.
- Activity modification
  - Avoidance of unnecessary microtrauma from repetitive motions or joint postures

CMC JOINT OF THE THUMB

- Also known as the **basal joint** or **trapeziometacarpal (TMC)** joint
- Second most commonly involved joint in OA
- Stability of TMC joint largely dependent on **anterior oblique ligament** or **volar "beak" ligament**[3]
  - Beak ligament: From volar-ulnar area of metacarpal to trapezium
  - Limits dorsal translation of thumb metacarpal (MC)
  - *Ligament stretched or severely attenuated in OA*
- **Signs and symptoms**
  - Pain
  - Swelling
  - Crepitus
  - Weak lateral pinch (pulling pants up or holding large objects)
- **Provocative tests during physical examination**
  - Compression grind test (crepitus plus pain)
  - TMC stress tests
  - Torque test
  - Resisted-opposition maneuvers
- **Eaton's four radiographic stages of CMC joint degeneration**[4]
  Stage I: Slight joint narrowing, possible ligament laxity
  Stage II: Slight joint narrowing and minimal sclerosis, osteophytes less than 2 mm
  Stage III: Significant joint narrowing, sclerosis, large osteophytes, and cysts (Fig. 73-1)
  Stage IV: Arthritic changes seen at scaphotrapezial joint

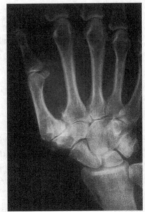

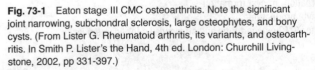

Fig. 73-1 Eaton stage III CMC osteoarthritis. Note the significant joint narrowing, subchondral sclerosis, large osteophytes, and bony cysts. (From Lister G. Rheumatoid arthritis, its variants, and osteoarthritis. In Smith P. Lister's the Hand, 4th ed. London: Churchill Livingstone, 2002, pp 331-397.)

THUMB CMC JOINT SURGICAL OPTIONS[3,5-9]

- **Indications for surgery**
  - Failure of conservative measures
  - Pain and joint instability disabling
  - First web space contracture
- **Goals of surgical treatment**
  - Excision of degenerated joint to establish a stable space between thumb metacarpal and scaphoid
  - Stability of thumb metacarpal joint during motions (e.g., lateral pinch)
- **Ligament reconstruction tendon interposition (LRTI) arthroplasty[5]**
  - **Most common** procedure performed today: 95% satisfaction rate[10]
  - Long-term outcomes (6 years): Pain relief and improved grip strength for 95% of patients[10]
  - **Principles**
    1. **Excision of degenerative surface:** Trapezium with or without MC base
    2. **Tissue interposition:** Tendon, rib allograft, or autograft to help maintain metacarpal scaphoid space
    3. **Beak ligament reconstruction:** Usually using distally based flexor carpi radialis (FCR) (radial half or whole tendon) or adductor pollicis longus (APL) as suspension ligament
  - **Current techniques[5]** (Fig. 73-2)
    - ▶ Modified Burton and Pellegrini technique[3]
      - ✦ Trapezial excision: Whole versus partial, based on extent of trapezial and/or scaphoid involvement
      - ✦ Beak ligament reconstruction with distally based, whole to half of FCR tendon
      - ✦ Remaining FCR, after tunneled through metacarpal, tied to itself and "anchovied" as a spacer
    - ▶ **Other variations**
      - ✦ APL used as suspending ligament
      - ✦ FCR brought through a "T-shaped bony tunnel" in MC for suspension
      - ✦ FCR anchored to metacarpal base with Mitek™ bone anchor suture (Mitek Surgical Products, Norwood, MA) to allow suspension
      - ✦ Other material (allograft, rib graft, or hematoma) to fill space

---

TIP: Choose a technique with which you are comfortable and that gives predictable results in your hands.

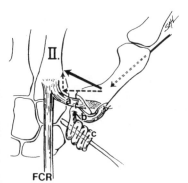

Fig. 73-2 Ligament reconstruction with tendon interposition arthroplasty. The distally based FCR tendon is tunneled through the first metacarpal base toward a dorsoradial exit hole, sutured back onto itself, and "anchovied" into the trapezial space. (From Burton RI, Pellegrini VD Jr. Surgical management of basal joint arthritis of the thumb. Part II: Ligament reconstruction with tendon interposition arthroplasty. J Hand Surg Am 11:324-332, 1986.)

FCR

- **Implant arthroplasty:** No longer used because of high complication rates
- **Ligament reconstruction (without interposition)**
  - For hypermobile CMC joints and beak ligament laxity in Eaton stage I and II disease, use distally based half of FCR strip.
- **Arthrodesis or metacarpal osteotomy**
  - Closing-wedge osteotomy of MC base with minimal instability in stage I or II: 30-degree volar and radial abduction (15-degree pronation)
  - **Indication**
    - ▸ Young, high-demand laborers
  - **Contraindications**
    - ▸ Pantrapezial OA
    - ▸ Stiff metacarpophalangeal (MP) or interphalangeal (IP) joints of thumb
    - ▸ Nonunion rates as high as 50%[8]
- **Trapezial excision alone**
  - K-wires used to maintain space but still lose approximately 50% of space
  - Perhaps better indicated for elderly, low-demand patients
  - Significant subsidence without LRTI combination
  - Dead space filled by hematoma and subsequent fibrosis

THUMB METACARPOPHALANGEAL JOINT

- *Most common digit requiring surgical intervention for OA*
- **Mechanism**
  - MC base subluxation caused by MP joint degeneration
  - First web space narrowed by MC adduction deformity
  - Hyperextension deformity or instability
- **Treatment goals**
  - Provide good pinch grip, resistance, and stability
  - If hyperextension is more than 30 degrees, then perform MP joint arthrodesis (15 degrees flexion and 10 degrees pronation), volar plate capsulodesis, or APL advancement
  - If hyperextension is less than 30 degrees, then use K-wire pin.

PIP JOINT

- **Mechanism:** Often posttraumatic
- **Treatment**
  - Conservative, standard modalities
  - **Surgical indication:** Pain, deformity, osteophyte impingement *(Bouchard's nodes)*
    - ▸ **Arthrodesis:** Especially for index finger, to provide solid post for pinch
    - ▸ **Arthroplasty:** Preferred in ring finger and small finger to assist with power grip
      - ♦ Requires adequate bone stock and intact, balanced flexion and extension mechanism

DIP JOINT

- *Most commonly affected joint in OA*
- Rarely disabling or painful if without mucous cyst and/or *Heberden's nodes*
- **Mucous cyst or ganglion**
  - Osteophyte spurs
  - Eccentric location (ulnar, or radial, to terminal tendon)
  - May compress germinal matrix (nail-grooving or deformity) or overlying thin skin
  - **Treatment**
    - ▸ **Excision:** For pain or impending rupture or cosmetic deformity (nail deformity)
    - ✦ Preserve at least half of the terminal tendon.
    - ✦ Must excise osteophytes or cyst will recur.
    - ✦ Use a rotation flap to improve skin healing.

HEBERDEN'S NODES
- Painful osteophytes of DIP joint
- Can enlarge and cause obvious deformity
- **Treatment**
  - NSAIDs, rest, and possible intraarticular steroid injection (often very painful), splinting possibly helpful otherwise
  - Joint fused in up to 20 degrees of flexion for pain, functional deformity, and instability

TIP: Do not cross K-wires at fusion site. Use H-shaped or Y-shaped incision or small rotation flap for better skin healing, and leave germinal matrix intact to prevent nail growth problems.

PISOTRIQUETRAL ARTHRITIS

SYMPTOMS
- Pain is felt over the volar-ulnar wrist area.
- One third of patients have ulnar neuropathy.
  - Symptoms elicited by hand resting on hard surfaces (writing, computer use)

EXAMINATION
- **Provocative maneuver:** Compression and side-to-side shucking elicits severe pain over the pisotriquetral joint.

TREATMENT
- Use steroid injection and splint wrist in slight flexion.
- If no relief is obtained after two injections, consider pisiform excision, with or without a minimal triquetral excision.

KEY POINTS

✔ Women are more commonly affected by trapeziometacarpal arthritis than men, usually after menopause.

✔ As for RA, treat with medical management, steroid injections, and splinting before considering surgical intervention.

✔ LRTI arthroplasty for thumb CMC arthritis treatment gives excellent long-term success; 95% of patients obtain significant pain relief and grip improvement.[10]

✔ LRTI is based on three principles:
 • Excision of degenerative surface (trapezial resection)
 • Tissue interposition (e.g., tendon, rib allograft, or autograft) to help maintain trapezial space
 • Beak ligament reconstruction, usually using distally based FCR (radial half or whole tendon)

REFERENCES

1. Bednar MS, Light TR. Degenerative arthritis. In Achauer BM, Eriksson E, Guyuron B, et al, eds. Plastic Surgery: Indications, Operations, and Outcomes, vol 4. St Louis: Mosby, 2000, pp 2235-2248.
2. Bettinger PC, Linscheid RL, Berger RA, et al. An anatomic study of the stabilizing ligaments of the trapezium and trapeziometacarpal joint. J Hand Surg Am 24:476-482, 1999.
3. Burton RI, Pellegrini VD Jr. Surgical management of basal joint arthritis of the thumb. Part II: Ligament reconstruction with interposition arthroplasty. J Hand Surg Am 11:324-332, 1986.
4. Davis TR, Brady O, Dias JJ. Excision of the trapezium for osteoarthritis of the trapeziometacarpal joint: A study of the benefit of ligament reconstruction or tendon interposition. J Hand Surg Am 29:1069-1077, 2004.
5. Day CS, Gelberman R, Patel AA, et al. Basal joint osteoarthritis of the thumb: A prospective trial of steroid injection and splinting. J Hand Surg Am 29:247-251, 2004.
6. Eaton RG, Glickel SZ. Trapeziometacarpal osteoarthritis: Staging as a rationale for treatment. Hand Clin 3:455-471, 1987.
7. Lister G. Rheumatoid arthritis, its variants, and osteoarthritis. In Smith P. Lister's the Hand, 4th ed. London: Churchill Livingstone, 2002, pp 331-397.
8. Tomaino MM. Ligament reconstruction tendon interposition arthroplasty for basal joint arthritis: Rationale, current technique, and clinical outcome. Hand Clin 17:207-221, 2001.
9. Tomaino MM, Pellegrini VD, Burton RI. Arthroplasty of the basal joint of the thumb: Long-term follow-up after ligament reconstruction with tendon interposition. J Bone Joint Surg Am 77:346-355, 1995.
10. Young SD, Mikola EA. Thumb carpometacarpal arthrosis. J Am Soc Surg Hand 4:73-93, 2004.

74. Vascular Disorders of the Hand and Wrist

George Broughton II*

DIAGNOSIS

Compared with vascular disorders elsewhere in the body, vascular disorders in the hand are very uncommon.

- Three methods are used to make a diagnosis of vascular disorders in the hand.
  - History and physical examination (see Chapter 50)
  - Noninvasive studies using Doppler imaging
  - Invasive imaging studies (Table 74-1)

Table 74-1 *Imaging Studies*

Test Name	Purpose	Comment
Magnetic resonance imaging (MRI)	MRI is the leading imaging modality in the diagnosis and follow-up of patients with vascular malformations. MRI should include T1- and T2-weighted spin-echo imaging in multiple planes, fat-saturated T1-weighted imaging with the intravenous administration of a gadolinium-based contrast agent, and gradient-recalled echo (GRE) imaging. For any vascular anomaly, the basic approach is to first evaluate fat-suppressed T2-weighted images to determine the extent of the anomaly, and then to evaluate the GRE images to decide whether the anomaly is a high-flow lesion.	MRI is commonly performed without a gradient-echo sequence or without the intravenous administration of contrast material. T2-weighted images are mainly used to evaluate the extent of the abnormality; GRE images are used to identify the hemodynamic nature of the condition (high- versus low-flow lesion); and contrast-enhanced images are used to determine the extent of the malformation and to distinguish slow-flow vascular anomalies (VM versus LM).
Magnetic resonance angiography (MRA)	Among the available MRA techniques (time-of-flight [TOF] imaging, phase-contrast [PC] imaging, and contrast-enhanced imaging), contrast-enhanced MRA has been gaining widespread clinical use. The advantage of this technique relative to conventional angiography is that MRA permits the production of multiangular reprojections; it uses no ionizing radiation, and its contrast materials are less toxic than those of other modalities.	The technique is not yet standardized, and imaging characteristics are not well documented.

Continued

Data from Lee BB, Do YS, Yakes W, et al. Management of arteriovenous malformations: A multidisciplinary approach. J Vasc Surg 39:590-600, 2004; Menzoian JO, Doyle JE, LoGerfo FW, et al. Evaluation and management of vascular injuries of the extremities. Arch Surg 118:93-95, 1983; Newmeyer W. Vascular disorders. In Green DP, ed. Operative Hand Surgery, 3rd ed. Philadelphia: Churchill Livingstone, 1993, pp 2251-2308.

AVF, Arteriovenous fistulas; *AVM,* arteriovenous malformations; *LM,* lymphatic malformation; *VM,* venous malformation.

---

*The opinions or assertions contained herein are the private views of the author and are not to be construed as official or as reflecting the views of the Department of the Army or the Department of Defense.

Table 74-1 *Imaging Studies—cont'd*

Test Name	Purpose	Comment
Magnetic resonance venography (MRV)	MRV is commonly used for patients with low-flow vascular anomalies to identify those involving the venous system. MRV can also be performed with either flow-dependent angiographic techniques (TOF or PC imaging) or contrast-enhanced angiographic techniques.	MRV is commonly used to demonstrate the patency of the deep veins in the extremities before surgical debulking procedures.
Magnetic resonance lymphangiography (MRL)	MRL is used to demonstrate malignant lymph nodes by using special contrast agents or to evaluate the lymphatic system by using presaturated, heavily T2-weighted sequences without the administration of contrast material.	MRL is promising as an adjunct to the conventional MRI protocol for vascular anomalies and edematous extremities; however, the technique has not been fully integrated into mainstream practice.
Ultrasound (US)	Portability and availability are the main advantages of US. Duplex US, continuous-wave Doppler US, color Doppler US, and Doppler spectral analyses all are useful in the evaluation of vascular malformations.	Doppler spectral analysis can be used to differentiate arterial from venous flow. An experienced sonographer or radiologist is necessary for appropriate sonographic evaluation.
Computed tomography (CT)	CT is particularly useful for detecting phleboliths in VMs and evaluating bone overgrowth or lysis that may accompany vascular anomalies.	CT can also be used for patients who cannot be sedated for MRI or for patients in whom MRI is contraindicated (e.g., presence of a pacemaker or aneurysm clip).
Angiography	Angiography includes arteriography, venography, and direct intralesional contrast agent injection. Arteriography is the criterion standard for the evaluation of high-flow vascular anomalies, particularly for AVMs and AVFs.	Arteriography has no diagnostic value for assessing low-flow anomalies. However, venography and direct intralesional contrast material injections usually are performed during interventional procedures for low-flow vascular anomalies (particularly VMs) to confirm the diagnosis and to tailor the procedure (sclerotherapy). Occlusive venography can be helpful for assessing the extent of low-flow vascular anomalies.
Radiography	Plain radiographs have limited value in the diagnostic workup for vascular anomalies.	Plain radiographs can demonstrate phleboliths (characteristic of VMs), and they are helpful for evaluating leg-length discrepancies and/or osseous involvement.

Data from Lee BB, Do YS, Yakes W, et al. Management of arteriovenous malformations: A multidisciplinary approach. J Vasc Surg 39:590-600, 2004; Menzoian JO, Doyle JE, LoGerfo FW, et al. Evaluation and management of vascular injuries of the extremities. Arch Surg 118:93-95, 1983; Newmeyer W. Vascular disorders. In Green DP, ed. Operative Hand Surgery, 3rd ed. Philadelphia: Churchill Livingstone, 1993, pp 2251-2308.
AVF, Arteriovenous fistulas; *AVM,* arteriovenous malformations; *LM,* lymphatic malformation; *VM,* venous malformation.

- Vascular disorders can be placed into **five general groups:**
  1. Arterial problems in the hand or wrist
  2. Vascular compression in the neck
  3. Raynaud's phenomenon and related disorders
  4. Vascular tumors
  5. Arteriovenous (AV) malformations

ARTERIAL PROBLEMS

ULNAR ARTERY AND OTHER LOCAL ARTERY THROMBOSES[1,2]

Thrombosis of the ulnar artery in Guyon's canal can occur from direct trauma.

- Patients with ulnar artery thrombosis at the wrist may present with **pain at night or with repetitive activity** and **cold intolerance.**
- **Exquisite tenderness** is present at the site of thrombosis.
- Eventually, patients may have **dependent rubor** or **ulceration** at the tips of the ring and little fingers.
- Excitation of the sympathetic fibers of the ulnar proper digital nerves is frequently noted.
- Diagnosis is confirmed with **Allen's test.**
- **Arteriography** is often helpful before a definitive treatment is decided.
- The standard treatment is **ligation and resection of the thrombosed segment.**
- Reconstructing the artery with a vein graft is necessary only when backflow from the radial side of the arch is insufficient.

UPPER EXTREMITY ANEURYSMS[1,3]

- Most caused by **trauma**
- **Mycotic aneurysms** generally caused by injecting drugs into hand with dirty needle, but also can be caused by septic emboli
- Atherosclerotic aneurysms very rare
- More common in the wrist and digital arteries
- **True versus false (pseudo) aneurysms**
  - **True aneurysms**
    - **All three layers** of arterial wall are involved.
    - Aneurysms usually result from arterial wall weakness, from either trauma or disease.
    - **Trauma** is the most common cause.
      - An aneurysm in the hand can result from a single episode of blunt trauma or from repetitive trauma, such as using a jackhammer.
      - Repetitive trauma can result in **hypothenar hammer syndrome.**
- **Hypothenar hammer syndrome**
  - Results from thrombosis of ulnar artery in the area of Guyon's canal from **repeated blunt trauma** to base of hypothenar eminence
  - Results in media damage followed by aneurysm formation and eventual thrombosis
  - If intima damaged first, then thrombosis occurs first
  - Syndrome associated with cold intolerance, pain, and sometimes ulceration of ring and small fingers

---

TIP: *True* aneurysms are usually *fusiform shaped,* and *false* aneurysms are *saccular shaped.*

■ **False aneurysms**
  • Much **more common** than true aneurysms in the hand
  • Result from arterial perforation
  • Blood leaks into surrounding tissue
  • Hematoma resolves and cavity replaced by scar tissue (usually takes weeks)
  • Does **not** involve all three layers of the arterial wall
■ **Diagnosis**
  • Perform a physical examination; frequently, a **pulsatile painful mass** is felt.
  • If the aneurysm is deep or small, the patient may complain of pain in the digits from emboli and show pallor of digits.
  • Allen's test should be performed, and any of the imaging studies in Table 74-1 can be used, although an arteriogram is rarely needed.
■ **Treatment**
  • Resection and primary repair or vein graft is used.
  • If there is sufficient collateral flow, an aneurysm involving the arch can be resected and ligated.

TRAUMATIC ARTERIAL INJURIES[1,4]

■ The **radial artery** is the most commonly used arterial cannulation site.
■ In a review of the literature published from 1978 to 2001,[5] a total of 19,617 patients had radial artery cannulation, and the incidences of permanent ischemic damage and pseudoaneurysm were each **0.09%**.
■ There are **seven physical findings** that alert for a possible arterial injury.
  1. Decreased or absent pulse
  2. History of persistent arterial bleeding
  3. Large or expanding hematoma
  4. Major hemorrhage with hypotension
  5. Bruit at or distal to the artery
  6. Injury to an anatomically related nerve
  7. Anatomic proximity of a wound to a named artery
■ If physical findings are equivocal for an arterial injury, but the wound is in proximity to a named artery, then angiography is indicated.
■ If the audible Doppler signal is different between two paired extremities, then angiography is also indicated.
■ **Treatment:**
  • Table 74-2 summarizes different injury scenarios and recommended treatment strategies.

TIP: One can never go wrong in safely repairing normal anatomy.

EMBOLI[3,7]

Emboli to the arm and hand are an unusual event; approximately **15%** of all emboli go to the upper extremity.
■ **Source:** The **heart is the most common source,** resulting from arterial fibrillation or a recent myocardial infarction (MI). Other sources include:
  • Thoracic outlet syndrome
  • Atherosclerotic plaques
  • Subclavian and axillary artery aneurysm (traumatic or atherosclerotic)
  • Takayasu's disease and giant cell arteritis

Table 74-2 *Treatment Strategies for Arterial Injuries*

Injury	Treatment	Comment
Forearm vessel: Single with no nerve injury	Ligation	Gelberman et al[4] found that single, unrepaired arterial injuries caused modest consistent changes in hand vascularity but few clinical signs of ischemia or cold intolerance.
Forearm vessel: Single with nerve injury	Repair	Gelberman et al[4] found that an arterial injury combined with a nerve injury (especially the median nerve) resulted in decreased vascularity of the hands (which could be disabling). Repairing the artery had no effect on nerve recovery. Leclercq et al[6] had a different result. In a study of ulnar nerve and artery injuries, nerve recovery (both motor and sensory) was superior when the artery was repaired compared with a ligated or thrombosed artery.
Radial and ulnar artery	Repair	At a minimum, attempt to repair at least one artery, preferably the ulnar, and suture ligate the other ends of the other vessel.
Superficial palmar arch	Ligation	If there is brisk flow from both cut ends.
Superficial palmar arch	Repair	If there is sluggish or no flow from one end or the other.

Data from Perry MO, Thal ER, Shires GT. Management of arterial injuries. Ann Surg 173:403-408, 1971; Gelberman RH, Blasingame JP, Fronek A, et al. Forearm arterial injuries. J Hand Surg Am 4:401-408, 1979; Leclercq DC, Carlier AJ, Khuc T, et al. Improvement in the results in sixty-four ulnar nerve sections associated with arterial repair. J Hand Surg Am 10:997-999, 1985; Katz SG, Kohl RD. Direct revascularization for the treatment of forearm and hand ischemia. Am J Surg 165:312-316, 1993.

- Mechanical problems in a graft, usually an AV fistula graft for dialysis or an axillofemoral bypass graft
- Penetrating trauma
- Catheter-related
- Supracondylar humeral fractures

■ **Clinical presentation**

- Emboli from the heart are *macroemboli* and produce immediate symptoms of acute arterial obstruction (**the five Ps:** **P**ain, **p**allor, **p**ulselessness, **p**aresthesia, **p**oikilothermia).
- Emboli originating from an artery are either *atheroemboli* or *thromboemboli,* and will result in multiple *microemboli* showering the distal end arteries of the hand. This may result in Raynaud's phenomenon (see later in this chapter).

■ **Diagnosis is made by arteriography.** The groin should always be accessed so the subclavian and distal arteries can be entirely evaluated.

■ **Treatment**

- Emboli in the arteries need **aggressive treatment.**
- **Proximal arteriotomy with embolectomy using a Fogarty catheter** (small enough to pass through the superficial and deep arches in the hand) is the treatment of choice.
- If the patient has severe pain that is not alleviated by the following treatment plans, a **stellate ganglion block** may relieve acute symptoms of pain.
- A **cervicodorsal sympathectomy** may give long-term relief for chronic pain caused by distal small-vessel occlusion.

- **Emboli from the heart**
  - ▶ Patients should be started on **immediate intravenous heparin therapy** and undergo embolectomy.
  - ▶ Arterial embolization recurs in up to 33% of patients who do not receive long-term anticoagulative therapy.[3]
  - ▶ After an embolectomy, all patients must receive maintenance therapy with intravenous heparin to keep the activated partial thromboplastin time at 1.5-2.5 times the control values.
  - ▶ Patients should also receive **outpatient anticoagulation therapy** with oral warfarin or low-molecular-weight heparin. Treatment duration depends on the cause of the emboli (e.g., chronic atrial fibrillation, acute MI, etc.). Treatment is 95% effective.[3]
- **Emboli from sources other than the heart**
  - ▶ **Trauma**
    - ◆ **Penetrating and catheter-related**[5]
      - Although embolectomy alone is effective in treating 95% of patients with emboli of cardiac origin, thrombectomy alone is successful in restoring circulation in only **20%** of patients with catheter-related brachial artery occlusions.
      - Underlying pathology includes arterial stenosis at the site of arteriotomy closure, and intimal disruption from catheter manipulation.
      - In one series of arterial traumas, 80% of patients required arterial repair as well as clot retrieval. Treatment included primary resection and repair, vein patch angioplasty, and interposition vein grafting.
      - Level of arterial injury is often localized to **the site of arterial cannulation,** and perioperative arteriography is rarely warranted.
      - **Heparin** is used preoperatively to prevent propagation of distal thrombus but is discontinued once the operative repair is complete. Long-term anticoagulation therapy is **not** required.
    - ◆ **Supracondylar humeral fractures**
      - These fractures usually are seen in **children.**
      - **Noninvasive Doppler studies** may be helpful in documenting abnormal perfusion in the injured extremity.
      - The persistence of abnormal Doppler pressures after fracture reduction warrants operative exploration.
      - Arteriography may occasionally be helpful, but the risk of potential iatrogenic catheter injury in children mandates judicious use.
      - Brachial artery injury repairs are indicated in virtually all pediatric patients.
      - Thrombectomy and adjunctive arterial repairs are usually required.
  - ▶ **Subclavian and axillary arteries**
    - ◆ Regardless of underlying pathology, exclude the diseased proximal artery, restore circulation, and, for patients with macroembolization, retrieve distal clot.
    - ◆ Carotid-subclavian, axillary-axillary, and carotid-axillary bypass grafts have been used to reconstruct proximal arterial circulation, with excellent long-term patency.
    - ◆ Because early intervention is crucial for achieving limb salvage, **brachiocephalic arteriography** is strongly encouraged for all unexplained cases of upper extremity ischemia.
  - ▶ **Takayasu's disease and giant cell arteritis**
    - ◆ Both conditions often respond to **nonoperative therapy** with corticosteroids.
    - ◆ Surgery remains the mainstay of treatment for severely symptomatic, chronic, upper-extremity ischemia.
    - ◆ Treatment of subclavian artery lesions includes carotid-subclavian, axillary-axillary, or carotid-axillary bypass grafts.

- Excellent results and low morbidity can be expected with either surgical procedure.
- Autogenous vein bypass remains the treatment of choice for diseases of axillary and brachial arteries.
► **Thrombosed grafts**
  - **Intravenous heparin** therapy should be started as soon as the clinical problem is recognized.
  - **Embolectomy** should be performed in conjunction with revision of the thrombosed graft if possible.
  - Multiple graft configurations can be used depending on the vascular anatomy.
  - Three common polytetrafluoroethylene (PTFE) graft configurations include **forearm loop, upper arm straight,** and **brachial–internal jugular vein graft.**
  - Optimally, a new graft might remain patent for an **average of 8-19 months.**
  - Traditionally, surgical thrombectomy and revision of the venous end of the graft have been used to restore function to a thrombosed graft.
  - With each successful revision, the subsequent period of patency decreases.
  - Percutaneous endovascular thrombectomy and angioplasty of the venous anastomosis have been used to restore perfusion with improved secondary patency rates.[8]

THORACIC OUTLET SYNDROME[3,9-11]

Thoracic outlet syndrome refers to compression of the neurovascular structures at the superior aperture of the thorax.
- Thoracic outlet syndrome represents a constellation of symptoms.
- The cause, diagnosis, and treatment are controversial.
- Affected structures include the brachial plexus (95%), subclavian vein (4%), and subclavian artery (1%).
- Most presentations are nonemergent and require only symptomatic treatment and referral.

INCIDENCE
- Overall incidence remains controversial in the United States, with reports ranging from **3:1000 to 80:1000.**

SEX
- The sex ratio varies depending on the type of thoracic outlet syndrome.
- Overall, the syndrome is approximately **three times more common in women than in men.**
  - **Neurologic:** Female/male ratio is approximately 3.5:1
  - **Venous:** More common in males than in females
  - **Arterial:** No sexual predilection

AGE
- The onset of symptoms usually occurs between the ages of **20 and 50 years.**
- It *never* occurs before puberty and *rarely* after age 50 years.

HISTORY
- Patients with venous compression complain of an **ache or dull pain** and **swelling** in the affected arm.
- Patients also may complain of **engorged veins** on their hands and arms.
- Patients with arterial compression complain of "ischemic-like" pain or pain brought on when exercising an arm **(upper extremity claudication).**

CAUSES

- The **three major causes** of thoracic outlet syndrome are **anatomy, traumatic or repetitive activities,** and **neurovascular entrapment** at the costoclavicular space.
  - **Anatomy**
    - ▸ **Scalene triangle:** Anterior scalene muscle anteriorly, middle scalene muscle posteriorly, and the upper border of the first rib inferiorly account for most neurologic and arterial thoracic outlet syndrome cases.
    - ▸ **Cervical ribs** are involved in most **arterial** cases but rarely in venous and neurologic cases.
    - ▸ **Congenital fibromuscular bands** occur in as many as 80% of patients with neurologic thoracic outlet syndrome.
    - ▸ The transverse process of C7 is elongated.
  - **Traumatic or repetitive activities**
    - ▸ **Motor vehicle accident:** Hyperextension injury with subsequent fibrosis and scarring
    - ▸ **Effort vein thrombosis:** Spontaneous thrombosis of the axillary veins following vigorous arm exertion
    - ▸ **Playing a musical instrument:** Musicians particularly susceptible because of need to maintain the shoulder in abduction or extension for long periods
  - **Neurovascular entrapment**
    - ▸ Occurs in the costoclavicular space between first rib and head of clavicle

PHYSICAL FINDINGS

NOTE: In most cases, the physical examination findings are completely normal.[10,11]

- **Provocative tests,** such as Adson's maneuver or the costoclavicular and hyperabduction maneuvers, are unreliable.
  - With interscalene compression of the subclavian artery, Adson's test is positive if the radial pulse is lost when the affected arm is held in extension and dependent while the patient looks toward the ipsilateral shoulder.
  - *Approximately 92% of asymptomatic patients have variation in the strength of the radial pulse during positional changes.*
- The **EAST** *(elevated arm stress test)* is of debatable use, but it may be the most reliable screening test. It evaluates **all three types** of thoracic outlet syndrome.
  - The patient sits with the arms abducted 90 degrees from the thorax and the elbows flexed 90 degrees. The patient then opens and closes the hands for 3 minutes.
  - Patients with thoracic outlet syndrome cannot continue this for 3 minutes because symptoms soon appear. Patients with carpal tunnel syndrome experience dysesthesia in the fingers, but do not have shoulder or arm pain.
- **Venous**
  - Edema
  - Cyanosis
  - Distended superficial veins of the shoulder and chest
- **Arterial**
  - Pallor and pulselessness
  - Coolness on the affected side
  - Lower blood pressure in affected arm (a reliable indicator of arterial involvement)
  - Multiple small infarcts on hand and fingers (embolization)

IMAGING STUDIES

- **Cervical radiographs:** May demonstrate skeletal abnormality
- **Chest radiographs**
  - Cervical or first rib
  - Clavicle deformity
  - Pulmonary disease
  - Pancoast's tumor
- **Color-flow duplex scanning** for suspected vascular thoracic outlet syndrome
- **Arteriogram indications**
  - Evidence of peripheral emboli in the upper extremity
  - Suspected subclavian stenosis or aneurysm (e.g., bruit or abnormal supraclavicular pulsation)
  - Blood pressure differential greater than 20 mm Hg
  - Obliteration of radial pulse during EAST
- **Venography indications**
  - Persistent or intermittent edema of the hand or arm
  - Peripheral unilateral cyanosis
  - Prominent venous pattern over the arm, shoulder, or chest

TREATMENT

- **Surgical removal of the offending structure** (first rib, cervical rib, and middle third of the clavicle, scalenus muscle, or fibrous band) should be performed.
- If arterial obstruction is present, **thromboendarterectomy** or an **interposition graft** may be done. If symptoms persist, then a **cervicodorsal sympathectomy** may help alleviate hand pain and ischemia.
- Rarely, an arterial bypass graft may be needed.
- Venous obstruction may require the additional step of thrombectomy.
- Nonoperative treatment can be tried, but should not be continued for longer than 4 months if it fails. Options include:
  - Postural reeducation
  - Activity modification
  - Weight loss

RAYNAUD'S PHENOMENON AND RELATED DISORDERS[3,12-14]

Raynaud's phenomenon refers to reversible ischemia of peripheral arterioles. This can occur in response to a variety of stimuli, but it is most commonly caused by exposure to cold or stress.

- Raynaud's phenomenon is related to Raynaud's disease. They are **distinct disorders** that share a similar name.
- **Raynaud's disease** is *vasospasm alone*, with no other associated illness.
- **Raynaud's phenomenon** is a *vasospasm associated with another illness*, most commonly an autoimmune disease.
- Other terms used for this distinction are **primary Raynaud's** phenomenon (the disease) and **secondary Raynaud's** phenomenon (the phenomenon).
  - Patients who have had Raynaud's phenomenon alone for more than 2 years, and have not developed any additional manifestations, are at low risk for developing an autoimmune disease. Most of these patients are considered to have primary Raynaud's phenomenon.

- Although Raynaud's phenomenon has been described with a variety of autoimmune diseases, the **most common association is with progressive systemic sclerosis** *(scleroderma)*. It is an almost universal association.
- Raynaud's phenomenon has also been described with such diseases as systemic lupus erythematosus and other disorders not classified as autoimmune, including frostbite, vibration injury, polyvinyl chloride exposure, and cryoglobulinemia.

PATHOPHYSIOLOGY

- One or more body parts experience intense vasospasm with associated pallor and, often, cyanosis.
- This is often followed by a hyperemic phase with associated erythema.
- The affected body parts are usually those **most susceptible to cold injury.**
  - It most commonly affects the digits of the fingers but may affect the toes, nose, and ears.
- A clear line of demarcation exists between the ischemic areas and unaffected areas.

> TIP: These effects are *reversible,* and they must be distinguished from irreversible causes of ischemia such as vasculitis or thrombosis. Rarely, tissue necrosis occurs distal to the affected vessel. This usually happens in the periphery of the vasculature.

INCIDENCE[3,14]

- **In the United States:** One survey reported a 5%-10% incidence of primary Raynaud's phenomenon in persons who are nonsmokers. However, the more accepted figure is **3%-4%.**
  - The frequency of secondary Raynaud's phenomenon depends on the underlying disorder. For example, it is **almost universal in patients with scleroderma** (progressive systemic sclerosis).
- **Internationally:** The prevalence of primary Raynaud's phenomenon varies among populations, ranging from 4.9%-20.1% in women to 3.8%-13.5% in men. The commonly accepted rate is about 3%-4%.
  - As in the United States, the prevalence of secondary Raynaud's phenomenon depends on the underlying disorder.

RACE

- Primary Raynaud's phenomenon shows **no racial predilection.**
- Secondary Raynaud's phenomenon approximates the **racial prevalence of the underlying disease.**

AGE

- Primary Raynaud's phenomenon usually occurs in the second or third decade of life.
- Secondary Raynaud's phenomenon begins simultaneously with the underlying disorder.

HISTORY

- **Numbness and pain** may be present in the affected areas.
- **Affected areas** show at least **two** color changes: White (pallor), blue (cyanosis), and red (hyperemia).
  - The color changes are usually in the order noted, but not always.
  - The affected body part usually changes colors at least twice during the episode.
  - These changes should be completely reversible.
- Any history of associated symptoms should raise a suspicion of an underlying disorder.

- **Obtain an occupational history.**
  - **Secondary Raynaud's** phenomenon has been associated with the **frequent use of vibrating tools** such as jackhammers and sanders.
  - Industrial exposure to **polyvinyl chloride** has been implicated.
  - Any history of **injury or frostbite** may leave the involved limb vulnerable to vasospasm.
- Syndromes associated with Raynaud's phenomenon are shown in the box on page 734.

DIFFERENTIAL DIAGNOSIS

Some syndromes may be confused with Raynaud's phenomenon.

- **Anatomic syndromes**
  - Carpal tunnel syndrome
  - Reflex sympathetic dystrophy syndromes
  - Thoracic outlet syndrome
- **Miscellaneous circulatory syndromes**
  - Atherosclerosis
  - Thromboangiitis obliterans
  - Vasculitis
  - Thromboembolic disease
- **Vasospastic syndromes**
  - Livedo reticularis
  - Acrocyanosis
  - Chilblains

LABORATORY STUDIES

- **Complete blood cell count:** To evaluate polycythemia disorders, underlying malignancies, or autoimmune disorders
- **Blood urea nitrogen:** To evaluate possible renal impairment or dehydration
- **Creatinine:** To evaluate possible renal impairment
- **Prothrombin time:** To detect any evidence of hepatic dysfunction
- **Activated partial thromboplastin time:** To detect any evidence of antiphospholipid antibody syndrome or hepatic dysfunction
- **Serum glucose:** To evaluate patient for diabetic disease
- **Thyroid-stimulating hormone:** To detect thyroid disorders
- **Optional laboratory tests**
  - **Antinuclear antibody:** May be positive in autoimmune disorders and should be ordered for patients with features of these disorders
  - **Serum viscosity:** Elevated with hyperviscosity syndromes such as paraproteinemia
  - **Serum creatine kinase:** Elevated with muscle damage such as polymyositis and dermatomyositis
  - **Rheumatoid factor:** May be elevated with rheumatoid arthritis, other autoimmune disorders, and some forms of cryoglobulinemia (monoclonal proteins in multiple myeloma and Waldenström's macroglobulinemia have an increased frequency of rheumatoid factor activity)
  - **Hepatitis panel:** Positive for B or C infection in many patients with cryoglobulinemia
  - **Cold agglutinins:** Present with *Mycoplasma* infections and lymphomas
  - **Heavy metal screen:** To detect patients with neuropathic pain resulting from poisoning
  - **Growth hormone:** To evaluate patients for acromegaly
  - **Serum vanillylmandelic acid:** To evaluate for pheochromocytoma

Autoimmune disorders
- Progressive systemic sclerosis (scleroderma) including diffuse and localized (formerly called CREST syndrome)
- Systemic lupus erythematosus
- Mixed connective tissue disease (and other overlap syndromes)
- Dermatomyositis and polymyositis
- Rheumatoid arthritis
- Sjögren's syndrome
- Vasculitis
- Primary pulmonary hypertension

Infectious syndromes
- Hepatitis B and C (especially associated with mixed or type 3 cryoglobulinemia)
- *Mycoplasma* infections (with cold agglutinins)

Neoplastic syndromes
- Lymphoma
- Leukemia
- Myeloma
- Waldenström's macroglobulinemia
- Polycythemia
- Monoclonal or type 1 cryoglobulinemia
- Lung adenocarcinoma
- Other paraneoplastic disorders

Environmental associations
- Vibration injury
- Vinyl chloride exposure
- Frostbite
- Lead exposure
- Arsenic exposure

Metabolic and endocrine syndromes
- Acromegaly
- Myxedema
- Diabetes mellitus
- Pheochromocytoma
- Fabry's disease

Hematologic syndromes
- Paroxysmal nocturnal hemoglobinuria

Drug-related associations
- Oral contraceptives
- Ergot alkaloids
- Bromocriptine
- β-adrenergic–blocking drugs
- Antineoplastics (e.g., vinca alkaloids, bleomycin, cisplatin)
- Cyclosporine
- α-interferon

From Wigley FM, Flavahan NA. Raynaud's phenomenon. Rheum Dis Clin North Am 22:765-781, 1996.

- **Metanephrine:** To detect pheochromocytoma in appropriate patients
- **Catecholamines:** To detect pheochromocytoma
- **Leukocyte alkaline phosphatase:** To evaluate for leukemias in appropriate patients

IMAGING STUDIES

- **Thermography** and **arteriography** both have been used, but neither has proved superior to clinical assessment.
- A fixed, nonreversible, cyanotic lesion is **not** Raynaud's phenomenon and may require further evaluation of the vasculature.

MEDICAL TREATMENT[12-14]

- **Primary Raynaud's phenomenon**
  - Use **calcium channel blockers,** especially those that cause vasodilation.
  - **The most commonly used drug is nifedipine.**
    - ▶ Use the lowest dose of a long-acting preparation and titrate up as tolerated.
    - ▶ If adverse effects occur, decrease dosage or use another agent such as nicardipine, amlodipine, or diltiazem.
  - The following have been advocated, but they are still experimental.
    - ▶ Angiotensin-converting enzyme inhibitors
    - ▶ Angiotensin receptor antagonists
    - ▶ Intravenous prostaglandins
  - Therapy with antiplatelet agents has been tried but has not been proved effective.
  - Anticoagulation is **not** indicated.
  - Losartan at 50 mg/day was effective in a 1999 study of patients with primary Raynaud's phenomenon and scleroderma by Dziadzio et al.[13]
- **Secondary Raynaud's phenomenon**
  - Therapy must be **tailored to the underlying disorder.**
  - If associated with occupational or toxic exposure, the patient should avoid the inciting environment.
  - Patients with hyperviscosity syndromes and cryoglobulinemia improve with treatments that decrease viscosity and improve the rheologic properties of their blood (e.g., plasmapheresis).
  - Patients with autoimmune disorders and associated Raynaud's phenomenon do **not** usually respond well to therapy.
  - Address the following:
    - ▶ Hepatitis B
    - ▶ Hepatitis C
    - ▶ *Mycoplasma* infections
  - In older patients with new-onset Raynaud's phenomenon and no obvious underlying cause, **malignancy** must be considered.

SURGICAL TREATMENT

- **Cervical sympathectomy** still is considered controversial and may offer only temporary relief.
- **Digital sympathectomy** has been gaining support for patients with severe or tissue-threatening disease.
  - May be used for patients with either primary or secondary disease
  - More commonly necessary with the secondary forms

- Flatt[15] described an alternative approach to digital sympathectomy.
  - He stripped a 3-4 mm length of the adventitia (without compromising the vessel).
  - Eight treated patients had relief of symptoms and an increase of skin hand temperature for 1-12 years.
  - Only one patient had a relapse.
- In a later 1999 report, seven patients underwent digital artery sympathectomy as a salvage procedure to prevent amputation. In six of the patients the digital ulcers healed, and amputation was avoided.

COMPLICATIONS
- Rarely, digital ulceration and tissue loss may result from primary Raynaud's phenomenon.
- The complications associated with secondary Raynaud's phenomenon are usually related to the underlying disease. The worst are loss of tissue pulp in the distal phalanx, ulceration, and digital gangrene.

PROGNOSIS
- Prognosis of **primary** Raynaud's phenomenon is usually **very good,** with no mortality and little morbidity.
- Prognosis of **secondary** Raynaud's phenomenon is **related to the underlying disease.**
  - Prognosis for the involved digit is related to the severity of the ischemia and the effectiveness of maneuvers to restore blood flow.

MORTALITY AND MORBIDITY
- **Primary Raynaud's** phenomenon does not usually cause death or serious morbidity. However, ischemia of the affected body part can result in necrosis; this is a very rare occurrence.
- **Secondary Raynaud's** phenomenon is important as a **possible marker for other diseases** that may lead to morbidity and mortality, such as:
  - Scleroderma (progressive systemic sclerosis)
  - Systemic lupus erythematosus
  - Hyperviscosity syndromes

OTHER VASOSPASTIC DISEASES[3]
- Buerger's disease *(thromboangiitis obliterans)*
  - Usually **not** seen in the upper extremities.
  - Inflammatory thrombosis mostly in **young men who smoke.**
  - Characterized by **progressive ischemic changes.**
  - The only practical treatment is for the patient to **stop smoking;** lesions are treated symptomatically as the local condition dictates.
- Giant cell arteritis
- Wegner's granulomatosis
- Polyarteritis nodosa
- Takayasu's arteritis
- Hyperparathyroidism
- Iron overload in dialysis patients
- Vinyl chloride exposure

VASCULAR TUMORS[3,16-20]

■ Vascular tumors in the hand are **not common.**
* Two studies show the incidence of vascular tumors at 5%-8% of all hand tumors, with hemangiomas making up 50%-70% of these.
■ **Vascular tumors include:**
* Hemangiomas (infantile and congenital subtypes)
* Glomus tumors
* Malignant vascular tumors
  ▶ Hemangiosarcoma
  ▶ Hemangioendothelioma
  ▶ Kaposi's sarcoma
  ▶ Less than 1% of hand vascular tumors are malignant.
* Lymphangioma

HEMANGIOMAS

Hemangiomas are often grouped with congenital arteriovenous fistulas (share many similarities), but they are technically a tumor. Table 74-3 shows the current classification schema of the two.
■ **Description**
* Mulliken and Glowacki[20] defined hemangiomas as **true tumors** seen in **the first 4 weeks of life.**
* Although 30% are seen at birth, 70%-90% are discovered by the fourth week of life.
* There are two types:
  ▶ Infantile hemangioma
  ▶ Congenital hemangioma
* Hemangiomas are **three times more common in females than in males.**

Table 74-3 *Classification of the International Society for the Study of Vascular Anomalies*

Vascular Tumors	Vascular Malformations
Hemangioma of infancy*	Simple malformation
(GLUT1-positive)	Capillary (port-wine stain)
Superficial	Venous
Deep	Lymphatic
Mixed	Microcystic (e.g., lymphangioma)
Congenital hemangioma	Macrocystic (e.g., cystic hygroma)
Rapidly involuting congenital	Arteriovenous malformation (AVM)
hemangioma (RICH)	Combined malformation
Noninvoluting congenital	Capillary-lymphatic-venous (includes most cases of Klippel-Trénaunay)
hemangioma (NICH)	Capillary-venous (includes mild cases of Klippel-Trénaunay)
Kaposiform	Capillary-venous with arteriovenous shunting and/or fistulas
hemangioendothelioma	(Parkes-Weber syndrome)
Tufted angioma	Cutis marmorata telangiectatica congenita
Pyogenic granuloma (lobular	
capillary hemangioma)	
Hemangiopericytoma	

Modified from Chang MW. Updated classification of hemangiomas and other vascular anomalies. Lymphat Res Biol 1:259-265, 2003; and the International Society for the Study of Vascular Anomalies, Brussels, Belgium, www.http://www.issva.org/
*The descriptors of *superficial, deep,* and *mixed* have replaced the archaic modifiers *strawberry, capillary,* and *cavernous.*

■ **Natural History**
- Classic infantile hemangiomas undergo **three phases of growth**.[3,17,18]
  1. The classic infantile hemangioma appears as a vascular stain or a small vascular papule at birth or during the first few weeks of life.
  2. The rapid growth phase starts in the first month and lasts approximately 10-14 months. During this time, the mass may develop from a reddish-purple lesion to a large, bright-red or bright-blue mass.
  3. During the last phase, the lesion involutes over many months or years. **By the age of 7 years, 70% of lesions have involuted.**

■ **Congenital hemangiomas**
- The growth phase is in utero, reaching peak size before birth.[16,17] Lesions are mature at birth.
- The appearance can be different from a classic infantile hemangioma. Congenital hemangiomas may be purplish, or have telangiectasias or peripheral blanching.
- Based on differences in natural history, congenital hemangiomas are divided into two subtypes.
  ▸ **RICH** *(rapidly involuting congenital hemangioma)*
  ▸ **NICH** *(noninvoluting congenital hemangioma)*
- **Diagnosis of RICH and NICH**
  ▸ **RICH is more common than NICH,** but both are rare vascular birthmarks.
  ▸ The diagnosis of **RICH** is confirmed when the hemangioma **involutes** by age 6-10 months.
  ▸ **NICH** is stable and does **not** involute.
  ▸ NICH can be identical in appearance to RICH at birth, and serial examinations are often required to confirm the diagnosis.
  ▸ Skin biopsy and/or imaging (MRI or sonography) may be needed to exclude other neoplasms.
  ▸ NICH and RICH are both glucose transporter isoform 1 (GLUT1) negative, compared with hemangiomas of infancy, which are GLUT1 positive.
    ◆ GLUT1 is an immunohistochemical marker that is normally restricted to endothelial cells with a blood-tissue barrier function, as in the brain and placenta.
    ◆ Specimens from infantile hemangiomas are universally GLUT1 positive. In comparison, biopsies of RICH, NICH, pyogenic granuloma, granulation tissue, vascular malformations, tufted angioma, and kaposiform hemangioendothelioma are GLUT1 negative.

■ **Imaging**
- Plain radiographs demonstrate that hemangiomas have a soft tissue shadow and may contain calcifications.
- Typically, hemangiomas have well-defined borders on CT scan images.
- With the increased use of MRI, the reliance on angiography has diminished.

■ **Treatment**[16,19]
- Traditional management has been based on the assumption that the birthmark will **involute spontaneously** by the age of 3-7 years.
  ▸ With our current understanding and the known history that the RICH subtype quickly involutes, this remains sound practice.
- **Surgical intervention** is indicated for **symptomatic problems** such as ulceration, infection, bleeding, obstruction of orifices, or psychosocial factors.
  ▸ Hemangiomas on the palm of the hand and some on the face are usually aggressively treated early, without a "wait and see" period.
- A number of alternative methods have been reported with varying results.

NOTE: It is difficult to attribute the efficacy of any of these modalities, because many hemangiomas involute spontaneously without any intervention.

TIP: Future treatment protocols will need to differentiate infantile from congenital hemangiomas (by GLUT1 testing) and RICH from NICH congenital hemangiomas.

▶ Cryotherapy with carbon dioxide snow and liquid nitrogen.
▶ Radiation therapy.
▶ Steroid therapy has been advocated for palliation of symptomatic hemangiomas.
▶ Interferon-α2a has been given in cases of rapidly expanding, life-threatening hemangiomas that have failed an initial trial of steroids and require early intervention.
▶ Compression therapy.
▶ Injection of sodium tetradecyl sulfate (Sotradecol® 3%) alone or with surgery.
▶ Laser therapy: Nd:YAG lasers are used for intralesional laser photocoagulation.

TIP: *Maffucci's syndrome* is a rare disorder characterized by multiple hamartomas, including enchondromas and subcutaneous hemangiomas. It is frequently included on written examinations.

GLOMUS TUMORS[3,16,21]

*Glomus tumors are **benign lesions** containing cells from the **glomus apparatus.***

■ The **glomus body** lies in the reticular layer and is responsible for **thermoregulatory control.**
■ The **glomus apparatus** contains an afferent vessel, a Sucquet-Hoyer canal (an arteriovenous shunt in the dermis that contributes to temperature regulation), and multiple shunts in the glabrous skin of the hand and beneath the nail beds.
■ Numerous nonmyelinated nerve fibers are seen histologically.
■ As many as **75%** of glomus tumors are found in the **hand,** and up to **65%** of these lesions are found in the **fingertip.**
■ **Classification:** Glomus tumors are classified into three groups:
  1. Solitary lesions
  2. Multiple painful lesions
  3. Multiple painless lesions
■ **Symptoms:** A **classic triad** is observed with glomus tumors.
  • Cold hypersensitivity
  • Paroxysmal pain
  • Pinpoint pain

TIP: This classical triad of symptoms for glomus tumors is frequently seen on written examinations.

  • The pain caused by glomus tumors is not primarily nocturnal, has a paroxysmal pattern, and is not usually relieved with salicylates. Localization can be done by applying pressure to the suspected area with the head of a pin, which elicits intense pain **(Love's sign).** If a blood pressure cuff is inflated proximally, the pain is abolished **(Hildreth's sign).**[21]
■ **Physical findings**
  • Painful subcutaneous nodules subungually
  • Bluish discoloration in the nail beds, with or without nail plate ridges

- **Imaging**
  - Imaging of glomus tumors includes **MRI,** which reveals a dark, well-defined lesion on T1-weighted images and a bright lesion on T2-weighted images.
  - Doppler ultrasound studies can be used to help detect the **high blood flow** that occurs in glomus tumors.
- **Treatment:** Excision
  - Following removal of the nail, the nail bed is exposed.
  - Careful examination of the matrix is necessary because recurrence rates reportedly are as high as **20%.**
  - Persistence of symptoms following exploration may require reexploration, secondary to the likelihood of **multiple lesions.**
  - Vasisht et al[21] describe an alternative technique that uses a lateral incision and raises a subperiosteal flap to gain full access to the subungual region in 19 patients with only a 15.4% recurrence rate.

MALIGNANT TUMORS[3,22]

Angiosarcoma and **Kaposi's sarcoma** are most common in adult white men and are seen in the extremities.

- **Angiosarcomas** are red vascular tumors and can metastasize; their behavior is variable. Wide excision is usually curative.
- **Kaposi's sarcoma (KS)** shows small bluish-red to dark brown plaques and nodules.
  - The clinical course is variable—it can be rapidly fatal or indolent for many years.
  - KS usually starts on the extremities and spreads to other cutaneous sites or to bowel viscera.
  - KS has become much more common since **AIDS** became prevalent and can be found in young men.
  - Highly active antiretroviral therapy (HAART) treatment for AIDS also treats KS. In lesions not treated with HAART, a variety of systemic and, sometimes, topical therapies have been used with variable results.
  - **Surgical treatment** of KS on the hand or extremities is **rarely indicated,** except for symptomatic complications (a KS-associated aneurysm of the ulnar artery has been reported).

LYMPHANGIOMAS

- These are a very rare subgroup of malignant hemangiomas. Table 74-4 summarizes the subtypes and treatment options.

Table 74-4   *Subtypes of Lymphangiomas*

Subtype	Description	Treatment
Simple lymphangiomas	Lesions are small and well-circumscribed with a wartlike appearance and little tendency to grow	Local excision
Cavernous lymphangiomas	Most common variety Appear within the first month of life Can grow to become massive Consist of dilated lymphatic sinuses	Usually excision or amputation is needed Radiation treatments are helpful for common recurrences
Cystic hygromas	Occur in the neck or rarely axilla Originate from primitive jugular sacs Present at birth and grow rapidly	Excision

From Sofocleous CT, Rosen RJ, Raskin K, et al. Congenital vascular malformations in the hand and forearm. J Endovasc Ther 8:484-494, 2001.

ARTERIOVENOUS MALFORMATIONS AND FISTULAS[3,16,19,20]

An arteriovenous malformation (AVM) is an abnormal communication between an artery and a vein.
- These communications are **congenital;** can occur at any point in the vascular system; and vary in size, length, location, and number.
- **Arteriovenous fistula (AVF)** is a **single communication** between an artery and a vein that usually has an acquired cause.
- Table 74-5 summarizes the differences between AVM and AVF.

Table 74-5   *Differences Between AVM and AVF*

	AVM	AVF
History		
Discovered early in life	Often	
Discovered after trivial injury	Often	
Seen after penetrating injury	No	Only mechanism
Symptoms		
Mass, fullness, discomfort	Often	Often
Signs		
Mass	Yes	Yes
Warm limb	Yes	Yes
Limb longer	Often	No
Distal ischemia	Sometimes	Sometimes
Bruit and thrill	Sometimes	Usually
Scar of trauma	No	Yes
Arteriogram		
Large, single feeder	Sometimes	Yes
Rapid shunting	Sometimes	Yes
Treatment		
Conservative often best	Yes	No
May need multiple stages	Yes	No
May require amputation	Yes	No
Single stage, straightforward	Rarely	Usually

Data from Lee BB, Do YS, Yakes W, et al. Management of arteriovenous malformations: A multidisciplinary approach. J Vasc Surg 39:590-600, 2004; Newmeyer W. Vascular disorders. In Green DP, ed. Operative Hand Surgery, 3rd ed. Philadelphia: Churchill Livingstone, 1993, pp 2251-2308.

PATHOPHYSIOLOGY
- Congenital vascular malformations are inborn errors in embryologic development.
- Most AVMs are developmental errors that occur between the **4th and 10th weeks** of embryogenesis.
- The causes of these errors are **unknown.**

- Potential exogenous causes, such as viral infections, toxins, and drugs, have been implicated but not proven.
- Almost all AVMs are sporadic and nonfamilial, although a few syndromes such as Sturge-Weber and Klippel-Trénaunay, include inherited vascular abnormalities.
- Although the pathogenetic mechanisms of AVMs are not understood yet, the hemodynamic alterations that lead to the clinical manifestations of AVMs have been described.
  - An abnormal communication causes shunting of blood from the high-pressure arterial side to the low-pressure venous side. This creates an abnormal low-resistance circuit that steals from the high-resistance normal capillary bed.
  - Blood follows the path of least resistance. Flow in the afferent artery and efferent vein increases, causing dilation, thickening, and tortuosity of the vessels.
  - If the resistance in the fistula is low enough, the fistulous tract will steal from the distal arterial supply, actually causing a reversal of arterial flow in the segment distal to the AVM. This is known as a **parasitic circulation.** The parasitic circulation causes decreased arterial pressures in the distal capillary beds and can cause tissue ischemia.
  - The increased flow into the venous circulation does not necessarily cause higher venous pressures. However, it can cause vessel wall abnormalities such as thickening of the media and fibrosis of the wall. These changes are known as **arterialization.**
  - The blood flow into the venous circulation causes turbulence, which is responsible for the **palpable thrill.** The thrill depends on the geometry of the fistula and does not represent volume of flow accurately.
  - In addition to the decreased distal arterial pressures, peripheral venous pressures are increased, leading to tissue ischemia and its sequelae.
  - The heart responds to the decreased peripheral vascular resistance by increasing stroke volume and cardiac output. This leads to tachycardia, left ventricular dilation, and, eventually, heart failure.

Sex
- AVMs occur with **equal frequency** among males and females.

Age
- All AVMs are present at birth, but they are not always evident clinically.
- A triggering stimulus during puberty or pregnancy or following minor trauma can precipitate clinical features of the malformation.

Symptoms
- Cutaneous malformations can present with a mass, pink stain, dilated veins, unequal limb length and girth, or skin ulceration.
- Patients may complain of limb heaviness that is aggravated with dependency and relieved with elevation.
- Fifty percent of patients complain of pain. The pain may be caused by tissue ischemia or by mass effect on local nerves.

Physical Findings
- The lesion may be **pulsatile.**
- **Branham's sign** (slowing of the heart rate during compression proximal to AVM) may be present.
- Patients may develop hyperhidrosis, hypertrichosis, hyperthermia, or a palpable thrill or bruit over the lesion.

- Patients may have functional impairment of limbs or joints from mass effect or gangrene from prolonged tissue ischemia.
- Visceral AVMs can present with hematuria, hematemesis, hemoptysis, or melena.
- Rarely, patients present with signs of congestive heart failure (e.g., dyspnea, leg edema).

LABORATORY STUDIES

- Blood gas analysis in an AVM case reveals a higher oxygen partial pressure in the venous blood immediately distal to the fistula, compared with normal venous blood.

IMAGING STUDIES

- Plain films may demonstrate soft tissue masses or abnormalities within bony structures.
- **Duplex ultrasonography** can be used to characterize the **direction and velocity of blood flow.** A Doppler scan can be used preoperatively and intraoperatively. However, ultrasound does not have any therapeutic use.
- **Contrast-enhanced CT scans** are useful to locate the abnormality, to evaluate for aneurysm formation, and to identify bony involvement.
- **Contrast angiography is the most important method for investigating AVMs.**
  - It is an excellent method to delineate the number, location, and extent of the arteriovenous connections.
  - Angiographic signs include early filling of veins, hypertrophied and tortuous arteries proximal to the malformation, and varicose and dilated veins distal to the fistula.
- **MRI** has become the new standard in the preoperative evaluation of patients with AVMs.
  - MRI generates multiplanar views and can be used to accurately define tissue planes and identify critical flow characteristics.
  - It is the best modality to define local soft tissue and adjacent organ involvement, which helps with preintervention planning.
  - Magnetic resonance (MR) sequences can be postprocessed into **MR angiogram images,** which help define the malformation more clearly.
- **Radiolabeled studies** can determine the shunt fraction, which is the proportion of blood being shunted through the fistulous tract.
- **Other tests**
  - Invasive and noninvasive cardiac evaluation may be indicated in patients with congestive heart failure because cardiac output can be markedly elevated in patients with large proximal AVMs.

CAUTION: Percutaneous biopsy is never indicated! Biopsy can be helpful if a lesion is suspected to be sarcomatous or if the clinical impression is unclear.

TREATMENT

- **Medical care**
  - Most arteriovenous malformations can be managed and controlled **medically.**
  - Only a few AVMs demonstrate progressive growth and require surgical intervention.
  - Most of the symptoms of AVMs (pain, heaviness, and swelling) are caused by venous hypertension.
  - The cornerstone approach in managing lower extremity symptoms is **elastic support hose.**
    - ▶ An elastic support stocking that provides **30-40 mm Hg** of compression usually is sufficient to relieve leg symptoms.
  - Arm and some hand lesions can also be managed with compressive garments.

- **Alcohol sclerotherapy** may shrink the size of the AVM, but this treatment also places the patient at risk for peripheral nerve injury.
  - ▸ The treatment of large AVMs with alcohol needs to be performed by an experienced interventional radiologist, and these risks must be explained to patients when they consent to undergo therapy.
- **Surgical care**
- **Indications for surgical intervention of AVMs:**
  - ▸ Hemorrhage
  - ▸ Painful ischemia
  - ▸ Congestive heart failure
  - ▸ Nonhealing ulcers
  - ▸ Functional impairment
  - ▸ Limb-length inequality
- **Embolization** is an option for treatment and should be considered when conservative measures have failed or when the vascularity of the malformation needs to be reduced before surgical resection.
  - ▸ The procedure involves the injection of particulate matter into the malformation.
  - ▸ The common adverse effects are pain and tenderness near the malformation, a transient fever, and leukocytosis.
  - ▸ Excision should be performed 48-72 hours after embolization.[23]
- Most AVMs are not amenable to complete surgical excision, and it is not required.
  - ▸ A lesion must be well localized for a chance of complete resection.
  - ▸ Resectability depends on the degree of extension into adjacent structures.
- Patients severely afflicted with malformations, who are not candidates for local extirpation, may be candidates for amputation and rehabilitation with a limb prosthesis.

PROGNOSIS

- Lee et al[16] reported their results with **nonsurgical management of AVMs.**
  - 32 patients with surgically inaccessible lesions were treated with embolism and sclerotherapy alone.
  - There were nine failures from a total of 171 sessions.
  - Interim results of embolism and sclerotherapy alone, with a mean of 19 months of follow-up, were excellent in most (25 of 32) and good to fair among the rest (7 of 32).
  - There were 31 complications, mostly minor (27 of 31), and four major.
    - ▸ Facial nerve palsy
    - ▸ Pulmonary embolism
    - ▸ Deep vein thrombosis
    - ▸ Massive necrosis of an ear cartilage
- Sofocleous et al[18] reported their results of **embolization** of hand and forearm AVMs.
  - In a 15-year period, 39 patients (22 men, mean age 22.5 years) had symptomatic vascular lesions diagnosed in the forearm and hand.
    - ▸ 21 AVMs
    - ▸ 17 primary venous malformations (PVMs)
    - ▸ One complex lesion with both AVM and PVM
  - Lesions were treated in 34 cases (87%), with immediate technical success achieved in 31 (91%); lesions were not amenable to percutaneous treatment in 5 (13%).

- There were no major complications, but three embolized AVMs had significant residual flow (81.6% technical success on intention-to-treat basis).
- Long-term follow-up ranging up to 5 years was available in 26 of the 34 treated patients; the mean symptom-free period was 30 months for the AVM patients and 30.5 months for the PVM group, with an average of 1.5 and 1.2 embolization procedures, respectively.

KEY POINTS

✔ MRI is the most useful imaging study for vascular disorders.

✔ Injuries to arteries of the hand (the arch) and forearm usually can be safely managed with ligation when there is sufficient backbleeding. An injured blood vessel should be repaired if there is an accompanying nerve injury, regardless of whether there is adequate bleeding.

✔ Emboli should be surgically treated with embolectomy, and the source of the emboli needs to be addressed.

✔ Diagnosis of vascular compression at the neck (thoracic outlet syndrome) is difficult, and physical examination findings are usually normal. Most provocative tests are unreliable; only the EAST test has some debatable usefulness.

✔ Raynaud's phenomenon is vasospasm that is associated with another illness (usually autoimmune), whereas Raynaud's disease is vasospasm that is not associated with other illnesses.

✔ Management of Raynaud's phenomenon and disease is difficult; medical therapy helps to manage the symptoms. Surgical therapy is used for failed medical therapy and includes cervical sympathectomy, which only offers temporary relief, and digital sympathectomy, which has some promising results.

✔ There are two types of hemangiomas. **Classic infantile hemangiomas** are characterized by three growth phases, being GLUT1 positive, and having 70% involution by the age of 7 years. **Congenital hemangiomas** are GLUT1 negative and are characterized by two subtypes, RICH and NICH; RICH rapidly involutes by age 6-10 months, but NICH never involutes.

✔ A glomus tumor is characterized by the classic triad of cold hypersensitivity, paroxysmal pain, and pinpoint pain. Treatment is excision.

✔ Most AVMs can be successfully treated with embolization and sclerotherapy. Lesions that require surgical excision (symptomatic or psychological symptomatic facial lesions) should have preoperative embolization, and the hemangioma should be excised within 48-72 hours.

REFERENCES

1. Menzoian JO, Doyle JE, LoGerfo FW, et al. Evaluation and management of vascular injuries of the extremities. Arch Surg 118:93-95, 1983.
2. Perry MO, Thal ER, Shires GT. Management of arterial injuries. Ann Surg 173:403-408, 1971.
3. Newmeyer W. Vascular disorders. In Green DP, ed. Operative Hand Surgery, 3rd ed. Philadelphia: Churchill Livingstone, 1993, pp 2251-2308.
4. Gelberman RH, Blasingame JP, Fronek A, et al. Forearm arterial injuries. J Hand Surg Am 4:401-408, 1979.
5. Scheer B, Perel A, Pfeiffer UJ. Clinical review: Complications and risk factors of peripheral arterial catheters used for haemodynamic monitoring in anaesthesia and intensive care medicine. Crit Care 6:199-204, 2002.

6. Leclercq DC, Carlier AJ, Khuc T, et al. Improvement in the results in sixty-four ulnar nerve sections associated with arterial repair. J Hand Surg Am 10:997-999, 1985.

7. Hood DB, Kuehne J, Yellin AE, et al. Vascular complications of thoracic outlet syndrome. Am Surg 63:913-917, 1997.

8. Savader SJ, Lund GB, Scheel PJ. Forearm loop, upper arm straight, and brachial-internal jugular vein dialysis grafts: A comparison study of graft survival utilizing a combined percutaneous endovascular and surgical maintenance approach. J Vasc Interv Radiol 10:537-545, 1999.

9. Franklin GM, Fulton-Kehoe D, Bradley C, et al. Outcome of surgery for thoracic outlet syndrome in Washington state workers' compensation. Neurology 54:1252-1257, 2000.

10. Plewa MC, Delinger M. The false-positive rate of thoracic outlet syndrome shoulder maneuvers in healthy subjects. Acad Emerg Med 5:337-342, 1998.

11. Oates SD, Daley RA. Thoracic outlet syndrome. Hand Clin 12:705-718, 1996.

12. McCall TE, Petersen DP, Wong LB. The use of digital artery sympathectomy as a salvage procedure for severe ischemia of Raynaud's disease and phenomenon. J Hand Surg Am 24:173-177, 1999.

13. Dziadzio M, Denton CP, Smith R, et al. Losartan therapy for Raynaud's phenomenon and scleroderma: Clinical and biochemical findings in a fifteen-week, randomized, parallel-group, controlled trial. Arthritis Rheum 42:2646-2655, 1999.

14. Wigley FM, Flavahan NA. Raynaud's phenomenon. Rheum Dis Clin North Am 22:765-781, 1996.

15. Flatt AE. Digital artery sympathectomy. J Hand Surg Am 5:550-556, 1980.

16. Lee BB, Do YS, Yakes W, et al. Management of arteriovenous malformations: A multidisciplinary approach. J Vasc Surg 39:590-600, 2004.

17. Chang MW. Updated classification of hemangiomas and other vascular anomalies. Lymphat Res Biol 1:259-265, 2003.

18. Sofocleous CT, Rosen RJ, Raskin K, et al. Congenital vascular malformations in the hand and forearm. J Endovasc Ther 8:484-494, 2001.

19. Achauer BM, Chang CJ, Vander Kam VM. Management of hemangioma of infancy: Review of 245 patients. Plast Reconstr Surg 99:1301-1308, 1997.

20. Mulliken JB, Glowacki J. Hemangiomas and vascular malformations in infants and children: A classification based on endothelial characteristics. Plast Reconstr Surg 69:412-422, 1982.

21. Vasisht B, Watson HK, Joseph E, et al. Digital glomus tumors: A 29-year experience with a lateral subperiosteal approach. Plast Reconstr Surg 114:1486-1489, 2004.

22. Noy A. Update in Kaposi sarcoma. Curr Opin Oncol 15:379-381, 2003.

23. Weinzweig N, Chin G, Polley J, et al. Arteriovenous malformation of the forehead, anterior scalp, and nasal dorsum. Plast Reconstr Surg 105:2433-2439, 2000.

PART VII

Aesthetic Surgery

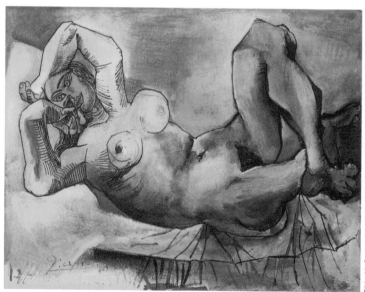

75. Nonoperative Facial Rejuvenation

Sacha I. Obaid
John L. Burns

CAUSES OF FACIAL AGING[1,2]

ACTINIC DAMAGE

- **Chronic sun exposure** causes changes in the skin.
  - Elastic fibers accumulate in abnormal arrangements.
  - The number of collagen fibers decreases, and the remaining fibers become increasingly disorganized.
  - A thin layer of dermis called the **grenz zone,** or **border zone,** forms between the abnormal dermis and the epidermis.
- **The net result of these changes causes several conditions to develop:**
  - Fine rhytids
  - Skin laxity
  - Dyschromia
  - Cutaneous malignancies

CHRONOLOGIC AGING

- **Skin changes occur with age**
  - Thinning of the dermis
  - Fewer fibroblasts, mast cells, and blood vessels
  - Fewer elastic fibers
- Dynamic forces from underlying mimetic muscles cause rhytids in the overlying skin.
- Gravitational forces cause deep wrinkles, because facial fat descends.

CHOICE OF PROCEDURE

- The surgeon and patient must decide together
  - Which aspects of facial appearance are most distressing
  - Realistic treatment goals
- Patients must understand
  - Nonoperative facial rejuvenation can restore a more youthful appearance.
  - Nonoperative facial rejuvenation is not as powerful as operative techniques, nor as long lasting.
- Resurfacing techniques
  - Cause dermal collagen reorganization and new collagen deposition
    - ▶ Reduce actinic damage
    - ▶ Improve dyschromias
    - ▶ Restore a more youthful appearance
- Downtime
  - In general, deeper and more aggressive resurfacing creates longer downtime, erythema, edema, and time to reepithelialization, but more dramatic results.

- The surgeon and the patient must balance treatment result desired with patient's tolerance for downtime.
- The patient and surgeon need to be willing to accept multiple treatments or less dramatic results to allow for faster recovery.
■ Fillers
  - Augment depressions in the soft tissue
  - Mask the appearance of fine lines and wrinkles

METHODS OF NONOPERATIVE TREATMENT

■ **Lasers**
■ **Chemical peels**
■ **Dermabrasion**
■ **Radiofrequency**
■ **Botulinum toxin**
■ **Soft tissue fillers**

LASERS

METHOD OF ACTION
■ Lasers produce **heat** in target tissue that rapidly dissipates by conduction.
■ The **energy wavelength** and the **exposure duration** determine the amount of heat transferred and the amount of collateral damage.
■ Selective tissue injury is produced by the selection of a wavelength of energy that is specific for a **chromophore** in the skin.
■ To prevent collateral damage, the duration of exposure of the laser must be **equal to or shorter than the thermal relaxation time** of the chromophore target.
■ Both **ablative** and **nonablative** lasers can be used for facial rejuvenation (see Chapter 7).

ABLATIVE LASERS
■ The goal is to vaporize superficial epidermal tissues and coagulate deeper tissues without causing scarring.
■ Thermal damage causes collagen remodeling, with the goal of tightening the skin and reversing actinic and chronologic changes seen with age.
■ There are various laser effects on skin.
  - The area of direct contact is vaporized.
  - A surrounding area of thermal damage is produced.
  - Areas of irreversible and reversible damage are produced, both of which produce inflammation and wound healing.
■ **Two most common types of ablative lasers**
  - CO_2 laser
  - Erbium:YAG laser

CO_2 LASERS
■ The CO_2 laser is one of the first and longest-used laser types in facial rejuvenation.
■ The wavelength is **10,600 nm.**

- The target chromophore is **water.**
- Studies have shown that 20-60 μm of vaporization can be produced with the first pass, and 20-150 μm of additional thermal injury can be produced, depending on the settings.[3-7]
- The **depth of ablation** depends on the **number of passes** and the **amount of cooling time** allowed between passes.
  - CO_2 **lasers** have a higher ablation threshold than erbium lasers, resulting in **deeper thermal heating.**

CAUTION: If insufficient cooling time is provided, less ablation and increased thermal damage will be produced.

- With each additional pass, vaporization decreases and thermal injury increases because of the reduced water content after the initial pass.
- The **clinical endpoint** is a pale yellow color of the skin surface (midreticular dermis).
- Ablated epidermis is replaced with normal healthy epidermal cells from adnexal structures.
- **The greatest effect is in the papillary dermis,** where disorganized damaged collagen masses are replaced with normal compact collagen bundles arranged parallel to the skin's surface.
- The mean time for reepithelialization is **8.5 days.**
- Patients experience **3-6 months** of erythema.
- The most common adverse reaction is **hypopigmentation.**
  - This can lead to obvious lines of demarcation if regional resurfacing is performed.
  - Stuzin et al[8] advocate limiting CO_2 laser resurfacing to when the entire face will be treated rather than just one area.
  - Hypopigmentation from CO_2 lasers is most pronounced in fair-skinned individuals (i.e., Fitzpatrick classes I and II).
    - ▶ The **Fitzpatrick classification** is a scale of a patient's ability to tan (Table 75-1).

Table 75-1 *Fitzpatrick Skin Type Classification*

Skin Type	Sun Exposure History/Skin Color
I	Never tans, burns easily and severely, extremely fair skin
II	Usually burns, tans minimally
III	Burns moderately, tans moderately
IV	Tans moderately and easily, burns minimally
V	Rarely burns, dark brown skin
VI	Never burns, dark brown or black skin

- Hypopigmentation has been reported to occur up to 1-2 years after treatment.
- **Other potential side effects**[9-13]
  - Erythema
  - Hyperpigmentation
    - ▶ In Burns' series of studies,[14] the incidence of hyperpigmentation was reduced from 43% to 6% by adding hydroquinone, kojic acid, and sunscreen to the postoperative regimen.
  - Milia formation
  - Acne exacerbation

- Contact allergies with soaps and moisturizers
- Superficial infection
- Stimulation of herpes simplex flare-ups
- Hypertrophic scarring
- Ectropion
- **Absolute contraindications**
  - Active viral, bacterial, or fungal infection
  - **Isotretinoin use** within the previous 6-12 months (because of its suppressive effects on adnexal structures)
- CO_2 laser resurfacing may be combined with surgical rhytidectomy, but the surgeon must be very cautious about the dual insult created to the skin flaps.[15]

ERBIUM:YAG LASER[16-26]

- The wavelength is **2940 nm.**
- The chromatophore is **water.**
- Energy is absorbed by water 12-18 times more efficiently than with CO_2 lasers.
- There is **less thermal diffusion** to the surrounding tissues than with CO_2 lasers.
- The ablated, desiccated tissue is ejected when hit by the laser, producing a popping sound.

TIP: The combination of less thermal diffusion and ejection of tissues may allow the Erbium:YAG laser to give a more consistent result with each pass, compared with the CO_2 laser.

- Because of the consistent penetration depth with each pass, surgeons initially favored multiple passes at lower fluences (5 J/cm^2). The current trend is to use higher fluences (e.g., 10-25 J/cm^2) and fewer passes to effect a deeper peel.[16]
- There is 3-5 μm of ablation per pass.
- There is 20-50 μm of thermal damage.[16-21]
- The **clinical endpoint** can be recognized by a punctate bleeding pattern and a fragmented appearance of the dermis.

TIP: Because the depth of penetration is much less than with a CO_2 laser, Erbium:YAG lasers should be reserved for treating problems that are located more superficially such as epidermal or dermal lesions, mildly atrophic acne scars, mild actinic damage, and subtle dyspigmentation.

- It does not stimulate continued collagen remodeling as a CO_2 laser does. Consequently, it does not function well as a tightening device.
- The primary advantage of using an Erbium:YAG laser is a shorter recovery time compared with a CO_2 laser.
  - 5.5 days for reepithelialization
  - 3-4 weeks of erythema[18-20]
  - Controversy exists about the shorter recovery time.
    - It may be caused by the **decreased thermal diffusion** in the surrounding tissue from an Erbium:YAG laser.
    - It may be because of the **lower depth of penetration** from an Erbium:YAG laser.

▶ Adrian[22,23] found that when the CO_2 laser and Erbium:YAG laser were adjusted to the same depth of penetration, there was **no difference in the duration of clinical erythema.**

▶ Because a decrease in penetration depth results in less inflammation and collagen remodeling, there is a less dramatic result. If the decreased erythema seen with Erbium:YAG lasers is the result of decreased penetration depth, the use of erbium over CO_2 means accepting a less dramatic result in exchange for less downtime.

■ The incidence of transient hyperpigmentation is 3.4%-24%.[16]

■ The incidence of hypopigmentation is 0%-12%.[16,24-26]

■ The potential side effects are similar to those seen for CO_2 lasers.

CAUTION: Erbium:YAG resurfacing has been safely performed at the same time as rhytidectomy. The surgeon who contemplates this must, however, consider the dual insult that is inflicted on the skin flaps with such a procedure.[15]

NONABLATIVE LASER

■ Epidermal vaporization is **not** produced. Consequently, **recovery is much easier** with nonablative lasers than with ablative lasers.

■ Nonablative lasers generate heat in the dermis and cause inflammation, collagen reorganization, and new collagen generation, thus tightening and rejuvenating the skin.

■ Nonablative lasers also can treat dyschromia.

FRACTIONAL RESURFACING

■ Fractional photothermolysis uses a light with a **1.5 μm** wavelength.[27]

■ Light penetrates **300 μm** into skin.

■ **Blue dye** is laid down on the skin, and it **functions as the target chromophore** for the laser.

■ The blue dye pattern is confined to small areas known as **microscopic thermal zones.** When the laser strikes the skin, it heats just these microscopic thermal zones and leaves the surrounding skin untreated.

■ The distance between microscopic thermal zones can be as little as **250 μm.**

• The blue dye can be laid down to treat various portions of the skin. Traditionally **13%-17%** of the skin is targeted at each application.

• Patients receive repeat treatments once a week with four or five treatments total.

• The net result is treatment of the entire face, with no more than 17% of the skin experiencing the inflammatory response at one time.

■ Fractional resurfacing represents a compromise.

• Downtime is minimized.

• Results are less dramatic with each treatment.

• Multiple treatments are needed to achieve the desired results.

■ Downtime is approximately 24 hours.

■ The treatment is excellent for dyschromia.

■ Fine wrinkles of the neck, chest, hands, and face can be treated safely.

ND:YAG LASER

■ It is also known as a **neodymium:yttrium-aluminum-garnet** laser.

■ Its **wavelength** is **1064 nm.**

■ Energy is nonspecifically absorbed by target tissue.

• Various proteins appear to be the main target.

• Blood vessels, red blood cells, collagen, and melanin are the most sensitive.

- Water is a secondary target.
- Because of the nonspecific target, there is **nonspecific heating of the tissue.**
- The scattering of laser energy by the tissues at the 1064 nm wavelength causes the area of greatest photon density to be 1-2 mm below the surface of the skin, in the dermis.[28-31]
- Transmission of energy causes photo damage and inflammation in the dermis, leading to collagen reorganization and neocollagenesis, which in turn may have a mild tightening effect on the skin.
- The epidermis is not ablated, because the energy is concentrated on the dermis.

TIP: Although the overall collagen remodeling and neocollagenesis is less than with ablative lasers, the Nd:YAG laser is attractive because the crusting, edema, and prolonged erythema of ablative lasers are avoided.

- A **1320 nm Nd:YAG** laser has been developed and marketed specifically for nonablative facial rejuvenation.
- The **1320 nm** wavelength targets **dermal water.**
- The greater water absorption and nonspecific dermal scatter of the 1320 nm laser increases dermal heating and requires a cooling agent to be placed on the epidermis to prevent blistering.
- Like the 1064 nm version, the 1320 nm laser produces much less dramatic results than ablative lasers. Patients must have realistic expectations before undergoing treatment.[32,33]

POSTTREATMENT CARE
Posttreatment care is critical to prevent complications. It is especially critical with ablative laser resurfacing.
- Patients will often be concerned.
- Moist wound healing is best.
- Prescribe valacyclovir (Valtrex®) or acyclovir (Zovirax®) for 1 week to prevent herpes simplex flare-up.
- Cephalexin (Keflex®), or other antibiotics aimed at skin flora, should be given for 1 week to prevent superficial infections.
- Fluconazole (Diflucan®) is given by some for 1 week to prevent fungal infections.
- A steroid dose pack may decrease inflammation or swelling.
- A 10% topical vitamin C cream may be used.

CAUTION: Avoid topical growth factors, because they may promote hypertrophic scarring.

- Use lipid-based ointments to provide a moist environment.
- **Occlusive** and **nonocclusive** dressings are acceptable alternatives.
- Hydroquinone, kojic acid, and sunscreen can help prevent hyperpigmentation.

INTENSE PULSED LIGHT (IPL)

- IPL is **not** a laser technique.
- IPL emits a spectrum of photons in the **500-1300 nm** range.
- **The chromophore is water and hemoglobin at 550-580 nm, superficial pigment at 550-570 nm, and deeper pigment at 590-755 nm.**
- Filters can be used to include or exclude particular wavelengths.
  - If filters are used that limit transmission to shorter wavelengths, such as 550-800 nm, superficial chromophores such as melanin and dermal oxyhemoglobin are treated.

- If a filter is used that allows transmission of higher wavelengths, dermal water will be nonspecifically targeted. This results in dermal heating and inflammation, which then can lead to collagen deposition and reorganization to provide a mild tightening effect.
- IPL can treat signs of hypervascularity, such as flushing, telangiectasias, or rosacea.
- IPL can be used to treat signs of hyperpigmentation, such as solar lentigines, melasma (chloasma), or freckling.
- IPL also can be used to improve skin texture and decrease pore size.
- **Contraindications**
  - Unrealistic expectations
  - Tanned skin
  - Hypersensitivity to sunlight
  - Photosensitizing medications
  - Active isotretinoin (Accutane®) treatment
  - Therapeutic anticoagulation medications
  - Pregnancy
  - Active lupus
  - History of wound healing problems
  - Skin cancer
  - Fitzpatrick VI skin type (Fitzpatrick V is a relative contraindication)
- **Potential side effects** include prolonged redness, transient speckling of pigmentation, scabbing, edema, hair loss, purpura, hyperpigmentation, hypopigmentation, herpes eruption, infection, and scarring.
- A series of treatments, usually 4-7, is needed to provide a long-lasting effect.
- The interval between treatments should be 2-3 weeks.
- One of the keys to IPL is **realistic expectations.** Reasonably, IPL can be expected to improve facial flushing or rosacea by **50%-75%** and dyschromia by **40%-60%.**[34-36]
- Pretreatment of the skin is **not** necessary.
- Patient should **not** be tanned when undergoing treatment.
- Topical anaesthesia can be placed before treatment.
- Patients should expect **24 hours** of slight redness and dermal edema.
- **Sunblock** should be used between treatments.
- If the goal is to treat superficial dyschromia, supplement IPL treatments with topical retinoids and/or bleaching creams such as hydroquinone.

MECHANICAL RESURFACING

DERMABRASION

Dermabrasion uses a handheld rotary device to remove superficial layers of the skin.
- It can be used to treat fine rhytids in the perioral region with good results.
- It is also very effective for reducing superficial acne scarring and scarring secondary to other surgical procedures.
- It can be used for minor skin tightening when larger areas are treated.
- The **depth of resurfacing** can be controlled by the **amount of pressure** the device applies to the skin, **speed** of rotation, **coarseness** of the tip, **length** of treatment, and patient's **skin type and texture.**
- The ability to manually control the depth of resurfacing is an advantage over other resurfacing methods where control is not as precise.

- The ability to manually control the depth of resurfacing is also a disadvantage because postoperative results are **highly technique- and operator-dependent.**
- If resurfacing is performed too deeply, scarring occurs. If resurfacing is too superficial, minimal or no results are seen.
- Mechanical factors limit the ability to treat periorbital wrinkling and wrinkles between the lower lip and chin.
- Cryoanaesthetic sprays can provide anaesthesia and reduce bleeding.
- **Paprika bleeding indicates penetration into the superficial papillary dermis and is a safe endpoint for treatment.**

TIP: As resurfacing proceeds deeper into the reticular dermis, the bleeding vessels become larger, and white parallel lines of frayed collagen may be seen if loupe magnification is used.

- Yellow globules of sebaceous glands should be avoided when treating deeply.

CAUTION: When treating deeper rhytids, avoid the upper lip, malar prominence, chin, and mandible, because these areas are prone to hypertrophic scarring.

TIP: When resurfacing a large area, two things can be done to produce a more consistent result. First, gentian violet can be applied topically. The pigment is removed as areas are treated, leaving a guide of what is left to treat. Second, plan the areas to be dermabraded first, based on the knowledge that dermabraded areas bleed, and the blood will flow downward, potentially obscuring your vision in untreated areas.

- The **reepithelialization time** depends on the depth of resurfacing but is generally **7-10 days.**
- Typically, treated skin is red for 1-2 weeks and pink for up to 2-3 months afterward.[37,38]
- Intradermal postoperative swelling improves over 3 months.
- Collagen remodeling takes 3-6 months.
- Milia formation may occur for several weeks postoperatively.
- Acne outbreaks may occur.
- Hypopigmentation can occur in **10%-20%** of patients.[39,40]
- Hyperpigmentation may complicate recovery, but it is almost always reversible with hydroquinone and sun avoidance.
- Antibacterial ointments, especially those with neomycin, can cause contact dermatitis and should be used with caution postoperatively.

MICRODERMABRASION
Microdermabrasion uses a handheld, particle-containing device applied to the skin to produce a superficial injury.
- A microdermabrator uses mild suction to pull skin into the handpiece, and then it removes dirt, oil, surface debris, and dead skin by sending a stream of particles toward the skin.
- The particles can be **aluminum oxide** or **sodium chloride.**
- Following microtrauma to the skin, the crystals are aspirated into a container within the machine.
- The **particle flow rate** and **strength of the suction** control the **depth of penetration.**

- **Repetitive intraepidermal injury is the result,** which may cause gradual improvement in damaged skin by stimulating fibroblast proliferation and generation of new collagen.
- Microdermabrasion can improve rough skin, texture irregularities, acne scarring, and mottled pigmentation resulting from photoaging. Its ability to treat fine rhytids is inconsistent.
- Because it penetrates only the epidermis, microdermabrasion can be repeated frequently with minimal erythema and does not require anaesthesia.
- 4-12 weekly or bimonthly treatments should be performed.[41-43]
- Avoid the sun for 1 week before the procedure.
- Refrain from retinoids and glycolic acid creams for a few days.
- Patients with darker color skin types should be treated with a less aggressive power setting.
- After the treatment, clean the skin and apply protective moisturizer and sunscreen.
- Skin recovery takes 7-10 days.
- Potential complications include excessive bleeding, infection, scarring, hypopigmentation, and infection.
- **Relative** contraindications include **rosacea** and **telangiectasias,** both of which may be exacerbated by treatment.[43-45]
- **Absolute** contraindications include **impetigo, flat warts,** and **active herpes simplex virus infection.**
- To prevent hypertrophic scarring, wait 1 year after isotretinoin (Accutane) treatment before considering microdermabrasion.

MONOPOLAR RADIOFREQUENCY DERMAL REMODELING (THERMAGE®)

Thermage is a relatively new technology that seeks to remodel the dermis using **radiofrequency.**
- Thermage is used to tighten and contour mild laxity of the skin on the lower face or neck for patients without underlying structural ptosis.
- **Radiofrequency** is applied to the skin with **simultaneous cryogenic cooling.**
- The radiofrequency changes polarity on the skin 6 million times per second.
- **Capacitive coupling** causes **uniform distribution of heat.**
- The **geometry** and **size** of the tip affect the **depth** of injury.
- The treatment energy is typically **85-135 J/cm²,** and it is usually titrated to patient's tolerance for pain.
- Typically there are 24-36 hours of erythema after the procedure.
- Treated skin shows preservation of epidermis with alteration in the underlying collagen.
- Increased collagen deposition occurs in the grenz zone, which is thought to be the mechanism behind the skin tightening.
- Patients typically experience mild edema and mild-to-moderate erythema immediately following the treatment. Rare dysesthesias are reported.
- Results are variable and not as dramatic as with a facelift or ablative resurfacing techniques.

TIP: Patients usually require multiple treatments to obtain noticeable results with Thermage. Patients must be educated before treatment about the possibility of obtaining moderate results at best.

Thermage is probably best reserved for patients who desire nonsurgical alternatives to rejuvenation and are willing to accept modest results with minimal downtime.

■ Disadvantages include potential pain, a potential for less dramatic results, or rare indentations. There is also a potential for **fat atrophy.**[46]

CHEMICAL PEELS

INDICATIONS
■ **Superficial peels**
  • Upper epidermal defects
  • Mild dyschromia
  • Melasma
■ **Medium-depth peels**
  • Superficial dermal defects
  • Mild dermatoheliosis
  • Superficial rhytids
■ **Deep peels**
  • Deeper dermal defects
  • Severe dyschromia
  • Deep rhytids

TYPES OF PEELS
■ **Superficial peeling agents**
  • Alpha hydroxy acid (AHA) peels
  • Jessner's solution
  • Salicylic acid
  • Dry ice
■ **Medium-depth peels**
  • Trichloroacetic acid (TCA) peels
  • Combination peels
■ **Deep peels**
  • Phenol
    ▸ Baker-Gordon formula
    ▸ Hetter's formula

PATIENT EVALUATION
An accurate assessment of a patient's skin type is essential to optimize the rejuvenation and avoid complications.
■ As with other types of nonsurgical rejuvenation, the key to success is **preoperative evaluation** and **patient selection.**
■ The first step is to assess the patient's ability to tan.

TIP: In general, the absence of tanning ability is closely related to a patient's sensitivity to a peel.

■ The second step is to assess the **amount of actinic damage.** In general, the worse the actinic damage, the thicker the skin, and the more aggressive the peel should be.
■ Glogau[47] developed a classification system to describe the degree of actinic damage in a patient.

GLOGAU'S CLASSIFICATION OF PHOTOAGING GROUPS

Group I: Mild (usually age 28-35 years)
No keratoses
Little wrinkling
No scarring
Little or no makeup

Group II: Moderate (usually age 35-50 years)
Early actinic keratoses: Slight yellow skin discoloration
Early wrinkling: Parallel smile lines
Mild scarring
Little makeup

Group III: Advanced (usually age 50-65 years)
Actinic keratoses: Obvious yellow skin discoloration with telangiectasia
Wrinkling: Present at rest
Moderate acne scarring
Wears makeup always

Group IV: Severe (usually age 60-75 years)
Actinic keratoses and skin cancers have occurred
Wrinkling: Much cutis laxa of actinic, gravitational, and dynamic origin
Severe acne scarring
Wears makeup that does not cover, but cakes

Modified from Glogau RG. Presentation at the Chemical Peel Symposium, American Academy of Dermatology, Atlanta, Dec 1990.

FACTORS AFFECTING THE DEPTH OF PENETRATION

- Concentration of acid
- Peeling formula used
- Skin preparation before peeling
- Degreasing
- Skin cleansing
- Abrasion or topical retinoic acid
- Sebaceous gland density
- Cutaneous anatomy
- Occlusion
- Method of application
- Acid neutralization (for alpha hydroxy acids)
- Repetition and frequency of peel
- Storage and age of peeling solution

COMPARISON WITH LASER RESURFACING

- Less dermal thinning
- Cheaper
- More effective in treating deep rhytids
- Redness lasts longer
- More swelling in first 5 days

- Can perform light peels—repeatable without scarring and with minimal erythema
- Deep peels: Take longer to heal with prolonged erythema and risk of hypopigmentation and dermal scarring[37,48,49]

PRETREATMENT REGIMEN

- **Pretreatment is key for preventing complications, optimizing the effect of the peel, and ensuring the most dramatic results.**
- Pretreatment begins with **avoidance of sun and cigarette smoke** and the **initiation of a daily skin care regimen** consisting of a buffing grain cleanser, an alpha hydroxy acid toner, and a vitamin A conditioning lotion.
  - Buffing grains strip off dead skin cells.
  - Alpha hydroxy acid toners strip off the upper layer of epidermal cells, forcing the skin to proliferate rapidly.
  - Vitamin A conditioning lotions are thought to help regenerate the skin.
  - The net result of this skin care regimen is to increase the cell turnover from the normal 28 days to 10-12 days.
  - Ideally, a rosy red hue should be produced, indicating rapid skin turnover.
  - This skin care regimen can be adjusted as needed.
  - For patients who will eventually need more aggressive treatments, this regimen still should be used as the first-line pretreatment of the skin for several weeks or months before deeper peels or resurfacing are performed.
- Patients who have more significant photoaging should have either microdermabrasion or a glycolic acid peel monthly, in addition to this skin care regimen.
- IPL therapy can be used for patients with moderate-to-severe actinic damage. Intermediate-to-deep resurfacing with a laser, dermabrasion, and TCA or phenol peels also can be used.
- **Sunscreen** should be used daily.
- **Tretinoin** (Vesanoid), a synthetic retinoic acid, should be prescribed.
  - Stimulates papillary dermal collagen synthesis and angiogenesis
  - Increases glycosaminoglycan (GAG) deposition
  - Exfoliates the stratum corneum, which makes the skin more sensitive to the peel

CAUTION: Users should be aware of increased photosensitivity during tretinoin use. Sunscreen should be worn during use.

- **Tyrosinase inhibitors,** such as **hydroquinone,** also should be used to block tyrosinase, a key enzyme in the production of melanin.
  - Tyrosinase inhibitors prevent new melanosome formation but do not lighten existing pigment.
  - Tyrosinase inhibitors help prevent postpeel hyperpigmentation.

NOTE: Significant controversy exists about the optimal duration of the prepeel regimen. As little as 2 weeks and as much as 3 months have been recommended.

SUPERFICIAL PEELING AGENTS

- **Alpha hydroxy acid peels**
  - AHA occurs naturally in many fruits including apples, grapes, and citrus fruits.
  - Lactic acid, glycolic acid, tartaric acid, and malic acid can be used.

- Concentrations range from 10%-70% with 50% or 70% the most common.
  - ▶ At **lower** concentrations, AHAs **decrease keratinocyte cohesion** above the stratum granulosum, causing desquamation.
  - ▶ At **higher** concentrations, AHAs can cause **epidermolysis.**
- The primary use of AHAs is as an **exfoliant.**
- Exfoliation occurs over a few days.
- The **pH** of the solution controls the effect.

CAUTION: A pH of less than 2 causes epithelial necrosis instead of exfoliation.

- The FDA has approved AHAs for consumer sale if the pH is greater than 3.5 and the acid concentration is no greater than 10%.
- The FDA has approved AHAs for use by cosmetologists, as long as the pH is greater than 3.0 and the concentration is no greater than 30%.
- Physicians can use higher concentrations of AHAs with a lower pH.
- Moy et al[50] have developed different concentrations and treatment times for various skin conditions (Table 75-2).

Table 75-2 *Recommended Duration of Glycolic Acid Peels for Different Skin Conditions*

Condition	Glycolic Acid (%)	Time (Minutes)
Melasma	50	2-4
Acne	50	1-3
Actinic keratosis	70	5-7
Wrinkles	70	4-8
Solar lentigines	70	4-6

Data from Moy LS, Murad H, Moy RL. Glycolic acid peels for the treatment of wrinkles and photoaging. J Dermatol Surg Oncol 19:243-246, 1993.

TIP: Pretreatment with tretinoin (Retin-A) increases the depth of penetration and accelerates wound healing.[51-53]

■ **Jessner's solution**
- Can be used as another superficial peel or as an intermediate peel
- Like alpha hydroxy acids, functions as a **keratolytic**
- **Solution consists of:**
  - ▶ Resorcinol: 14 g
  - ▶ Salicylic acid: 14 g
  - ▶ Lactic acid: 14 cc
  - ▶ qs ethanol: 1000 cc
- Can be used to perform a **superficial peel** or as a **keratolytic** to prepare the skin for a TCA peel, as it produces keratolysis that allows the TCA peel to have a deeper and more profound effect.
- **Depth of penetration determined by number of coats**

- Can be applied in six or seven coats for an intermediate peel
  - The skin will slough, starting with the central face area in 3 days, progressing to the midcheek in 5 days, and toward the ears in 7 days.
- Peel repeatable every 2-3 months

> TIP: Jessner's solution is easy to use, with no timing necessary. Neutralize with water after creating a light frost.

- **Salicylic acid**
  - Use at concentrations of **20%-30%.**
  - It is lipid soluble, and therefore good for comedonal acne.
  - Antiinflammatory and anaesthetic effects result in decreased erythema and pain.
- **Carbon dioxide ice (dry ice)**
  - Apply with an alcohol-acetone mixture.
  - Apply for 5-15 seconds, depending on the desired depth.
  - Dry ice is applied at $-78°$ C versus $-196°$ C for liquid nitrogen.

MEDIUM-DEPTH PEELS

- **Trichloroacetic acid**
  - TCA is derivative of acetic acid used for **intermediate to deep peels.**
  - TCA is commonly used at concentrations of 15%-50%.
    - At concentrations of **20%-35%,** functions as an **intermediate** peel
    - At concentrations of **45%-55%,** can penetrate the skin irregularly and cause **scarring**
  - TCA causes **coagulative necrosis** of cells through extensive protein denaturation and cell death.
  - Over 5-7 days, the epidermis and superficial dermis slough.[54-57]
  - The skin slough usually begins centrally and proceeds laterally.

> TIP: If the TCA peel is performed midweek, most of the skin sloughing will occur over the weekend.

- **Depth of penetration** is directly related to **strength of the solution** and to **pretreatment of the skin.**

> TIP: Retin-A can be used to pretreat the skin, causing dekeratinization and allowing for a greater depth of penetration. It also can accelerate the postoperative healing process.

- **Penetration can be improved** and made more uniform by using the following procedure immediately before the TCA peel.
  - **Wash** and **degrease** the skin to remove oil.
  - **Mechanically remove** surface debris.
  - **Chemically disrupt the skin barrier** with mild acid solutions such as **Jessner's solution.**

- When using Jessner's solution before the TCA peel, apply 3-4 coats. Then follow with a 20%-35% TCA peel.
- The **endpoint** for an intermediate-depth peel, using Jessner's solution and TCA, is the production of Obagi's level 1 frost, which is a **foggy white frost on an erythematous base.**
- A **second endpoint** is an epidermal slide, which is produced if a cotton tip applicator is applied to the surface of the skin.
  - ▸ This has also been given the name *accordion sign.*
  - ▸ The epidermal slide disappears as the peel penetrates deeper.
- As a peel is made deeper, an intense white to yellow blanch is produced, indicating a peel at Obagi's level 2 or 3.[49,58]
- The wounds are healed by secondary intention, during which the epidermis is repopulated and the disorganized, damaged collagen of the superficial dermis is replaced by orderly, newly formed collagen.

CAUTION: Dingman et al[59] have shown that TCA peels can be used safely in conjunction with a deep-plane facelift. Peeling in the setting of undermined skin in the facelift patient is nevertheless worrisome because of the potential development of postoperative skin slough.

DEEP PEELS
- **Phenol peel**
  - **Phenol** is a derivative of **coal tar** that causes rapid denaturation and coagulation of surface keratin.
  - Phenol produces a new zone of collagen.
  - Phenol is effective for wrinkles and severe dyschromia.
  - Phenol penetrates to the **middle reticular dermis.**
  - Similar to TCA peels, the **depth of penetration** can be greatly affected by preparing the skin with **washing** and **degreasing** before peel application.

CAUTION: Cardiac monitoring is required, because phenol can cause arrhythmias.

  - Occluding methods prevent evaporation, resulting in deeper penetration.
  - Significant controversy exists about the concentration required for optimal results.
    - ▸ Mackee and Karp[60] have used 88% phenol to produce superficial peels that were repeatable every month for 4-6 months.
    - ▸ 50% concentrations of phenol were found by Spira et al[61] to be as effective as stronger concentrations, with fewer complications.
  - Today the most common formulation is the **Baker-Gordon peel.**[62-64]
    - ▸ **Phenol:** 3 cc
    - ▸ **Tap water:** 2 cc
    - ▸ **Liquid soap:** Eight drops
      - ✦ Soap acts as a surfactant to lower surface tension. It also emulsifies and aids in penetration.
    - ▸ **Croton oil:** Three drops
      - ✦ **Croton oil** is a skin irritant that causes inflammation, vesication, and secondary collagen formation.
- **Hetter's croton oil peel**
  - Hetter[65-68] believes that the true active ingredient in phenol peels is the **croton oil, not the phenol,** and that minute changes in the concentration of the croton oil can cause very different results.

- Hetter has published the **"heresy phenol formulas,"** which give the concentrations of ingredients needed for different levels of peeling in different anatomic regions (Table 75-3).
- **Hetter has suggested the following order for mixing the solution:**
  1. Croton oil is added to undiluted phenol.
  2. After this mixture dissolves completely, water is added.
  3. Finally, Septisol soap is added.
- Truppman and Ellenby[69] found a significant incidence of cardiac arrhythmias when 50% of the face was treated with a phenol–croton-oil peel in less than 30 minutes. If this treatment was spread out over 60 minutes, no arrhythmias were seen.

> TIP: Cardiac monitoring should be employed whenever phenol peels are used.

- To avoid arrhythmias, Binstock[70] advises peeling the face by small sections 15-20 minutes apart, preparing the skin with washing, and degreasing the skin before peel application.

Table 75-3 *Formulas Varying the Concentration of Phenol and Croton Oil*

35% Phenol Vehicle*

	Croton Oil (%)			
	0.4	0.8	1.2	1.6
Water	5.5	5.5	5.5	5.5
USP phenol 88%	3.0	2.0	1.0	0.0
Stock solution containing croton oil	1.0	2.0	3.0	4.0
Septisol	0.5	0.5	0.5	0.5
TOTAL	10	10	10	10

48.5% Phenol Vehicle†

	Croton Oil (%)				
	0.4	0.8	1.2	1.6	2.0
Water	4.0	4.0	4.0	4.0	3.5
USP phenol 88%	4.5	3.5	2.5	1.5	1.0
Stock solution containing croton oil	1.0	2.0	3.0	4.0	5.0
Septisol	0.5	0.5	0.5	0.5	0.5
TOTAL	10	10	10	10	10

From Hetter GP. An examination of the phenol-croton oil peel. Part IV. Face peel results with different concentrations of phenol and croton oil. Plast Reconstr Surg 105:1061-1083, 2000.
*For eyelids and neck, take 1 ml of the 0.4% solution and mix it with 1.2 ml of USP phenol 88% and 1.8 ml of water for a 0.1% solution of croton oil in 35% phenol.
†For eyelids and neck, take 1 ml of the 0.4% solution and mix it with 1.7 ml of USP phenol 88% and 1.3 ml of water for a 0.1% solution of croton oil in 50% phenol.

- **Comparison of TCA peel with phenol–croton-oil peel**
  - Phenol–croton-oil peels produce **less hypertrophic scarring** than TCA peels for every layer of wrinkle depth.
  - All deep phenol peels cause some degree of hypopigmentation.
  - Phenol–croton-oil peels tend to produce less hypopigmentation than TCA peels.

COMPLICATIONS OF RESURFACING

- **Infection:** Bacterial, viral, or fungal
  - Antiviral prophylaxis is indicated for those with a history of herpes simplex.
- **Prolonged erythema**
  - Topical hydrocortisone can improve erythema.
- **Acne:** Possible between days 3 and 9
- **Scarring**
  - Avoid resurfacing for patients with a history of keloid scars.
- **Pigmentary change**
  - Hyperpigmentation usually resolves.
  - Hypopigmentation can be permanent.
- **Milia:** Sometimes appear 2-3 weeks after reepithelialization
  - May be aggravated by ointments because of occluded sebaceous glands.

BOTULINUM TOXIN

- Botulinum toxin is derived from the bacterium *Clostridium botulinum*.[71]
  - *C. botulinum* produces seven distinct neurotoxins.
- Botulinum toxins A and B are both commercially available.
- The FDA has approved type A for treatment of glabellar frown lines and for hyperhidrosis. Type B is approved for treatment of cervical dystonia.
- Type A typically is used for aesthetic rhytid reduction.
- Different preparations are commercially available. To standardize methodology, dosages should be in **cosmetic units.**
- The **lethal dose 50** of botulinum toxin A is **2700 units** for a **70 kg** human.[72]
- Botox® (Allergan Corp., Santa Barbara, CA) comes in vials, each consisting of 100 units of dry powder. This powder is typically diluted with 2.5 to 4 cc of normal saline for a final concentration of 2.5 to **4 units/0.1 cc.**
- Preserved or nonpreserved normal saline may be used for reconstitution.
  - Preserved saline may be associated with decreased pain from injections.[73]
- When reconstituted, Botox should be clear, colorless, and free from particulate matter.
- The manufacturer recommends using Botox within 4 hours of reconstitution.
  - The literature reports use of Botox up to 6 weeks after reconstituting it with nonpreserved saline and storing it at 4° C.[73]
- Bruising can be decreased by stopping medications that inhibit clotting 10-14 days before treatment. These include aspirin, nonsteroidal antiinflammatory drugs (NSAIDs), and vitamin E.
- Botox is contraindicated by active infection at the proposed treatment sites and by hypersensitivity to any of the ingredients contained within the diluent, including albumin.

- **Use Botox cautiously with:**
  - Patients who have a peripheral motor neuropathic disease such as **myasthenia gravis** or **Eaton-Lambert syndrome**
  - **Coadministration of aminoglycoside antibiotics** or other agents that interfere with neuromuscular transmission
  - **Inflammatory skin disorders** at the injection site
  - **Pregnancy**
  - **Lactation**[73]
- Reassess the patient at 14 days and consider any touch-ups at that time.
- The typical interval for treatment is 3-4 months.

GLABELLAR COMPLEX AND VERTICAL FOREHEAD LINES[73]

- The targeted muscles include the **corrugator supercilii, procerus,** and **orbicularis oculi.**
- The starting dose for women is 20-30 U and 30-40 U for men.
- 5-7 injection points are recommended (Fig. 75-1).
- Avoid injecting too low around the orbit—all injections should be directed outside the orbital rim.

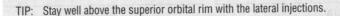

Fig. 75-1 From Carruthers J, Fagien S, Matarasso SL, et al. Consensus recommendations on the use of botulinum toxin type A in facial aesthetics. Plast Reconstr Surg 114(Suppl 6):S1-S22, 2004.

TIP: Stay well above the superior orbital rim with the lateral injections.

HORIZONTAL FOREHEAD LINES

- The target muscle is the **frontalis.**
- The starting dose for women is 10-20 U and 20-30 U for men.
- 4-8 injection points may be used.
- Stay at least **2 cm** above the brow.
- Look for brow asymmetry before injecting. This may be partially corrected by additional injections on the side where the brow is the most depressed.

CAUTION: If injections are too centralized, a "quizzical" eyebrow appearance results, with lateral brow elevation and central depression.

- Avoid low, lateral brow injections. A high, lateral brow injection results in a significant alteration of the lateral brow.

CROW'S FEET (LATERAL ORBITAL WRINKLES)[73]

- The target is the **lateral portion of the orbicularis oculi muscle.**
- The total starting dose is 12-30 U.
- Use 2-5 injection points per side (Fig. 75-2).
- Before injecting this area, perform a snap test to the lower lids. If they are lax, there is significant risk for postinjection ectropion, and low injections must be avoided.

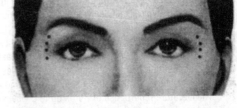

Fig. 75-2 From Carruthers J, Fagien S, Matarasso SL, et al. Consensus recommendations on the use of botulinum toxin type A in facial aesthetics. Plast Reconstr Surg 114(Suppl 6):S1-S22, 2004.

- Use caution around the lower one third of the canthal area.
- **Do not inject below the zygomatic arch** or in the region of the **zygomaticus muscle,** because this can cause lip and cheek ptosis.

CAUTION: To prevent postoperative bruising, take care to search for veins and avoid injuring them.

- Use caution if the patient has a history of dry eyes, recent blepharoplasty, or has had LASIK surgery.

BUNNY LINES
Bunny lines appear on the sides of the nose and radiate downward.[73]

- Targets include the **nasalis** and **procerus** muscles.
- The typical starting dose is 3-6 U.
- Typically, three injection points are used, one in the midline and one on each side (Fig. 75-3).
- Keep injections in this area superficial to prevent bruising.
- To prevent drooping of the upper lip, take care **not to inject the levator labii superioris alaeque nasi** and **levator labii superioris.** To prevent Botox from diffusing into these muscles, take care not to massage too vigorously or in a downward direction.

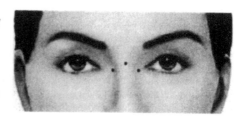

Fig. 75-3 From Carruthers J, Fagien S, Matarasso SL, et al. Consensus recommendations on the use of botulinum toxin type A in facial aesthetics. Plast Reconstr Surg 114(Suppl 6):S1-S22, 2004.

PERIORAL WRINKLES[73]

- Use Botox to decrease the appearance of fine vertical wrinkles of the upper lip.
- Use Botox to produce a fuller upper lip by relaxing the orbicularis, causing slight eversion of the upper lip.
- The target is the **orbicularis oris** muscle.
- The usual starting dose is 4-10 U, evenly divided among the two sides.
- 2-7 injection points can be used (Fig. 75-4).
- Do **not** use in patients who use their lips for their professions, such as musicians, singers, or public speakers.
- Always inject symmetrically.
- Avoid the corners of the lips (to prevent drooling).
- Avoid the midline (to prevent flattening of the lip).
- Stay within 5 mm of the vermilion border.
- Lower lip injections have a more significant effect on muscle function and should be limited or avoided.

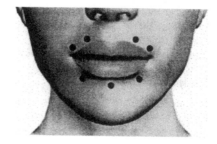

Fig. 75-4 From Carruthers J, Fagien S, Matarasso SL, et al. Consensus recommendations on the use of botulinum toxin type A in facial aesthetics. Plast Reconstr Surg 114(Suppl 6):S1-S22, 2004.

DIMPLED CHIN[73]

- The target is the **mentalis** muscle.
- The usual starting dose is 2-6 U in women and 2-8 U in men.
- One injection site in the midline, or two laterally, are recommended.

- Avoid injecting too high (to prevent affecting orbicularis function in the lower lip).
- Avoid the depressor labii.

PLATYSMAL BANDS[73]

- Treatment with botulinum toxin may be effective for patients who have platysmal banding but have retained their skin elasticity or those who have banding and previously had skin tightening from a rhytidectomy.
- The target is the **platysma** muscle.
- The usual starting dose is 10-30 U in women and 10-40 U in men.
- Women receive 2-12 injections per band, and men receive 3-12 injections.
- Patient selection and expectations are critical. Botox is **not** an alternative to surgery, and it **will not correct skin laxity or fat deposits.**
- **Strap muscles should be avoided.** To ensure that the treatment is limited to the platysma, grasp the bands and pull them toward the injecting hand, and then inject.
- Horizontal "necklace" lines also may be treated.

SOFT TISSUE FILLERS

IDEAL SOFT TISSUE FILLER[74]

- Safe and nontoxic
- Nonallergenic
- Easy to use
- Minimal downtime
- Predictable
- Potentially reversible
- Ages appropriately with the patient
- Nonpalpable
- Readily available

NOTE: The perfect soft tissue filler has yet to be created. The fillers that we have now incorporate many of the ideal characteristics but do not encompass them all.

CLASSES OF SOFT TISSUE FILLERS

- Autologous materials
- Biologic materials
- Synthetic materials
- Off-label materials

AUTOLOGOUS MATERIALS

- **Safety** is perhaps the biggest advantage of using autologous materials.
- Toxicity, allergic reactions, immunogenicity, carcinogenicity, and teratogenicity are not concerns.
- **Potential pitfalls** with autologous materials include infection, migration, inflammatory reactions, impermanence, technique dependence, and lack of reproducibility and reliability.
- Examples include fat, dermis, fascia, cartilage, subcutaneous musculoaponeurotic system (SMAS), Autologen® (collagen prepared from the patient's own skin; Collagenesis, Beverly, MA), and Isolagen® (tissue-culture–derived fibroblasts from a patient's own fibroblasts; Isolagen, Exton, PA).

BIOLOGIC MATERIALS

- Biologic materials are derived from **organic sources.**
- Primary **advantages** include ready, off-the-shelf availability and ease of use.
- **Disadvantages** include sensitization to foreign animal or human proteins, transmission of disease, and immunogenicity.
- Longevity is limited.
- Collagen products and hyaluronic acid products are the two major types.

SYNTHETIC MATERIALS

- **Advantages** include potential permanence, reduced concerns of disease transmission, and sensitization to foreign animal or human proteins.
- **Disadvantages** include potential for granuloma formation, acute and delayed infections, migration or displacement, and deformities that can result from complications or removal of the material.
- PTFE (polytetrafluoroethylene) is currently FDA approved for facial augmentation.
- Artecoll® (Canderm Pharma Inc., St. Laurent, Quebec) and Bioplastique™ (Ingenta, Providence, RI) are currently under FDA consideration.
- The FDA approval process limits the availability of synthetic materials for use as a soft tissue filler. Many more products are available outside the United States.

OFF-LABEL MATERIALS

- Many synthetic fillers are FDA approved for use with conditions unrelated to plastic surgery.
- The FDA limits and prevents manufacturers from marketing these products for other uses; however, plastic surgeons have found alternative uses for some of these products off-label.
- Liability is a concern if potential complications arise.
- Calcium hydroxyapatite (Radiesse™; BioForm Medical, Inc., San Mateo, CA) is perhaps the best example of this class. It is currently FDA approved for vocal cord injections but is used by plastic surgeons for soft tissue augmentation.

CHARACTERISTICS OF SPECIFIC COMMON SOFT TISSUE FILLERS

AUTOLOGOUS FAT

- Autologous fat can be injected for soft tissue augmentation.
- It does not act as a dermal filler, but subcutaneous volume is enhanced.
- It can be used in facial or body contouring.

CAUTION: Do not use in the breast, because the microcalcifications that result may raise suspicions of malignancy.

- Common areas of use include the infraorbital hollow, malar region, angle of the mandible, anterior or posterior jaw line, chin, nasolabial fold, and supraorbital or temporal region.
- It is also used to fill iatrogenic deformities after liposuction.
- **Fat survival is technique dependent.**
  - Peer[75,76] found a 50% survival of autologous fat grafts.

- Coleman[77] demonstrated long-term survival of fat with his "structural fat-grafting technique" and provided the following principles and guidelines for structural fat grafting:
  - Fatty tissue is more fragile than most other human tissues and is damaged easily outside the body by mechanical insults.
  - To survive harvesting, transport, and implantation with cannulas and syringes, fat must be harvested in intact parcels, small enough to be inserted through a small cannula but large enough so that the tissue architecture is maintained.
  - Fat is living tissue that must be in close proximity to a nutritional and respiratory source to survive.
  - Placement by keeping the fat parcels separate from one another encourages longevity and stability.
  - It is essential to maximize the contact surface area of each fatty tissue parcel with the surrounding host tissues for successful integration and anchoring of newly placed tissue.
  - Whenever possible, incisions are placed in wrinkle lines, folds, or hair-bearing areas to facilitate placement of the fat grafts in at least two directions when indicated.
  - To strengthen bony or underlying support, the fat can be layered against bone or cartilage in the deeper levels.
  - To support the skin, fat is layered immediately under the skin.
  - For filling and plumping or restoring fullness, tissues are placed in the intermediate layers between skin and the appropriate underlying layers.
- **Technique**
  - Harvest with a Coleman 14-gauge harvesting cannula or a Lambros 3 mm cannula.[78-80]
  - Harvesting should be done with a 10-20 cc syringe held at 1-2 cc of negative pressure to minimize trauma to the fat.
  - **The site of fat harvest does not alter success or longevity.[81]**
  - After fat harvest, spin for 1 minute at 1500 RPM to remove blood, oil, and local anaesthetic.
  - Inject fat in the facial region using a 1 cc syringe, with 0.1 cc of fat placed during each pass.[82]
  - The fat that survives transfer can be permanent, and it gains and loses volume with fluctuations in the weight of the patient.
  - **Great care must be taken when injecting fat into the eyelids.**
    - ▸ Small injection amounts should be used with each pass to prevent fat emboli to the eye or brain.
    - ▸ If the fat is injected too superficially, such as just below the thin eyelid skin or at the junction of the muscle and subcutaneous tissue, palpability or irregularities may be seen.

BOVINE COLLAGEN

- Bovine collagen was initially approved by the FDA in 1977.
- Multiple formulations of bovine collagen are commercially available.
  - **Zyderm I®** (Inamed Corp., Santa Barbara, CA): **35 mg/ml**
  - **Zyderm II®: 65 mg/ml**
    - ▸ **Zyderm** should be injected in the **dermal-epidermal** junction.
    - ▸ Zyderm is used to correct fine lines such as glabellar lines that remain after Botox treatment.
    - ▸ Zyderm can be layered, in addition to Zyplast, to give a more sculpted and potentially longer-lasting look.
    - ▸ Zyderm can be used in conjunction with Botox to treat vertical lines of the lips, crow's feet, and other fine lines in the face and neck.[74]

- **Zyplast®** (Inamed Corp.): Glutaraldehyde is used to cross-link the collagen moieties so that it is less immunogenic and lasts longer.
  - ▸ **Zyplast** should be used in the **middle dermis.**
  - ▸ Zyplast is best used for deeper folds or lines such as the nasolabial folds, melolabial and mental folds, angles of the mouth, vermilion border, and body of the lip.
- Histologic studies show disappearance of injected collagen by 6-9 months.[83]
- **3.5%** of the population has a **localized hypersensitivity** reaction.[84,85]
  - 1%-5% of patients with a negative skin test will still have an allergic reaction when collagen is injected into the face.
  - Because of hypersensitivity reactions, two skin tests should be performed. The first should be 5-6 weeks before injection followed by a second test 2 weeks after the first.
  - Even after two negative tests, there is a **0.1%** chance of a reaction to bovine collagen injections.[85,86]
  - Hypersensitivity reactions can be severe, lasting up to 1 year.
  - Hypersensitivity reactions to bovine collagen may manifest as redness, plaques, and scaling dermatitis.
  - Hypersensitivity reactions may be unresponsive to steroids.
- Inject with a 30-gauge needle and **overcorrect by 10%-20%.**

CAUTION: Use care when injecting Zyplast into the glabellar region, because there are reports of skin necrosis in this region following injection.

- There is no need to massage after collagen injection unless there are obvious lumps. Some believe that vigorous massage actually decreases the longevity of the injection.
- Ice the face for 15-20 minutes after injection.
- Compared with other fillers, there is limited swelling. Swelling that does occur usually resolves within 24 hours.

HUMAN COLLAGEN
- **CosmoDerm™** (Inamed Corp.) is purified human-based collagen in phosphate-buffered saline with 0.3% lidocaine.
  - CosmoDerm may last up to **4 months.**
  - CosmoDerm should be injected in the **superficial dermis.**
  - CosmoDerm can be used in conjunction with Botox to treat vertical lines of the lips, crow's feet, and other fine lines in the face and neck.
- **CosmoPlast™** (Inamed Corp.) is purified human-based collagen that is cross-linked with glutaraldehyde to decrease immunogenicity and increase longevity.
  - CosmoPlast can be used to treat deeper lines or folds such as the nasolabial folds or mental folds; it may also be used to augment the lips or vermilion border.
  - CosmoPlast will last anywhere from **4 weeks to 3 months.**
  - CosmoPlast should be injected in the **middle to deep dermis.**

TIP: Human collagen is favored by most, rather than bovine collagen, because there is no concern for hypersensitivity reactions.

NOTE: **No skin test is required.**

> TIP: When correcting smile lines at the corners of the mouth, inject CosmoPlast deeply and CosmoDerm more superficially. This tends to be a difficult area, and a 50% correction is a very good result.[74]

- Use a 30-gauge needle and **overcorrect by 10%-20%.**
- Collagen tends to be easier to inject than hyaluronic acids.
- There is no need to massage after collagen injection, unless there are obvious lumps. Some believe that vigorous massage actually decreases the longevity of the injection.
- Ice the face for 15-20 minutes after injection.
- Compared with other fillers, there is limited swelling. The swelling that does occur usually resolves within 24 hours.

HYALURONIC ACID (HA) DERIVATIVES

- HA is a normal component of the ground substance responsible for dermal hydration.
- HA is a linear polysaccharide composed of repeating disaccharide units of N-acetyl-glucosamine and N-acetyl-glucuronic acid. It belongs to a larger class of molecules called **glycosaminoglycans.**
- HA was approved by the FDA in 2003.
- It is a polysaccharide with no species specificity, so there is **no immunologic activity** and **no need for a skin test.**
- HA absorbs water and **expands after injection.**
- **Injections can be painful.** Topical and/or injectable anaesthesia should be used to make the patient comfortable.
- **Potential complications** include erythema, edema, ecchymosis, and acneiform dermatitis.
- HA lasts approximately **6-9 months.**
- Hyaluronic acid products include Restylane® (Q-Med AB, Uppsala, Sweden), Restylane Touch® (Q-Med AB), Perlane® (Q-Med AB), Hylaform® (Inamed Corp.), Hylaform Plus® (Inamed Corp.), Juvederm® (Inamed Corp.), and Captique™ (Inamed Corp.).
- The various HA products available are differentiated based on their source (bacterial or avian), the cross-linking agent, particle size, and HA concentration.
- **Perlane, Juvederm 30,** and **Hylaform Plus** are the **largest hyaluronic acid** particles and should be injected into the **deepest layer of the dermis.**
- **Restylane, Juvederm 24,** and **Hylaform** are **midsized particles** and should be injected at the **middle dermis level.**
- **Restylane Fine Lines, Juvederm 18,** and **Hylaform Fine Lines** are the **smallest particles,** and should be injected at the **dermal-epidermal junction.**

> TIP: Combining different particle sizes allows tailoring the therapy to treat a range of conditions, from deeper folds, such as the nasolabial folds, to finer lines.

CAUTION: Injection of HA too superficially can lead to a bluish discoloration.

- The higher viscosity of the material makes HA injection more difficult than collagen injection.
- Inject with an even flow to prevent lumps or irregularities.
- If lumps are noted at the time of injection, **massage** immediately.
- **Inject to the final desired volume.**

- HA derivatives cause much more swelling and bruising than collagen injections.
- After injection, patients should cool the area with ice packs for the first 24 hours; and they should take oral antihistamines.
- Patients should expect 3-5 days of swelling, which can cause worry of overcorrection.
- Bruising may last up to 1.5 weeks.
- With repeated injections of HA, the product lasts longer, and less volume is required.
- With larger injection volumes, abscesses may occur, which can be drained with an 18-gauge needle.
- Intermittent swelling may occur for the first 2-6 weeks in rare cases.
- If massive swelling occurs, consider using a steroid dose pack.
- Telangiectasias may form, especially in response to larger injections or in patients with either preexisting telangiectasias in the injection region, or rosacea.
- Rarely, patients may develop erythema of the overlying skin, which can be treated with a light topical steroid.
- **Lip augmentation**
  - Use midsized HA products such as Restylane, or a combination of a midsized HA and another filler.
  - Use infraorbital and mental nerve blocks or a topical anaesthetic.
  - Lidocaine with epinephrine can be used to decrease bruising.
  - If lip shape is good initially, then augmenting the vermilion border alone may be enough to produce a good result.
  - Note preexisting asymmetries between the right and left sides of the lips before injecting.
  - Long, thin lips tend to have a higher resting tension and experience less dramatic results.
  - In patients with lips that are tight to the dentition or with an Angle class II occlusion, augmentation should be conservative to prevent irregularities of the dentition to be reflected in the lips and to prevent the lips from appearing too prominent.
  - Use viral prophylaxis in patients with a history of herpes to prevent herpetic outbreak and scarring.
  - Begin with augmentation of the vermilion border.
  - If desired, proceed to augmentation of the philtral columns.
  - Injection within the lip itself should be performed in the substance of the orbicularis oris.
  - Limit injection of the skin above the upper lip vermilion border because augmentation of this region lengthens the upper lip skin.
  - HA can be combined with Botox to limit pinching of the lip and the formation of vertical lines.
    - ▸ Two units of Botox are used per side in the upper lip.
    - ▸ Take care to avoid the midline.
    - ▸ Botox should be placed within 5 mm of the vermilion border. The closer it is placed to the vermilion border, the greater the resulting lip projection.
- **Effacement of nasolabial folds**
  - A reasonable goal is **50% correction** of the depth of the nasolabial fold.
  - Place HA at angles to the fold, and layer to enhance longevity.
  - If the fold has a superficial line etched into it, use small-sized HA particles to address the condition.
  - Taping the fold for a few days after injection can prevent lateral displacement of the product when the patient smiles.
  - **Do not completely correct the fold,** because this will give the patient an odd appearance.
  - Too much filler in the areas over the dentition can appear as a bump.
- **Scar correction**
  - More than one treatment may be required to achieve full correction.
  - Using an 18-gauge needle to release the scar improves results.

- **Glabellar folds**
  - Treat in combination with Botox.
  - Use either a small or midsize HA product.
  - Use a cross-radial tunneling injection technique.
- Restylane and Perlane are ideal for correcting lipoatrophy secondary to antiretroviral therapy for HIV.
  - The areas most frequently treated are the inframalar hollow, concavities adjacent to the zygomatic temporal bone, and the zygomatic arch.
  - In the temple and adjacent to the arch, place the filler deep within or under the periosteum.
- The goal of lipoatrophy correction should be to soften the contours but not totally correct them.[74]

CALCIUM HYDROXYAPATITE (CAHA)

- Calcium hydroxyapatite (Radiesse™; BioForm Medical, Inc.) is a pure synthetic made primarily of calcium and phosphate ions.
- The particles are identical to the mineral portion of human bone.
- CaHA particles have a consistent, uniform, smooth, spherical shape with a narrow size range of 25-45 μm.
- CaHA particles are suspended in an aqueous gel composed of sodium carboxymethyl cellulose, glycerin, and sterile water.
- The carrier gel is replaced with the patient's own connective tissue over 3-6 months.
- The carrier gel is 70% of the product's volume.
- Fibrous tissue grows on the spheres and holds them in place. The manufacturer reports no evidence of fibroblastic encapsulation or particle migration.
- **No sensitivity testing** is required.
- Currently, the FDA has approved CaHA for oral or maxillofacial defects and vocal cord insufficiency.
- Clinical trials for use in nasolabial folds are under way.
- The **effect is permanent.**
- CaHA is used best for nasolabial folds, lips, radial lip lines, white rolls, glabellar lines, acne scars, facial lipoatrophy, posttraumatic or poststeroid atrophy, and cheek, chin, or mandibular borders.[74]
- Place CaHA in the **deep dermis.**
- Place the material as the needle is withdrawn with a linear injection technique.
- Layer the product for deep folds.
- Postinjection massage is important to smooth out any irregularities.
- The maximum volume occurs at 4-6 weeks.
- There is an 8%-10% incidence of lumps.[87-89]
- Treat irregularities monthly with dilute triamcinolone (Kenalog) until resolved.
- Use intermittent icing for 24 hours and avoid blood thinners before injecting.

POLY-L-LACTIC ACID (PLLA)

- **Sculptra™** (Dermik Laboratories, Berwyn, PA) is injectable poly-L-lactic acid.
- Sculptra is a synthetic polymer that is biodegradable, biocompatible, and immunologically inert.
- Because it is neither human nor animal derived, **no skin test is required.**
- Microparticles are broken down by nonenzymatic hydrolysis into lactic acid monomers, which are then metabolized into CO_2 or incorporated into glucose.
- The initial tissue reaction to PLLA is inflammatory, involving mononuclear macrophages and proliferating fibroblasts with capsule formation around the microspheres.
- **The PLLA eventually degrades and is replaced with collagen.**
- PLLA is currently FDA approved for restoration and/or correction of lipoatrophy associated with HIV.

- Because it must be injected **deeply,** Sculptra is **not** indicated for correction of perioral, periorbital, and facial lines requiring superficial deposition.
- **Reconstitute at least 2 hours before injection.**
- Once reconstituted, it may be stored at room temperature for 72 hours.
- Before use, the vial must be rolled or agitated to ensure a uniform translucent suspension.
- Reconstitute each vial with 3-5 cc of sterile water.
- The more water that is used for reconstitution, the less dense and viscous the injection product will be.
- 1%-2% lidocaine (Xylocaine) may be added to solution to reduce pain.[74]
- Injection requires a relatively large needle (**a 26-gauge needle is the smallest that can be used).**
- Inject into deep dermal, subcutaneous tissues, or directly over the periosteum.
- Multiple injections in a crisscross pattern produce the best results.
- If the product is injected over bone, place the needle on the periosteum and inject an aliquot. Then use fingers to massage and spread the filler over the bone.
- After injection, place moisturizer on the area, massage the area for at least 5 minutes, and then place ice packs.
- The patient should massage the injected area at home every day.
- If patients require significant volume correction, it is best not to do it all at once.
- Edema will give the initial appearance of a full correction, but it will resolve over several hours to several days, causing the contour defect to reappear.
- If facial fat loss is severe, 3-6 treatments may be required.
- The final effect may last up to **2 years.**[90-92]
- **Side effects** include delayed occurrence of subcutaneous papules, bleeding from the injection site, discomfort, erythema or inflammation, ecchymosis, granulation formation, and edema.[74]

POLYMETHYLMETHACRYLATE (PMMA)

- Artefill® (Artes Medical, Inc., San Diego, CA) and Artecoll are collagen-covered polymethylmethacrylate beads.
- The collagen is a transport vehicle and is absorbed over a 4-6–week period.
- The volume of the tissue is increased by the body making connective tissue around the PMMA beads.
- PMMA is a **permanent filler.**
- The safest areas of injection are the nasolabial folds and deep marionette lines.
- PMMA works well for deep soft acne scars.

CAUTION: Rhytids in the glabellar and periorbital region can thin with age, eventually causing the permanent filler to become visible.

- Do **not** use for superficial rhytids.
- Use caution and **preinjection testing** for patients with known collagen allergies.
- Use a 26-gauge needle for injection.
- Inject as the needle is withdrawn from the deep dermal plane.
- After injection, massage the area to ensure that there are no lumps.
- Immediately after injection into mobile areas, such as the lips or nasolabial folds, place tape on them to limit movement and filler migration.
- If filling depressed scars, release the scar before injecting the PMMA. In the case of scars, serial injections every 8 weeks should be used for complete correction.
- Although Artecoll and Artefill are considered permanent fillers, more volume may be required after approximately 1.5 years.[93]

- Because of its viscosity, Artecoll is the most difficult filler to inject. In addition, the syringes may contain air because of collagen evaporation, which may cause irregularities in the pressure and delivery of the filler.
- Inform patients that initial results are not seen for 6-8 weeks, because collagen is absorbed during this time and replaced with tissue growth into the PMMA beads.[93]
- Irregularities discovered soon after injection should be treated with injection of a dilute dose of a steroid (Kenalog, 0.2 mg/ml) to soften the irregularity. If this is unsuccessful, surgical excision of the irregularity may be required.
- Rare granulomas may form in response to the PMMA beads.[74,94,95]

KEY POINTS

- ✔ Successful rejuvenation of an aging face requires thorough analysis of both actinic and chronologic damage.
- ✔ A variety of options are available to treat an aging face nonsurgically. These include resurfacing, paralysis of underlying musculature, and soft tissue augmentation.
- ✔ When considering resurfacing, patients and physicians must balance the desire for dramatic results with the desire for minimal recovery.
- ✔ Botox requires a thorough understanding of the anatomy of the facial muscles. Successful injections can provide dramatic results, but poorly located injections can cause deformities.
- ✔ A variety of soft tissue fillers exist, each with its own profile of sensitivity and longevity. Patients and physicians must understand the limitations and potential benefits of each filler.

REFERENCES

1. Sauermann K, Clemans S, Jaspers S, et al. Age related changes of human skin investigated with histometric measurements by confocal laser scanning microscopy in vivo. Skin Res Technol 8:52-56, 2002.
2. West MD. The cellular and molecular biology of skin aging. Arch Dermatol 130:87-95, 1994.
3. Burkhardt BR, Maw R. Are more passes better? Safety versus efficacy with the pulsed CO_2 laser. Plast Reconstr Surg 100:1531-1534, 1997.
4. Walsh JT Jr, Deutsch TF. Pulsed CO_2 laser tissue ablation: Measurement of the ablation rate. Lasers Surg Med 8:264-275, 1988.
5. Stuzin JM, Baker TJ, Baker TM, et al. Histologic effects of the high-energy pulsed CO_2 laser on photoaged facial skin. Plast Reconstr Surg 99:2036-2050, 1997.
6. Smith KJ, Skelton HG, Graham JS, et al. Depth of morphologic skin damage and viability after one, two, and three passes of a high-energy, short-pulse CO_2 laser (Tru-Pulse) in pig skin. J Am Acad Dermatol 37:204-210, 1997.
7. Grossman AR, Majidian AM, Grossman PH. Thermal injuries as a result of CO_2 laser resurfacing. Plast Reconstr Surg 102:1247-1252, 1998.
8. Stuzin JM, Baker TJ, Baker TM. CO_2 and erbium:YAG laser resurfacing: Current status and personal perspective. Plast Reconstr Surg 103:588-591, 1999.
9. Weinstein C, Ramirez OM, Pozner JN. Postoperative care following CO_2 laser resurfacing: Avoiding pitfalls. Plast Reconstr Surg 100:1855-1866, 1997.
10. Williams EF III, Dahiya R. Review of nonablative laser resurfacing modalities. Facial Plast Surg Clin North Am 12:305-310, 2004.
11. Jacobson D, Bass LS, VanderKam V, et al. Carbon dioxide and ER:YAG laser resurfacing. Results. Clin Plast Surg 27:241-250, 2000.

12. Chajchir A, Benzaquen I. Carbon dioxide laser resurfacing with fast recovery. Aesthetic Plast Surg 29:107-112, 2005.
13. Brunner E, Adamson PA, Harlock JN, et al. Laser facial resurfacing: Patient survey of recovery and results. J Otolaryngol 29:377-381, 2000.
14. Schwartz RJ, Burns AJ, Rohrich RJ, et al. Long-term assessment of CO_2 facial laser resurfacing: Aesthetic results and complications. Plast Reconstr Surg 103:592-601, 1999.
15. Alster TS, Doshi SN, Hopping SB. Combination surgical lifting with ablative laser skin resurfacing of facial skin: A retrospective analysis. Dermatol Surg 30:1191-1195, 2004.
16. Bass S. Erbium:YAG laser skin resurfacing: Preliminary clinical evaluation. Ann Plast Surg 40:328-334, 1998.
17. Pozner JM, Goldberg DJ. Histologic effect of a variable pulsed Er:YAG laser. Dermatol Surg 26:733-736, 2000.
18. Goldman MP, Marchell N, Fitzpatrick RE. Laser skin resurfacing of the face with a combined CO_2/Er:YAG laser. Dermatol Surg 26:102-104, 2000.
19. Zachary CB. Modulating the Er:YAG laser. Lasers Surg Med 26:223-226, 2000.
20. Weinstein C. Erbium laser resurfacing: Current concepts. Plast Reconstr Surg 103:602-616, 1999.
21. Perez MI, Bank DE, Silvers D. Skin resurfacing of the face with the Erbium:YAG laser. Dermatol Surg 24:653-658, 1998.
22. Adrian RM. Pulsed carbon dioxide and erbium-YAG laser resurfacing: A comparative clinical and histologic study. J Cutan Laser Ther 1:29-35, 1999.
23. Adrian RM. Pulsed carbon dioxide and long pulse 10-ms erbium-YAG laser resurfacing: A comparative clinical and histologic study. J Cutan Laser Ther 1:197-202, 1999.
24. Tanzi EL, Alster TS. Side effects and complications of variable-pulsed erbium:yttrium-aluminum-garnet laser skin resurfacing: Extended experience with 50 patients. Plast Reconstr Surg 111:1524-1529, 2003.
25. Ross EV, Miller C, Meehan K, et al. One-pass CO_2 versus multiple-pass Er:YAG laser resurfacing in the treatment of rhytids: A comparison side-by-side study of pulsed CO_2 and Er:YAG lasers. Dermatol Surg 27:709-715, 2001.
26. Jimenez G, Spencer JM. Erbium:YAG laser resurfacing of the hands, arms, and neck. Dermatol Surg 25:831-834, 1999.
27. Manstein D, Herron GS, Sink RK, et al. Fractional photothermolysis: A new concept for cutaneous remodeling using microscopic patterns of thermal injury. Lasers Surg Med 34:426-438, 2004.
28. Trelles MA, Alvarez X, Martin-Vasquez MJ, et al. Assessment of the efficacy of nonablative long-pulsed 1064-nm Nd:YAG laser treatment of wrinkles compared at 2, 4, and 6 months. Facial Plast Surg 21:145-153, 2005.
29. Carniol PJ, Farley S, Friedman A. Long-pulse 532-nm diode laser for nonablative facial skin rejuvenation. Arch Facial Plast Surg 5:511-513, 2003.
30. Papadavid E, Katsambas A. Lasers for facial rejuvenation: A review. Int J Dermatol 42:480-487, 2003.
31. Friedman P, Skover GR, Payonk G, et al. Quantitative evaluation of nonablative laser technology. Semin Cutan Med Surg 21:266-273, 2002.
32. Trelles MA. Short and long-term follow-up of nonablative 1320 nm Nd:YAG laser facial rejuvenation. Dermatol Surg 27:781-782, 2001.
33. Trelles MA, Allones I, Luna R. Facial rejuvenation with a nonablative 1320 nm Nd:YAG laser: A preliminary clinical and histologic evaluation. Dermatol Surg 27:111-116, 2001.
34. Mark KA, Sparacio RM, Voigt A, et al. Objective and quantitative improvement of rosacea-associated erythema after intense pulsed light treatment. Dermatol Surg 29:600-604, 2003.
35. Huang L, Liao YL, Lee SH, et al. Intense pulsed light for the treatment of facial freckles in Asian skin. Dermatol Surg 28:1007-1012, 2003.
36. Raulin C, Greve B, Grema H. IPL technology: A review. Lasers Surg Med 32:78-87, 2003.
37. Fulton JE Jr. Dermabrasion, chemabrasion, and laserabrasion. Historical perspectives, modern dermabrasion techniques, and future trends. Dermatol Surg 22:619-628, 1996.
38. Branham GH, Thomas JR. Rejuvenation of the skin surface: Chemical peel and dermabrasion. Facial Plast Surg 12:125-133, 1996.

39. Fulton JE Jr, Rahimi AD, Mansoor S, et al. The treatment of hypopigmentation after skin resurfacing. Dermatol Surg 30:95-101, 2004.
40. Kunachak S, Leelaudomlipi P, Wongwaisayawan S. Dermabrasion: A curative treatment for melasma. Aesthetic Plast Surg 25:114-117, 2001.
41. Grimes PE. Microdermabrasion. Dermatol Surg 3:1160-1165, 2005.
42. Spencer JM. Microdermabrasion. Am J Clin Dermatol 6:89-92, 2005.
43. Shpall R, Bedingfield FC III, Watson D, et al. Microdermabrasion: A review. Facial Plast Surg 20:47-50, 2004.
44. Koch RJ, Hanasono MM. Microdermabrasion. Facial Plast Surg Clin North Am 9:377-382, 2001.
45. Shim EK, Barnette D, Hughes K, et al. Microdermabrasion: A clinical and histopathologic study. Dermatol Surg 27:524-530, 2001.
46. Abraham MT, Vic Ross E. Current concepts in nonablative radiofrequency rejuvenation of the lower face and neck. Facial Plast Surg 21:65-73, 2005.
47. Glogau RG. Aesthetic and anatomic analysis of the aging skin. Semin Cutan Med Surg 15:134-138, 1996.
48. Kauvar AN, Dover JS. Facial skin rejuvenation: Laser resurfacing or chemical peel: Choose your weapon. Dermatol Surg 27:209-212, 2001.
49. Fulton JE, Porumb S. Chemical peels: Their place within the range of resurfacing techniques. Am J Clin Dermatol 5:179-187, 2004.
50. Moy LS, Murad H, Moy RL. Glycolic acid peels for the treatment of wrinkles and photoaging. J Dermatol Surg Oncol 19:243-246, 1993.
51. Kim IH, Kim HK, Kye YC. Effects of tretinoin pretreatment on TCA chemical peel in guinea pig skin. J Korean Med Sci 11:335-341, 1996.
52. Vagotis FL, Brundage SR. Histologic study of dermabrasion and chemical peel in an animal model after pretreatment with Retin-A. Aesthetic Plast Surg 19:243-246, 1995.
53. Hevia O, Nemeth AJ, Taylor JR. Tretinoin accelerates healing after trichloroacetic acid chemical peel. Arch Dermatol 12:678-682, 1991.
54. Monheit GD. The Jessner's + TCA peel: A medium-depth chemical peel. J Dermatol Surg Oncol 15:945-950, 1989.
55. El-Domyati MB, Attia SK, Saleh FY, et al. Trichloroacetic acid peeling versus dermabrasion: A histometric, immunohistochemical, and ultrastructural comparison. Dermatol Surg 30:179-188, 2004.
56. Chiarello SE, Resnik BI, Resnik SS. The TCA masque. A new cream formulation used alone and in combination with Jessner's solution. Dermatol Surg 22:687-690, 1996.
57. Glogau RG, Beeson WH, Brody HG, et al. Re: Obagi's modified trichloroacetic acid (TCA)–controlled variable depth peel: A study of clinical signs correlating with histological findings. Ann Plast Surg 38:298-302, 1997.
58. Tse Y, Ostad A, Lee HS, et al. A clinical and histologic evaluation of two medium-depth peels. Glycolic acid versus Jessner's trichloroacetic acid. Dermatol Surg 22:781-786, 1996.
59. Dingman DL, Hartog J, Siemionow M. Simultaneous deep-plane face lift and trichloroacetic acid peel. Plast Reconstr Surg 93:86-93, 1994.
60. Mackee GM, Karp FL. The treatment of postacne scars with phenol. Br J Dermatol 64:456-459, 1952.
61. Spira M, Gerow FJ, Hardy SB. Complications of chemical face peeling. Plast Reconstr Surg 54:397-403, 1974.
62. Butler PE, Gonzalez S, Randolph MA, et al. Quantitative and qualitative effects of chemical peeling on photoaged skin: An experimental study. Plast Reconstr Surg 107:222-228, 2001.
63. Stuzin JM, Baker TJ, Gordon HL. Chemical peel: A change in the routine. Ann Plast Surg 23:166-169, 1989.
64. Kligman AM, Baker TJ, Gordon HL. Long-term histologic follow-up of phenol face peels. Plast Reconstr Surg 75:652-659, 1985.
65. Hetter GP. An examination of the phenol-croton oil peel. Part 4. Face peel results with different concentrations of phenol and croton oil. Plast Reconstr Surg 105:1061-1083, 2000.
66. Hetter GP. An examination of the phenol-croton oil peel. Part 3. The plastic surgeons' role. Plast Reconstr Surg 105:752-763, 2000.

67. Hetter GP. An examination of the phenol-croton oil peel. Part 2. The lay peelers and their croton oil formulas. Plast Reconstr Surg 105:240-248, 2000.

68. Hetter GP. An examination of the phenol-croton oil peel. Part 1. Dissecting the formula. Plast Reconstr Surg 105:227-239, 2000.

69. Truppman ES, Ellenby JD. Major electrocardiographic changes during chemical face peeling. Plast Reconstr Surg 63:44-48, 1979.

70. Binstock JH. Safety of chemical face peels. J Am Acad Dermatol 7:137-138, 1982.

71. Carruthers J, Stubbs HA. Botulinum toxin for benign essential blepharospasm, hemifacial spasm and age-related lower eyelid entropion. Can J Neurol Sci 14:42-45, 1987.

72. Gill DM. Bacterial toxins: A table of lethal amounts. Microbiol Rev 46:86-94, 1982.

73. Carruthers J, Fagien S, Matarasso SL. Botox Consensus Group. Consensus recommendations on the use of botulinum toxin type a in facial aesthetics. Plast Reconstr Surg 114(Suppl 6):S1-S22, 2004.

74. Nahai F. The Art of Aesthetic Surgery: Principles and Techniques. St Louis: Quality Medical Publishing, 2005.

75. Peer LA. The neglected free fat graft, its behavior and clinical use. Am J Surg 92:40-47, 1956.

76. Peer LA. The neglected free fat graft. Plast Reconstr Surg 18:233-250, 1956.

77. Coleman SR. Structural Fat Grafting. St Louis: Quality Medical Publishing, 2005.

78. Coleman WP III. Autologous fat transplantation. Plast Reconstr Surg 88:736, 1991.

79. Coleman SR. Long-term survival of fat transplants: Controlled demonstrations. Aesthetic Plast Surg 19:421-425, 1995.

80. Coleman WP III. Fat transplantation. Dermatol Clin 17:891-898, 1999.

81. Rohrich RJ, Sorokin ES, Brown SA. In search of improved fat transfer viability: A quantitative analysis of the role of centrifugation and harvest cite. Plast Reconstr Surg 113:391-395; discussion 396-397, 2004.

82. DeLustro F, Smith ST, Sundsmo J, et al. Reaction to injectable collagen: Results in animal models and clinical use. Plast Reconstr Surg 79:581-594, 1987.

83. Homicz MR, Watson D. Review of injectable materials for soft tissue augmentation. Facial Plast Surg 20:21-29, 2004.

84. Cukier J, Beauchamp RA, Spindler JS, et al. Association between bovine collagen dermal implants and a dermatomyositis or a polymyositis-like syndrome. Ann Intern Med 118:920-928, 1993.

85. Somerville P, Wray RC Jr. Asymmetrical hypersensitivity to bovine collagen. Ann Plast Surg 30:449-450, 1993.

86. Baumann LS, Kerdel F. The treatment of bovine collagen allergy with cyclosporin. Dermatol Surg 25:247-249, 1999.

87. Sklar JA, White SM. Radiance FN: A new soft tissue filler. Dermatol Surg 30:764-768, 2004.

88. Flaharty P. Radiance. Facial Plast Surg 20:165-169, 2004.

89. Tzikas TL. Evaluation of the Radiance FN soft tissue filler for facial soft tissue augmentation. Arch Facial Plast Surg 6:234-239, 2004.

90. Woerle B, Hanke CW, Sattler G. Poly-L-lactic acid: A temporary filler for soft tissue augmentation. J Drugs Dermatol 3:385-389, 2004.

91. Sterling JB, Hanke CW. Poly-L-lactic acid as a facial filler. Skin Therapy Lett 10:9-11, 2005.

92. Borelli C, Kunte C, Weisenseel P, et al. Deep subcutaneous application of poly-L-lactic acid as a filler for facial lipoatrophy in HIV-infected patients. Skin Pharmacol Physiol 18:273-278, 2005.

93. Lemperle G, Romano JJ, Busso M. Soft tissue augmentation with Artecoll: 10-year history, indications, techniques, and complications. Dermatol Surg 29:573-587, 2003.

94. Alcalay J, Alkalay R, Gat A, et al. Late-onset granulomatous reaction to Artecoll. Dermatol Surg 29:859-862, 2003.

95. Lombardi T, Samson J, Plantier F, et al. Orofacial granulomas after injection of cosmetic fillers. Histopathologic and clinical study of 11 cases. J Oral Pathol Med 33:115-120, 2004.

76. Hair Transplantation

Jeffrey E. Janis

HAIR[1,2]

EMBRYOLOGY
■ Hair follicles originate from **ectoderm** and **mesoderm**
■ Arise in the **third gestational month**

ANATOMY (Fig. 76-1)
■ Hair shaft made of **keratinized protein**
  • Several layers, including melanocytes
  • Hair bulb
  • Papilla
■ Sebaceous glands
■ Sweat glands
■ Erector pili muscle
■ Follicular unit
  • One to four terminal hairs
  • One vellus hair
  • Nine sebaceous glands
  • Insertions of erector pili muscles
  • Perifollicular vascular plexus
  • Perifollicular neural net
  • Perifolliculum
■ Average human scalp has approximately **100,000-150,000 hairs**
  • **Blondes,** on average, have slightly **more** hair.
  • **Redheads,** on average, have slightly **less** hair.
■ There are as many hair follicles in a bald scalp as a nonbald scalp (histologically)

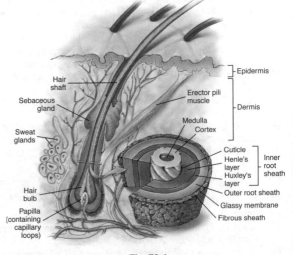

Fig. 76-1

PHYSIOLOGY OF HAIR GROWTH[2,3]

THREE PHASES (Fig. 76-2)
■ Anagen
  • *Active growth*
  • Follicular cells actively multiplying and becoming keratinized
  • **90%** of hairs normally in this phase
  • Lasts approximately **1000 days in men** and **2-5 years longer in women**

- **Catagen**
  - Also called *degradation phase*
  - Keratinization of hair base (i.e., forms a club)
  - Separation of base from dermal papilla
  - Moves toward the surface
  - Lasts **2-3 weeks**
- **Telogen**
  - Also called *resting phase*
  - Hair is shed
  - Follicle **inactive** and hair growth stops
  - Lasts **3-4 months**
  - Approximately **10%** of hairs normally in this phase
  - On average, **50-100 telogen hairs** fall out every day

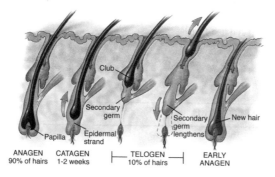

Fig. 76-2

NOTE: When the anagen phase shortens and the telogen phase is prolonged (i.e., rate of hair loss exceeds hair growth), thinning and eventual baldness develop.

TIP: Hair physiology is frequently covered on in-service examinations and written Boards.

ALOPECIA

INCIDENCE[4,5]

- It is estimated that 35,000,000 men and 21,000,000 women in the United States experience hair loss.
- It is so common in men that it is actually accepted as **normal.**
  - Of men seeking hair replacement surgery, approximately **33%** have variable amounts of alopecia by their **mid-30s.**
  - **50%** have variable amounts of alopecia by age 50 years.
  - **66%** have variable amounts of alopecia by their mid-60s.

ETIOLOGIC FACTORS[2,4,5]

- **Androgenic alopecia**
  - Male pattern baldness is the conversion of healthy, thick terminal hairs to clear, microscopic vellus hairs.
  - It is an **X-linked, dominant condition.**
  - **5α-reductase,** which is in the cells of susceptible hair follicles and the skin, is responsible for converting testosterone to dihydrotestosterone (DHT).
  - Normal circulating amounts of testosterone may be excessively converted to DHT, or the hair follicle may be abnormally sensitive to DHT, which creates androgenic alopecia.
- The donor follicles from **occipital regions** have decreased or absent DHT and thus are **not** influenced by hormonal factors, making them attractive for use as donor grafts.

NOTE: In general, the earlier the onset of alopecia, the more severe it will be.

- **Discoid lupus erythematosus**
- **Lichen planopilaris**
  - Lichen planus of skin and hair follicles
- **Alopecia areata**
- **Cicatricial alopecia**
- **Traumatic alopecia**

HAIR TRANSPLANTATION

INDICATIONS

- Androgenic alopecia
- Cicatricial alopecia
- Traumatic alopecia
- Traction alopecia

CONTRAINDICATIONS

- Diffuse female pattern baldness
- Non–donor-dominant alopecia
- Alopecia areata
- Active scarring alopecias (discoid lupus erythematosus, lichen planopilaris, and other cicatricial alopecia)

PATIENT EVALUATION

MALE CLASSIFICATION (Fig. 76-3)

- **Hamilton[6]** described **seven major types** of male pattern baldness.
- The **Norwood modification** is most commonly used.[4,5,7]
  - **Type I:** Minimal or no hairline recession at the frontotemporal areas
  - **Type II:** Symmetric triangular frontotemporal recessions extend posteriorly no more than 2 cm anterior to the coronal plane drawn between the external auditory canals
  - **Type III:** Symmetric triangular frontotemporal recessions extend posteriorly more than 2 cm
  - **Type III$_{vertex}$:** Primarily vertex hair loss; may be accompanied by frontotemporal recession that conforms to type III guidelines

- **Type IV:** Sparse or absent vertex hair with more severe frontotemporal recession; areas separated by a band of moderately dense hair that extends across the top of the head
- **Type V:** Same as type IV, but more severe hair loss; band of hair narrower and sparser
- **Type VI:** Band is absent and two areas interconnect
- **Type VII:** Most severe form; only a narrow horseshoe-shaped band of fine, sparse hair

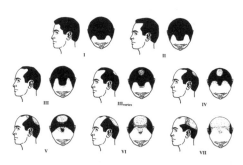

Fig. 76-3 (From Norwood OT, Shiell R, eds. Hair Transplant, 2nd ed. Springfield, IL: Charles C. Thomas, 1984.)

FEMALE CLASSIFICATION (Fig. 76-4)
- The **Ludwig classification**[8] is most commonly used.
- The following patient characteristics must be taken into account.
  - **Hair density:** A natural result is more difficult to achieve with poor density.
  - **Thickness of hair follicles:** Fine, thin hair is harder to disguise than curly, thicker hair.
  - **Stringent versus curly hair:** Natural curl produces a better result.
  - **Hair color:** Light-colored, gray, or salt-and-pepper hair is more natural than thin, straight, black hair.

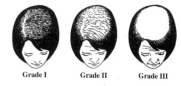

Grade I   Grade II   Grade III

Fig. 76-4 (From Ludwig E. Ludwig's Classification of female androgenic alopecia. Br J Dermatol 97:247, 1977.)

TREATMENT[2,9]

MEDICAL THERAPY
- Frequently used in conjunction with hair restoration surgery
- **Minoxidil (Rogaine®)**
  - Available in 2% and 5% topical solutions
  - Used on scalp twice daily
  - Cosmetically useful hair obtained only in about **one third** of cases
  - Must be used indefinitely to maintain a response
- **Finasteride (Propecia®)**
  - **5α-reductase inhibitor**
  - Promotes conversion of hair follicles to the anagen phase
  - Available in 1 mg tablets and given once daily
  - Lowers the dihydrotestosterone on the scalp and serum of treated patients
  - Effective in **preventing further hair loss** and **increasing hair counts** to the point of cosmetically appreciable results
  - Hair loss on temples is **not** improved (although vertex and frontal hair counts are increased)
  - Side effects rare (less than 1%)
  - Must be used indefinitely to maintain a response

SURGICAL THERAPY[2]

PRINCIPLES
- Provide a natural look.
- Reconstitute a normal anterior hairline with normal hair growth patterns.
- Minimize scalp scars in both the donor and recipient sites.

PREOPERATIVE CARE
- Ensure that the patient has discontinued the use of medications that may result in excessive bleeding (e.g., NSAIDs, anticoagulants, herbal medications).
- Assess for allergies to medications, including local anaesthetics, anxiolytics, and narcotic pain medication.

PREOPERATIVE PLANNING
- Average scalp measures **500 cm²** (50,000 mm²)
- Average **200 hairs/cm**
- **One follicular unit/mm²** for normal nonbalding scalp
  - Each unit contains **2 hairs** (therefore 2 hairs/mm²)
- Approximately **12.5%** of scalp available for hair transplantation in type V or type VI male pattern baldness
  - Equivalent to 12,500 hairs or 6250 follicular units (two hairs each)
  - Can be transplanted in two megasessions of 3000-4000 micrografts or minigrafts (see later)
- Donor site location
  - **Occipital** and **temporal** areas best donor sites
  - Optimal donor site varies with **age**
    - **In patients older than 40 years:** Donor site is half the vertical distance from the posterior upper healthy fringe to the lower hairline (Fig. 76-5, *A*).
    - **In patients younger than 40 years:** Donor site is at the junction of the middle third and caudal thirds of the same vertical distance described previously (Fig. 76-5, *B*).

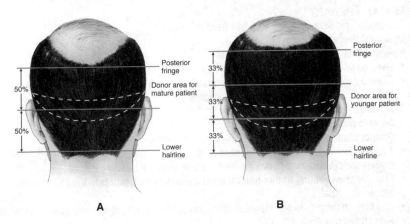

A

B

Fig. 76-5

MINIGRAFTS AND MICROGRAFTS (Fig. 76-6)

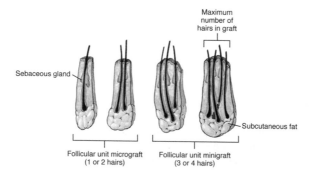

Fig. 76-6

- **Micrografts** contain one or two hairs per graft.
- **Minigrafts** contain three to eight hairs per graft.
- When properly placed, smaller grafts provide a more natural, less abrupt hairline than punch grafts (usually 4 mm).
- It is best to place grafts into incision sites, called *slits,* which are arranged in horizontal rows along the frontal hairline.
  - Slit techniques represent a simpler method for placing hair grafts.
  - Large numbers of one- to three-hair micrografts are placed in slit incisions without using recipient punches to remove bald scalp.
  - Fine micrograft hairs are placed in the front line and are backed up by larger micrografts and minigrafts.
  - Slits can be used for younger patients with thinning hair without sacrificing existing hair follicles in the recipient area.
  - Slits may require more than one session to complete.

TECHNIQUE
- **Harvesting the grafts**
  - **Strip excision (elliptical excision)**
    - ▶ Can be subdivided into minigrafts or micrografts
    - ▶ Less follicular loss
  - **Triple or quadruple blade knives**
    - ▶ Used to make 2 mm parallel excisions across the scalp
    - ▶ Easier and more precise
    - ▶ Allow the surgeon to accurately trim 1 mm and 2 mm grafts with no waste and little follicular damage
    - ▶ Donor excision site then reapproximated by sutures or staples

TIP: It is extremely helpful to have an assistant trained in harvesting and processing to drastically shorten the procedure time.

- **Recipient sites: Slits versus holes**
  - Slit grafts compress with healing to a single stalk from which 2-5 hairs grow.
    - ▸ Can give an artificial or tufted look when only slit minigrafts are used
  - Similar minigrafts placed in holes seem to remain spread out and do not have a compressed, artificial appearance.
  - Some doctors mix slits with holes and varying graft size to obtain a more natural result.
- **Proper orientation**
  - **Natural angles** (Fig. 76-7)
    - ▸ **Frontal hairline:** 45-60 degrees
    - ▸ **Posterior to hairline:** 75-80 degrees
    - ▸ **Crown/vertex:** 90 degrees (i.e., perpendicular to scalp)
    - ▸ **Posterior to crown:** 45-60 degrees downward
    - ▸ **Lateral fringes:** Follow direction of existing hair

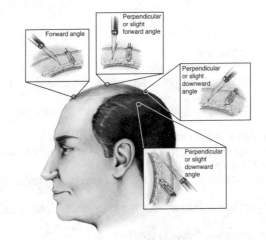

Fig. 76-7

TIP: It is helpful to wear loupes during the harvesting and transplantation.

POSTOPERATIVE CARE

- Cover the donor grafts with a nonstick dressing (Telfa®; Kendall Co, Mansfield, MA) and wrap patient's head in a turban.
- Keep the patient for approximately 1 hour after surgery and give oral fluids and a light snack.
- The patient should be accompanied home.
- The patient should not engage in strenuous exercise or heavy lifting.
- The patient should avoid direct sunlight.
- The patient should wash hair using the "pour method" (i.e., mix light shampoo with warm water and pour over the scalp without massaging).
- The patient may resume normal hair washing at postoperative day 14.
- The patient should follow up in the clinic 1 week after surgery.

COMPLICATIONS

INTRAOPERATIVE
- Hemorrhage
- Lidocaine toxicity

POSTOPERATIVE
- Hemorrhage
- Infection
- Scarring (including keloids)
- Poor hair growth
- Unnatural hairline
- Doll's head appearance

CAUTION: Be sure to plan for future hair loss when designing the donor incisions and recipient sites. Further hair loss may eventually expose donor site incisions or result in unnatural tufts of hair.

KEY POINTS

- ✔ Balding occurs when more hair follicles are in the telogen phase rather than the anagen phase.
- ✔ The temporal and occipital hair follicles are usually resistant to the effects of DHT and therefore are excellent as donors.
- ✔ Minigraft and microgroft techniques produce more natural results than punch grafts.
- ✔ Minigrafts and micrografts should be inserted at the proper angle and orientation to prevent an unnatural appearance.
- ✔ The anterior hairline is the most important location to reconstruct.
- ✔ Medical treatment, such as minoxidil and finasteride, are useful adjuncts to surgical treatment and have minimal side effects.
- ✔ Complete restoration may require more than one procedure.

REFERENCES

1. Orentreich N, Durr NP. Biology of scalp hair growth. Clin Plast Surg 9:197, 1982.
2. Barrera A. Hair Transplantation. The Art of Micrografting and Minigrafting. St Louis: Quality Medical Publishing, 2002.
3. Orentreich N. Scalp hair replacement in man. In Oregon Regional Primate Research Center, Montagna W, Dobson RL, eds. Advances on Biology of Skin, vol 9. Proceedings of the University of Oregon Medical School Symposium on the Biology of Skin. New York: Pergamon Press, 1969.
4. Norwood OT. Male pattern baldness: Classification and incidence. South Med J 68:1359, 1975.
5. Norwood OT, Shiell RC. Hair Transplant Surgery, 2nd ed. Springfield, IL: Charles C Thomas, 1984.
6. Hamilton JB. Patterned loss of hair in man: Types and incidence. Ann NY Acad Sci 53:708, 1951.
7. Norwood OT. Patient selection, hair transplant design, and hairstyle. J Dermatol Surg Oncol 18:386, 1992.
8. Ludwig E. Classification of the types of androgenic alopecia (common baldness) arising in the female sex. Br J Dermatol 97:247, 1977.
9. Beran S. Hair restoration. Sel Read Plast Surg 9(15):29, 2001.

77. Brow Lift

Jason E. Leedy

ANATOMY (Fig. 77-1)

MUSCULATURE

- **Frontalis muscle**
  - **Origin:** Galea aponeurosis
  - **Insertion:** Supraorbital dermis by interdigitating with orbicularis oculi
  - **Innervation:** Frontal branch of facial nerve
  - **Action:** Brow elevator; creates transverse forehead rhytids
  - **Galea aponeurosis:** Splits into two sheaths, which encapsulate the frontalis
    - ▶ Posterior sheath extends to the periosteum at the superior orbital rim

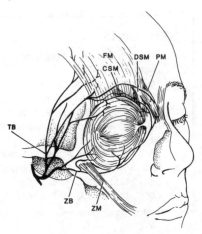

Fig. 77-1 Brow anatomy: Periorbital motor nerves and the muscles they activate. *CSM,* Corrugator muscle; *DSM,* depressor supercilii muscle; *FM,* frontalis muscle; *PM,* procerus muscle; *TB,* temporal branch of facial nerve; *ZB,* zygomatic branch of facial nerve; *ZM,* zygomaticus major muscle. (From Knize DM. Muscles that act on glabellar skin: A closer look. Plast Reconstr Surg 105:350, 2000.)

- **Corrugator supercilii muscle**
  - **Oblique head**
    - ▶ **Origin:** Superior-medial orbital rim
    - ▶ **Insertion:** Dermis at medial eyebrow
    - ▶ **Innervation:** Zygomatic branches
    - ▶ **Action:** Brow depressor; creates oblique glabellar lines
  - **Transverse head**
    - ▶ **Origin:** Medial-superior orbital rim
    - ▶ **Insertion:** Dermis just superior to the middle third of the eyebrow
    - ▶ **Innervation:** Frontal branch
    - ▶ **Action:** Moves the brow medially; creates oblique and vertical glabellar lines
- **Depressor supercilii muscle**
  - **Origin:** Superior-medial orbital rim
  - **Insertion:** Medial brow dermis
  - **Innervation:** Zygomatic branches
  - **Action:** Brow depressor; creates oblique glabellar lines

- **Procerus muscle**
  - **Origin:** Superior-medial orbital rim
  - **Insertion:** Dermis of medial brow
  - **Innervation:** Superior portion by frontal branch, inferior portion by zygomatic branches
  - **Action:** Brow depressor; creates oblique glabellar and transverse nasal root lines
- **Orbicularis oculi**
  - **Medial orbital portion** can cause medial brow depression
    - ▶ Insignificant contributor to glabellar rhytids
  - **Lateral orbital portion** can cause lateral brow depression
    - ▶ Creates lateral orbital rhytids (i.e., crow's feet)
  - Innervated by **zygomatic branch of facial nerve**

SENSATION
- **Supratrochlear nerve**
  - Exits orbit **medially** and usually arborizes
  - Enters corrugator then frontalis to supply the forehead
- **Supraorbital nerve**
  - Exits through foramen or notch **lateral to supratrochlear nerve**
  - Divides into **superficial** and **deep** branches
  - **Superficial branch** enters frontalis 2-3 cm above rim; supplies forehead
  - **Deep branch** supplies scalp posterior to the hairline
  - Runs 0.5-1.5 cm medial to the superior temporal line

> TIP: Transection of the deep branch with subgaleal dissection and coronal incisions is believed to be responsible for postoperative scalp paresthesias.[1]

BROW-RETAINING LIGAMENTS
- **Orbital ligament:** Fibrous band connecting the orbital rim and the superficial temporal fascia deep to the lateral eyebrow[2]
- **Temporal and supraorbital ligamentous adhesions and lateral brow and lateral orbital thickening of the periorbital septum:** Periorbital attachments released for brow elevation[3]
- **Brow-retaining ligament and upper lid-retaining ligament:** Zones of attachment from bone to overlying skin that require release for brow elevation[4]

AESTHETICS

YOUTHFUL APPEARANCE
- Absence of forehead and glabellar rhytids
- Absence of dyschromia
- Appropriately positioned hairline
- Pleasing eyebrow shape and position

AESTHETIC MEASUREMENT GUIDELINES[5] (Fig. 77-2)
- **Anterior hairline to brow:** 5 cm in women; 6 cm in men
- **Eyebrow position at lateral limbus:** On orbital rim in men; 1 cm above orbital rim in women

- **Medial brow** club-shaped, and **lateral brow** tapers; ends lie at approximately same level, but lateral end may be slightly elevated
- **Gentle arch:** Peak at junction of the medial two thirds and the lateral one third, lying halfway between lateral limbus and lateral canthus
- **Medial brow:** Lies in vertical line with medial orbital fissure and alar base
- **Lateral brow:** Lies on oblique line from alar base through lateral orbital fissure
- **In midpupillary line:** Anterior hairline to brow, 5-6 cm; brow to superior orbital rim, 1 cm; brow to supratarsal crease, 1.6 cm; and brow to midpupil, 2.5 cm

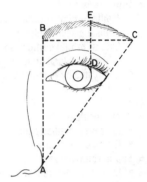

Fig. 77-2   Spatial relationships of the ideal brow. **A,** Nasal alar base. **B,** Medial eyebrow. **C,** Lateral eyebrow. **D,** Lateral limbus. **E,** Brow peak. (From Ellenbogen R. Transcoronal eyebrow lift with concomitant upper blepharoplasty. Plast Reconstr Surg 71:490, 1983.)

STIGMATA OF FOREHEAD AGING
- Transverse forehead rhytids
- Glabellar rhytids
- Brow ptosis
- Skin dyschromia

PREOPERATIVE EVALUATION

OUTLINE AESTHETIC GOALS
- Brow position
- Shape
- Symmetry

TIP: The brow should always be evaluated in patients seeking periorbital rejuvenation.

ASSESS HAIRLINE POSITION AND QUALITY OF ANTERIOR HAIR
- **High hairline**
  - Considered when brow to hairline distance is greater than 5 cm in women and greater than 6 cm in men
  - Alternatively considered when the anterior hairline lies on more oblique aspect of forehead from lateral view
- **Low hairline**
  - Brow to hairline distance less than 5 cm in women and less than 6 cm in men, with anterior hairline on vertical portion of forehead from lateral view
  - Fine, sparse anterior hair less likely to conceal a coronal incision than thicker, dark hair

ASSESS QUALITY OF RHYTIDS
- **Dynamic rhytids**
  - **Present only during animation**
  - Amenable to botulinum toxin
  - Surgical improvement with weakening of the involved muscles
- **Static rhytids**
  - *Present at rest; result of sustained muscle hyperactivity*
  - In general, partially improved with surgical muscle weakening but require redraping soft tissue
  - **Superficial rhytids:** Amenable to fillers and resurfacing procedures
  - **Deep rhytids:** Require extensive soft tissue redraping (e.g., subcutaneous dissection)

ASSESS POSITION AND SHAPE OF BROW
- Use aesthetic guidelines, mentioned previously.

TIP: Note that brow may be artificially elevated secondary to plucking and makeup.

ASSESS SKIN QUALITY
- Improvement in dyschromia and skin texture dramatically improves surgical result.

TIP: Consider skin care, dyschromia treatments, and resurfacing procedures as adjuncts.

SURGICAL TECHNIQUE

There are multiple variables to consider; therefore the surgical approach should be individualized for each patient.

INCISIONS
- **Direct, superciliary**
  - Removal of ellipse of skin and subcutaneous tissue at supraorbital rim, concealing scar above the eyebrow
  - **Useful in men with thick skin and alopecia,** thereby making coronal and temporal incisions less favorable
- **Transblepharoplasty**
  - Involves tacking brow to periosteum or deep temporal fascia to obtain lift
  - Can also perform simultaneous corrugator and procerus excision for glabellar rhytids[6] (Fig. 77-3)

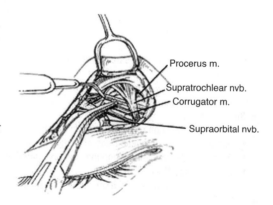

Procerus m.
Supratrochlear nvb.
Corrugator m.
Supraorbital nvb.

Fig. 77-3 Transblepharoplasty corrugator excision. (From Paul MD. The evolution of the brow lift in aesthetic plastic surgery. Plast Reconstr Surg 108:1409, 2001.)

- **Midbrow**
  - Removal of midforehead skin strip, concealing incision in transverse rhytid
  - **Useful in men with thick skin, deep rhytids, and alopecia,** thereby making coronal or temporal incisions less favorable
  - Advances hairline downward
- **Coronal**
  - **Useful for low hairline:** 1.5 mm of anterior hairline retrodisplacement required for every 1 mm of eyebrow elevation
  - Incision placed at least **3 cm posterior to hairline** for better scar camouflage

---

TIP: In bald men place the incision further posteriorly to make it less visible from the frontal view.

- Greater scalp excision (up to 3-4 cm) performed laterally than medially to preferentially correct lateral brow descent
- **Temporal** (Fig. 77-4)
  - One of the oldest techniques
  - Similar to coronal but spares midline vertex incision
- **Anterior hairline**
  - Useful if high hairline (hairline on oblique portion of forehead from lateral view)
  - Use extreme bevel to allow hair to grow through incision for camouflage
  - Temporal portion of incision follows coronal incision
- **Endoscopic**
  - Usually small central incision with two temporal incisions
  - Argued to limit morbidity of coronal and hairline incision
- **Combined**
  - Temporal with transpalpebral incisions (Knize[2])

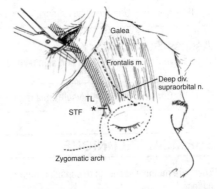

Fig. 77-4 Temporal approach. *TL,* Temporal fusion line; *STF,* superficial temporal fascia. (From Knize DM. Limited-incision forehead lift for eyebrow elevation to enhance upper blepharoplasty. Plast Reconstr Surg 97:1334-1342, 1996.)

PLANE OF DISSECTION

- **Subcutaneous**
  - Allows preservation of posterior scalp sensation
  - Useful for improving deep transverse rhytids
  - Decreases flap vascularity and **may be associated with increased wound complications**
  - Tedious dissection
  - Difficult to perform medial brow depressor muscle excision
- **Subgaleal**
  - Rapid, easy dissection
  - Allows direct excision or scoring of muscle

> **TIP:** Some surgeons argue that fixation of galea to periosteum is quicker than periosteum to bone, which may improve durability of the lift.[7]

- **Subperiosteal**
  - Some surgeons believe lifting the pericranium provides more sustained lift[8]
  - Requires release of arcus marginalis for effective lift

  NOTE: Troilius[8] evaluated 1-year results of subgaleal and subperiosteal lifts: Subperiosteal lifts had 7 mm of elevation compared with no elevation for subgaleal lifts. (This may be attributed to a fixation issue rather than an issue with the dissection plane.)

- **Biplanar** (Fig. 77-5)
  - Subcutaneous with endoscopic subperiosteal approach; allows improvement in forehead rhytids with suprabrow muscle excision[9]

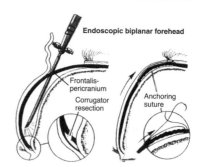

Fig. 77-5 Endoscopic biplanar forehead lift. (From Ramirez OM. Endoscopically assisted biplanar forehead lift. Plast Reconstr Surg 96:323, 1995.)

MUSCLE WEAKENING

- **Direct muscle excision**
  - Can remove corrugators and frontalis
  - Preserve suprabrow frontalis (at least 2 cm) to maintain brow animation
  - Can graft glabella with fat after removal of corrugators to correct depression deformities after resection of muscle bulk[10]
- **Muscle scoring**
  - Corrugators and frontalis
- **Chemical paralysis**
  - Botulinum toxin

SECURING BROW ELEVATION

- **Elastic band principle:** *The farther away the suspension point is from the brow, the less effective the lift*[7]
- **Skin excision:** Open technique
  - 2:1 ratio of skin excision to brow elevation, or 3:1 if frontalis removed for brow elevation[11]
  - Some authors recommend up to 5:1 skin excision to achieve longer-lasting results
- **Suture techniques**
  - **Endoscopic techniques**
    - ▸ **Cortical tunnel:** Suture secured to tunnel made in outer table of calvarium
    - ▸ **Lateral spanning suspension sutures**

DEVICES

- **Percutaneous or internal screw placement with attached suture:** Screws can be removed at later follow-up
- **K-wire placement:** May be left permanently or removed
- **Endotine™** (Coapt Systems, Palo Alto, CA): Dissolvable, fan-shaped anchoring device
- **DePuy Mitek** (Raynham, MA): Bone anchor with attached suture

COMPLICATIONS

- **Sensory nerve deficit:** Results from injury to supraorbital or supratrochlear nerves; requires careful preservation during corrugator excision
- **Posterior scalp dysesthesias:** Results from transection of deep branch of supraorbital nerve
- **Frontalis muscle paralysis:** Results from frontal branch injury in temporal dissection
- **Skin necrosis:** Results from excessive tension
- **Alopecia:** Results from excessive tension or thermal injury
- **Infection**
- **Hematoma and bleeding**
- **Abnormal hair part or visible scar:** Excessive tension
- **Chronic pain:** Supraorbital nerve dysesthesias; more likely if history of migraines
- **Permanent overcorrection**
- **Abnormal soft tissue contour:** Can occur with muscle excision
- **Asymmetry, poor cosmesis, or lateral displacement of brow:** Results from excessive corrugator excision

---

KEY POINTS

- ✔ Frontalis muscle action is antagonized by corrugators, procerus, depressor supercilii, and orbicularis oculi muscles.
- ✔ High hairline occurs when hairline is on the superior, oblique portion of frontal bone.
- ✔ Coronal incisions cause posterior scalp paresthesias, which may trouble patients postoperatively.
- ✔ Endoscopic approaches require fixation techniques.

REFERENCES

1. Knize DM. Reassessment of the coronal incision and subgaleal dissection for foreheadplasty. Plast Reconstr Surg 102:478, 1998.
2. Knize DM. Limited-incision forehead lift for eyebrow elevation to enhance upper blepharoplasty. Plast Reconstr Surg 97:1334, 1996
3. Moss CJ, Mendelson BC, Taylor GI. Surgical anatomy of the ligamentous attachments in the temple and periorbital regions. Plast Reconstr Surg 105:1475, 2000.
4. Byrd HS, Burt JD. Achieving aesthetic balance in the brow, eyelids, and midface. Plast Reconstr Surg 110:926, 2002.
5. Ellenbogen R. Transcoronal eyebrow lift with concomitant upper blepharoplasty. Plast Reconstr Surg 71:490, 1983.
6. Fodor PB. Subperiosteal transblepharoplasty forehead lift. Plast Reconstr Surg 99:605, 1997.
7. Flowers FS, Caputy GC, Flowers SS. The biomechanics of brow and frontalis function and its effect on blepharoplasty. Clin Plast Surg 20:255-268, 2003.
8. Troilius C. A comparison between subgaleal and subperiosteal brow lifts. Plast Reconstr Surg 104:1079, 1999.
9. Ramirez OM. Endoscopically assisted biplanar forehead lift. Plast Reconstr Surg 96:323, 1995.
10. Guyuron B. Corrugator supercilii resection through blepharoplasty incision. Plast Reconstr Surg 107: 606-607, 2001.
11. Ortiz Monasterio F. Aesthetic sugery of the facial skeleton: The forehead. Clin Plast Surg 18:19, 1991.

78. Blepharoplasty

Jason E. Leedy

ANATOMY[1,2] (Fig. 78-1)

LAYERS
- **Anterior lamella:** Skin and orbicularis muscle
- **Middle lamella:** Septum
- **Posterior lamella:** Tarsus and conjunctiva

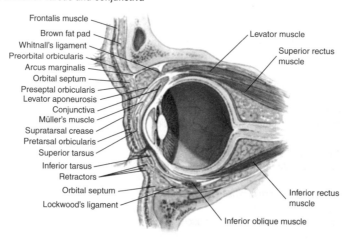

Frontalis muscle
Brown fat pad
Whitnall's ligament
Preorbital orbicularis
Arcus marginalis
Orbital septum
Preseptal orbicularis
Levator aponeurosis
Conjunctiva
Müller's muscle
Supratarsal crease
Pretarsal orbicularis
Superior tarsus
Inferior tarsus
Retractors
Orbital septum
Lockwood's ligament
Levator muscle
Superior rectus muscle
Inferior rectus muscle
Inferior oblique muscle

Fig. 78-1   Cross section of the upper and lower eyelids.

ORBICULARIS MUSCLE[3] (Fig. 78-2)
- **Three portions**
  1. **Orbital**
     - ▸ Outermost portion
     - ▸ Superficial to corrugators and procerus
     - ▸ Voluntary
     - ▸ Allows for tight closure of eye
  2. **Preseptal**
     - ▸ Overlies septum
     - ▸ Both voluntary and involuntary
     - ▸ Assists with blinking
  3. **Pretarsal**
     - ▸ Adherent to tarsus
     - ▸ Involuntary

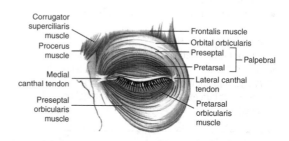

Corrugator superciliaris muscle
Procerus muscle
Medial canthal tendon
Preseptal orbicularis muscle
Frontalis muscle
Orbital orbicularis
Preseptal ⎱ Palpebral
Pretarsal ⎰
Lateral canthal tendon
Pretarsal orbicularis muscle

Fig. 78-2   Orbicularis oculi. (From Achauer BH, Eriksson E, Guyuron B, et al, eds. Plastic Surgery: Indications, Operations, and Outcomes. St Louis: Mosby, 2000, p 2528.)

795

- Assists with blinking
- Innervation primarily from the zygomatic branch, inferolateral on the deep surface

TARSOLIGAMENTOUS COMPLEX

- **Upper tarsus**
  - 7-11 mm wide
  - Müller's muscle: Inserts onto superior border
  - Anterior fibers of levator aponeurosis: Insert onto superior border but less so than Müller's muscle
- **Lower tarsus**
  - 4-5 mm wide
  - Capsulopalpebral fascia (lower lid retractor): Inserts onto lower border
- **Lateral raphe**
  - Lateral extension of the orbicularis oculi muscle along the lateral orbital rim and zygoma
  - Lies superficial to lateral canthal tendon
  - Component of the **lateral orbital thickening**[4]
- **Lateral canthal tendon**
  - **Formed by:**
    - Lateral horn of levator palpebrae superioris
    - Lockwood's ligament
    - Check ligament of the lateral rectus muscle
    - Deep preseptal and pretarsal orbicularis muscles

MEDIAL CANTHAL TENDON

- **Tripartite structure** (anterior horizontal, posterior horizontal, and vertical components)
- **Formed by:**
  - Deep head of pretarsal orbicularis
  - Medial Lockwood's ligament
  - Check ligaments of the medial rectus muscle
  - Whitnall's ligament

PRESEPTAL FAT

- Located between septum and orbicularis muscle
- Can be a significant factor in upper lid hooding and puffiness
- **Upper lid:** Retroorbicularis oculi fat **(ROOF)**
- **Lower lid:** Suborbicularis oculi fat **(SOOF)**

ORBITAL SEPTUM

- Septum is an extension of orbital periosteum.
- Upper septum extends from superior orbital rim to insertion on levator aponeurosis at varying levels (10-15 mm above superior tarsal border).
- Lower septum extends from inferior orbital rim to the capsulopalpebral fascia (5 mm below lower tarsal border).

TIP: Attenuation of the septum results in pseudoherniation of intraorbital fat.

LEVATOR AND RETRACTOR MUSCLES
- **Levator palpebrae**
  - **Origin:** Lesser wing of the sphenoid
  - **Insertion:** Dermis and superior edge of upper tarsus
  - **Innervation** by CN III
  - **Action:** 10-15 mm of upper lid excursion and sustained lid elevation from contractile tone
  - **Whitnall's ligament:** A fascial condensation 14-20 mm from superior edge of tarsus; translates posterior vector of pull into superior vector
    ▸ Inserts into dermis superior to superior edge of upper tarsus creating supratarsal crease (in Asians this insertion is much lower)
- **Müller's muscle**
  - **Origin:** Levator muscle
  - **Insertion:** Superior edge of tarsus
  - **Innervation:** Sympathetics
  - **Action:** 2-3 mm of upper lid lift

TIP: At the fornix the levator muscle splits into superficial and deep layers. The superficial layer continues as the levator aponeurosis, but the deep layer is Müller's muscle.

- **Capsulopalpebral fascia**
  - *Lower lid equivalent of levator muscle*
  - **Origin:** Inferior oblique muscle fascia
  - **Insertion:** Septum 5 mm below tarsus
  - **Action:** 1-2 mm of downward lower lid migration with downward gaze

ORBITAL FAT
- **Physiologically different from normal body fat**
  - Smaller cells
  - Fat more saturated
  - Less lipoprotein lipase
  - Less metabolically active
  - Minimally affected by diet
- **Distinct compartments** (Fig. 78-3)
  - **Two** in **upper** lid (medial and middle)
  - **Three** in **lower** lid (medial, central, and lateral)

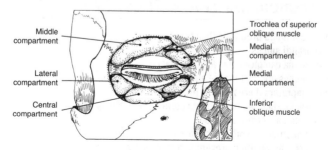

Fig. 78-3 Orbital fat pads.

> TIP: The medial compartment fat is more vascular than the others and pale with smaller lobules and more fibrous tissue.
>
> The trochlea of the superior oblique muscle separates the medial and middle compartments in the upper lid.
>
> The inferior oblique muscle separates the medial and central compartments in the lower lid.

LACRIMAL APPARATUS

- **Palpebral** and **orbital** portions separated by **levator aponeurosis.**
- Located beneath and behind lateral portion of superior orbital rim, it is normally not visible externally.
- **Lacrimal drainage system**
  - Punctum drains to canaliculus, which drains to lacrimal sac, which drains to the nasolacrimal duct
  - **Active pump mechanism**
    - ▶ Blinking creates negative pressure in lacrimal sac, allowing tears to pass through the punctum and canaliculus into the sac.
    - ▶ Eye opening increases sac pressure and passes tears into nasolacrimal duct.

TEARS

- **Functions**
  - Lubrication for lid movement
  - Antibacterial properties
  - Oxygenation of corneal epithelium
  - Maintains a smooth refractive globe surface
- **Three layers**
  1. **Lipid layer:** Superficial, thin; reduces evaporative losses; secreted by meibomian glands and accessory sebaceous glands of Zeiss and Moll
  2. **Aqueous layer:** Thick; from main lacrimal gland as well as accessory glands of Wolfring and Krause within the conjunctival tissue
  3. **Mucoid layer:** Maintains contact with the globe; hydrophilic; produced by mucin goblet cells
- **Basic secretion:** Accessory lacrimal glands of Wolfring and Krause, mucin goblet cells, and meibomian glands
- **Reflex secretion:** Main lacrimal gland, parasympathetic innervation

AESTHETIC PERIORBITAL CHARACTERISTICS[5,6]

- **Aesthetically positioned brow** (see Chapter 77)
- **Full superior orbital sulcus**
  - Aging and trauma can give hollowed appearance.
  - Excessive volumes are unattractive and can cause blepharoptosis.
- **Crisp, precise supratarsal crease with pretarsal show**
  - Formed by levator muscle insertion into dermis above tarsus
  - 3-6 mm of pretarsal show favorable
- **Appropriate lid position:** No ptosis or ectropion
- **Lower lid pretarsal bulge often present in attractive eyes**
  - Results from pretarsal orbicularis muscle fullness

- **Smooth lid-cheek junction**
  - Stigmata of aging: Excess skin, pseudoherniation of intraorbital fat, malar pad descent, nasojugal groove, visible inferior orbital rim
  - Hollowed appearance from paucity of intraorbital fat

AESTHETIC MEASUREMENTS[5]

- **Palpebral fissure:** 12-14 mm vertically, 28-30 mm horizontally
- **Upper lid:** At level of upper limbus, highest point just medial to pupil
- **Lower lid:** At level of lower limbus, lowest point slightly temporal, forms "lazy-S"
- **Visible pretarsal skin:** 3-6 mm
- **Lash line to supratarsal crease:** 8-10 mm
- **Lateral canthus:** 1-2 mm above medial canthus
- **In midpupillary line**
  - **Anterior hairline to brow:** 5-6 cm
  - **Brow to orbital rim:** 1 cm
  - **Brow to supratarsal crease:** 16 mm, minimum 12 mm
  - **Brow to midpupil:** 2.5 cm

EYELID CONDITIONS AND DEFORMITIES

- **Dermatochalasis:** Excess eyelid skin
- **Steatoblepharon:** Excess or protruding fat through a lax septum
- **Blepharochalasis:** Thin excessive upper and lower lid skin
  - Caused by repeated bouts of painless edema
  - 80% of cases have onset before age 20 years; edema refractory to antihistamines and steroids
- **Blepharoptosis:** Drooping of the upper eyelid; disorder of eyelid levator mechanism
- **Pseudoblepharoptosis:** Eyelid in normal position but appearance of ptosis as a result of a ptotic brow and brow skin
- **Ptosis adipose:** Extreme attenuation of the canthus and septum

PREOPERATIVE EVALUATION[7]

HISTORY

- **Patient expectations**
  - Functional versus aesthetic
  - Mirror examination
  - Assessment of potentially unrealistic expectations
- **Dry-eye symptoms**
  - Itching
  - Scratching
- **Epiphora**
- **Causation**
- **Frequency**
- **Inquire about:**
  - Coagulopathies
  - Thyroid dysfunction

- Hypertension
- Renal or cardiac abnormalities that may predispose to edema
- Allergies
- Anticoagulant or antiplatelet medications

PHYSICAL EXAMINATION

FOREHEAD AND BROW
- **Frontalis crease:** May indicate unconscious effort to keep brows elevated
- **Brow ptosis** (Fig. 78-4)
  - With eyes closed and brow relaxed, immobilize frontalis function with gentle pressure on forehead; have patient open eyes.
    - ▸ If the brow position is lower than when the patient is looking straight forward, **compensated brow ptosis** is diagnosed (i.e., the brow is ptotic but is compensated by frontalis hyperactivity).

> TIP: Identify compensated brow ptosis preoperatively because upper blepharoplasty alone may exacerbate brow ptosis and failure to identify brow ptosis in artificially positioned brows before blepharoplasty may result in excessive skin resection.

- **Glabellar frown lines:** Indicate corrugator hyperactivity

UPPER LID
- **Redundant skin:** Lateral hooding
- **Position of supratarsal fold**
  - 7-11 mm from lash line
  - Examine during downward gaze
  - High supratarsal fold indicative of **levator dehiscence** (see Chapter 79)
- **Fat herniation** (pseudohernia)
- **Soft tissue excess**
  - Subcutaneous fat
  - Preseptal fat
  - Lacrimal gland ptosis
- **Lid position:** Should be at the superior border of the limbus

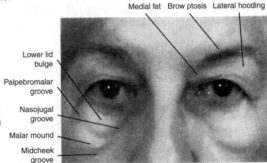

Medial fat   Brow ptosis   Lateral hooding

Lower lid bulge

Palpebromalar groove

Nasojugal groove

Malar mound

Midcheek groove

Fig. 78-4   Aging eye. (From Muzaffar AR, Mendelson BC, Adams WP Jr. Surgical anatomy of the ligamentous attachments of the lower lid and lateral canthus. Plast Reconstr Surg 110:881, 2002.)

> TIP: If upper lid ptosis is acquired, consider myasthenia gravis as a potential underlying etiologic factor.

LOWER LID
- **Redundant skin**
  - **Rhytids:** Fine and deep (crow's feet)
- **Tarsal laxity**
  - **Pinch test** (snap-back): If slow to conform to eye, indicative of tarsal laxity

- **Skin pigmentation** (blepharomelasma)
  - Possibly thin skin with underlying muscle or hyperpigmentation of skin
- **Redundant, ptotic orbicularis oculi muscle** (festoons)
  - **Squinch test** (also called squint test; forcible eye closure): Improvement of festoon if caused by ptotic orbicularis muscle
  - **Malar bag:** Shelving of orbicularis over orbital retaining ligament with excess intraorbital fat
    - ▸ Correction involves improving lid-cheek junction (Loeb procedure, septal reset, midface lift)
- **Fat herniation:** Three compartments
- **Tear trough**
  - Created by herniation of orbital fat, tight attachment of the orbicularis along the arcus marginalis, and malar retrusion (Fig. 78-5)
- **Scleral show**
  - Lower lid should be up to 2 mm below inferior limbus
  - Can be present with tarsal laxity, negative vector orbit, exophthalmos, or middle lamellar contracture of lower lid

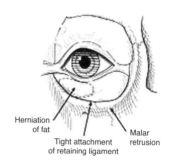

Herniation of fat

Tight attachment of retaining ligament

Malar retrusion

Fig. 78-5 Tear trough. (From Barton FE, Ha R, Awada M. Fat extrusion and septal reset in patients with the tear trough triad: A critical appraisal. Plast Reconstr Surg 113:2116, 2004.)

GLOBE POSITION
- **Proptosis:** Thyroid disease
- **Enophthalmos:** Posttraumatic
- **Negative vector:** If anterior portion of globe is anterior to most projecting portion of the zygoma

> TIP: A patient undergoing lower lid procedures is at risk of scleral show and ectropion, because tightening of the lower lid can cause downward migration of the lower lid on a prominent globe.

OCULAR EXAMINATION
- Record the best corrected visual acuity for each eye.
- If there is a visual field defect, refer to ophthalmologist or optometrist.
- **Bell's phenomenon:** If lids are forcibly held open while patient attempts to close them, the globe rotates upward.
  - When condition is **not** present, the patient may be **more susceptible** to dry-eye symptoms with postoperative lagophthalmos.
- Evaluate for eyelid ptosis.

> TIP: Suspect ptosis if supratarsal fold is high or asymmetric.

LACRIMAL FUNCTION TEST
- Useful for **elderly patients** and all patients with **dry-eye symptoms;** consider ophthalmologic consultation
- **Schirmer's test I:** Basic and reflexive secretion
  - Whatman filter paper (Whatman Inc, Florham Park, NJ) (5 by 35 mm, distal 5 mm folded) placed on lateral sclera: More than 10 mm of wetting after 5 minutes is normal

- **Schirmer's test II:** Basic secretion
  - Perform after topical anaesthetic applied; usually less than 40% of Schirmer's I
- **Advanced tests:** Tear film breakup, rose bengal staining, tear lysozyme electrophoresis

UPPER BLEPHAROPLASTY PRINCIPLES AND TECHNIQUES[5,8]

Objective: To create a well-defined supratarsal fold, exposing smooth pretarsal skin, while refining volume of the supratarsal lid

MARKINGS
- **Lower line**
  - Mark in upright position with upper lid under "closing tension"; that is, mark while applying gentle upward traction on upper lid to smooth the pretarsal skin as desired postoperatively.
  - Usually made 9-11 mm above the lash line; be meticulous about making symmetric bilateral lower marks.

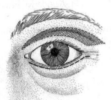

Fig. 78-6   Blepharoplasty markings. (Loeb R. Fat pad sliding and fat grafting for leveling lid depressions. Clin Plast Surg 8:774, 1981.)

- **Upper line**
  - Mark varies depending on the amount and location of redundancy.
  - Extend the lateral excision by canting upward from lower line to upper line so that closure will lie within a rhytid; avoid medial extension (Fig. 78-6).

TECHNIQUE

NOTE: Anaesthetic choice depends on surgeon preference, length of procedure, and whether concomitant procedures are to be performed.

- Excise skin (can use knife or CO_2 laser).
- Open/excise orbicularis muscle (if desired): Must maintain pretarsal orbicularis to preserve blink; excision is usually performed concurrently with skin excision.
  - Excision of muscle can decrease bulk of upper lid and allow for adherence of skin to septum, thereby creating supratarsal fold.
  - Preservation of muscle maintains upper lid fullness; the literature varies on treatment of the muscle.
- Incise orbital septum: Must incise high to avoid injury to levator palpebrae.
  - Use separate stab incisions rather than opening widely.
- Excise redundant intraorbital fat, if indicated.
  - Medial fat has more compact, dense fat lobules that are more pale than in central compartment. It is also more vascular.
  - Central compartment has more loosely organized yellow fat lobules.

CAUTION: Avoid overresection of intraorbital fat to prevent a hollowed appearance with advancing age. Conservative resection involves removal of only the excess fat that comes easily through the septal perforation.

- Excise the retroorbicularis fat, if indicated. This fat lies anterior to the septum but posterior to the orbicularis and creates lateral fullness.[9]
- Assess the lacrimal gland: If lacrimal gland ptosis is contributing to lateral fullness, consider glandulopexy rather than resection to avoid dry-eye symptoms.
- Recognize a prominent superolateral bony orbit preoperatively; bony reduction can be performed.
- Close skin: Multiple techniques and suture types are practiced (subcuticular Prolene pull-out sutures to running fast-absorbing gut); in general, single-layer closure is all that is needed; permanent sutures should be removed early (4 days) to help prevent inclusion cyst.

TARSAL FIXATION TECHNIQUES

- Techniques designed to help create a **high supratarsal fold**
- **Indicated in:**
  - Asian eyelids
  - Preoperative lid fold less than 4-7 mm from lid margin
  - Secondary blepharoplasty
  - Men with brow ptosis
- Principles
  - **Flowers et al**[10]**:** *"Anchor blepharoplasty"* uses a permanent suture from skin to tarsus and then levator
  - **Sheen et al**[11]**:** Sutures pretarsal orbicularis to levator
  - **Baker et al**[12]**:** No suture, excise at least 5 mm of orbicularis, and allow skin to scar to septum overlying levator

LOWER BLEPHAROPLASTY PRINCIPLES AND TECHNIQUES

Objective: Restore youthful appearance with lower lid just touching inferior edge of limbus and lateral canthus being elevated approximately 1-2 mm above the medial canthus; recontour or excise redundant fat, tighten skin, and smooth lid-cheek interface.

APPROACHES TO LOWER LID

- **Skin flap**[13]
  - Subciliary incision to create a skin flap over preseptal orbicularis
  - Removal of excess skin possible without disturbing the orbicularis
  - Useful for removing a large amount of skin
  - Tedious dissection with risk of skin perforation
  - Can result in scarring of skin with muscle
- **Skin-muscle flap**[14]
  - Subciliary incision with skin-muscle flap, pretarsal muscle left undisturbed
  - Allows resection of skin and muscle together, up to 3-5 mm
  - Easier dissection
- **Transconjunctival**[15]
  - Incision made in palpebral conjunctiva, just above fornix, through capsulopalpebral fascia, thereby giving access to intraorbital fat
- **Fat resection**
  - Can be removed through transcutaneous and transconjunctival preseptal and postseptal approaches

- **Fat manipulation**
  - **Loeb procedure:** Medial fat slid out of compartment into tear trough, sutured to angular muscles[16]
  - **Arcus marginalis release:** Lower compartment fat redraped over rim[17,18]
  - **Septal reset:** Lower compartment fat redraped over rim with repositioning of orbital septum by suturing it to periosteum[19-21] (Fig. 78-7)

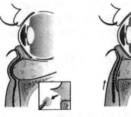

Fig. 78-7 Septal reset. (From Hamra ST. The role of the septal reset in creating a youthful eyelid-cheek complex in facial rejuvenation. Plast Reconstr Surg 113:2127, 2004.)

LOWER LID LAXITY

- **Tarsal shortening**
  - **Kuhnt-Szymanowski procedure:** Pentagonal excision lateral to lateral limbus to avoid visible notching
    - ▶ Useful for patients with **true lower lid tarsal excess**
- **Canthoplasty**
  - Involves division of commissure with repositioning of the lower canthal tendon (tarsal strip procedure) and the lateral canthus
  - Can correct more lower lid laxity than tarsal wedge excision because of repositioning the lateral canthus[23] (Fig. 78-8)
  - Synechia of upper and lower lid can occur at commissure
- **Canthopexy/retinacular suspension: Suture suspension to orbital rim**[23]
  - Involves tightening the lateral canthus or lateral retinaculum to periosteum using sutures; does not involve disinsertion of the lateral canthus
  - Provides for mild lid tightening and canthal elevation, mainly to counteract downward scar forces during healing from lower lid procedures (Fig. 78-9)

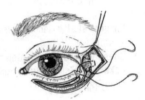

Fig. 78-8 Canthoplasty. (From Fagien S. Algorithm for canthoplasty: The lateral retinacular suspension: A simplified suture canthopexy. Plast Reconstr Surg 103: 2042-2053, 1999.)

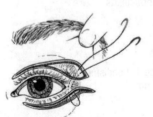

Fig. 78-9 Lateral retinacular suspension. (From Fagien S. Algorithm for canthoplasty: The lateral retinacular suspension: A simplified suture canthopexy. Plast Reconstr Surg 103:2042-2053, 1999.)

COMPLICATIONS[24]

ASYMMETRY

- **Most common complication,** may require corrective surgery.

RETROBULBAR HEMATOMA
- Related to fat excision
- **Signs/symptoms**
  - Pain
  - Proptosis
  - Lid ecchymosis
  - Decreased vision and extraocular movements
  - Dilated pupils
  - Scotomas
  - Increased intraocular pressure
- **Treatment**
  - Elevate head of bed
  - Release surgical incisions
  - Lateral cantholysis
  - Mannitol (12.5 g IV bolus over 3-5 minutes)
  - Acetazolamide (Diamox) (500 mg IV bolus)
  - Steroids (Solu-Medrol) (100 mg IV)
  - Rebreathe in bag (elevates CO_2)
  - Topical beta blockers (Betopic)
  - Emergent ophthalmologic consultation
  - Reoperation

BLINDNESS
- 0.04% incidence, usually only occurs if there is bleeding after fat removal
- **Pathophysiology**
  - Retrobulbar hematoma leading to central retinal artery occlusion or optic nerve ischemia
  - Considered irreversible after 100 minutes

ECTROPION
- **Causes**
  - Excessive skin resection
  - Scar contracture
  - Cicatricial adhesion to orbital septum
  - Dystonia of the orbicularis
  - Contraction of the capsulopalpebral fascia
  - Disinsertion of lateral canthus
  - Midfacial descent
- **Predisposing factors**
  - Lower lid laxity
  - Proptosis
  - Unilateral high myopia (increase anterior-posterior eye dimension)
  - Thyroid disease
- **Early treatment**
  - Taping
  - Frost sutures
  - Massage (Carraway exercises)[25]
  - Steroid injection

- **Late treatment**
  - **Skin loss:** Midface lift or skin graft
  - **Hypotonic lid:** Wedge resection or canthoplasty
  - **Posterior/middle lamella scarring:** Release and spacer graft (Alloderm [LifeCell Corp, Branchburg, NJ], palatal mucosa)

LAGOPHTHALMOS
- Usually temporary, but if not may require skin grafting

KERATOCONJUNCTIVITIS SICCA (DRY-EYE SYNDROME)
- If identified preoperatively should approach very conservatively, if at all
- Postoperatively treat with topical moisturizers

CORNEAL INJURY
- Confirm with **fluorescein testing**
  - Superficial injury treated with **topical antibiotics** and **eye patching**
  - Should resolve in 24-48 hours

DIPLOPIA
- **Inferior oblique muscle most commonly injured** followed by superior oblique muscle
- Usually resolves spontaneously but may require corrective muscle surgery

PTOSIS
- Often present preoperatively but not identified by surgeon and patient until postoperatively
- Can occur from direct injury to levator

KEY POINTS
- ✔ Pretarsal muscle is the most important for blink.
- ✔ The upper eyelid has two fat compartments; the lower lid has three.
- ✔ Avoid aggressive fat resection in upper and lower lid blepharoplasty.
- ✔ Lower lid blepharoplasty techniques should limit orbicularis denervation and limit cicatricial adhesions between lamellae.
- ✔ Retrobulbar hematoma is a surgical emergency.

REFERENCES
1. Baker TJ, Gordon HL. Surgical Rejuvenation of the Face, 2nd ed. St Louis: Quality Medical Publishing, 1998.
2. Carraway JH. Surgical anatomy of the eyelids. Clin Plast Surg 14:693-701, 1987.
3. Furnas DW. The orbicularis oculi muscle. Clin Plast Surg 8:687-715, 1981.
4. Muzaffar AR, Mendelson BC, Adams WP Jr. Surgical anatomy of the ligamentous attachments of the lower lid and lateral canthus. Plast Reconstr Surg 110:873-884, 2002.
5. Flowers RS, DuVal C. Blepharoplasty and periorbital aesthetic surgery. In Aston SJ, Beasley RW, Thorne HM, et al. Grabb and Smith's Plastic Surgery, 5th ed. Philadelphia: Lippincott, 1997, pp 609-631.
6. Guyuron B. Blepharoplasty and ancillary procedures. In Achauer BH, Eriksson E, Guyuron B, et al, eds. Plastic Surgery: Indications, Operations, and Outcomes. St Louis: Mosby, 2000, pp 2527-2547.

7. Jelks GW, Jelks EB. Preoperative evaluation of the blepharoplasty patient: Bypassing the pitfalls. Clin Plast Surg 20:213-223, 1993.

8. Rohrich RJ, Coberly DM, Fagien S, et al. Current concepts in aesthetic upper blepharoplasty. Plast Reconstr Surg 113:32-42, 2004.

9. May JW, Feron J, Zingarelli P. Retro-orbicularis oculi fat (ROOF) resection in aesthetic blepharoplasty: A 6 year study in 63 patients. Plast Reconstr Surg 86:682, 1990.

10. Flowers RS. Upper blepharoplasty by eyelid invagination: Anchor blepharoplasty. Clin Plast Surg 20:193-207, 1993.

11. Sheen JH. A change in the technique of supratarsal fixation in upper blepharoplasty. Plast Reconstr Surg 59:831-834, 1977.

12. Baker TJ, Gordon HL, Mosienko P. Upper lid blepharoplasty. Plast Reconstr Surg 60:692-698, 1977.

13. Casson P, Siebert J. Lower lid blepharoplasty with skin flap and muscle split. Clin Plast Surg 15:299-304, 1988.

14. Aston SJ. Skin-muscle flap lower lid blepharoplasty. Clin Plast Surg 15:305-308, 1988.

15. Tomlinson F, Hovey L. Transconjunctival lower lid blepharoplasty for removal of fat. Plast Reconstr Surg 56:314-318, 1978.

16. Loeb R. Fat pad sliding and fat grafting for leveling lid depressions. Clin Plast Surg 8:757-776, 1981.

17. Hamra ST. Arcus marginalis release and orbital fat preservation in midface rejuvenation. Plast Reconstr Surg 96:354-362, 1995.

18. McCord CD, Codner MA, Hester TR. Redraping the inferior orbicularis arc. Plast Reconstr Surg 102:2471, 1998.

19. Hamra ST. The role of orbital fat preservation in facial aesthetic surgery. Plast Reconstr Surg 23:17-28, 1996.

20. Hamra ST. The role of the septal reset in creating a youthful eyelid-cheek complex in facial rejuvenation. Plast Reconstr Surg 113:2124-2142, 2004.

21. Barton FE, Ha R, Awada M. Fat extrusion and septal reset in patients with the tear trough triad: A critical appraisal. Plast Reconstr Surg 13:2115-2121, 2004.

22. Kawamoto HK, Bradley JP. The tear "TROUF" procedure: Transconjunctival repositioning of orbital unipedicled fat. Plast Reconstr Surg 112:1903-1907, 2003.

23. Fagien S. Algorithm for canthoplasty: The lateral retinacular suspension: A simplified suture canthopexy. Plast Reconstr Surg 103:2042-2053, 1999.

24. Lisman RD, Hyde K, Smith B. Complications of blepharoplasty. Clin Plast Surg 15:309-335, 1988.

25. Carraway JH, Mellow CG. The prevention and treatment of lower lid ectropion following blepharoplasty. Plast Reconstr Surg 85:971-981, 1990.

79. Blepharoptosis

Jason E. Leedy

DEFINITION

Drooping of the upper lid margin to a position that is lower than normal

ANATOMY (Fig. 79-1)

LEVATOR APONEUROSIS
- **Origin:** Lesser wing of the sphenoid
- **Insertion:** Orbicularis oculi, dermis, tarsus
- **Innervation:** Superior division of oculomotor nerve (CN III)
- **Action:** Provides 10-12 mm of eyelid elevation
- **Embryology:** Develops in the third gestational month from the superior rectus muscle
- **Anterior lamella:** Forms aponeurosis
- **Posterior lamella:** Forms Müller's muscle
- Approximately 2-5 mm above the tarsus the levator aponeurosis joins the septum

MÜLLER'S MUSCLE
- **Origin:** Posterior lamella of levator muscle
- **Insertion:** Superior border of tarsus
- **Innervation:** Sympathetics
- **Action:** Provides 2-3 mm of eyelid elevation

FRONTALIS MUSCLE
- **Origin:** Galeal aponeurosis
- **Insertion:** Suprabrow dermis
- **Innervation:** Frontal branch of facial nerve
- **Action:** Elevates brow and upper eyelid skin

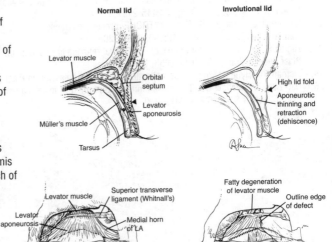

Fig. 79-1 Anatomy. (From McCord CD. The evaluation and management of the patient with ptosis. Clin Plast Surg 15:173, 1988.)

ETIOLOGIC FACTORS/PATHOPHYSIOLOGY[1,2]

TRUE PTOSIS
- Intrinsic drooping of the affected eyelid

PSEUDOPTOSIS: CONDITIONS THAT MIMIC TRUE PTOSIS
- **Grave's disease:** Retraction of contralateral lid can give appearance of ptosis on unaffected side
- **Hypotropia:** Downward rotation of the globe with accompanying lid movement
- **Duane's syndrome:** Extraocular muscular fibrosis giving globe retraction
- **Posttraumatic enophthalmos**
- **Contralateral exophthalmus:** Gives impression of ptosis on the unaffected side
- **Chronic squinting** from irritation

CONGENITAL PTOSIS[1,2]
- Developmental dysgenesis in the levator muscle
- Idiopathic persistent ptosis noticed shortly after birth
- Usually not progressive
- Signs confined to the affected eyelid(s)
- Decreased palpebral aperture with reduction of the pupil reflex to upper eyelid margin measurement
- Decreased levator excursion
  - Poor or absent levator function is reflected in the absence of the eyelid crease
- Ptotic eyelid is generally higher than the normal eyelid during downgaze
- Inheritance pattern unclear
- Levator biopsies in congenital ptosis show absence of striated muscle fibers with fibrosis

> TIP: History alone usually can discern congenital from acquired ptosis, but if there is a question, lagophthalmos on downward gaze is characteristic of congenital ptosis because levator fibrosis prevents downward lid migration.

- **Associated ocular abnormalities**
  - **Coexistent strabismus and amblyopia**
    - ▶ Caused by pupil occlusion
  - **Marcus Gunn's jaw-winking syndrome**
    - ▶ Synkinesis of upper lid with chewing
    - ▶ Seen in 2%-6% of congenital ptosis
    - ▶ Caused by aberrant innervation from fifth cranial nerve
  - **Blepharophimosis syndrome**
    - ▶ Triad of **ptosis, telecanthus,** and **phimosis** of lid fissure
  - **Congenital anophthalmos or microphthalmos**
    - ▶ Hypoplasia of the lids, globe, and orbital bones
  - **Coexistent eyelid hamartoma**
    - ▶ Neurofibromas
    - ▶ Hemangiomas
    - ▶ Lymphangiomas

ACQUIRED PTOSIS[1,2]

- **Myogenic**
  - **Involutional myopathic (senile ptosis)**
    - ▸ *Most common type*
    - ▸ Stretching of the levator aponeurosis attachments to the anterior tarsus
    - ▸ Dermal attachments are maintained and therefore the supratarsal crease rises
    - ▸ Levator function is usually good
  - **Chronic progressive external ophthalmoplegia**
    - ▸ Progressive muscular dystrophy affecting the extraocular muscles and levator
    - ▸ 5% of cases involve the facial and oropharyngeal muscles
- **Traumatic**
  - *Second most common*
  - Allow for recovery of myoneural dysfunction, resolution of edema, and softening of scar (approximately 6 months)
  - Can occur after cataract surgery from dehiscence of levator aponeurosis
- **Neurogenic**
  - **Third nerve palsy:** Paralyzes levator muscle
  - **Horner's syndrome:** Paralyzes Müller's muscle
  - **Myasthenia gravis**
    - ▸ Primarily affects young women and old men
    - ▸ Ptosis worsening with fatigue, at the end of the day
    - ▸ Improvement with neostigmine or edrophonium is characteristic
- **Mechanical**
  - Upper lid tumors
  - Severe dermatochalasis, brow ptosis

EVALUATION[1,2]

DETERMINATION OF CAUSE
- Congenital or acquired

> TIP: Evaluate for lagophthalmos during downward gaze, which indicates levator fibrosis, more commonly seen with congenital cases.

DEGREE OF PTOSIS (Table 79-1)
- Compare with contralateral side if unilateral
- Measure amount of descent over upper limbus
  - 1-2 mm: Mild
  - 3 mm: Moderate
  - 4 mm or more: Severe
- Record palpebral fissure height

Table 79-1 *Degree of Ptosis*

Degree of Ptosis	Mild	Moderate	Severe
Lid descent over upper limbus	1-2 mm	3 mm	>4 mm

Table 79-2 *Levator Function*

Levator Function	Good	Fair	Poor
Levator excursion	>10 mm	5-10 mm	0-5 mm

LEVATOR FUNCTION (Table 79-2)
- Measure from extreme downward gaze to extreme upward gaze while immobilizing the brow
- More than 10 mm: Good
- 5-10 mm: Fair
- Less than 5 mm: Poor

PREOPERATIVE EVALUATION FOR DRY-EYE SYMPTOMS
- **Schirmer's tests I and II** (see Chapter 78)
- **Bell's phenomenon:** Upward rotation of globe when eyes forcibly opened, corneal protective mechanism during sleep
- **Tear film breakup and tear lysozyme electrophoresis:** Advanced ophthalmologic tests useful to further characterize causes of dry-eye symptoms

> TIP: General rule: If contact lenses can be worn, then tear production is adequate.

- **Assess lower lid position:** Scleral show or lower lid laxity—patient more prone to postoperative dry-eye symptoms and may benefit from lower lid procedure to improve position or tone in conjunction with ptosis correction

> TIP: All ptosis procedures cause lagophthalmos, therefore dry-eye symptoms must be evaluated preoperatively.

ASSESS CONTRALATERAL EYE
- **Hering's law**[3]
  - Levator muscles receive equal innervation bilaterally.
  - Severe ptosis on one side creates impulse for bilateral lid retraction. Therefore if the severely affected side is corrected, innervation impulse for lid retraction diminishes, which may reveal ptosis of the contralateral side.[3]
- **Hering's test**
  - Attempt to reveal contralateral ptosis.
  - With brow immobilized in straightforward gaze, elevate affected lid with cotton-tipped applicator to alleviate ptosis; then examine for contralateral ptosis.

LID CONTOUR AND LID CREASE

- Evaluate contralateral lid contour and lid crease to determine proper postoperative lid crease on affected side.

OCULAR EXAMINATION

- Assess general ocular visual function and consider ophthalmologic consultation for formal examination.
- Consult with ophthalmologist preoperatively for baseline visual field testing.

COMPLICATING ISSUES[4,5]

- **Dry eyes**
  - Postoperative lagophthalmos with corneal exposure may threaten vision.
- **Hypoplastic tarsus**
  - Seen in congenital cases, ptosis repair can cause lid eversion.
- **Floppy upper lid**
  - Medial horn of levator aponeurosis is commonly dehisced and creates temporal shift of tarsus. Ptosis repair must recenter tarsus.
- **Asymmetric ptosis**
  - Correcting ptosis in the severe eye can unmask ptosis in the contralateral eye.
- **Widened intercanthal distance**
  - Ptosis gives illusion of narrower intercanthal distance; if widened preoperatively, patient should be informed for possible appearance of telecanthus postoperatively.

ANAESTHESIA FOR PTOSIS REPAIR

- IV sedation with local anaesthetic
- Useful for mild to moderate degrees of ptosis correction in cooperative patients
- Most amenable to anterior-approach levator surgery
- Allows for active patient participation with eye opening and closure so that precise correction can be achieved

TECHNIQUE

- Inject local anaesthetic (use sparingly).
- Expose aponeurosis.
- Place key sutures.
- Have patient sit upright and focus on premarked spot on distant wall.
- Adjust key sutures until ptosis is corrected at appropriate level.

TIP: Excess local anaesthetic may impair levator function, which can markedly affect results.

CHOICE OF SURGICAL PROCEDURE

- If **more than 10 mm** of levator excursion (excellent), then **aponeurotic surgery** or **müllerectomy**
- If **5-10 mm** of excursion (moderate), then **levator resection** or advancement
- If **0-5 mm** of excursion (poor), then need **frontalis suspension**

TIP: If there is mechanical ptosis, address contributing factor(s) (e.g., brow ptosis, upper lid tumor).

The most important factor is the amount of levator excursion.

Limit use of epinephrine in local anaesthetic, because it stimulates Müller's muscle, which gives 0.5 to 1 mm of temporary lid elevation. If using epinephrine with monitored anaesthesia care, the operated side should be slightly overcorrected to account for postoperative relaxation of Müller's muscle.

FASANELLA-SERVAT PROCEDURE (Fig. 79-2)
- Conjunctival approach to excise tarsus, Müller's muscle, and conjunctiva
- Should be considered only when levator function is excellent with minimal ptosis
- Avoids external incision—therefore unable to alter supratarsal crease
- Somewhat less predictable than external approaches
- Resection of tarsus can result in postoperative floppy lid with lid peaking and eversion
- **Putterman's procedure:** Similar, except conjunctivomüllerectomy only

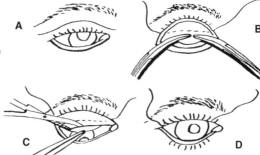

Fig. 79-2   Fasanella-Servat procedure. (From Carraway JH. Cosmetic and function considerations in ptosis surgery: The elusive "perfect" result. Clin Plast Surg 15:186, 1988.)

MUSTARDE'S SPLIT-LEVEL APPROACH (Fig. 79-3)
- Anterior resection of skin, conjunctival resection of tarsus and conjunctiva, retention of levator and Müller's muscle
- Not frequently described, perhaps of historical significance only

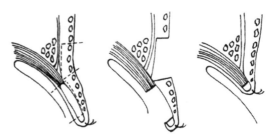

Fig. 79-3   Mustarde split-level ptosis repair. (From Carraway JH. Cosmetic and function considerations in ptosis surgery: The elusive "perfect" result. Clin Plast Surg 15:186, 1988.)

LEVATOR APONEUROSIS ADVANCEMENT[6] (Fig. 79-4)

■ Useful for mild to moderate ptosis
■ Amenable to monitored anaesthesia technique
■ **Technique**
  • Incise skin at desired supratarsal fold.
  • Expose orbital septum and distal levator aponeurosis beneath orbicularis fibers.
  • Incise septum and retract the preaponeurotic fat to expose the aponeurosis, which can be identified by the vertically oriented vessels on its superior surface.
  • Incise distal aponeurosis at the superior tarsal border, and dissect it free from Müller's muscle.
  • Place a central-lifting suture: Double-arm 6-0 suture passed into superior tarsus and levator aponeurosis; tarsus will need to be recentered in cases of temporal displacement.

TIP: In general, 4 mm of levator advancement is needed for every 1 mm of ptosis correction.

If patient is under general anaesthesia, a gapping method can be applied, in which an advancement is performed until upper and lower eyelids are separated by an amount corresponding to preoperative levator excursion.

  • If levator excursion is 8-10 mm, then upper lid should be slightly lower than the upper limbus after advancement; if 6-8 mm, then it should be at the limbus; if 4-6 mm, then slightly higher than limbus.
  • Additional medial and lateral sutures are placed.
  • Perform supratarsal crease fixation—"anchor blepharoplasty" or resection of orbicularis.

TIP: Alternatively, levator aponeurosis advancement can be performed by exposing levator muscle above Whitnall's ligament and resecting muscle in ratio of 4:1 for desired correction.[6]

Levator plication has also been described using a 3:1 ratio without incision of aponeurosis, performed concurrently with aesthetic facial procedures under general anaesthesia.[7]

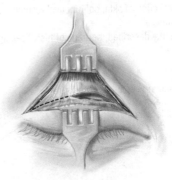

Fig. 79-4   Dissection of the levator aponeurosis.

EXTERNAL LEVATOR RESECTION (Fig. 79-5)[8]
- Best used when levator function is fair
- Sacrifices the viable levator muscle

TIP: Carraway and Vincent[6] espouse levator advancement over external levator resection because of improved results with less morbidity.

- **Technique**
  1. Incise skin and orbicularis muscle at the desired supratarsal crease.
  2. Expose superior border of the tarsus.
  3. Incise full thickness through superior tarsal attachments and place ptosis clamp.
  4. Dissect levator and Müller's muscle complex from conjunctiva and orbital septum/preaponeurotic fat; cut medial and lateral horns as necessary.
  5. Remove full thickness levator aponeurosis/muscle and Müller's muscle.
  6. **Beard method:** If there are 1-2 mm of ptosis with 8-10 mm of levator function, resect 10-12 mm; if there are 2 mm of ptosis with 5-7 mm of levator function, resect 18 mm.
  7. **Berke method:** Use the gapping method (see previous description).

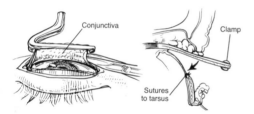

Conjunctiva · Clamp · Sutures to tarsus

Fig. 79-5 Levator resection. (From McCord CD, Codner MA, Hester TR. Eyelid Surgery: Principles and Techniques. New York: Raven, 1995, p 124.)

LEVATOR REINSERTION
- Only useful in true levator dehiscence, which is likely only after trauma
- Involves resuturing the dehisced end to the tarsus
- Uncommon procedure because of uncommon indication

FRONTALIS SUSPENSION (Fig. 79-6)
- Required if levator function **poor** (congenital cases, neurogenic cases)
- Can give 1 cm of excursion; good result in straightforward gaze; gives lagophthalmos while asleep, which requires ointment or nighttime patching
- Incorporates a sling (fascia lata, temporalis fascia, homograft fascia, silicone strips, Gore-Tex) from frontalis to lid
  - If eyes are dry preoperatively, use alloplastic material so level can be adjusted.
- For unilateral congenital cases, bilateral suspension performed to improve symmetry
- **Crawford's technique**
  - Harvest 3 mm fascia lata strip.
  - Use three supralash incisions at medial, central, and lateral limbus and three brow incisions.
  - Thread fascia submuscularly from upper lid to brow.
- **Direct tarsal suturing with lid crease formation**
  - Creates supratarsal crease and fixation of sling material to tarsus to prevent late entropion seen with Crawford's procedure

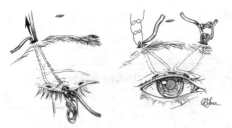

Fig. 79-6 Frontalis suspension, Crawford technique. (From McCord CD. The evaluation and management of the patient with ptosis. Clin Plast Surg 15:182, 1988.)

COMPLICATIONS[7]

- Undercorrection
- Overcorrection
- Excessive lagophthalmos
- Corneal exposure or keratitis, dry-eye syndrome
- Eyelid contour abnormality, temporal overcorrection
- Eyelid crease asymmetry
- Eyelash ptosis or lash abnormalities
- Entropion or ectropion/eversion of the upper lid
- Extraocular muscle imbalance
- Conjunctival prolapse

> ## KEY POINTS
> ✔ Congenital ptosis usually requires frontalis suspension.
> ✔ Acquired ptosis is most often involutional.
> ✔ For correction of involutional ptosis use levator advancement with monitored anaesthesia and advance approximately 4 mm for every 1 mm of desired lid elevation.

REFERENCES

1. McCord CD. The evaluation and management of the patient with ptosis. Clin Plast Surg 15:169-184, 1988.
2. McCord CD. Evaluation of the ptosis patient. In McCord CD, Codner MA, Hester TR. Eyelid Surgery: Principles and Techniques. New York: Raven, 1995, pp 99-112.
3. Parsa FD, Wolff DR, Parsa MM, et al. Upper eyelid ptosis repair after cataract extraction and the importance of Hering's test. Plast Reconstr Surg 108:1527-1536, 2001.
4. Carraway J. Correction of blepharoptosis. In Achauer BM, Eriksson E, Guyuron B, et al, eds. Plastic Surgery: Indications, Operations, and Outcomes, St Louis: Mosby, 2000, pp 2549-2561.
5. Carraway JH. Cosmetic and function considerations in ptosis surgery: The elusive "perfect" result. Clin Plast Surg 15:185-193, 1988.
6. Carraway JH, Vincent MP. Levator advancement technique for eyelid ptosis. Plast Reconstr Surg 77:394-402, 1986.
7. de la Torre JI, Martin SA, De Cordier BC, et al. Aesthetic eyelid ptosis correction: A review of technique and cases. Plast Reconstr Surg 112:655-660, 2003.
8. McCord CD. Complications of ptosis surgery and their management. In McCord CD, Codner MA, Hester TR. Eyelid Surgery: Principles and Techniques. New York: Raven, 1995, pp 144-155.

80. Face Lift

Sumeet S. Teotia

ANATOMY

A thorough grounding in facial anatomy is crucial when attempting to deliver consistent, safe, and reproducible results in rhytidectomy.

MUSCLES OF THE FACE
- Facial mimetic muscles control the movement of the midface and lips, and the size and shape of the mouth. **Four layers of muscles have been described (from superficial to deep).**[1]
  1. Depressor anguli oris, zygomaticus minor, orbicularis oris
  2. Depressor labii inferioris, risorius, platysma
  3. Zygomaticus major, levator labii superioris alaeque nasi
  4. Mentalis, levator anguli oris, buccinator
- The muscles of the **first three layers** are innervated by the facial nerve on their **deep** surfaces, and the muscles of the **fourth layer** are innervated by the facial nerve on their **superficial** surfaces.

BLOOD SUPPLY[1,2]
- The vascular territory of the face and scalp is supplied primarily by the branches of the external carotid artery, with small contributions to the eyelid, brow, forehead, and scalp through ophthalmic division of the internal carotid artery.
  - **Anterior face arteries:** Facial, superior and inferior labial, supratrochlear, and supraorbital
  - **Lateral face arteries:** Transverse, submental, zygomaticoorbital, anterior auricular
  - **Scalp and forehead:** Superficial temporal, frontal and temporal branches of the superficial temporal, posterior auricular, occipital
- Facial vessels lie in the deepest plane with the parotid duct and buccal and zygomatic branches of the facial nerve.
- Blood supply of the facial skin is through a network of musculocutaneous perforators located along the oral commissures and nasolabial folds.
  - The **anterior region** of the face is supplied by a dense network of **musculocutaneous** perforators.
  - The **lateral face** is supplied by a network of sparsely populated **fasciocutaneous** perforators.
- Skin undermining during face lift divides the fasciocutaneous perforators located laterally; thus the blood supply of the facial flap is dependent on the medially based musculocutaneous perforators.

SENSORY NERVE INNERVATION[1]
- The face is supplied by branches of the trigeminal (maxillary and mandibular division) and cervical spinal nerves, with a small contribution to the auditory canal through CN VIII and CN X.
  - **Great auricular nerve** (C2-3)
    - *Most common nerve injured during face lifts (symptomatic).*
    - It is at greatest risk in its superficial location on the sternocleidomastoid muscle, 6.5 cm inferior to the tragus.
    - Division of the nerve leads to numbness of portions of the ear.

- **Auriculotemporal nerve**
  - Courses with the superficial temporal artery
  - Can be divided during a face lift
  - **Frey's syndrome:** Sympathetic reinnervation of facial skin flap after division of auriculotemporal nerve fibers causing gustatory sweating
- **Lesser occipital nerve**
  - Travels mostly over the sternocleidomastoid muscle, running between the muscle fascia and superficial facial fascia
  - Innervates the superior third of the ear and mastoid region in about 60% of cases.
  - Occasionally supplies two thirds of the superior ear.
  - **Skin of midface supplied by branches of the maxillary division**
  - Zygomaticotemporal, zygomaticofacial, and infraorbital nerves
  - Knowing the locations of these nerves prevents division during face lifts

MOTOR NERVE SUPPLY: THE FACIAL NERVE[1]

- The facial nerve emerges through the stylomastoid foramen and is immediately protected by the parotid gland.
- It divides into an upper and lower portion within the parotid gland, and then divides into **five major branches:**
  1. Temporal (frontal)
  2. Zygomatic
  3. Buccal
  4. Marginal mandibular
  5. Cervical
- *The frontal and marginal mandibular branches are most at risk during rhytidectomy.*[3,4]
  - **Frontal branch**
    - Courses superficially after crossing the zygomatic arch (at midpoint between the tragus and lateral canthus) within the sub-SMAS fat just deep to the temporoparietal fascia
    - Travels superiorly, approximately along a trajectory from the tragus to a point 1.5 cm above the lateral brow
  - **Marginal mandibular branch**
    - Protected by the thick SMAS platysma layer after exiting the parotid gland
    - Follows the mandibular border, and before crossing the facial vessels may extend 1 to 2 cm below the mandibular border
    - Runs above the mandibular border after crossing the facial vessels
    - Runs deep to platysma throughout its course
    - Dissection above platysma laterally, and deep to platysma centrally, avoids injury to the nerve
- **Buccal branches**
  - Emerge from the anterior parotid
  - Lie in the loose areolar tissue and fat superficial to the masseter and deep to the SMAS
- **Buccal and zygomatic branches**
  - Injuries are rare and result from their multiple interconnections.
  - These branches are deep to the SMAS and deep facial fascia.
  - Injury to one or more branches may yield only a temporarily noticeable deficit.

FACIAL DANGER ZONES[5]

- Fig. 80-1 outlines the zones of the face where motor branches of the facial nerves and sensory nerves are at greatest risk during face lift.

FACIAL DANGER ZONES: MOTOR AND SENSORY NERVES

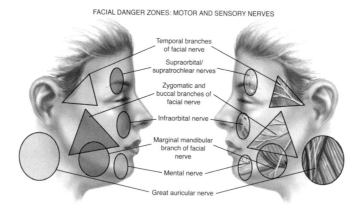

Temporal branches
of facial nerve

Supraorbital/
supratrochlear nerves

Zygomatic and
buccal branches of
facial nerve

Infraorbital nerve

Marginal mandibular
branch of facial
nerve

Mental nerve

Great auricular nerve

Fig. 80-1

FASCIAL LAYERS OF THE FACE (Fig. 80-2)[1]

■ **The layers of the facial soft tissues can be conceptualized as a series of concentric layers from superficial to deep.**
  • Skin
  • Subcutaneous tissue
  • Superficial facial fascia
  • Facial mimetic muscles
  • Deep facial fascia (parotidomasseteric fascia)
■ **Deepest plane contains the following:**
  • Facial nerve
  • Parotid duct
  • Buccal fat pad
  • Facial vessels

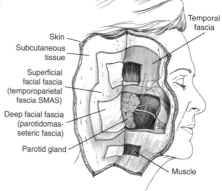

Skin
Subcutaneous
tissue

Superficial
facial fascia
(temporoparietal
fascia SMAS)

Deep facial fascia
(parotidomas-
seteric fascia)

Parotid gland

Temporal
fascia

Muscle

Fig. 80-2

■ **Superficial musculoaponeurotic system (SMAS)**[1,6,7]
  • The SMAS is a well-defined portion of the superficial facial fascia.
  • SMAS thickness varies by patient and region of the face.
  • The superficial facial fascia is a discrete fascial layer.
    ▸ Forms a continuous sheath through the face and neck
    ▸ Extends into malar region, lip, and nose, covering the mimetic muscles
  • The SMAS is an upward extension of the superficial cervical fascia into the face.
  • The fascia of the platysma muscle is part of the superficial cervical fascia and is continuous with the SMAS.
  • The temporoparietal fascia (superficial temporal fascia) is an extension of the SMAS over the temporal region.
  • There are **three fascial layers** in the temporal region.
    1. Temporoparietal fascia
    2. Superficial layer of the deep temporal fascia
    3. Deep layer of the deep temporal fascia
  • From the level of the superior orbital margin and to the zygomatic arch, the superficial and deep layers of the deep temporal fascia are separated from each other by the **superficial temporal fat pad.**

TIP: Dissect in the area beneath the superficial layer of the deep temporal fascia to protect the
frontal branch.

- The galea is an extension of the SMAS over the scalp.
- **Fixed SMAS**
  - ▸ Adherent to and lies over the parotid.
- **Mobile SMAS**
  - ▸ Lies beyond the parotid gland, directly over the mimetic muscles, facial nerves, and parotid duct
  - ▸ Not adherent and highly mobile
- Traction and mobilization of the mobile SMAS permits the movement of the midface and lower
  face during rhytidectomy
  - ▸ Allows proper elevation, repositioning, and rotation for optimal outcome
- ■ **Deep facial fascia (parotidomasseteric fascia)**[8]
- Deep facial fascia is a continuation of the superficial layer of the deep cervical fascia on the face.
- Over the parotid, it is called the *investing fascia of the parotid*.
- Over the masseter, it is called the *masseteric fascia*.
- Above the zygomatic arch, it is called the *deep temporal fascia*.
- The deep facial fascia contains the facial nerve branches, buccal fat pad, parotid duct, and facial
  artery and vein.
- ■ **Relationship between superficial and deep facial fascia** (Fig. 80-3)[1,8]
- Separated by loose areolar tissue. Within this areolar plane lies the frontal branch of the facial
  nerve and the temporal artery.
- The two layers are firmly attached in certain areas.
  - ▸ The zygomatic arch is over the parotid and along the anterior border of the masseter.
- Over the masseter there is also an areolar plane between the SMAS (superficial) and the parotido-
  masseteric (deep) fascia.

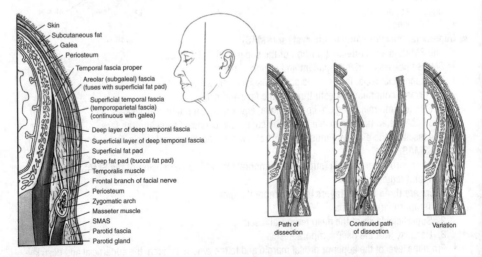

Skin
Subcutaneous fat
Galea
Periosteum
Temporal fascia proper
Areolar (subgaleal) fascia
(fuses with superficial fat pad)
Superficial temporal fascia
(temporoparietal fascia)
(continuous with galea)
Deep layer of deep temporal fascia
Superficial layer of deep temporal fascia
Superficial fat pad
Deep fat pad (buccal fat pad)
Temporalis muscle
Frontal branch of facial nerve
Periosteum
Zygomatic arch
Masseter muscle
SMAS
Parotid fascia
Parotid gland

Path of
dissection

Continued path
of dissection

Variation

Fig. 80-3

LIGAMENTS AND ADHESIONS OF THE UPPER FACE (Fig. 80-4)[1,9-12]

- Various names given to these anatomic structures have created confusion.
- It is important to be reminded of their role in mobilization of the brow and periorbital tissues as part of facial rejuvenation.

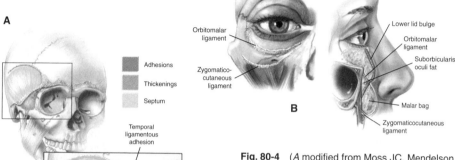

A

B

Orbitomalar ligament

Adhesions

Thickenings

Septum

Zygomatico-cutaneous ligament

Lower lid bulge

Orbitomalar ligament

Suborbicularis oculi fat

Malar bag

Zygomaticocutaneous ligament

Temporal ligamentous adhesion

Temporalis muscle

Sentinel vein

Zygomatico-temporal nerve

Inferior temporal septum

Temporal branches of facial nerve

Zygomatic branch of facial nerve

Supraorbital ligamentous adhesion

Lateral brow thickening of periorbital septum

Lateral orbital thickening of periorbital septum

Periorbital septum

Fig. 80-4 (*A* modified from Moss JC, Mendelson BC, Taylor GI. Surgical anatomy of the ligamentous attachments in the temple and periorbital regions. Plast Reconstr Surg 105:1475-1490, 2000.)

LIGAMENTS AND ADHESIONS OF THE MIDDLE AND LOWER FACE[1,13]

- The retaining ligaments of the face anchor the underlying fixed bony structure to the overlying dermis, supporting the facial skin in its normal position.
- **Two types** of retaining ligaments have been described.
  1. **Osteocutaneous ligaments**
     - ▶ **Zygomatic osteocutaneous ligament**
       - ✦ Extends from the zygomatic arch and body, through the malar fat pad, to the overlying dermis
       - ✦ **McGregor's patch:** Part of the ligament over the zygomatic body
     - ▶ **Mandibular osteocutaneous ligament**
       - ✦ Extends from the parasymphyseal mandibular region to the overlying dermis
  2. **Parotid and masseteric cutaneous ligaments** (Fig. 80-5)
     - ▶ Formed by coalescence of the superficial and deep facial fascia
     - ▶ Fixes these facial layers to the parotid and masseter, and attaches to the overlying dermis by fibrous septa

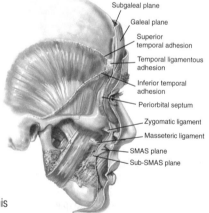

Subgaleal plane

Galeal plane

Superior temporal adhesion

Temporal ligamentous adhesion

Inferior temporal adhesion

Periorbital septum

Zygomatic ligament

Masseteric ligament

SMAS plane

Sub-SMAS plane

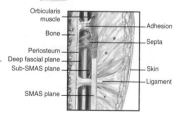

Orbicularis muscle

Bone

Periosteum

Deep fascial plane

Sub-SMAS plane

SMAS plane

Adhesion

Septa

Skin

Ligament

Fig. 80-5

- The functional significance of these ligaments is important for understanding the pathophysiology of the aging face.[1]
  - These ligaments attenuate and relax with age, causing creases by pivoting facial tissue.
  - The characteristics of aging are the result of these ligaments relaxing along with loss of skin elasticity and atrophy of soft tissues.
    ▸ Weakening of the zygomatic ligaments, which suspend the malar soft tissues and fat pad
      ✦ Causes downward migration of the malar soft tissues
      ✦ Creates redundant skin that hangs over the fixed nasolabial fold (not deepening of the nasolabial fold)
    ▸ Weakening of the masseteric ligaments
      ✦ Causes downward migration of the cheek tissues below the mandibular margin
      ✦ **Jowls** formed from tethering by the **mandibular ligament** (Fig. 80-6)

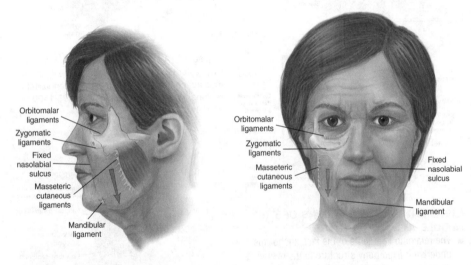

Fig. 80-6

MALAR FAT PAD[1]

A youthful cheek prominence is related to the zygoma and the malar fat pad.
- The malar fat pad is located superficial to the SMAS and mimetic muscles.
- Triangular, its base is along the nasolabial sulcus and its apex toward the zygomatic prominence.
- It is an area of thickened subcutaneous tissue, and with age the fat pad descends and loses volume.
- The descent of the malar fat pad creates fullness and deepening of the nasolabial sulcus

BUCCAL FAT PAD[14]

The buccal fat pad is an important structure contributing to cheek and facial contour.
- Buccal fat pad consists of a **central body and three extensions:** Temporal, pterygoid, and buccal.
- Central body and buccal extensions contribute to cheek contour.
- Buccal fat pad is similar to an egg yolk in color, size, and consistency.
- The zygomatic and buccal branches of the facial nerve lie superficial to the buccal extension, with the parotid duct passing through it.
- In select cases, the buccal extension can be removed using an intraoral approach with a longitudinal incision in the buccal sulcus to reduce cheek fullness and enhance the malar eminence.

ASSESSING THE AGING FACE

WRINKLES AND HISTOLOGY

Wrinkling occurs as a result of aging, actinic damage, or genetic disorders. Normal aging is a process of atrophy.

- **Three types of creases occur in the skin.**[15]
  1. Animation creases from mimetic muscle insertions
  2. Fine, shallow wrinkles (caused by disruption of skin elastic structures)
  3. Coarse, deep wrinkles resulting from solar elastosis and epidermal atrophy
- **Histologic changes**[15]
  - Loss of dermoepidermal papillae
  - Fewer melanocytes and Langerhans cells
  - Less dermal collagen, leading to thinning of the skin
  - Loss of reticular dermis with reduced dermal organization
  - Decreases in ground substance (elastic fibers, collagen, glycosaminoglycan gel)
  - Larger sebaceous glands

PHOTOAGING[15]

- **Actinic-damaged skin is different from normal aging skin.**
  - Elastic fibers thicken in the dermis.
  - Ground substance increases.
  - Collagen decreases, with an increase in collagen type III.
  - Histologically this process is also called *basophilic degeneration,* or *elastosis.*

MORPHOLOGY[15]

The aging face is characterized by volume changes of the skeletal and soft tissues. Deflation of facial structures occurs, which is as important as gravitational laxity of the tissues.

- There is loss of soft tissue volume.
- There is a skeletal remodeling with aging, resulting in clockwise rotation of the midface relative to the cranial base.
- The adult facial skeleton continues to grow throughout life in the absence of tooth loss or bone demineralization.
- Facial structures rotate downward and inward with respect to the cranial base.

PATIENT SELECTION

- The entire face should be evaluated and an algorithm developed to correct aspects of aging.
- History is obtained to exclude high-risk patients: Smokers, patients with poorly controlled hypertension, diabetics, chronic NSAID users, and those with other medical conditions.
- The entire face should be addressed to prevent a patchwork appearance.
- Divide the face into zones when examining the patient, and develop a checklist.

PERIORBITAL ZONE: UPPER THIRD OF FACE (FOREHEAD, BROW, AND UPPER MIDFACE)[1]

- **Brow position:** Assess the medial and lateral brow position and the relationship of the brow to the upper lid.
- **Forehead height:** Note the distance from the hairline to the brow; the brow is not an exact point, but measuring between fixed points, such as hairline to pupil, is exact.
- **Glabellar creases:** Assess for corrugator (vertical) wrinkling, procerus (horizontal) wrinkling, and depth of rhytids.
- **Temporal region:** Evaluate the presence of crow's feet and excess skin.
- **Upper eyelid:** Assess the skin, the effect of brow ptosis (pseudoptosis), lid ptosis (congenital or senile), and fat (mostly medial).
- **Lower eyelid:** Observe the lower lid–cheek junction; assess lid tone; look for festoons and tear-trough deformity with orbital fat herniation.
- **Lateral canthal position:** Note the canthal relationship and lid tone.

PERIORAL ZONE: MIDDLE THIRD OF FACE (LOWER FACE)[1]

- **Nasolabial folds and marionette grooves:** Assess depth at rest and animation.
- **Angle of the mouth:** Aging lowers the angle of the mouth.
- **Upper lip:** Note presence of perioral rhytids, length of upper lip, and volume loss with increased distance from nose to vermilion border of upper lip, leading to loss of definition of philtral columns.
- **Lower lip:** Assess volume loss.
- **Chin:** Assess the depth of labiomental fold, chin ptosis, and jowls.
- **Nose:** Assess the aging, ptotic nose.
- **Ear position:** Assess for lobular ptosis and elongation; observe increased vertical height of the ear.

NECK ZONE: LOWER THIRD OF FACE[1]

- The neck is addressed in detail in Chapter 81.
- Examine for excess skin, platysmal banding causing transverse cervical creases, subcutaneous and subplatysmal fat.
- Assess the jawline and the submandibular gland.

VARIATIONS IN TECHNIQUE

INCISION PLACEMENT

- Scar location depends on location of hairline and sideburns, Fitzpatrick skin classification, and ear topography.
- **Temple incision**[1] (Fig. 80-7)
  - Widening the distance between the lateral canthus and the anterior part of the temporal hairline creates an unnatural appearance.
  - **Prehairline:** Ideal with short sideburns, secondary face lifts, and when excision of excess skin would widen the distance from the lateral canthus.
  - **Posthairline:** Often used in continuation with an open-coronal brow-lift procedure, and also when minimal excess temporal skin is recruited.

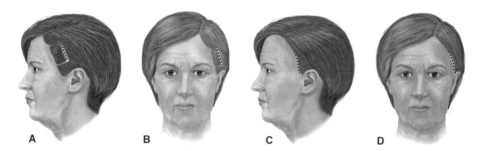

Fig. 80-7 A and **B,** Incision behind the temporal hairline; **C** and **D,** Prehairline incision.

■ **Preauricular incision**[1] (Fig. 80-8)
  • Incision is made between the anatomic margin of the face and ear, taking notice of the width of the root of the helix.
  • The incision is curved along the anterior border of the helix to the upper tragus.
  • An intratragal incision along its posterior border is best suited to hide the scar.
■ **Postauricular incision**[1] (Fig. 80-9)
  • The incision is best placed at the retroauricular sulcus.
  • The horizontal limb is based on the amount of skin excised and the redundancy of neck skin.
    ▶ **High retroauricular incision:** Moderate neck skin redundancy
    ▶ **Low retroauricular incision:** Moderate to excessive neck skin
    ▶ **Occipital (hairline) incision:** Excessive neck skin

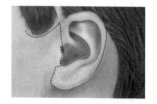

Fig. 80-8

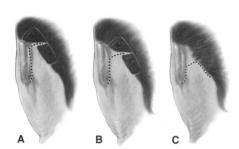

Fig. 80-9 A, A high retroauricular crossing to the hairline is best suited to individuals with modest redundancy of neck skin. **B,** A lower retroauricular crossing to the hairline is best suited to individuals with modest to excessive redundancy of neck skin. **C,** An occipital hairline incision is best suited to individuals with excessive or massive skin redundancy, especially in the lower neck.

VECTORS AND FIXATION[1]

■ The SMAS should ideally be fixed and elevated in a more vertical or diagonally vertical vector.
■ Skin fixation should be more posterior and vertical.
■ The vertical vector on the SMAS is critical and improves the jawline, the perioral areas and, with high SMAS, the midface.
■ The diagonal vector on the platysma improves the neck and submental areas.

- Permanent sutures are mostly used to suspend the SMAS, and absorbable sutures are used for the skin.
- Some propose the use of Vicryl mesh to suspend the SMAS for added support and fixation.[16]

OPERATIVE TECHNIQUES

Most techniques involve some degree of subcutaneous dissection in combination with methods to address the SMAS. Techniques include surgical endoscopy, various degrees of sub-SMAS dissection, SMAS plication and imbrication, and attempts to restore a youthful lower eyelid–cheek junction.

- **Subcutaneous face lift**[15]
  - The standard subcutaneous face lift with variable skin undermining is rarely performed today.
  - A thicker flap may be developed by releasing the osteocutaneous ligaments and redraping the skin.
  - The persistence of this face lift is shortened by recurring signs of aging.
  - The SMAS is not addressed.
- **Subcutaneous face lift with plication and/or imbrication**[15,17]
  - SMAS *plication* (suture infolding) is the elevation of a subcutaneous flap and placement of direct sutures to tighten the SMAS without elevating it as a discrete layer.
  - SMAS *imbrication* involves incision, advancement, and overlapping with suture fixation.
  - The fatty tissues of the cheek and neck are suspended upward and laterally without SMAS undermining.
- **Skoog face lift**[18]
  - In 1974 Skoog described skin and SMAS elevation as a single unit, advancing the entire skin-SMAS unit posteriorly onto the cheek and neck.
  - Skoog's method identified SMAS as a discrete layer that could be used to augment skin suspension.
  - Procedure fails to improve nasolabial folds and anterior neck pull.
  - Skoog's procedure was modified further by Barton[19] and by Hamra[20] to address the nasolabial fold.
- **Subcutaneous dissection and deep SMAS advancement with several variations**
  - The term *deep plane or sub-SMAS or deep SMAS* refers to dissection that lifts the SMAS layer.
  - A **low SMAS** technique (inferior to the zygomatic arch) addresses the lower face only and has no effect on tissues of the midface or perioral and infraorbital regions.
  - A **high SMAS** technique (superior to the zygomatic arch) addresses the midface and periorbital area in combination with the lower face.
    - ▶ Refined, perfected, and popularized by Barton.
  - **Composite face lift** of Hamra[20-27]
    - ▶ Carries not only the platysma and subcutaneous fat but also the lower lid orbicularis muscle as a single dissected unit.
    - ▶ The malar and periorbital areas are directly suspended in the upper face with this rhytidectomy.
    - ▶ The skin and subcutaneous tissues are not elevated as an independent layer.
  - **Short-scar face lift with lateral SMASectomy** of Baker[28]
    - ▶ Excises a strip of SMAS in the region overlying the anterior edge of the parotid gland parallel to the nasolabial fold.
    - ▶ The vector of elevation is perpendicular to the nasolabial fold.
  - **Lamellar SMAS face lift**
    - ▶ The skin and SMAS are dissected as two separate lamellae (layers).
    - ▶ They are advanced to different degrees along separate vectors and suspended under different tension.
    - ▶ Each layer is addressed separately.
  - **Minimal access cranial suspension (MACS) short-scar face lift** of Tonnard and Verpaele[29]
    - ▶ Dissects subcutaneous tissues from the underlying SMAS-platysma layer and then suspends the tissue from the deep temporal fascia.

- The **foundation face lift** of Pitman[30]
  - ▶ Separates the SMAS-platysma only from the underlying tissues while simultaneously raising a composite flap of SMAS-platysma, subcutaneous fat, and skin.
- **Subperiosteal face lift**[15]
- A subperiosteal face lift does not dissect the SMAS or skin as an independent layer.
- The midface periosteum is elevated as a single unit, and then this layer is redraped and affixed to achieve tissue repositioning.
- A combined **temporal and perioral subperiosteal midface release** is advocated by Little; it stacks the entire cheek–soft tissue unit to further accentuate the malar eminence.
- This technique allows adequate redraping of the forehead and malar areas
  - ▶ The perioral and neck region requires an additional procedure for suspension.
  - ▶ Additional procedure may involve skin, SMAS, or a combination.
- Patients with great skin redundancy of the nasolabial folds, jawline, and neck are not candidates for the isolated subperiosteal face lift.
- **Temporal supraperiosteal dissection**
- An **endoscopic method** is described by Byrd et al.[31,32]
  - ▶ Addresses the bony and soft tissues in the upper face as a single unit approached from the temporal region
- Subperiosteal plane is abandoned, and dissection is made supraperiosteally around the lateral orbital rim and into the malar region.
- Dissection is superficial to origin of zygomaticus major.
- The malar fat pad is suspended independently by sutures from the temporal fascia.
- The dissection involves an avascular plane between the SMAS and the periosteum around the zygomatic arch.

SPECIAL CONSIDERATIONS

JOWLS
- The best correction of jowls is achieved by SMAS-platysma rotation.
- Rarely, the buccal fat pad may be partially excised using an intraoral approach.

NASOLABIAL FOLDS[19,33-36]
- Many methods exist to attempt correction of deep nasolabial folds.
- A subSMAS face lift that goes through the SMAS to the subcutaneous plane at the level of the belly of the zygomaticus major muscle can stretch out the nasolabial fold if sufficient tension is placed on the anterior cheek skin.
- Dermal attachments of the fold can be released and filled with fat or dermal fat grafts.
- Soft tissue fillers can be used to attempt smoothing out the fold but have variable longevity and are not appropriate for all patients.
- Adjunctive suction can be applied to thick folds, but success is variable.

MALAR ENHANCEMENT[15]
A youthful face has high cheekbones, with concavity in the buccal area. The goal of a face lift is to accentuate the zygomatic body, and several methods are available.
- Malar augmentation can be provided by implants, fillers (fat, hydroxyapatite), or autogenous tissues (SMAS).
- The goal is to resuspend or reposition the ptotic malar fat pad.

- Redundant dissected SMAS can enhance the malar prominence by folding it onto itself and suturing it to the zygomatic body.
- The cheek mass can be anchored to the lateral orbital rim using materials such as permanent suture, tendon, fascia, or Gore-Tex.
- Transblepharoplasty techniques have been described that suspend the cheek mass to the temporal fascia at its insertion near the lateral orbital rim.[37,38]
- Temporal supraperiosteal approaches for elevating the cheek flap also exist (see previous discussion).[31,32,39]
- Methods exist that address the ptotic orbicularis oculi muscle.
- The **malar septum** is the basis of malar mounds and malar edema. Adequate release of this septum may be necessary to smooth out the lower orbital and malar soft tissues.[35,40]

THE AGING LIP[15]

- **Signs**
  - Longer distance between the columellar base and upper vermilion border
  - Less exposed vermilion (thin lips)
  - Loss of vermilion bulk (pout)
- **Vermilion advancement technique**
  - Directly and precisely positions the Cupid's bow.
  - A visible scar is left on the lip margin.
- **Skin removal along the alar and columellar bases**
  - Can shorten the aging upper lip
  - Hidden scar along the base of the nose
- Can add bulk to vermilion volume using fat injections, fillers, AlloDerm, or dermal grafts (using redundant SMAS)

JAWLINE[15]

- Slings and sutures may be placed along the mandibular border in an attempt to smooth out the jawline, but caution must be exercised.
- **Submandibular gland** and **digastric muscle excision** has been advocated by some surgeons but is not widely accepted.
- Suction may be applied with caution along the submandibular border, but only after a face lift has been performed to prevent contour hollowing.

FAT INJECTIONS[1]

- The purpose of fat injections is to attempt to restore age-associated volume loss and tissue atrophy.
- Fat can be placed in the lips, nasolabial folds, chin, jawline, tear trough and periorbicular deformities, zygomatic prominence, and labiomandibular folds.
- Aim for slight overcorrection with much expected loss over time.
- Repeat injections are almost always necessary.
- Dermal fat grafts can also be used adjunctively.
- Injections must be deep and contour irregularities corrected by massaging.
- Fat must be placed in 1 cc syringes and injected using a 19-gauge long needle.
- Fat can be harvested periumbilically or from the thighs using a 60 cc syringe attached to a 3 mm short-suction cannula.
- Generally aim for about 3 cc in the upper lip and 2 cc in the lower lip; expect a 50% loss over several months.

- The injected fat can be filtered first using a sieve (a double-overlap gauze) and can also be centrifuged.
- The viability of fat injections is highly variable.

CHIN PTOSIS[15]

- Occasionally, an aging lower face may have a "witch's chin" (prominent submental crease and a hanging soft tissue mass below the lower mandibular border).
- Corrected most effectively by resuspension of chin mass and insertion of a chin implant.
- Cutaneous dissection to release the mental crease and retaining ligaments is important when redraping.

PERIOPERATIVE MANAGEMENT AND ASSESSMENT

PREOPERATIVE ASSESSMENT AND PATIENT INTERVIEW

- All NSAIDs must be stopped at least 2 weeks before surgery.
- If the patient is on other anticoagulants (such as Plavix or Coumadin), then a face lift is high risk and not medically advisable.
- A thorough interview process with adequate time for questions and decision making should be allowed.
- Patient selection is critical in delivering results.
- Unrealistic expectations should be assessed; do not operate if they are present.
- Evaluate psychological and social issues of the patient, and learn why a face lift is wanted; if unusual, do not operate.
- Contraindications for a face lift include smoking, obesity, skin disorders, systemic medical problems such as diabetes, uncontrolled hypertension, history of angina.
- Consider the patient's general appearance.
- If you feel any "sixth-sense" indication that something is wrong, do not operate.
- Avoid angry or rude patients, those who require multiple preoperative visits, and those who do not seem to understand the face lift you are offering.

INTRAOPERATIVE CONSIDERATIONS

- Have an exact plan of execution, and be surgically precise and decisive.
- Time injection of local anaesthetic with epinephrine to allow at least 10 minutes before incision so that you will not have to wait for the anaesthetic to take effect and waste precious time.
- Repeat injections should rarely be needed if the timing is accurate.
- Have strict guidelines on how to manage intraoperative hypertension, and discuss expectations with the person administering anaesthesia.
- The face should not be dependent during surgery to prevent venous pooling.
- The patient's body should remain warm and covered.
- Hair should be washed, braided, or clustered with rubber bands before incision is made.
- Wearing a headlamp eliminates need for frequent and annoying adjustments of overhead lighting.
- Note that a face lift is performed with the patient in a recumbent position, and the final vectors will have gravitational effects not realized in the operating room.

POSTOPERATIVE MANAGEMENT

- Prevention of hematoma is the most important factor immediately after a face lift.
- The head of the bed must be elevated at all times.
- Pain control and sedation should be balanced with pulse oximetry.

- Strict **blood pressure control** is necessary; the degree of intraoperative blood pressure control predicts postoperative management.
- A clonidine (Catapres) patch is used as necessary, along with intravenous labetalol (Normodyne, Trandate).
- All incisions must be examined, and the hair must be washed with soap on postoperative day 1.
- **Drains:** Neck drains should be used to collect large hematomas and prevent airway compromise; usually removed on postoperative day 1.
- **Dressings:** Dressing is vital and should not be too tight, especially over the forehead and on undermined skin flaps. Ideally, no dressing should be placed under the chin to monitor the patient for fluid collection in the neck.
- Small fluid collections can occur in the temporal region and should be aspirated with a 19-gauge needle attached to a 3 cc syringe.
- Hematomas and continued bleeding should be treated by returning the patient to the operating room for an immediate evacuation procedure.
- Small hematomas or fluid collections beyond 3 or 4 days can also be treated with needle aspiration.

COMPLICATIONS

HEMATOMA

- One of the most dreaded complications is development of hematoma.
- Meticulous intraoperative hemostasis and adequate postoperative blood pressure control are the most important factors of prevention.
- The reported rate of hematoma is about **4% in female patients.**
- **Males** have a higher rate of about **8%.**
- Development of hematoma requires a surgical evacuation.
- Fibrin glue has **not** been shown to be an effective preventive measure.
- **Risk factors for hematoma development**
  - Male patient
  - Preoperative systolic blood pressure greater than 150 mm Hg
  - Rebound hypertension after low intraoperative blood pressure
  - Use of NSAIDs and smoking

NERVE INJURY[3,15]

- The buccal branch is *most often injured* during a face lift, and the injury can go unnoticed because of overlapping territories in the upper lip.
- The great auricular nerve, however, is the *most often recognized* nerve injury after a face lift.
- The marginal mandibular branch suffers *more* trauma than the temporal branch.
- Paralysis from the marginal mandibular branch results in a "full denture smile."
- Deeper dissections increase the chances of nerve injuries.
- Platysma "pseudoparalysis" is asymmetrical lower lip movement or a full-toothed grin as a result of injury to the cervical branches innervating the platysma. Patients recover completely from this injury.
- Dissection near facial nerve branches can create mild neurapraxia, which resolves in several weeks.
- Permanent nerve injuries have been reported to occur more commonly with the use of the classic subcutaneous dissections than with sub-SMAS dissections.

Skin Dehiscence and Necrosis[15]

- Subcutaneous dissection has higher rates of skin sloughing (4%) than sub-SMAS dissections (1%).
- Skin sloughing is preceded by hematoma or infection and most commonly occurs in the **retroauricular region.**
- Prevention: Active smokers should not be operated on.
- Undue tension on the skin should be avoided during suturing.
- If skin perfusion is questionable postoperatively, then release of skin sutures may be indicated to prevent loss of skin flaps. It is more practical to return to the operating room at a later date for scar revision than to lose a potentially devastating area of the facial skin flap.
- All areas of compromised skin perfusion should be kept moist with triple antibiotic ointment and impregnated gauze (such as Xeroform).
- Postoperative visits should be frequent to monitor progress of healing.

Hypertension[15]

- Systolic blood pressure is important postoperatively to prevent hematoma.
- Chlorpromazine (Thorazine) (25 mg) 1 hour and 3 hours postoperatively can be very effective for rebound hypertension. This dose can be repeated at 4-hour intervals up to 24 hours to keep systolic blood pressure at less than 150 mm Hg.
- A clonidine (Catapres) patch (0.2 mg) can be placed for sustained intraoperative or postoperative hypertension.
- Preoperatively clonidine, 0.1-0.3 mg, can be given before surgery to patients who are prone to hypertension.
- Alternatively, labetalol (Normodyne, Trandate) (5 mg/ml IV) can be given in 1-2 ml boluses, which will lower blood pressure for 1-2 hours.

Other Complications

- Infection is very rare, but if it does occur antibiotics are necessary.
- Parotid fistulas rarely occur and usually respond to aspiration, which can be repeated.
- Prolonged edema, chronic pain, salivary cysts, hypertrophic scars, and pigment changes have been reported but are rare.

UNFAVORABLE RESULTS AND THEIR PREVENTION

- **An *unnatural* or *"pulled"* appearance**
  - Usually results from excessive tension on the skin layer or improper vectors of tension on the SMAS layer.
  - **Tension should be on the deep (SMAS) layer, not on the skin.**
  - Tension on the SMAS should be uniform to avoid an abnormal facial appearance during animation.
- ***Visible scars***
  - Are usually too far anterior or too wide.
  - Commonly caused by excessive tension on skin flaps or improper planning of incision placement.
- **The *tragus deformity***
  - Is either blunting of the pretragal depression or anterior displacement of the tragus.
  - Can occur as a result of excessive tension on the skin closure or because the incision was not placed right at the tragal border.

■ **Movement of the hairline**
- Movement lateral to the orbit should be avoided.
- The temporal hair should ideally be 3-4 cm from the lateral orbit.
- If preoperative assessment indicates that significant superolateral movement of the midfacial skin is expected, then a sideburn component of the incision should be planned.
■ Unrecognized *contour irregularity,* such as buccal fat pseudoherniation, a prominent parotid, submandibular gland ptosis, or digastric muscle hypertrophy can occur as a result of inadequate preoperative analysis.
■ **"Pixie ear" deformity**
- Results from the lobule insertion migrating inferiorly as wound healing progresses
- Occurs as a result of insetting the lobule under tension
- Lobule must be inset without tension
■ **Alopecia**
- Can be prevented by proper placement of temporal incision, being parallel to the hair fibers and deep to the follicles, and by preventing tension on closure.

KEY POINTS

✔ A solid foundation of facial anatomy with attention to all fascial layers and suspensory ligaments is necessary to execute a successful face lift.

✔ Accurate diagnosis of the aging face begins with accurate assessment during physical examination.

✔ When evaluating a patient during a face consultation, address all components independent of a patient's self-assessment.

✔ No single technique addresses all varieties of facial aging.

✔ It is a rare patient who benefits from a midface correction only.

✔ Aging is characterized by loss of volume, skin changes, and fascial attenuation.

✔ An ideal face-lift procedure stands the test of time, avoids hollow orbits and lateral sweep, achieves a youthful harmony of the entire face, and avoids a mosaic appearance by addressing all components of the face; it rebuilds the face in layers and avoids distortion of anatomy while minimizing complications and delivering consistent results.

✔ A successful face lift requires a logical and thoughtful preoperative plan that properly applies anatomy knowledge to the aging face.

✔ A face lift mentally begins during proper patient selection and accurate patient evaluation; it leads to an appropriately selected surgical procedure that fits the patient, and carries into assisting the patient during convalescence by proactively preventing complications.

✔ Excessive reliance on adjunctive procedures to deliver the goals of a face lift should be reconsidered.

✔ Addressing the skin is an important part of delivering a successful face lift.

✔ A smooth lower eyelid and cheek junction is perhaps one of the most challenging aspects of a face lift.

✔ Performing a face lift is a privilege not extended to many; hence there can be no compromise of excellent results concomitant with utmost safety for the patient.

REFERENCES

1. Nahai F. The Art of Aesthetic Surgery: Principles and Techniques. St Louis: Quality Medical Publishing, 2005.
2. Whetzel TP, Mathes SJ. Arterial anatomy of the face: An analysis of vascular territories and perforating cutaneous vessels. Plast Reconstr Surg 89:591, 1992.
3. Baker DC, Conley J. Avoiding facial nerve injuries in rhytidectomy. Anatomic variations and pitfalls. Plast Reconstr Surg 64:781, 1979.
4. Stuzin JM, Wagstrom L, Kawamoto HK, et al. Anatomy of the frontal branch of the facial nerve: The significance of the temporal fat pad. Plast Reconstr Surg 83:265, 1989.
5. Seckel BR. Facial Danger Zones: Avoiding Nerve Injury in Facial Plastic Surgery. St Louis: Quality Medical Publishing, 1994.
6. Gosain AK, Yousif NJ, Madiedo G, et al. Surgical anatomy of the SMAS: A reinvestigation. Plast Reconstr Surg 92:1254, 1993.
7. Mitz V, Peyronie M. The superficial musculo-aponeurotic system (SMAS) in the parotid and cheek area. Plast Reconstr Surg 58:80, 1976.
8. Stuzin JM, Baker TJ, Gordon HL. The relationship of the superficial and deep facial fascias: Relevance to rhytidectomy and aging. Plast Reconstr Surg 89:441, 1992.
9. Knize DM. An anatomically based study of the mechanism of eyebrow ptosis. Plast Reconstr Surg 97:1321, 1996.
10. Mendelson BC, Muzaffar AR, Adams WP. Surgical anatomy of the midcheek and malar mounds. Plast Reconstr Surg 110:885, 2002.
11. Moss JC, Mendelson BC, Taylor GI. Surgical anatomy of the ligamentous attachments in the temple and periorbital regions. Plast Reconstr Surg 105:1475, 2000.
12. Muzaffar AR, Mendelson BC, Adams WP. Surgical anatomy of the ligamentous attachments of the lower lid and canthus. Plast Reconstr Surg 110:873, 2002
13. Furnas DW. The retaining ligaments of the cheek. Plast Reconstr Surg 83:11, 1989.
14. Dubin B, Jackson IT, Hahm A, et al. Anatomy of the buccal fat pad and its clinical significance. Plast Reconstr Surg 83:257, 1989.
15. Gonyon DL, Barton FE. The aging face: Rhytidectomy and adjunctive procedures. Sel Read Plast Surg 10, 2005.
16. Stuzin JM, Baker TJ, Baker TM. Refinements in face lifting: Enhanced facial contour using Vicryl mesh incorporated into SMAS fixation. Plast Reconstr Surg 105:290, 2000.
17. Owsley JQ. Platysma-fascial rhytidectomy. Plast Reconstr Surg 60:843, 1977.
18. Skoog T. Plastic Surgery: New Methods. Philadelphia: WB Saunders, 1974.
19. Barton FE. Rhytidectomy and the nasolabial fold. Plast Reconstr Surg 90:601, 1992.
20. Hamra ST. Composite rhytidectomy. Plast Reconstr Surg 90:1, 1992.
21. Hamra ST. The deep-plane rhytidectomy. Plast Reconstr Surg 86:53, 1990.
22. Hamra ST. The zygorbicular dissection in composite rhytidectomy: An ideal midface plane. Plast Reconstr Surg 102:1646, 1998.
23. Hamra ST. Prevention and correction of the "face-lifted" appearance. Fac Plast Surg 16:215, 2000.
24. Hamra ST. Frequent face lift sequelae: Hollow eyes and the lateral sweep: Cause and repair. Plast Reconstr Surg 102:1658, 1998.
25. Hamra ST. Arcus marginalis release and orbital fat preservation in midface rejuvenation. Plast Reconstr Surg 96:354, 1995.
26. Hamra ST. Repositioning the orbicularis muscle in the composite rhytidectomy. Plast Reconstr Surg 90:14, 1992.
27. Hamra ST. A study of the long-term effect of malar fat repositioning in face lift surgery: Short-term success but long-term failure. Plast Reconstr Surg 110:940, 2002.
28. Baker DC. Minimal incision rhytidectomy (short scar face lift) with lateral SMASectomy: Evolution and application. Aesthetic Surg J 21:14, 2001.

29. Tonnard PL, Verpaele AM. The MACS-Lift Short-Scar Rhytidectomy. St Louis: Quality Medical Publishing, 2004.
30. Pitman GH. Foundation face lift. In Nahai F, ed. The Art of Aesthetic Surgery: Principles & Techniques, vol II. St Louis: Quality Medical Publishing, 2005, p 1195.
31. Byrd HS, Andochick SE. The deep temporal lift: A multiplanar, lateral brow, temporal, and upper face lift. Plast Reconstr Surg 97:928, 1996.
32. Hunt JA, Byrd HS. The deep temporal lift: A multiplanar lateral brow, temporal, and upper face lift. Plast Reconstr Surg 110:1793, 2002.
33. Barton FE. The SMAS and the nasolabial fold. Plast Reconstr Surg 89:1054, 1992.
34. Owsley JQ. Lifting the malar fat pad for correction of prominent nasolabial folds. Plast Reconstr Surg 91:463, 1993.
35. Pessa JE, Brown F. Independent effect of various facial mimetic muscles on the nasolabial fold. Aesthetic Plast Surg 16:167, 1992.
36. Yousif NJ, Gosain A, Matloub HS, et al. The nasolabial fold: An anatomic and histologic reappraisal. Plast Reconstr Surg 93:60, 1994.
37. Hester TR Jr, Codner MA, McCord CD, et al. Evolution of technique of the direct transblepharoplasty approach for the correction of lower lid and midfacial aging: Maximizing results and minimizing complications in a 5-year experience. Plast Reconstr Surg 105:393, 2000.
38. Gunter JP, Hackney FL. A simplified transblepharoplasty subperiosteal cheek lift. Plast Reconstr Surg 103:2029, 1999.
39. Seify H, Jones G, Bostwick J, et al. Endoscopic-assisted face lift. Review of 200 cases. Ann Plast Surg 52:234, 2004.
40. Pessa JE, Garza JR. The malar septum: The anatomic basis of malar mounds and malar edema. Aesthetic Surg J 17:11, 1997.

81. Neck Lift

Ricardo A. Meade

ANATOMY[1] (Figs. 81-1 through 81-3)

SKIN

- Each patient's neck should be evaluated for **cervical rhytids** and **skin excess**.
- There is a varying amount of fat in the subcutaneous layer between the skin and the platysma muscle.
- Additional fatty tissue may be found in the interplatysmal submental region.
- Although a fatty layer maintains the soft appearance of the neck, it may be molded to help address contours.
- The **anterior jugular veins** course within the fatty layer and should be respected when working in the deep interplatysmal area. There are other veins of significant caliber that can present difficulties if dissection is made in the wrong plane (Fig. 81-3).

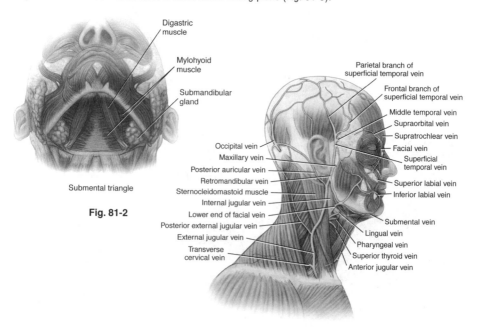

Fig. 81-1

Fig. 81-2

Fig. 81-3

MUSCLE

- The **platysma** is a broad, thin muscle that spans the neck and is a key instrument for controlling neck contour.
  - **Origin:** Pectoralis and deltoid muscle fascia
  - **Insertion**
    - ▸ **Anterior fibers:** Symphysis of the mandible and slightly laterally
    - ▸ **Posterior fibers:** Cross the mandible and insert into the superficial musculoaponeurotic system (SMAS)
  - **Blood supply**
    - ▸ Major: Branch of the submental artery
    - ▸ Minor: Branch of the suprasternal artery
  - **Innervation:** Cervical branch of the facial nerve
  - **Action:** Drawing on the lower lip and angle of the mouth causing oblique wrinkling of the skin of the neck[2]
- The **superficial cervical fascia** is a thin, aponeurotic lamina that immediately covers the platysma on its surface.
- The **deep cervical fascia** lies under the platysma and constitutes a complete investment for the neck.
  - In the midline this fascia is attached to the symphysis and body of the hyoid bone.
  - It divides laterally to enclose the sternocleidomastoid, and the investing portion is attached to the ligamentum nuchae and to C7 (Fig. 81-4).
  - **Three classic decussation and interdigitation patterns**[5] (Fig. 81-5)
    - ▸ **Type I** (75%): Decussates 1-2 cm below the mandibular symphysis
    - ▸ **Type II** (15%): Decussates to the thyroid cartilage
    - ▸ **Type III** (10%): No interdigitation

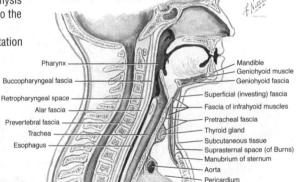

Pharynx
Buccopharyngeal fascia
Retropharyngeal space
Alar fascia
Prevertebral fascia
Trachea
Esophagus

Mandible
Geniohyoid muscle
Geniohyoid fascia
Superficial (investing) fascia
Fascia of infrahyoid muscles
Pretracheal fascia
Thyroid gland
Subcutaneous tissue
Suprasternal space (of Burns)
Manubrium of sternum
Aorta
Pericardium

Fig. 81-4 Sagittal section. (From Netter FH. Atlas of Human Anatomy. Summit, NJ: CIBA-GEIGY, 1989.)

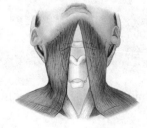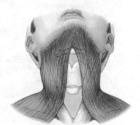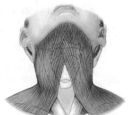

Fig. 81-5

NERVES

- **Inframaxillary** or **cervical nerve branches**
  - Run beneath the platysma across the side of the neck over the suprahyoid region
- **Marginal mandibular nerve**
  - Located at the tail of the parotid in a subplatysmal plane.
  - Posterior to the facial artery, it runs above the inferior border of the mandible (81%) or up to 1 cm below it (19%).[3]
  - Anterior to the facial artery, all of the branches are above the inferior border of the mandible.
  - Innervates the **depressor anguli oris,** the **depressor labii inferioris,** the **mentalis,** part of the **orbicularis oris,** and the **risorius**[3,4]

SUBMANDIBULAR GLANDS

- Located in the **submental triangle** with the facial artery imbedded in a groove along their posterior and upper border
- Crossed superficially by the **marginal mandibular branch** of the facial nerve
- Covered by skin, platysma, deep cervical fascia, and the body of the lower jaw
- **Intracapsular resection of the superficial lobe** sometimes recommended because it is well away from the facial vessels, facial nerve, and lingual nerve *(dissecting beyond this increases risk of injury to these structures)*

DIGASTRIC MUSCLES

- Each muscle consists of **two muscles** joined by a tendon forming the **submental triangle.**
  - The **posterior muscle,** the longer of the two, courses from the mastoid process on the temporal bone down, forward, and medial.
    - ▶ **Innervation:** CN7
  - The **anterior muscle** courses near the symphysis, down and posteriorly.
    - ▶ **Innervation:** CN5
  - Both bellies terminate in the **central tendon.**[5]

RETAINING LIGAMENTS (Fig. 81-6)

- **Retaining ligaments** help support facial soft tissues in their normal location. As these attenuate, the stigmata of aging appear.
- The **zygomatic** and **mandibular** ligaments are examples of true osteocutaneous ligaments. (They go from bone to overlying skin.)
- The mandibular ligaments are found in the parasymphyseal region of the mandible just lateral to the chin pad.

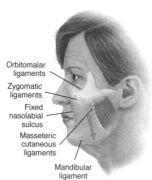
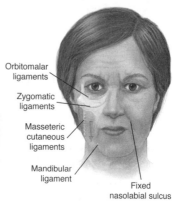

Orbitomalar ligaments

Zygomatic ligaments

Fixed nasolabial sulcus

Masseteric cutaneous ligaments

Mandibular ligament

Orbitomalar ligaments

Zygomatic ligaments

Masseteric cutaneous ligaments

Mandibular ligament

Fixed nasolabial sulcus

Fig. 81-6

PREOPERATIVE ASSESSMENT

SKIN

- Skin quality, with rhytids **at rest** and **during animation,** must be evaluated in detail.
- Skin excess may suggest elasticity of the skin, or lack thereof.
- The quality of the skin elasticity is inversely related to the length of the incision required.
  - Normal skin elasticity is essential for all short-scar procedures.
  - Skin damage and actinic changes alone require a full-length retroauricular incision because of the increased need to redrape.
- Evaluation of skin excess can help determine which direction to redrape the skin flap. Hairline distortion is unacceptable after rhytidectomy.
  - The direction of pull is slightly cephalad and mostly lateral. This vector is parallel to the cervical creases.
- **Apparent** skin excess redrapes after neck contouring. **Real** skin excess usually extends below the thyroid cartilage and posteriorly beyond the sternocleidomastoid (SCM).

FAT

- Evaluate for subcutaneous and preplatysmal fat.
- Differentiate this from subplatysmal fatty excess by pinching the submental area at rest and then after contraction of the platysma muscles.

PLATYSMA[6] (Fig. 81-7)

- Look for **static or dynamic banding** of the platysma.
- Evaluate imperfections in the neck and jaw shadows.
- Assess the neck and face interface and see how facial soft tissue ptosis affects the jawline.

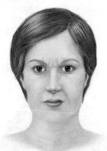 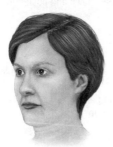 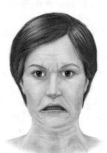 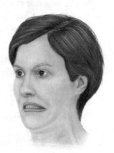

Evaluation of excess skin of the neck and platysma bands with the patient at rest

Evaluation of platysma bands on animation

Fig. 81-7

DIGASTRIC MUSCLES[7]

- These bulge below the inferior border of the mandible.

TIP: Often persistent bulging following fat removal from the neck is caused by prominence of the digastric muscles.

SUBMANDIBULAR GLAND
- Look for a bulge below the mandibular rim within the submandibular triangle.

TIP: It can be helpful to accentuate this deformity by having the patient flex his or her neck.

MANDIBULOCUTANEOUS LIGAMENT
- Tethering of the relaxing facial tissues at this ligament produces the appearance of **jowls.**
- Feel the volume of jowling tissue with the patient in a supine position to evaluate the need for liposuction of the fat pad or simple tightening of the SMAS-platysma laterally.

CHIN
- Assess the projection of the chin relative to all facial proportions.

TIP: An alloplastic chin implant or osseous genioplasty may complement neck contours.

VISUAL CRITERIA OF A YOUTHFUL NECK[8]

- Distinct inferior mandibular border
- Visible subhyoid depression
- Visible thyroid cartilage bulge
- Visible anterior border of the SCM muscle
- Cervicomental angle of 105-120 degrees

OPTIONS FOR NECK REJUVENATION

PROCEDURES
- **Options to address superficial, intermediate, and deep tissues**
  - **Superficial tissues:** Skin and fat
  - **Intermediate tissues:** Muscle
  - **Deep tissues:** Includes the anterior belly of the digastric muscles, the submandibular gland, and the suprahyoid fascia
- **Surgical approaches**
  - Suction lipectomy only
  - Submental cervicoplasty
  - Endoscopic cervicoplasty
  - Short-scar face lift without submental incision (lateral pull)
  - Short-scar face lift with submental incision (direct view)
  - Full-scar face lift without submental incision (lateral pull)
  - Full-scar face lift with submental incision (direct view)

LIPOSUCTION ALONE
- **Indications**
  - Young patients
  - Good dermal quality
  - Localized fat
- **Technical tips**
  - Incision in the submental neck area or behind earlobes
  - 2-3 mm single-hole cannula recommended for suction-assisted liposuction (SAL)
  - 50% energy ultrasound-assisted lipectomy (UAL) with a 2 mm solid probe for no longer than 3 minutes recommended, if using UAL
  - No drains required if the sole procedure

TIP: Small quantities of aspirate can create big differences.

NOTE: After suctioning the neck, platysmal banding or other underlying irregularities may become evident.

CAUTION: Avoid oversuctioning. Leave 5 mm of fat on the skin to give it a soft contour and prevent scarring and tethering to the underlying platysma.

TIP: Avoid repeat passes within tunnels—crisscross strokes.

SUBMENTAL NECK LIFT[9]
- **Indications**
  - Direct viewing of the internal neck anatomy is indicated by findings from neck examination (e.g., platysmal banding).
  - Undermining is required to recontour the neck.
- **Technical tips**
  - Extend the patient's neck.
  - Make incision just posterior to the submental crease. (Do not deepen the existing crease.)
  - Release the crease anteriorly from underlying tissues.
  - **Interplatysmal fat excision** may be performed in addition to subcutaneous defatting. If a lymph node is seen in this fatty layer, include it in the resection.
  - The mandibular ligaments can be released as the dissection is continued forward and laterally.
  - Tangential (partial) digastric resection can be performed through this incision.[7] Use a hemostat to partially divide it halfway through the thickness of the muscle.
  - Piecemeal intracapsular submandibular gland resection can be considered with this approach.

CAUTION: Be sure to discuss complications with the patient (i.e., increased risk of bleeding, nerve injury, dry mouth, or salivary fistula).

  ► If the submandibular gland is removed partially, a drain is usually placed deep to the platysma after layered closure.

ENDOSCOPIC NECK LIFT[10]
- This procedure has generally been replaced by the submental neck lift procedure.
- Fiberoptic light helps with viewing and hemostasis.

Short-Scar Face and Neck Lift[11]

- **Indications**
  - No excess neck skin
  - Presence of jowling
  - Aged neck-face interface
- **Technical tips**
  - Technique involves prehairline incision below the sideburn and a preauricular retrotragal incision ending at the earlobe.
  - Neck recontouring through a submental approach or liposuction may be performed at the same time.
  - Skin flap is elevated extending to the posterior border of the SCM muscle.
  - A SMAS-platysma flap is then dissected and pulled up in the face and posteriorly in the neck.

Full-Scar Face and Neck Lift

- **Indications**
  - Patients with aging changes in the face and neck with inelastic and excess lower and posterior neck skin
- **Technical tips**
  - If the patient has unusually lax skin with significant excess in the lower neck, the retroauricular incision can be continued along the hairline to avoid notching the occipital hairline and to remove more excess skin.
  - First align the hairline, then remove the excess skin.
  - Close the retroauricular sulcus with three-point suture technique, incorporating the deep fascia to prevent migration of the scar.

OPERATIVE TECHNIQUES

Skin Flap Procedures

- In general, a **vertical vector** of pull is required for a youthful, harmonious lift of the neck.
- A **posterior and diagonal vector** is required when using a **retroauricular approach.**
- Managing neck skin differs from managing facial skin. Avoid removal of skin before considering redraping and redistributing it.
  - If excision is necessary, one must consider a retroauricular incision or a hairline incision according to the amount to be removed.
- Cronin and Biggs[12] excised excess skin in the severe "turkey gobbler" neck deformity using a **T-Z incision,** restoring a youthful contour to the cervical angle
  - The scarring that remains is only occasionally acceptable in the male neck that presents with a generous redundancy of skin.
  - This has become a particularly popular option for patients who have experienced massive weight loss.

Platysmal Procedures

- The platysma may be imbricated, plicated, incised, lengthened, or suspended.[7,13]
  - Once the platysmal diastasis is plicated, the surrounding skin is recruited toward the midline. Any areas that are tethered must be released from their attachments to the platysmal fascia.

- **Platysmal flap cervical rhytidoplasty**[14]
  - Sectional myotomy of the medial edge of the platysma allows lateral rotation and advancement of the flap edges.
  - Suture the flaps to the mastoid fascia laterally to avoid recurrence of vertical banding.
  - Consider the thyroid cartilage's capability for masculinization of the neck when performing a myotomy. Some describe controlling the effect by performing the platysmal transection above or below the cartilage to camouflage or accentuate it.
- **Suspension sutures** (Fig. 81-8)
  - Suspension sutures running along the inferior border of the mandible over the superficial fascia on the platysma can help define the jawline.
  - Sutures are interlocked at the midline and tacked to the mastoid fascia as described by Guerrero-Santos[14] and later popularized by Giampapa.[15]
- **Platysma muscle sling**[7] (Fig. 81-9)
  - A sling is made by dividing the platysma horizontally across the entire width.
  - A wide gap is created that is potentially visible, which made the procedure lose its popularity.
  - Muscle tissue bunches on the cephalad portion of the platysma. This phenomenon is known as the *window-shading* effect.

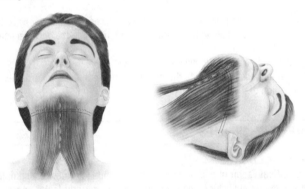

Fig. 81-8 Suspension sutures, interlocked at midline, run along the inferior mandibular border.

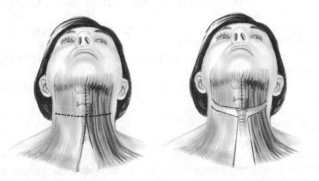

Fig. 81-9 Full transection of platysma, which creates a wide gap and "window-shading" effect.

- **Corset platysmaplasty**[16] (Fig. 81-10)
  - The neck skin is shifted posteriorly, but the platysma pull is forward toward the anterior midline.
  - The anterior pull of the platysma is a key element that is called *corset platysmaplasty*.
  - No muscle is resected. Occasionally a very low, 3 cm transection from the medial edge allows comfortable rotation of the flaps to the midline for multilayered approximation.
  - The procedure is performed through a 4 cm submental incision.
  - A multilayered seam approximates the full height of the midline platysma muscle edges, creating a "waistline" to the neck from an anterior platysmal shift.
  - Plication continues to 2 fingerbreadths above the suprasternal notch.
  - Crisscrossing and backtracking is advocated to keep the seam tight.

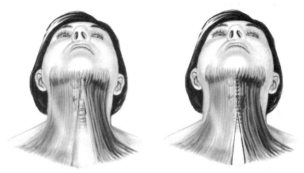

Fig. 81-10   Coaptation of decussated platysmal fibers in the midline creates a "corset-type" effect.

TIP: This technique is highly effective in recontouring the submental area.

- If combined with lateral plication, midline plication of the platysma can define the jawline and neck-jaw angle nicely. This is done with an occasional second row of running vertical oblique sutures.
- Additional submandibular suturing may be performed to treat bulging in this area by creating a strong, flat pleat.

POSTOPERATIVE CARE[1]

- Provide oral analgesics, sleeping pills, antiemetics, and specific instructions for their use.
- Instruct patients to avoid pillows that flex the neck to keep the cervicomental angle open.
- Avoid folding the neck skin flaps, because this contributes to edema by obstructing the neck lymphatics.
- Although drains are a personal preference, they help eliminate serum and small amounts of blood oozing, potentially reducing postoperative edema.
- Remove drains on the first postoperative day after examining the patient.
- Without applying pressure, place cotton dressings or foam tape and an elastic garment on the wound overnight to absorb wept fluids.

- On the first postoperative day, remove the operative dressing and replace it with a neck strap for no longer than 4 weeks.
- Some surgeons do not place dressings on the neck to avoid pressure necrosis.
- Instruct the patient to maintain an open neck angle similar to how it would be if they had their elbows on their knees while sitting.
- Antibiotics are used routinely for 3-5 postoperative days.
- Wounds are cleaned with half-strength hydrogen peroxide and coated with a topical antibiotic ointment.
- Remove all sutures by day 7. (Some sutures are removed as early as postoperative day 4.)
- Alcohol is prohibited until patients stop taking pain medications.
- Recommend that patients avoid strenuous activities for 6 weeks.
- The teaching of "if it hurts, don't do it" has been adopted by many surgeons.

COMPLICATIONS[17]

- Overall hematoma rate is about 4% in women and 8% in men.
- A higher incidence of hematoma has been associated with preoperative systolic blood pressure greater than 150 mm Hg.
- The buccal branch of the facial nerve is injured most often during rhytidectomy. In neck-lift procedures, the marginal mandibular ramus may incur damage with upward pulling on the superior platysmal flap.
- Idiopathic trauma to the great auricular nerve may cause temporary loss of sensation of a portion of the ear, scalp, or face.
- Skin slough often preceded by hematoma or infection is most common in the retroauricular area.
- Overresecting the fat superficially does not correct a problem that is in the deeper layers.
- Underestimating submental fat removal is often caused by fatty deposits deep to the platysma.

KEY POINTS

- ✔ When evaluating a neck for cervicoplasty, evaluate the midface for an ideal combined result.
- ✔ Rarely does a patient need a cervicoplasty only. Diligently examine facial proportions, including chin projection.
- ✔ If the skin is sun damaged and inelastic, a full periauricular incision is required.
- ✔ Do not overresect fat; leave 3-5 mm of a subcutaneous cushion on the flap.
- ✔ Look and gently pinch the neck to consider the need for fat removal.
- ✔ Evaluate muscles and banding.
- ✔ With an anterior platysmaplasty the neck is better consolidated, but this does not suffice to treat banding. A myotomy must be performed on the platysma to solve the problem.
- ✔ The height of the myotomy is usually at the level of the cricoid cartilage.
- ✔ The best result is in harmony between all facial proportions.

REFERENCES

1. Nahai F, ed. The Art of Aesthetic Surgery: Principles and Techniques. St Louis, Quality Medical Publishing, 2005.
2. Gray H. Gray's Anatomy: Anatomy, Descriptive, and Surgical 1901 Edition. Philadelphia: Running Press, 1974.
3. Dingman RO, Grabb WC. Surgical anatomy of the mandibular ramus of the facial nerve based on the dissection of 100 facial halves. Plast Reconstr Surg 29:266, 1962.
4. Netter FH. Atlas of Human Anatomy. Summit, NJ: CIBA-GEIGY, 1989.
5. Cardoso de Castro C. The anatomy of the platysma muscle. Plast Reconstr Surg 66:680, 1980.
6. Connell BF. Contouring the neck in rhytidectomy by lipectomy and a muscle sling. Plast Reconstr Surg 61:376, 1978.
7. Connell BF, Shamoun JM. The significance of digastric muscle contouring for rejuvenation of the submental area of the face. Plast Reconstr Surg 99:1586, 1997.
8. Ellenbogen R, Karlin JV. Visual criteria for success in restoring the youthful neck. Plast Reconstr Surg 66:826, 1980.
9. Knize DM. Limited incision submental lipectomy and platysmaplasty. Plast Reconstr Surg 101:473, 1998.
10. Eaves FE, Nahai F, Bostwick J III. The endoscopic neck lift. Op Tech Plast Reconstr Surg 2:145, 1995.
11. Baker DC. Lateral SMASectomy. Plast Reconstr Surg 100:509, 1997.
12. Cronin TD, Biggs TM. The T-Z-plasty for the male "turkey gobbler" neck. Plast Reconstr Surg 47:534, 1971.
13. Fuente del Campo A. Midline platysma muscular overlap for neck restoration. Plast Reconstr Surg 102:1710, 1998.
14. Guerrero-Santos J. Neck lift: Simplified surgical techniques, refinements, and clinical classification. Clin Plast Surg 10:379, 1983.
15. Giampapa VC, Di Bernardo BE. Neck recontouring with suture suspension and liposuction: An alternative for the early rhytidectomy candidate. Aesthetic Plast Surg 19:217, 1995.
16. Feldman JJ. Corset platysmaplasty. Plast Reconstr Surg 85:333, 1990.
17. Gonyon DL, Barton FE. The aging face: Rhytidectomy and adjunctive procedures. Sel Read Plast Surg 10(11), 2005.

82. Rhinoplasty

Sacha I. Obaid

ANATOMY

SKIN
- Skin is thinner and relatively more mobile in the upper two thirds of the nose.
- Skin is more adherent and thicker in the lower third of the nose.

MUSCLES
- Only two muscles are clinically significant:
  - Levator labii superioris alaeque nasi
  - Depressor septi nasi
- The **levator labii superioris alaeque nasi** functions to keep the external nasal valve open.

> TIP: In cases of facial paralysis, a nonfunctional levator labii superioris alaeque nasi may be the cause of functional nasal obstruction.

- The **depressor septi nasi** can be hyperactive in certain patients and cause shortening of the upper lip and decreased tip projection with smiling.[1]

> TIP: In cases where the depressor septi is hyperactive, dividing it at the time of rhinoplasty will improve projection of the nasal tip and relative lengthening of the upper lip.

BLOOD SUPPLY (Fig. 82-1)
- Arterial supply to nose is located superficial to the nasal musculature in the subcutaneous plane
- **Ophthalmic artery**
  - Supplies the proximal portion of the nose
  - Branches: Anterior ethmoidal artery, dorsal nasal artery, and external nasal artery
- **Facial artery**
  - Branches: Superior labial artery and angular artery, which combine to supply the nasal tip area
  - Columellar branch, which supplies columella, given off by superior labial artery
- **Angular artery**
  - Gives off lateral nasal branch, which arises 2-3 mm above the alar groove
    - Primary blood supply to the nasal tip after transcolumellar incision in open rhinoplasty

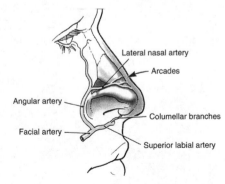

Fig. 82-1

- Cadaveric study by Rohrich et al[2,3]
  - ► Lateral nasal branch supplies the subdermal plexus at the nasal tip area either unilaterally or bilaterally in 100% of patients.
  - ► The superior labial artery gives off a columellar branch, which supplies the columella.

TIP: To avoid jeopardizing the blood supply to the nasal tip, the surgeon must be aware of the location of the lateral nasal branch. Excessively defatting the nasal tip area jeopardizes the subdermal plexus supplying the nasal tip.

NASAL VAULTS (Fig. 82-2)

- **Three vaults of nose:** Bony vault, upper cartilaginous vault, and lower cartilaginous vault
- **Bony vault**
  - Consists of paired nasal bones and the ascending frontal process of the maxilla
  - Makes up the proximal one third to one half of the nose
- **Upper cartilaginous vault:** Outlined by the paired upper lateral cartilages
  - Upper lateral cartilages
    - ► Underlie the nasal bones for approximately 6-8 mm at their junction.
      - ◆ This is known as the *keystone area*, and it represents the widest portion of the nasal dorsum.
    - ► The junction of the upper lateral cartilages and the lower lateral cartilages occurs at the *scroll area*.
    - ► Upper lateral cartilages join the septum to form a "T."
      - ◆ This relationship is responsible for production of the dorsal aesthetic lines.

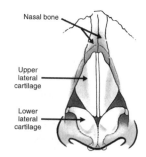

Fig. 82-2

TIP: When reducing a dorsal hump more than 1-2 mm, the upper lateral cartilages must be separated from the septum and preserved to prevent disruption of the critical relationship between the upper lateral cartilages and the septum.[4]

- **Lower cartilaginous vault:** Made of paired lower lateral cartilages
  - Lower lateral cartilages: Each has medial, middle, and lateral crus (Fig. 82-3)

NASAL TIP

- Nasal tip is given support and projection by the following.[5]
  - Lower lateral cartilages and their abutment with the piriform aperture
  - Domal suspensory ligament
  - Fibrous intercartilaginous connections between the upper and lower lateral cartilages
  - Medial crural ligaments
  - Anterior septal angle

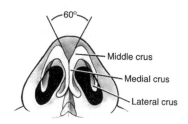

Fig. 82-3

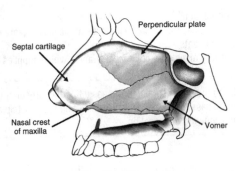

Fig. 82-4

SEPTUM
- Composed of septal cartilage, perpendicular plate of the ethmoid, and vomer (Fig. 82-4)

> TIP: The perpendicular plate of the ethmoid is in continuity with the cribriform plate. As a result, whenever it must be fractured (e.g., for cartilage harvest or correction of nasal deviation), it must be fractured sideways to prevent disruption of the cribiform plate and resultant cerebrospinal fluid rhinorrhea.

INTERNAL NASAL VALVE
- Internal nasal valve provides half of total airway resistance.[6]
- Internal valve is formed by junction of caudal upper lateral cartilages and nasal septum.
- Normal angle between upper lateral cartilages and nasal septum is **10-15 degrees.** If angle is less than this, nasal airway obstruction results.[7]

> TIP: To prevent internal nasal valve obstruction in primary rhinoplasty or to correct it in secondary rhinoplasty, spreader grafts can be placed to restore this critical angle between the upper lateral cartilages and the septum.

EXTERNAL NASAL VALVE
- External nasal valve is formed by the caudal edge of the lateral crus of the lower lateral cartilages, soft tissue of the alae, membranous septum, and sill of the nostril.
- It can be the site of nasal airway obstruction in secondary rhinoplasty with pinched alae deformity.

TURBINATES
- The three turbinates (superior, middle, and inferior) are extensions of the lateral wall of the nasal cavity.
- The anterior aspects of the middle and inferior turbinates project into the airway.
- The inferior turbinate can provide up to two thirds of the total airway resistance in the region of the internal nasal valve.[8]

ANALYSIS AND PLANNING[9]

- The key to a successful rhinoplasty lies in accurate preoperative assessment of the nose and identification of the deformities to be corrected.
- Preoperative assessment requires anteroposterior, lateral, and basilar nasal views.
- Once the surgeon identifies the defect to be corrected, an accurate and comprehensive surgical plan can be developed.

ANTEROPOSTERIOR VIEW
- Define the skin type and thickness.

> TIP: Thicker skin requires more dramatic alterations to the osteocartilaginous framework for them to be noticeable.

- Assess proportions and symmetry of upper, middle, and lower thirds of the face.
- Evaluate for nasal deviation by drawing a line from the midglabellar area to the menton.
  - Line should bisect nasal ridge, upper lip, Cupid's bow, and central two incisors if there is no deviation.
- Evaluate the width of the bony base.
  - This should be 75%-80% of the width of the normal alar base.
- Evaluate the presence, symmetry, and any deviation in the dorsal aesthetic lines.
  - The dorsal aesthetic lines are two slightly curved, divergent lines extending from the medial superciliary ridges to the tip-defining points.
- Examine the width of the alar base, which should be the same as the intercanthal distance.
  - If the alar base is wider than the intercanthal distance, the degree of alar flare should be determined.
    - ▸ Compare the maximum alar width with the width of the ala at the alar base.
    - ▸ If the difference between these two widths is greater than 2 mm, the problem is excessive alar flaring.
    - ▸ If the difference is less than 2 mm, the problem is an excessively wide alar base.
- The alar rims should be symmetrical and should have a slight outward flare in the inferior and lateral direction. The outline of the alar rims and columella should resemble a gull in gentle flight.
- The tip should have four defining points: One on each side, a supratip break (more important in women), and the columellar-lobular angle.
- Symmetry of the tip-defining points is assessed by drawing lines connecting the points with the supratip break and the columellar lobular angle. These lines should form two equilateral triangles.

BASILAR VIEW
- The alar rims and tip should form an equilateral triangle with a ratio of one third to two thirds lobule to columella.
- The nostril should have a slight teardrop shape with the apex slightly medial to the base.

LATERAL VIEW
- The nasofrontal angle should lie between the upper lash line and the supratarsal fold.
- In women, the aesthetic nasal dorsum should lie 2 mm behind and parallel to a line from the nasofrontal angle to the nasal tip. In men, it should be slightly higher.

- Tip projection should be assessed by drawing a line from the alar-cheek junction to the nasal tip. The aesthetic tip has 50%-60% of the length of this line anterior to the upper lip.
- Women should have a slight supratip break, but men should not.
- Tip rotation is assessed.
  - Draw a line from the anterior and posterior edges of the nostril.
  - A plumb line is then drawn that is perpendicular to the natural horizontal facial plane.
  - The angle that is formed between these two lines is the **nasolabial angle.**
  - In **women** it should be **95-100 degrees,** and in **men** it should be **90-95 degrees** (Fig. 82-5).
- The **columellar-labial angle** is at the junction of the columella with the upper lip. Fullness in this region is the result of a prominent caudal septum.
- The **columellar-lobular angle** is formed by the junction of the columella with the infratip lobule. It should be **30-45 degrees** (Fig. 82-6).

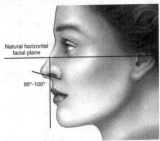
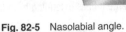
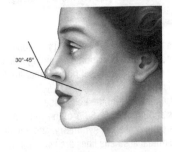

Fig. 82-5   Nasolabial angle.   **Fig. 82-6**   Columellar lobular angle.

ENDONASAL (CLOSED) VERSUS OPEN (EXTERNAL) APPROACH

ENDONASAL APPROACH
Endonasal rhinoplasty involves no external incisions. The guiding principle is to limit dissection to areas of interest.
- **Advantages** (as listed by Sheen[10,11])
  - No external scar
  - Dissection limited to areas of interest
  - Precise pockets can be created for insertion of graft material without fixation
  - Allows for percutaneous fixation when large pockets are made
  - Minimizes postsurgical edema
  - Decreases operative time
  - Faster recovery
  - Creates an intact tip graft pocket
  - Allows for composite grafting to the alar rim
- **Disadvantages**
  - Need for experience and great reliance on preoperative diagnosis
  - Does not allow simultaneous viewing of surgical fields by surgeons and students
  - Does not allow for direct viewing of nasal anatomy
  - Difficult dissection of alar cartilages, especially if they are malpositioned

- **Principles[9,12]**
  - Accurate preoperative diagnosis is essential because a different incision must be made for each deformity.
  - Placement of the incisions depends on the deformity that is to be corrected.
  - **Alar cartilage incisions**
    - ▶ Incisions may be *intercartilaginous* (between the upper and lower lateral cartilages), *transcartilaginous* (at the level of the lower lateral cartilages), or *marginal* (caudad to the lower lateral cartilages) (Fig. 82-7).

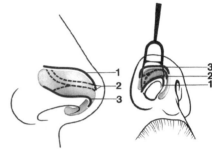

Fig. 82-7 Preferred incisional approaches: *1*, Intercartilaginous; *2*, transcartilaginous; *3*, marginal.

  - ▶ If an intercartilaginous incision is made, the lower lateral cartilages can be delivered through the incision using a retrograde or eversion approach.
  - ▶ If a transcartilaginous incision is made, the lower lateral cartilages are accessed using a cartilage-splitting approach.
  - ▶ If a marginal incision is made, often an intercartilaginous incision must also be made to deliver the lower lateral cartilages into the wound.
  - **Septal incisions**
    - ▶ Septal transfixion incisions can be made in a *complete, partial (limited), hemi-, or high fashion.*
    - ▶ **Complete transfixion incision**
      - ✦ Is usually made as a continuation of the intercartilaginous or transcartilaginous incision.
      - ✦ Separates the caudal end of the septum from the membranous septum and medial crura.
      - ✦ Can sweep posteriorly, then all the way to the nasal spine.
      - ✦ Frees the tip completely, exposes the nasal spine and depressor septi muscles, and exposes the septum to allow elevation of mucoperichondrial flaps.

CAUTION: This incision disrupts the attachments of the medial crural footplate to the caudal septum. This results in significant loss of tip support and potential loss of tip projection.

  - ▶ **Limited partial transfixion incision**
    - ✦ Indicated if less tip access is required with preservation of attachments between medial crural footplates and caudal septum
  - ▶ **Partial transfixion incision**
    - ✦ Begins caudal to anterior septal angle and continues to just short of the medial crural attachment to the caudal septum
  - ▶ **Hemitransfixion incision**
    - ✦ Made unilaterally at the junction of the caudal septum and columella
    - ✦ Typically used for procedures in which the caudal septum is deviated or needs resection for tip rotation or columellar adjustment
  - ▶ **High septal transfixion incision** (Fig. 82-8)
    - ✦ Does not violate the junction of the caudal septum and the medial crura
    - ✦ Does not violate the junction of the caudal septum and the membranous septum

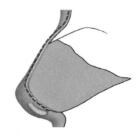

Fig. 82-8 Transfixion incision.

REASONS TO AVOID CLOSED RHINOPLASTY

- For patients with a "cocaine nose," an open approach may lead to improved integrity and vascularity of the nasal mucosa.
- A cantilevered graft needs to be affixed to the bony arch.
- Excess skin needs to be excised.
- There is extreme cephalic malposition of the lateral crura that makes dissection of the lower lateral cartilages difficult from an endonasal approach.

OPEN APPROACH

The open approach to rhinoplasty allows for complete exposure and viewing of the anatomic support structures of the nose.

- **Advantages** (as listed by Gunter et al[9])
  - Binocular vision
  - Evaluation of the complete deformity without disruption
  - Precise diagnosis and correction of deformities
  - Use of both hands
  - Increased options with original tissues and cartilage grafts
  - Direct control of bleeding with electrocautery
- **Disadvantages**
  - External nasal incision
  - Prolonged operative time
  - Increased tip edema
  - Columellar incision separation and delayed wound healing
  - Suture stabilization of grafts may be needed
- **Technique**[9]
  - Bilateral marginal incisions are made at the caudalmost edge of the lower lateral cartilages.
  - Marginal incisions are continued medially to the narrowest part of the columella.
  - A stair-step incision is then carried across the columella at this level (Fig. 82-9).
  - The stair-step incision is connected to the marginal incision from the other side.
  - Crosshatches are marked on the columellar incision to ensure accurate repositioning postoperatively.
  - The skin is elevated off the caudal edge of the medial crura.
  - Dissection continues over the lateral crura and cartilaginous-bony dorsum to the root of the nose.
  - Retraction is used to expose the entire cartilaginous framework.

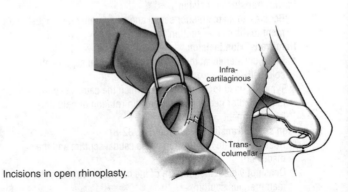

Fig. 82-9 Incisions in open rhinoplasty.

NASAL TIP

PREOPERATIVE ANALYSIS

- During preoperative analysis, the surgeon must evaluate tip projection, definition, symmetry, and rotation.
- Tip projection is evaluated by drawing a line from the alar-cheek junction to the nasal tip; 50%-60% of this line should lie anterior to the upper lip.
- Tip definition is assessed by looking for the four tip-defining points.
- Symmetry of the tip is assessed by drawing lines connecting the four tip-defining points. These should form two equilateral triangles.
- Tip rotation is assessed by evaluating the nasolabial angle, which should be 90-95 degrees in men and 95-100 degrees in women.

TIP PROJECTION

- **Tip projection depends on the support structures**[5] (Fig. 82-10)
  - Length and strength of the lower lateral cartilages
  - Suspensory ligaments that span the crura over the anterior septal angle of the upper and lower lateral cartilages
  - Fibrous connections between the upper and lower lateral cartilages
  - Abutment of the lower lateral cartilages with the piriform aperture
  - Anterior septal angle

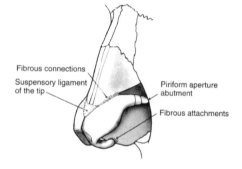

Fibrous connections

Suspensory ligament of the tip

Piriform aperture abutment

Fibrous attachments

- **Increasing tip projection**
  - **Graduated approach**
    - ▸ Begin with placement of columellar strut grafts and suture techniques (both of which are nonpalpable).
    - ▸ Progress if needed to cartilage grafting techniques (which run the risk of palpability in thinner-skinned patients).[13]

Fig. 82-10 Support structures of the nasal tip.

  - **Columellar strut grafts**[9,14]
    - ▸ Floating columellar strut grafts are made from cartilage (Fig. 82-11).
      - ✦ Placed 2-3 mm anterior to the nasal spine
      - ✦ Secured in a pocket between the medial crura
      - ✦ Used to maintain tip projection after the open rhinoplasty technique or to increase tip projection by 1-2 mm
    - ▸ If 3 mm or more of projection is required, a fixed columellar strut graft is fashioned from rib cartilage.
      - ✦ It is placed on top of the nasal spine.
      - ✦ Of note, this graft can be moved from side to side by the patient, which may be distressing.
  - **Suture techniques:** Can be used to increase tip projection an additional 1-2 mm, and can help refine the tip and provide definition[13]

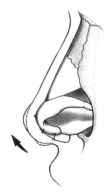

Fig. 82-11 Floating columellar strut graft with resultant increase in tip projection.

- **Medial crural sutures** (Fig. 82-12)
  - Horizontal mattress sutures placed between the medial crura
  - Unify the lower lateral cartilages and can stabilize the columellar strut either in front of or between the medial crura
- **Interdomal sutures** (Fig. 82-13)
  - Placed between the domes of the two lower lateral cartilages
  - Create increased infratip columellar projection and refinement of the nasal tip
- **Transdomal sutures** (Fig. 82-14)
  - Placed between the medial and lateral portions of a single lower lateral cartilage
  - Allow for correction of domal asymmetry in addition to providing tip projection

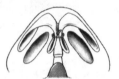 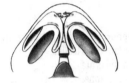 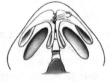

Fig. 82-12 Medial crural sutures.   **Fig. 82-13** Interdomal sutures.   **Fig. 82-14** Transdomal sutures.

- **Medial crural septal sutures** (Fig. 82-15)
  - Placed between the medial crura and the septum
  - Cause rotation of the nasal tip, which increases tip projection and corrects rotation from a drooping nasal tip or aging nose
- **Tip grafts:** Used if columellar strut grafts and suture techniques are insufficient to create desired tip projection

CAUTION: Be careful when placing tip grafts in thin-skinned patients, because they may become visible through the skin.

- **Infralobular graft** (Sheen[15]) (Fig. 82-16)
  - Enhances the infratip lobular contour and increases tip projection.
  - A hexagonal or diamond shape may be used.
  - Care must be taken to bevel or morselize the sharp edges.
- **Onlay graft** (Peck[16]) (Fig. 82-17)
  - Primary function is to increase tip projection.
  - An additional effect is to create some tip refinement.
  - If additional tip projection is required, the graft can be double or even triple layered.
- **Combined columellar, infratip lobular, and onlay tip graft** (Gunter[14]) (Fig. 82-18)
  - This graft can enhance tip projection, refine the tip, and alter tip rotation.
- **Cap graft** (cephalic trim graft)[13]
  - This graft is fashioned from extra cartilage derived from the cephalic trim.
  - Because of its thin nature, the cap graft is not likely to become visible even in thin-skinned patients.

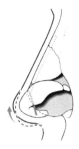

Fig. 82-15   Medial crural septal sutures.

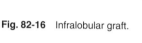

Fig. 82-16   Infralobular graft.

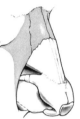

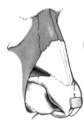

Fig. 82-17   Onlay graft (Peck).

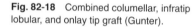

Fig. 82-18   Combined columellar, infratip lobular, and onlay tip graft (Gunter).

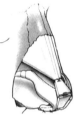

- **Decreasing tip projection**[9,17,18]
  - **Graduated approach**
    - ▸ Begin with releasing the ligamentous and fibroelastic attachments of the lower lateral crura.
    - ▸ Progress to transection of the lateral crus of the lower lateral cartilages.
    - ▸ Finish with transection of the medial crura of the lower lateral cartilages if needed.
  - **Closed approach**
    - ▸ If used, a transfixion incision is needed, taking care to separate the lower lateral cartilages from the cartilaginous septum.
  - **Open rhinoplasty approach**
    - ▸ If used, the attachments of the feet of the medial crura to the caudal septum should be resected submucosally.
    - ▸ This procedure eliminates the support of the nasal tip that is provided by the intercartilaginous ligaments.
  - **If further decrease in tip projection required**
    - ▸ Undermine the vestibular skin and transect the lateral crura.
    - ▸ Then overlap the two transected ends an amount that provides the desired tip projection.
  - **If even further decrease in tip projection required**
    - ▸ Transect the medial crura 2 mm posterior to the junction of the medial crura with the intermediate crura.
    - ▸ Overlap the two transected ends and suture together an amount that will provide the desired change in tip projection.

TIP: In most cases, the tip can be moved backward only about 2 mm before flaring of the alar bases or downward bowing of the columella occurs that needs correction.

■ **Correcting the boxy nasal tip**

A boxy nasal tip is one that appears broad and rectangular in the basilar view. It lacks definition. Three different anatomic variations can lead to a boxy nasal tip.

Type I: There is an increased angle of divergence (>30 degrees) between the two domes. Domal and middle crural cephalic trim should be performed with interdomal sutures placed to narrow the angle of divergence. Transdomal sutures may also be added in thick-skinned patients.

Type II: There is a wide dome arc but a normal angle of divergence. Domal cephalic trim and transdomal sutures are placed with possible addition of intradomal sutures in thick-skinned patients.

Type III: There is an increased angle of divergence between the domes and a wide arc to the domes. Domal and middle crural cephalic trim should be performed. In addition, placement of interdomal and transdomal sutures is necessary.[19]

NASAL DORSUM

PREOPERATIVE ANALYSIS
■ Begin by assessing for deviation.
  • Draw a line from the midglabellar area to the menton.
  • This line should bisect nasal ridge, upper lip, Cupid's bow, and two central incisors.
■ Next, analyze the dorsal aesthetic lines.
  • These should appear as two slightly curved, divergent lines extending from the medial superciliary ridges to the tip-defining points.
■ Finally, the height of the nasal dorsum should be evaluated in the lateral view.
  • In women the aesthetic nasal dorsum should lie 2 mm behind and parallel to a line from the nasofrontal angle to the nasal tip.
  • In men it should be slightly higher.

DORSAL HUMP REDUCTION[4]
■ Dorsal hump reduction should be performed before tip refinement.
■ The dorsal osteocartilaginous framework is exposed with skeletonization of the bony and cartilaginous framework.
■ Care must be taken not to disrupt the periosteum of the nasal bones and not to detach the upper edge of the upper lateral cartilages.
■ The upper lateral cartilages are separated from the septum proper.
■ The septum is serially shaved using a No. 15 blade.
■ The upper lateral cartilages are preserved and are not reduced (Fig. 82-19).
■ The osseous hump is reduced using a sharp downbiting rasp, taking care not to avulse the upper lateral cartilages from the nasal bones.
■ If the bony hump is very large, an 8 mm osteotome or guarded power burr can be used for further reduction.
■ After reduction of the cartilaginous septum and bony dorsal components, the dorsum must be palpated to assess for irregularities.

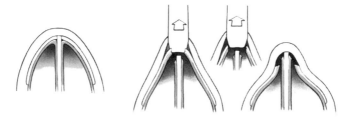

Fig. 82-19 Preservation of the upper lateral cartilages during reduction of the septum.

- After reduction of the cartilaginous and bony septum, conservative upper lateral cartilage resection is performed only in select patients.
  - Patient selection for this is key because overresection of the upper lateral cartilages leads to internal nasal valve collapse and irregularity of the dorsum.
- If necessary, dorsal spreader grafts of cartilage can be placed between the upper lateral cartilages and the cartilaginous septum.
  - Grafts help maintain the internal nasal valve, straighten or buttress the deviated septum, or maintain the dorsal aesthetic lines.
  - Spreader grafts are 5-6 mm in height and 30-32 mm in length.
- Medial and lateral osteotomies of the nasal bones can be performed to correct wide nasal bones, to reposition asymmetrical nasal bones, or to close an open-roof deformity where there is a gap between the nasal bones and the nasal septum.

DORSAL AUGMENTATION

- Dorsal augmentation can be performed using septal cartilage grafts, autologous rib cartilage, or Allo-Derm® (LifeCell Corp, Branchburg, NJ).
- In the case of septal cartilage, partial-thickness incisions can be made through the cartilage to create a dorsal onlay graft in the shape of a V, U, or A (Fig. 82-20).[20]
- An inverted V-shaped graft fits well over the arched contour of the dorsum, but because it is only one layer thick, it provides only minimal dorsal augmentation.
- Greater augmentation can be created with an A-shaped graft that is essentially an inverted V-shaped graft with a crossbar of cartilage underneath.
- Thin-skinned patients may have problems with the visibility of inverted V-shaped or A-shaped cartilage grafts. In these patients an inverted U-shaped graft provides a more natural contour.
- Dorsal augmentation can also be performed with costal cartilage grafts that are stabilized with a 0.028 K-wire drilled into the nasal root.
  - Suture fixation to the nasal septum just above the septal angle and just below the bony cartilaginous junction should also be performed to assist in stabilization.
  - The K-wire is removed at 1 week.[9]

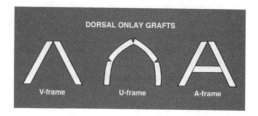

DORSAL ONLAY GRAFTS

V-frame   U-frame   A-frame

Fig. 82-20

OSTEOTOMIES

- The bony vault is pyramidal and composes the upper third of the external nose.
  - It consists of an ascending process of the maxilla and the paired nasal bones.
  - The bony vault also supports the upper nose and the upper lateral cartilages.
- Nasal bones articulate with each other medially, the frontal bone superiorly, the maxilla laterally, and the perpendicular plate of the ethmoid posteriorly.
- Nasal bones average 2.5 cm in length.
- Nasal bones are much thicker and denser above the level of the medial canthus at the radix and get thinner toward the tip.
- Nasal bones are widest at the nasofrontal suture and then become narrowest at the nasofrontal angle before becoming wider again inferior to the radix and then narrow again at their inferior margin.
- The key to successful osteotomies is **control.**

> TIP: The nasal bones are thickest at anatomic suture lines. The nasal bones require greater force
> (with resultant decreased control) to fracture in these areas. As a result, osteotomies
> should be designed to cut through thinner areas such as the intermediate or transition
> zones. This will optimize control and precision.

- Transition zones with thinner bones are found along the ascending process of the maxilla beginning at the piriform aperture and continuing up to the radix just along the nasal side wall.
- The thickness of the bones in this region is 2.5 mm.
- **Relative contraindications to osteotomies include:**
  - Elderly patients with thin bones
  - Heavy eyeglasses
  - Ethnic noses that are low and broad
  - Short nasal bones with a distal border less than 1 cm below the intercanthal line
    - ▶ Osteotomies in these patients may cause upper lateral cartilage collapse.
- Lateral osteotomies are performed to narrow the widened lateral nasal side wall, close an open-roof deformity, and straighten the deviated nasal pyramid.
- **Three types of lateral osteotomies**[21,22] (Fig. 82-21)
  - **Low-high:** Use to mobilize a medium-wide nasal base or small open-roof deformity. The osteotomy begins low (lateral) at the piriform aperture and extends cephalad to the intercanthal line ending high (medial) on the dorsum.
  - **Low-low:** Use to mobilize bony roof to correct an excessively wide nasal base or a large open-roof deformity. The osteotomy begins low (lateral) at the piriform aperture and continues low (lateral) to the dorsal region near the intercanthal line.
  - **Double-level:** Use for excessive lateral wall convexity and symmetrical or asymmetrical lateral nasal deformities. A lateral osteotomy is performed first along the nasal side wall roughly approximating the nasomaxillary suture. This is then combined with a low-low osteotomy.

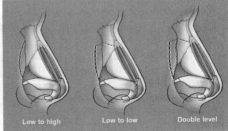

Fig. 82-21   Types of lateral osteotomies.

- **Technique**[21]
  - ► Infiltrate with lidocaine with epinephrine
  - ► At the level of the inferior orbital rim and nasofrontal junction, a 2 mm osteotome is introduced.
  - ► The osteotome should be parallel to the surface of the maxilla and positioned at the midportion of the bony nasal pyramid.
  - ► Gentle pressure is exerted on the nasal bones with the osteotome, and the osteotome is swept down the lateral nasal wall and laterally along the frontal process of the maxilla in a subperiosteal plane until the site of the first osteotomy is reached. This effectively displaces the angular artery, which is critical to prevent bleeding.

> TIP: Angle the osteotome so that just one edge contacts the bone. This increases the force per square centimeter.

  - ► Multiple 2 mm osteotomies are carried out in the paths described previously, taking care to leave 2 mm of normal bone between each osteotomy.
  - ► It is important when moving the osteotome from one position to the next to keep it against the maxilla to prevent the angular artery from returning to its previous position and potentially being injured.
  - ► Once the osteotomies have been made, the thumb and index finger are used to gently reposition the bones.
- Medial osteotomies involve a separation of the nasal bones and the bony septum.[23,24]
- Medial osteotomies can help reduce a traumatically narrowed upper vault.
- Medial osteotomies can also be helpful for patients with excessively thick and/or wide nasal bones or if the upper bony septum is wide and deviated; in these cases medial osteotomies can be performed to provide a medial shift of the bones.
- The two most common medial osteotomies are the medial oblique and the paramedian (Fig. 82-22).
- Medial osteotomies must be kept below the intercanthal line because of the thickness of the bones in this region.
- Medial osteotomies must be performed **before** lateral osteotomies if medial osteotomies are to be successful.
  - • This will allow for stable upper vault bones on which the medial osteotomies can be performed.
  - • If lateral osteotomies are performed first, the bones will have little support, making them a moving target during the performance of the medial osteotomies.

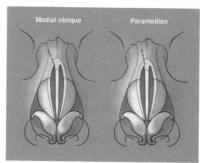

Fig. 82-22 The two most common medial osteotomies.

NASAL ALAE

Anatomy and Aesthetics[25-27]
- The width of the alae should be the same as the intercanthal distance.
  - • If they are wider than the intercanthal distance, then consideration should be given to correction of the widened nasal alae.

- In this case, the surgeon must decide if the widened alae are caused by excessive alar flaring or excessively wide alar bases.
- The alar rim should also have a smooth oval contour from the lateral view.
- The greatest distance from the long axis of the nostril to either the columella or alar rim should be 1-2 mm.
- The outline of the alar rims from the basilar view should resemble an equilateral triangle with slight alar flaring toward the alar base.
- The lower lateral cartilages are the primary support for the alae.
- The lower lateral cartilages can be divided into medial, middle, and lateral crura.
- It is the lateral crura of the lower lateral cartilages that provide the primary support for the alae.
- The lateral crus runs parallel to the alar rim for half the distance from the tip toward the piriform aperture.
- The lateral crus attaches to the accessory cartilages, which then attach to the piriform aperture.
- The lateral crus shares a common perichondrium with the accessory cartilages; this perichondrium allows the lateral crus and the accessory cartilages to function as a single unit, called the *lateral crural complex.*
- The lateral crural complex is supported by three things:
  1. Suspensory ligaments of the tip
  2. Fibrous connections to the upper lateral cartilage
  3. Abutment with the piriform aperture
- The posterior 50% of the alar rim has no cartilage and is composed of fibrofatty areolar tissue and overlying skin.
- If a patient has poor cartilaginous support, the alar rim appears collapsed or notched, typically between the superior third and middle of the alar rim.
- Alar deformity can also appear with alar retraction causing increased columellar show.
- Because the alar rim forms the external nasal valve, collapse of the alar rim can have functional as well as aesthetic sequelae, such as nasal airway obstruction.

ALAR RIM DEFORMITIES
- Deformities of the alar rim may be acquired or congenital.
- Acquired defects are usually secondary to overzealous resection of the lateral crus during a previous rhinoplasty.
- Nonanatomic alar contour grafts can be used to lend structural support to the alar rim.
- **Indications for placement of nonanatomic alar contour grafts**[28]
  - Secondary rhinoplasty patients with minimal vestibular lining loss and at least 3 mm of residual lower lateral cartilage
  - Primary rhinoplasty patients with congruent alar rim notching
  - Primary or secondary rhinoplasty patients with malpositioning of the lower lateral cartilages
- **Nonanatomic alar contour grafts are *not* effective for:**
  - Patients with alar rim retraction secondary to significant vestibular lining loss
  - Severe alar scarring
  - No lower lateral cartilage remnant
- **Principles for nonanatomic alar contour graft placement**[28]
  - This graft requires an open rhinoplasty approach.
  - 6 by 2 mm cartilage graft is fashioned.
  - Septal cartilage is preferred for this technique.
  - Use long sharp Stevens scissors to create a pocket immediately above the alar rim.

- Place cartilage graft in this pocket and confirm that alar notching is corrected and that the graft is not visible.
- In patients with severe scarring from previous rhinoplasty, a wider or second additional graft may be necessary.

TIP: It is essential at the end of every rhinoplasty to take a close look at the basilar view of the nose. If there is any hint of alar notching, a nonanatomic alar contour graft can be placed to prevent postoperative alar notching.

- An alternative to the nonanatomic alar contour graft is the **lateral crural strut graft.**
- The lateral crural strut graft is a cartilage graft placed on the deep surface of the lateral crus to reshape, reposition, or reconstruct the lateral crura.
- **Indications for placement of a lateral crural strut graft.**
  - Correction of the boxy nasal tip
  - Malpositioned lateral crura
  - Alar retraction
  - Alar rim collapse
  - Concave lateral crura
- **Principles of lateral crural strut graft placement.**[29]
  - Perform cephalic trim of lateral crura using an open rhinoplasty approach.
  - Undermine the vestibular skin off the lateral crura.
  - Carve a cartilage graft 3-4 mm by 15-25 mm, preferably of septal cartilage.
  - Place the lateral crural strut graft on the deep surface of the lateral crus in the undermined pocket.
  - Secure cartilage graft with two or three 5-0 Vicryl sutures.
  - Be sure to place the lateral end of the graft caudal to the alar groove to prevent visibility.
  - These lateral crural strut grafts will be thicker and longer than the lower lateral cartilages, and the lateral crura will assume the shape of the grafts.
  - If the alar rim is severely deformed, the lower lateral cartilages may need to be separated from the accessory chain of cartilages to allow the lateral crural strut graft to extend further laterally (Fig. 82-23).

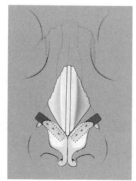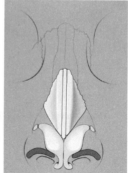

A

B

Fig. 82-23 **A,** Lateral crural strut graft. **B,** Nonanatomic alar contour graft.

CORRECTION OF WIDENED NASAL ALAE

- During preoperative analysis, the width of the alar base should be the same as the intercanthal distance.
- If the width of the alar base is wider than the intercanthal distance, then the degree of alar flare should be determined.
  - Alar flare is determined by comparing the maximum alar width with the width of the ala at the base.
  - If the difference between these two widths is greater than 2 mm, the problem is excessive alar flaring.
  - If the difference is less than 2 mm, the problem is excessively wide alar bases.[9]
- To correct alar flaring with preservation of the alar bases, the alar flare should be wedge excised.
  - The inferior portion of this wedge should preserve 1-2 mm of alar base to prevent alar notching.
  - The incision should not be carried into the nasal vestibule.

TIP: When correcting alar flaring by wedge excision of the alar flare, the alar groove incision is longer than the incision on the alar surface. To prevent postoperative irregularities, close the wound by the halving principle (Fig. 82-24).

- If the problem is excessively wide alar bases, a complete wedge should be excised with an excision that extends into the nasal vestibule 2 mm above the alar groove.
- A No. 11 blade should be used to make the medial incision at the sill.
- The No. 11 blade should be angled 30 degrees laterally. This results in a small flap medially, which is important to prevent notching postoperatively (Fig. 82-25).

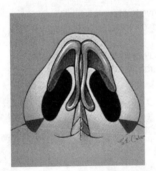

Fig. 82-24 Correction of alar flaring.

Fig. 82-25 Correction of excessively wide alar bases.

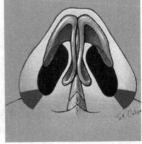

NASAL AIRWAY

- The nose is more than just an aesthetic organ; it is also functional.
  - It plays a key role in regulating air flow, humidification, olfaction, and filtration of inspired air.
  - The rhinoplasty surgeon must not forget the importance of the nose in regulating air flow and will often be called on to address issues of airway obstruction.
- The nasal airway contributes 50% of the overall airway resistance.[8]
- Engorgement of the nasal mucosa produces a significant decrease in the lumen of the relatively fixed volume of the nasal cavity.
- The internal nasal valve is bounded by the nasal septum, the caudal margin of the upper lateral cartilages, the anterior end of the inferior turbinate, and the floor of the nose.
- The internal nasal valve is the narrowest segment of the nasal airway and provides two thirds of the airway resistance in the nose.
- The junction between the caudal end of the upper lateral cartilages and the nasal septum forms the internal nasal valve angle. This should be 10-15 degrees.[8]
- The external nasal valve is a dynamic structure made of the mobile alar side walls and the caudal septum.
- Poiseuille's law says that airflow through the nose, similar to fluid through a tube, increases to the fourth power as the radius increases.
- During inspiration a negative pressure is generated, and the internal nasal valve narrows as the upper lateral cartilages are brought closer to the septum. In addition, the nostrils enlarge.
- The length and stability of the upper lateral cartilages and their relationship to the septum determine the function of the internal nasal valve.
- The size, shape, strength, and orientation of the lower lateral cartilages determine the strength of the external nasal valve.
- Flaccid lower lateral cartilages, slit-like nostrils, and thin alar side walls may have a tendency to allow collapse from the negative pressure generated during inspiration, causing external nasal valve obstruction.
- The nasal cycle is a normal phenomenon whereby there is alternating constriction and dilation of the mucosa on each side of the nose. The normal cycle takes 4 hours to complete.[8,32]
- Nasal obstruction is a frequent complaint of patients seeking cosmetic rhinoplasty.
- Problems associated with nasal obstruction include:
  - Nasal crusting
  - Dry mouth
  - Frequent sore throats
  - Sinus problems
- History should include:
  - Time of onset
  - Duration of obstruction
  - Precipitating or relieving factors
  - Rhinorrhea
  - Epistaxis
  - History of trauma or surgery
  - History of headaches, visual disturbances, and middle-ear symptoms
  - Use of medications, especially vasoactive nasal sprays
  - Use of tobacco, alcohol, or drugs
  - Seasonal obstruction

- Seasonal obstruction or obstruction related to dust, mold, pollen, etc. may suggest allergic rhinitis.
- Bilateral obstruction that changes in severity suggests mucosal disease.
- Constant obstruction is usually associated with a fixed structural abnormality such as septal deviation.
- Physical examination should discover the following:
  - Patients with allergic rhinitis often have conjunctivitis or dark circles under the eyes ("allergic shiners").
  - Patients who have internal nasal valve collapse may have supra-alar pinching or a narrow middle vault (inverted-V deformity).
  - Perform a **Cottle maneuver** by pulling the cheek laterally to displace the lateral nasal wall.
    - ▸ If this maneuver alleviates nasal airway obstruction, the site of airway obstruction can be localized to the lateral wall of the nose, indicating a collapse of the internal nasal valve during inspiration.
  - Assess the alar rims.
    - ▸ If they are notched or everted when the patient inspires, it may be the patient reflexively trying to flare the nostrils in a response to external nasal valve collapse.
  - Perform the intranasal examination with and without a speculum before and after administering a vasoconstrictive agent.
    - ▸ Examination with and without a vasoconstrictive agent allows the physician to check for congestion and rhinorrhea.
  - Evidence of crusting, ulceration, or polypoid changes should be reasons to postpone elective surgery and prompt a medical workup for a systemic condition.
  - Examine the septum for deviation, perforation, or spurs.
  - A narrow blunt-tipped instrument or nasal speculum can stabilize the lateral nasal wall during inspiration to determine whether this improves the airway (suggesting internal nasal valve collapse).
- Several medical therapies exist for nasal airway obstruction.[8,9,30]
  - Mucosal disease is the most common cause of nasal airway obstruction.
  - Viral rhinitis, the common cold, is the most common cause of mucosal disease.
    - ▸ Bacterial sinusitis may develop as a complication of viral rhinitis.
    - ▸ Acute or chronic rhinosinusitis may be treated with oral antibiotics or a combination of mucolytic-decongestant medication and topical nasal steroid spray.
  - Treat allergic rhinitis with avoidance of specific allergens, environmental control, antihistamines, and topical intranasal corticosteroids.
  - *Rhinitis medicamentosus* is a condition of rebound vasodilatation and engorgement of the nasal mucosa.
    - ▸ It is in response to overuse of topical nasal decongestants such as Neo-Synephrine® or Afrin®.
    - ▸ Often the patient is using the decongestants because of an undiagnosed nasal disorder such as nasal polyposis, septal deviation, or allergic rhinitis.
    - ▸ Treatment includes stopping use of the offending agent, patient education, a combination of oral antihistamines and decongestants, topical nasal steroid sprays, and possibly a steroid taper.
  - *Ozena* is primary atrophic rhinitis.
    - ▸ It is associated with aggressive submucous septal resection and total inferior turbinectomy.
    - ▸ The normal columnar epithelium undergoes squamous metaplasia.
    - ▸ Treatment can range from isotonic saline irrigation to high-dose vitamin A.
    - ▸ Some have even advocated surgical closure of the nostril to allow the mucosa time to heal and regenerate.
  - Submucosal corticosteroid injection may also help with inferior turbinate hypertrophy.

- Surgical treatment for nasal airway obstruction
  - Septal deviation can lead to airway obstruction at either the internal nasal valves or external nasal valves or both.
  - Septoplasty requires elevating the mucoperichondrium and mucoperiosteum with reshaping or resecting the deviated septum and midline mobilization of the quadrangular cartilage.
  - The membranous septum and columella may appear widened as a result of splaying of the medial crural feet.
    - ▸ This can be corrected using a small stab incision through the vestibular skin on both sides of the medial crural footplates.
    - ▸ A pocket is dissected on both sides, and a 5-0 clear nylon suture can be placed to bring the footplates together.
  - Internal nasal valve collapse is usually seen when the lateral crura are overresected or the upper lateral cartilages collapse inferomedially.
  - Internal nasal valve collapse can be corrected by placing spreader grafts or lateral wall grafts such as the alar batten graft.
    - ▸ Spreader grafts are the most effective way to correct internal nasal valve collapse (Fig. 82-26).
    - ▸ They can be placed by creating submucosal pockets at the most dorsal point of the nasal septum.
    - ▸ Spreader grafts are placed between the septum and the upper lateral cartilages, creating a cantilever effect and stenting the lateral nasal wall outward, which opens up the airway and prevents collapse of the internal nasal valve.[7]
  - Patients with internal nasal valve obstruction often have noticeable supra-alar pinching.
    - ▸ In addition to the placement of spreader grafts, alar batten grafts can be placed.
    - ▸ The alar batten graft extends internally from the area of overresection of the lateral crura down toward the alar base.
    - ▸ The graft should span the site of maximal collapse of the lateral nasal wall.
  - In cases of external nasal valve collapse, the key is to add support to the alar rim.

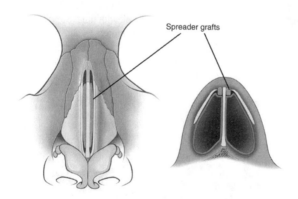

Spreader grafts

Fig. 82-26

▸ If the alar cartilages are cephalically positioned, they can be repositioned caudally to support the weak alar side walls.
▸ Convex autologous alar batten grafts (usually 4-8 mm wide and 10-15 mm long) can be placed by creating a pocket that extends from the piriform aperture to the approximate midpoint of the lower lateral cartilages (Fig. 82-27).
▸ Lateral crural grafts are anatomic grafts that can replace previously overresected lateral crura.
  ◆ Often, an external valve collapse requires more support than just a lateral crural graft.
  ◆ This can be done in the form of an alar batten graft.
▸ Lateral crural strut grafts are carved from curved septal or auricular cartilage and sandwiched between the vestibular skin and the weak lateral crura to strengthen the alar sidewall and resist collapse.

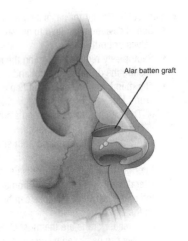

Alar batten graft

Fig. 82-27

TURBINATE HYPERTROPHY

• Hypertrophied inferior turbinates can cause significant airway obstruction.
• If a patient has a severely deviated septum, the contralateral inferior turbinate undergoes hypertrophy in an attempt to even out the resistance in both airways.
• After correcting septal deviation, it is critical to evaluate the inferior turbinates, because correction of the septal deviation may lead to airway obstruction on the side of hypertrophic inferior turbinate.
  ▸ Beekhuis[31] reviewed 1000 rhinoplasty patients and found 10% had nasal obstruction after the procedure. Most of this obstruction was the result of turbinate hypertrophy.
• Turbinate hypertrophy has some ability to correct itself with time. Steroid nasal sprays and decongestants can provide symptomatic relief in the interim.
• To prevent postoperative nasal airway obstruction, the inferior turbinate can be outfractured laterally or reduced with submucosal electrocautery. Outfracture of the inferior turbinate is performed using a long Vienna speculum (Fig. 82-28).

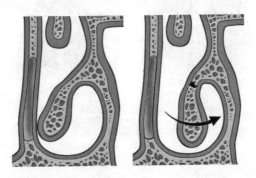

Fig. 82-28 Outfracture of the inferior turbinate.

- Submucous resection of the hypertrophic inferior turbinate can remove a larger portion of the inferior turbinate. Most of the mucosa is left intact to humidify nasal airflow.
  - Excessive resection of the inferior turbinate decreases its ability to regulate airflow.
    - It also exposes areas of the nasal mucosa that are not used to the drying effects of inspired air.
    - This causes mucous evaporation, causing it to become more viscous and crusty.
    - This also causes bleeding and dysfunction of the nasal cilia.
  - To perform a submucous resection, use a Bovie electrocautery with a Colorado pointed tip.
    - Incise a full-thickness portion of the anterior medial one third to one half of the inferior turbinate. (The incision should be 1.5-2 cm long.)
    - A Joseph periosteal elevator is used to elevate mucoperiosteal flaps.
    - Takahashi forceps are used to resect the exposed bone.
    - A long Boies elevator or a long Vienna speculum is used to outfracture the remaining inferior turbinate.[8]
- Total inferior turbinectomy has a tendency to cause crusting, ozena, and atrophic rhinitis. Therefore it is rarely indicated.

DEVIATED NOSE[32,33]

- Nasal deviation may be caused by a deviated septum, upper lateral cartilage-deforming forces, or asymmetrical nasal bones.
- Obtain wide exposure of the deviated structures.
- Release all of the mucoperichondrial attachments to all deviated portions of the deviated septum.
- Release all deforming forces, including the lower and upper lateral cartilages from each other, and the upper lateral cartilages from the septum.
- If the deviation is caused by asymmetry of the upper lateral cartilages, the septal deviation can be corrected by the release of the upper lateral cartilages from the lower lateral cartilages.
- If the deviation is the result of septal deviation, the septum must be straightened by addressing and correcting the intrinsic deforming forces.
- To do this, the deviated portion of the septum should be resected taking care to leave an 8-10 mm dorsal and caudal L-strut to provide structural support to the nasal dorsum. If less than 8-10 mm is left, the dorsum will be unstable and prone to collapse.
- The caudal septum must be anatomically reduced onto the nasal spine.
  - Reduction of the caudal septum may require a vertical sectioning to create a "swinging door."
  - If this is insufficient, small wedges of cartilage can be excised from the convex side of the deviation with cartilage scoring being performed on the concave side to destroy the cartilage memory and straighten the septum.
  - The caudal septum is sutured to the periosteum of the nasal spine and held reduced with a graft of septal cartilage.
- If septal deviation occurs higher up in the nose, correction should first be attempted by shaving the convex side of the deviation with addition of cartilage dorsal spreader grafts to the concave side of the dorsum to camouflage the deformity.
  - If this is unsuccessful in correcting the deformity, cartilage-scoring techniques such as those described for caudal defects can be attempted.

- If high dorsal deviation persists after these maneuvers, a series of full-thickness cuts can be made through the deviated portion of the dorsal septum.
  - ▸ These full-thickness cuts must be made only through 50% of the dorsal L-strut.
  - ▸ If the cuts are thicker than this, the L-strut will not be able to support the dorsum and collapse will occur.
- If full-thickness cuts need to be made, then bilateral cartilage spreader grafts should be placed for support and better definition of the dorsal aesthetic lines.
- Straightening the septum narrows the nasal airway in patients with preexisting inferior turbinate hypertrophy.
  - These patients may not have had airway obstruction preoperatively because the deviation of the septum away from the side of hypertrophy may have allowed for a preserved airway.
  - Submucous resection of the hypertrophied inferior turbinate must be performed to prevent postoperative airway obstruction.
- Asymmetrical nasal bones are addressed next.
  - Correction begins with asymmetrical oblique rasping of the nasal bones.
  - If this fails to correct the deviation or asymmetry, osteotomies should be performed to correct the deviation.
- If the nasal bones are symmetrical, lateral osteotomies alone will be sufficient.
- If the nasal bones are asymmetrical, then medial osteotomies should be added as well.

KEY POINTS

- ✔ The key to a successful rhinoplasty is a thorough understanding of nasal anatomy and nasal aesthetics.
- ✔ Planning begins with an in-depth analysis of nasal form using anteroposterior, lateral, and basilar views.
- ✔ The endonasal approach to rhinoplasty avoids any external incisions at the expense of a better view. The open approach to rhinoplasty uses a small external incision at the columella but affords a completely unobstructed view of the nasal anatomy.
- ✔ A graduated approach to increasing nasal tip projection should be taken. This should begin with columellar strut grafts, then proceed to tip suturing, and finish with tip grafts if needed.
- ✔ Dorsal hump reduction begins with shaving the cartilaginous septum after first separating the upper lateral cartilages from the septal cartilage. A downbiting rasp is then used to reduce the bony dorsum. Careful examination is then made of the internal nasal valve. If there is fear of collapse, dorsal spreader grafts are placed.
- ✔ Alar rim deformities may be congenital or may be the result of surgical alteration of the nose. A nonanatomic alar contour graft can be used to correct preexisting notching of the alar rim or prevent notching of the alar rim postoperatively.
- ✔ Three types of lateral osteotomies are common. Use the low-high osteotomy for small open-roof deformities. Use the low-low osteotomy to correct an excessively wide nasal base or a large open-roof deformity. Use a double-level osteotomy for excessive lateral wall convexity.
- ✔ Nasal airway obstruction may be caused by reversible medical conditions or by surgically correctible conditions such as internal or external nasal valve collapse, septal deviation, or inferior turbinate hypertrophy.

REFERENCES

1. Rohrich RJ, Huynh B, Muzaffar AR, et al. Importance of the depressor septi nasi muscle in rhinoplasty: Anatomic study and clinical application. Plast Reconstr Surg 105:376-383; discussion 384-388, 2000.
2. Rohrich RJ, Gunter JP, Friedman RM. Nasal tip blood supply: An anatomic study validating the safety of the transcolumellar incision in rhinoplasty. Plast Reconstr Surg 95:795-799; discussion 800-801, 1995.
3. Rohrich RJ, Muzaffar AR, Gunter JP. Nasal tip blood supply: Confirming the safety of the transcolumellar incision in rhinoplasty. Plast Reconstr Surg 106:1640-1641, 2000.
4. Rohrich RJ, Muzaffar AR, Janis JE. Component dorsal hump reduction: The importance of maintaining dorsal aesthetic lines in rhinoplasty. Plast Reconstr Surg 114:1298-1308; discussion 1309-1312, 2004.
5. Adams WP Jr, Rohrich RJ, Hollier LH, et al. Anatomic basis and clinical implications for nasal tip support in open versus closed rhinoplasty. Plast Reconstr Surg 103:255-261; discussion 262-264, 1999.
6. Toriumi DM, Josen J, Weinberger M, et al. Use of alar batten grafts for correction of nasal valve collapse. Arch Otolaryngol Head Neck Surg 123:802-888, 1997.
7. Rohrich RJ, Hollier LH. Use of spreader grafts in the external approach to rhinoplasty. Clin Plast Surg 23:255-262, 1996.
8. Rohrich RJ, Krueger JK, Adams WP Jr, et al. Rationale for submucous resection of hypertrophied inferior turbinates in rhinoplasty: An evolution. Plast Reconstr Surg 108:536-544; discussion 545-546, 2001.
9. Gunter JP, Rohrich RJ, Adams WP. Dallas Rhinoplasty: Nasal Surgery by the Masters. St Louis: Quality Medical Publishing, 2002.
10. Sheen JH. Closed versus open rhinoplasty—and the debate goes on. Plast Reconstr Surg 99:859-862, 1997.
11. Sheen JH. Rhinoplasty: Personal evolution and milestones. Plast Reconstr Surg 105:1820-1852; discussion 1853, 2000.
12. Sheen JH, Sheen AP. Aesthetic Rhinoplasty, 2nd ed. St Louis: Quality Medical Publishing, 1997.
13. Rohrich RJ, Griffin JR. Correction of intrinsic nasal tip asymmetries in primary rhinoplasty. Plast Reconstr Surg 112:1699-1712; discussion 1713-1715, 2003.
14. Gunter JP, Rohrich RJ. External approach for secondary rhinoplasty. Plast Reconstr Surg 80:161-174, 1987.
15. Sheen JH. Tip graft: A 20-year retrospective. Plast Reconstr Surg 91:48-63, 1993.
16. Peck GC Jr, Michelson L, Segal J, et al. An 18-year experience with the umbrella graft in rhinoplasty. Plast Reconstr Surg 102:2158-2165; discussion 2166-2168, 1998.
17. Tardy ME Jr. Graduated sculpture refinement of the nasal tip. Facial Plast Surg Clin North Am 12:51-80, 2004.
18. Johnson CM Jr, Godin MS. The tension nose. Plast Reconstr Surg 97:246, 1996.
19. Rohrich RJ, Adams WP Jr. The boxy nasal tip: Classification and management based on alar cartilage suturing techniques. Plast Reconstr Surg 107:1849-1863; discussion 1864-1868, 2001.
20. Gunter JP, Rohrich RJ. Augmentation rhinoplasty: Dorsal onlay grafting using shaped autogenous septal cartilage. Plast Reconstr Surg 86:39-45, 1990.
21. Rohrich RJ, Krueger JK, Adams WP Jr, et al. Achieving consistency in the lateral nasal osteotomy during rhinoplasty: An external perforated technique. Plast Reconstr Surg 108:2122-2130; discussion 2131-2132, 2001.
22. Rohrich RJ, Minoli JJ, Adams WP, et al. The lateral nasal osteotomy in rhinoplasty: An anatomic endoscopic comparison of the external versus the internal approach. Plast Reconstr Surg 99:1309-1312; discussion 1313, 1997.
23. Guyuron B. Nasal osteotomy and airway changes. Plast Reconstr Surg 102:856-860; discussion 861-863, 1998.
24. Harshbarger RJ, Sullivan PK. The optimal medial osteotomy: A study of nasal bone thickness and fracture patterns. Plast Reconstr Surg 108:2114-2119; discussion 2120-2121, 2001.
25. Gunter JP, Rohrich RJ, Friedman RM. Classification and correction of alar-columellar discrepancies in rhinoplasty. Plast Reconstr Surg 97:643-648, 1996.

26. Guyuron B. Alar rim deformities. Plast Reconstr Surg 107:856-863, 2001.
27. Guyuron B, Behmand RA. Alar base abnormalities. Classification and correction. Clin Plast Surg 23:263-270, 1996.
28. Rohrich RJ, Raniere J Jr, Ha RY. The alar contour graft: Correction and prevention of alar rim deformities in rhinoplasty. Plast Reconstr Surg 109:2495-2505; discussion 2506-2508, 2002.
29. Gunter JP, Friedman RM. Lateral crural strut graft: Technique and clinical applications in rhinoplasty. Plast Reconstr Surg 99:943-952; discussion 953-955, 1997.
30. Howard BK, Rohrich RJ. Understanding the nasal airway: Principles and practice. Plast Reconstr Surg 109:1128-1146; quiz 1145-1146, 2002.
31. Beekhuis GJ. Nasal obstruction after rhinoplasty: Etiology, and techniques for correction. Laryngoscope 86:540-548, 1976.
32. Gunter JP, Rohrich RJ. Management of the deviated nose. The importance of septal reconstruction. Clin Plast Surg 15:43-55, 1988.
33. Rohrich RJ, Gunter JP, Deuber MA, et al. The deviated nose: Optimizing results using a simplified classification and algorithmic approach. Plast Reconstr Surg 110:1509-1523; discussion 1524-1525, 2002.

83. Genioplasty

Ashkan Ghavami

ANATOMY

RELEVANT MUSCLES (Fig. 83-1)

- Mentalis
  - Conelike geometry
  - Vertical fibers from incisor fossa to overlying skin
    - ▸ Can cause wrinkling
    - ▸ If hyperdynamic, may be visible under lower lip
    - ▸ Midline void between fibers seen when chin dimple is present
- Orbicularis oris (lower fibers)
- Depressor anguli oris
- Quadratus (depressor) labii inferioris
- Geniohyoid, genioglossus, mylohyoid, and anterior belly of digastric
  - Attach to lingual (posterior) aspect of chin

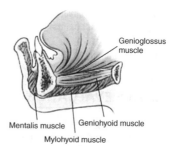

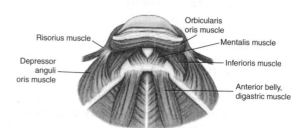

BONY LANDMARKS

- Mental foramen
- Digastric fossa
- Mental protuberance
- Mental spines
- Submandibular fossa

Fig. 83-1 (From Cohen SR. Genioplasty. In Achauer BH, Eriksson E, Guyuron B, et al, eds. Plastic Surgery: Indications, Operations, and Outcomes, vol 5. St Louis: Mosby, 2000.)

NERVE SUPPLY

- Inferior alveolar nerve
- Mental nerve (terminating branch exiting mental foramen)
  - Genioplasty procedures carry risk of injury.
  - Osteotomies should be 5-6 mm below mental foramen to avoid injury to nerve branches or tooth apices.
  - Nerve can be absent or distorted in patients with hemifacial microsomia or other facial deformities.

871

BLOOD SUPPLY

■ Labial branch of facial artery
■ Inferior alveolar artery

SIGNIFICANT CEPHALOMETRIC POINTS (Fig. 83-2)

■ **Pogonion (Pog):** Most projecting portion of mandible. Indicates chin excess or deficiency in relation to other structures (e.g., nasion and lip position)
■ **Menton (Me):** Lowest (most caudal) portion of chin
■ **Subspinale (A):** Columella-labial junction
■ **Supramentale (B):** Deepest point between pogonion and incisor
■ **Nasion (N):** Nasofrontal junction

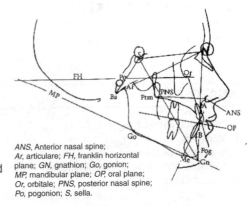

ANS, Anterior nasal spine; Ar, articulare; FH, franklin horizontal plane; GN, gnathion; Go, gonion; MP, mandibular plane; OP, oral plane; Or, orbitale; PNS, posterior nasal spine; Po, pogonion; S, sella.

Fig. 83-2 Significant cephalometric points. (From Wolfe SA, Spiro SA, Wider TM. Surgery of the jaws. In Aston SJ, Beasley RW, Thorne HM, et al. Grabb and Smith's Plastic Surgery, 5th ed. Philadelphia: Lippincott, 1997, p 322.)

PREOPERATIVE EVALUATION

MEDICAL COMORBIDITIES

■ Patients with diabetes and immunosuppression are not good candidates for implantation.
  • May also have poorly healed osteotomy site(s) postoperatively

OCCLUSION TYPE (Fig. 83-3)

■ **Angle class I**
  • Mesiobuccal cusp of maxillary first molar occludes in the buccal groove of the mandibular first molar (see Fig. 83-3, A).
■ **Angle class II**
  • Mesiobuccal cusp of maxillary first molar occludes **mesial** to the buccal groove (see Fig. 83-3, B).
  • This is the **most common malocclusion in North American Caucasians.**
  • Further evaluation is often indicated, as well as possible orthognathic surgery with maxillary and mandibular osteotomies.

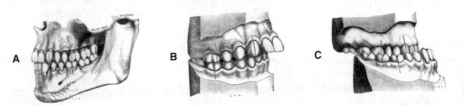

Fig. 83-3 Occlusion types. **A,** Angle class I. **B,** Angle class II. **C,** Angle class III. (From Angle EH. Treatment of malocclusion of the teeth and fractures of the maxillae. Angle's system. Philadelphia: SS White Dental Manufacturing System, 1898, p 6.)

- **Angle class III**
  - Mesiobuccal cusp of the maxillary first molar occludes **distal** to the buccal groove of the mandibular first molar (see Fig. 83-3, *C*).

TIP: Obtaining previous orthodontic history is important because occlusion may have been corrected without adjusting for maxillary and mandibular disharmonies (deformity is masked).

DENTITION

- Before age of 15: Dentition may not be fully erupted
  - Greater risk of injury during osteotomies
- Elderly patients: May have retruded alveolar ridge (if edentulous) that contributes to chin pad ptosis
  - Little bone stock present
  - Better candidates for alloplastic augmentation
- Patients with poor dentition or infected dentition: Very poor candidates for any form of genioplasty until fully treated

LIFE-SIZE PHOTOGRAPHS[1]

- Bilateral sagittal view, frontal views, and bilateral oblique (three-quarter) views

MIDFACE HEIGHT

- Watch for vertical maxillary excess: Especially important when accompanied by a deep labiomental fold
  - Patient better served with formal orthognathic correction

NOSE-CHIN EVALUATION

- Nasal aesthetic harmony linked with chin balance and vice versa
- Chin projection: Should be 3 mm posterior to nose-lip-chin plane[2]
- Nasal length: Two thirds of midfacial height and exactly equal to vertical length of chin[1]

SYMMETRY OF LOWER THIRD OF FACE

- Right-to-left asymmetries of the mandible and chin may require multiple osteotomy configurations to centralize the chin.

SOFT TISSUE ANALYSIS

- **Soft Tissue Pad:** Normally 9-11 mm thick
  - Palpated at pogonion and off midline in repose and when patient is smiling
  - Soft tissue contribution can predict effects of augmentation (see the following)
- **Stomion:** Junction between upper and lower lips in repose
- **Upper/lower lips:** Lower lip eversion from deep bite, excess lip bulk, or excess overjet may deepen labiomental fold[3]
- **Labiomental fold**

Indentation or crease between lower lip and lowest point of mandible (the menton). Best seen from sagittal view.

  - Fold aesthetics dependent on **vertical proportion of mandible and facial length**[7]
    - Example: Deep fold may look good on longer faces[4]
  - Evaluate for **height** (if dividing stomion to menton into thirds, fold often falls at junction of upper and middle thirds)
    - If fold is too low, augmentation may only address chin pad.[3]

- **Depth**
  - ▸ Fold depth should be approximately 4 mm in men and 6 mm in women.[5]
  - ▸ If fold is deep, horizontal vector chin augmentation may result in an awkward exaggerated deep fold and an overprojected chin.
  - ▸ If shallow, it may be effaced further by vertical augmentation.
- ■ **Riedel's line**

A line drawn vertically down the facial plane in the sagittal view, tangential to anterior upper and lower lip (Fig. 83-4).
  - Lower lip should be 2-3 mm posterior to the upper lip.
  - Pogonion should never project beyond this line and should fall slightly posterior to it or just touching it.

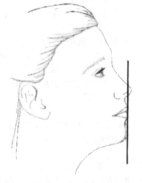

Fig. 83-4. Riedel's plane is a simple line connecting the most prominent portion of the upper and lower lip, which, on a balanced face, should touch the pogonion (the most prominent anterior portion of the chin). (From Guyuron B. Genioplasty. Boston: Little, Brown, 1993, p 44.)

DYNAMIC AND STATIC CHIN PAD ANALYSIS[3]

- ■ A **thin** chin pad when smiling: Potential for increased pad effacement with increased bony prominence (can be native or caused by augmentation).
  - Burr reduction or osteotomy setback may be required.
- ■ A **thick** pad may increase submental soft tissue fullness and worsen the cervicomental angle if bony setback is performed.

"WITCH'S CHIN"

Ptosis of soft tissue caudal to menton and an exaggerated submental crease.
- ■ Correction requires soft tissue/muscle resection and/or repositioning.
- ■ Augmentation can exaggerate deformity.

TIP: Mentalis muscle fixation superiorly is key for preventing soft tissue descent. Secondary cases may require soft tissue fixation to prevent ptosis recurrence.[6]

CERVICOMENTAL ANGLE

Angle between chin and neck in sagittal view.
- ■ Angle should be 105-120 degrees.
- ■ Adjunct neck soft tissue contouring techniques can further enhance chin aesthetics.
  - Submental lipectomy, platysmaplasty, or anterior digastric resection
  - Submandibular gland resection or suspension

IMAGING
- **Cephalograms and/or panoramic radiographs (Panorex)**
  - Required to properly evaluate chin deficiency or excess
  - Always indicated for secondary cases or if maxillary/mandibular imbalance or malocclusion is present
  - Obtain panoramic radiograph if any concern about nerve malposition, apical teeth location, or pathology

CLASSIFICATION OF CHIN DEFORMITIES (Table 83-1)
- **Microgenia:** Small chin
- **Macrogenia:** Large chin
- **Combined deformities:** Short or long macrogenia/microgenia
  - Horizontal (off center) asymmetries can also exist.
- Classification system proposed by Guyuron et al[7] can guide surgical planning (see Table 83-1)

Table 83-1 *Classification System*

Type	Deformity	Vector and Surgical Treatment
Class I	Macrogenia	Horizontal: Osteotomy with setback or ostectomy Vertical: Osteotomy and resection Both horizontal and vertical: Osteotomy, resection, and setback
Class II	Microgenia	Horizontal: Osteotomy with advancement, autogenous or alloplastic Augmentation Vertical: Osteotomy and lengthening, with or without graft Both horizontal and vertical: Osteotomy, lengthening, and advancement, with or without graft
Class III	Combined	Horizontal macrogenia: With vertical microgenia: Osteotomy with lengthening and setback Horizontal microgenia with vertical macrogenia: Osteotomy with resection of horizontal segment and advancement
Class IV	Asymmetrical chin	Short anterior lower face: Add wedge of bone to short side Normal lower facial height: Removal of wedge of bone from long side; add to short side Long anterior facial height: Removal of wedge of bone based on long side
Class V	Witch's chin	Soft tissue correction
Class VI	Pseudomacrogenia	Soft tissue adjustment (not predictable)
Class VII	Pseudomicrogenia	Maxillary osteotomy

SURGICAL PRINCIPLES

OSSEOUS GENIOPLASTY
- **Indications**
  - Horizontal asymmetries of any magnitude
  - Excess deficiency or excess in both vertical and sagittal planes
    - Moderate-to-severe microgenia

- Secondary cases
- Adjunct to formal orthognathic surgery
■ **Contraindications**
  - Inadequate bone stock (e.g., elderly patient)
  - Abnormal dentition
  - Patient prefers to not have osteotomies
■ Can be quick procedure
■ More versatile than alloplastic augmentation

ALLOPLASTIC AUGMENTATION
■ **Indications**
  - Mild isolated sagittal deficiencies
  - Need to only increase labiomental fold depth
  - Relative: Concomitant neck lift/face lift
■ **Contraindications**
  - Excessive horizontal deficiency
  - Vertical deficiency
  - Mandibular asymmetry
  - Secondary cases with bony erosion
  - Malocclusion: Orthognathic surgery required

TIP: In general, alloplastic augmentation should be used only for patients with mild-to-moderate chin deficiency in the sagittal plane and a shallow labiomental fold.[1,3,4,8]

■ **Caveat:** Cosmetic surgery patients seem to prefer alloplastic augmentation and shy away from osteotomies.

TIP: Face lift/neck lift procedures often include a submental incision that can easily be used for placing a chin implant.

■ **Malocclusion requires consideration of orthognathic surgery and a more extensive workup (e.g., cephalometric analysis, occlusion models).**
  - Significant microgenia usually requires an osseous genioplasty.

IMPLANT TYPES
■ **Synthetic**
  - **Silicone** (smooth or textured)
  - **Porous polyethylene (Porex®):** Contains 100-250 μm diameter pores that cause tissue ingrowth and incorporation of implant rather than encapsulation (as with silicone and nonporous implants).
    ► Infection rate may be lower for porous implants, but removal is much more challenging.
  - Custom-made implants based on three-dimensional modeling (perhaps more useful if multiple facial implants required).
  - Comprehensive approach: Large implants for lateral augmentation combined with mandibular angle implants or other facial implants.[9]

■ **Biologic**
  • Autogenous cranial bone
  • Rib or conchal cartilage grafts
  • Irradiated cartilage sources

SOFT TISSUE RESPONSE: OSSEOUS MOVEMENT RATIO
■ **Osteotomy and alloplastic augmentation:** Approximately 0.8-0.9:1
■ **Ostectomy:** Approximately 0.25-0.50:1

OSSEOUS GENIOPLASTY (Fig. 83-5)

REDUCTION GENIOPLASTY
■ **Indication:** Increased vertical height or sagittal excess
■ Osteotomy angled inferiorly to produce vertical reduction

NOTE: Excess vertical height of the mandible requires formal orthognathic procedures, commonly with a simultaneous genioplasty.

> TIP: Genioplasty results can be enhanced with submental soft tissue procedures such as liposuction, lipectomy, and platysmaplasty.

SLIDING GENIOPLASTY
■ **Indication:** Horizontal (sagittal) deficiency (standard operation)
■ **Two-tier genioplasty:** Two segments advanced anteriorly
  • Rarely necessary—for extreme sagittal and/or vertical deficiency

> TIP: Dissection carried oblique anterior or at right angle to the bone provides a small cuff of intact mentalis muscle to facilitate soft tissue approximation when closing.

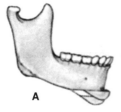 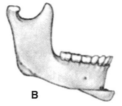 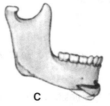

A   B   C

Fig. 83-5 Types of genioplasty. **A,** Reduction genioplasty. **B,** Sliding genioplasty. **C,** Jumping genioplasty. (From Cohen SR. Genioplasty. In Achauer BH, Eriksson E, Guyuron B, et al, eds. Plastic Surgery: Indications, Operations, and Outcomes, vol 5. St Louis: Mosby, 2000.)

JUMPING GENIOPLASTY
- **Indication:** Very minor chin height excess
- Inferior fragment "jumped" over superior segment as an onlay

> **TIP:** Excess inferior/posterior stripping may devascularize the lower bone segment after osteotomy is performed. Only lateral exposure is required to view the mental nerves.

OSTECTOMY
- **Indication:** Significant height reduction

INTERPOSITIONAL BONE GRAFTS (OR HYDROXYAPATITE)
- **Indication:** To add more vertical length
- Added to osteotomy segment that has been angled superiorly

CENTRALIZING GENIOPLASTY
- **Indication:** To correct horizontal asymmetries
- Wedges of autogenous bone graft or hydroxyapatite often needed

IMPLANT GENIOPLASTY[8]

APPROACH
- **Extraoral**
  - **Submental exposure** allows more precise placement.
  - Possibly fewer cases of malposition and mental nerve injury.
  - Soft tissue/muscle closure should be strong to prevent soft tissue ptosis.
- **Intraoral**
  - No visible scars
  - Similar infection rate
  - Can lead to improper implant position (often too superior): No direct view of pocket

FIXATION
- **Methods**
  - Screws[10]
  - Sutures[3,6,11]
  - Mitek®
- If no fixation: Precise pocket dissection and soft tissue approximation becomes even more important

IMPLANT POSITION
- **Proper position:** Directly over pogonion
- **Superior positioning**
  - Can get increased bone and/or tooth root resorption/erosion, movement, and asymmetries
- **Superficial placement**
  - Implant may be visible, palpable, and show irregularities

TIP: Creating too large a pocket can increase malposition rates.

IMPLANT REMOVAL/SECONDARY CASES
- **Often requires:**
  - Replacement with a smaller implant and fixation
  - Osseous genioplasty to fill the soft tissue void
  - Soft tissue/muscle manipulations (resection, repositioning) to prevent:
    - ▸ Soft tissue pad balling
    - ▸ Chin pad ptosis
    - ▸ Fasciculations: Not preventable, but can be treated with botulinum toxin type A injections (Botox®)[6]

COMPLICATIONS

POOR AESTHETIC RESULTS
- **Most common complication**
  - However, dissatisfaction rate very low
    - ▸ **Satisfaction rates**[12]
      - ✦ **Osseous genioplasty:** 90%-95%
      - ✦ **Alloplastic augmentation:** 85%-90%
- **Overcorrection:** More common in women; may result in overprojection and masculinization
- **Implant versus osseous genioplasty aesthetics:** Very controversial with limited reports
  - One study shows slightly higher satisfaction and self-esteem improvement rates with osseous genioplasty.[12]
- **Asymmetries:** Related to technique of improper soft tissue/muscle (mentalis) dissection and fixation/reapproximation
  - Bony asymmetries with osseous genioplasty: Increased chance if osteotomy is not posterior enough

HEMATOMA
- Rare
- Commonly at lateral osteotomy site
- Responds to simple aspiration and antibiotics: Cover for oral flora

INFECTION
- Uncommon (<5% for implants [Proplast], approximately 3% for osseous genioplasty)[8,12]
- More likely with hematomas in osseous techniques
- Overall may be more common in **alloplastic implantation** (may require implant removal)
- Some surgeons report no infections[10]
- Implant extrusion: Very rare; related to infection and high placement

MALPOSITION
- Perhaps more common with **intraoral** implant placement
- Leads to increased bone resorption rates

NERVE INJURY
- **Neurapraxia:** Often a retraction injury and resolves in 2-6 weeks

---

TIP: Limit retraction and manipulation of mental nerves as much as possible.

- **Lower lip paresthesias**
  - 5%-6% rate incidence
  - Possible temporary drooling
    - ▶ If it lasts longer than 6 weeks, consider removal, trimming of implant.
  - Permanent deficits extremely rare
    - ▶ Often related to improper osteotomy technique and damage of inferior alveolar nerve as it courses caudally

---

KEY POINTS

✔ Chin should never project beyond a line drawn from the anterior upper and lower lips (Riedel's line).

✔ Lower lip, chin pad (dynamic and static), nose-lip-chin relationship, and labiomental fold (depth and height) should be incorporated into preoperative analysis.

✔ Malocclusion and/or midface deficiency or excess warrant workup for orthognathic surgery.

✔ Osteotomy must be made at least 5 mm below the mental foramen to avoid inferior alveolar nerve injury.

✔ Soft tissue-to-bone response to osseous and alloplastic genioplasty is approximately 0.8:1.

✔ Alloplastic augmentation genioplasty is the most common genioplasty technique used today.

✔ Chin implant positioning is critical and should rest directly over pogonion.

✔ Alloplastic genioplasty cannot correct vertical deficiencies.

REFERENCES

1. Guyuron B. Genioplasty. Boston: Little, Brown, 1993.
2. Byrd HS, Hobar PC. Rhinoplasty: A practical guide for surgical planning. Plast Reconstr Surg 91:642-654, 1993.
3. Zide BM, Pfeifer TM, Longaker MT. Chin surgery. I. Augmentation—The allures and the alerts. Plast Reconstr Surg 104:1843-1853, 1999.
4. Rosen HM. Osseous genioplasty. In Aston SJ, Beasley RW, Thorne HM, et al. Grabb and Smith's Plastic Surgery, 5th ed. Philadelphia: Lippincott, 1997, pp 705-710.
5. Michelow BJ, Guyuron B. The chin: Skeletal and soft tissue components. Plast Reconstr Surg 95:473-478, 1995.
6. Zide BM, Boutros S. Chin surgery. III. Revelations. Plast Reconstr Surg 111:1542-1550; discussion 1551-1552, 2003.
7. Guyuron B, Michelow BJ, Willis L. Practical classification of chin deformities. Aesthetic Plast Surg 19:257-264, 1995.

8. Cohen SR. Genioplasty. In Achauer BH, Eriksson E, Guyuron B, et al, eds. Plastic Surgery: Indications, Operations, and Outcomes, vol 5. St Louis: Mosby, 2000, pp 2683-2703.

9. Terino EO. Alloplastic facial contouring by zonal principles of skeletal anatomy. Clin Plast Surg 19:487-510, 1992.

10. Yaremchuk MJ. Improving aesthetic outcomes after alloplastic chin augmentation. Plast Reconstr Surg 112:1422-1432, 2003.

11. Zide BM, Longaker MT. Chin surgery. II. Submental ostectomy and soft-tissue excision. Plast Reconstr Surg 104:1854-1860; discussion 1861-1862, 1999.

12. Guyuron B, Raszewski RL. A critical comparison of osteoplastic and alloplastic augmentation genioplasty. Aesthetic Plast Surg 14:199-206, 1990.

84. Liposuction

Jose L. Rios

ANATOMY

SUBCUTANEOUS LAYERS (Fig. 84-1)
- **Superficial**
  - Fat is dense and adherent to overlying skin.
  - **Suction with caution to avoid surface irregularities.**
- **Intermediate**
  - **Safest** layer
  - Most commonly suctioned layer
- **Deep**
  - Loose and less compact
  - Can be removed safely in most areas except the buttocks

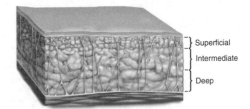

Fig. 84-1

ZONES OF ADHERENCE (Fig. 84-2)
- Distal iliotibial tract
- Gluteal crease
- Lateral gluteal depression
- Middle medial thigh
- Distal posterior thigh

CAUTION: Do not violate the zones of adherence during liposuction. This will result in contour deformities.

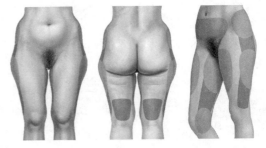

Fig. 84-2

PREOPERATIVE EVALUATION

PHYSICAL EXAMINATION
- Check for deviation from the ideal contour.
- **Note any of the following:**
  - Asymmetries
  - Dimpling/cellulite
  - Location of fat deposits
  - Areas of adherence
- Examine spine for **scoliosis** (may cause asymmetry).
- Check **laxity** of skin.
- Assess for **hernias/diastasis.**

PHOTOGRAPHS
- Standard photographs of areas to be treated should be obtained (see Chapter 9).

PERIOPERATVIE CONSIDERATIONS

PREOPERATIVE
- Complete blood count if expecting to perform **large-volume** procedure
- Intravenous antibiotics
- Deep venous thrombosis prophylaxis

HYPOTHERMIA
- Forced warm air over areas not being suctioned
- Warm intravenous fluid solutions
- Warm wetting solution
- Warm room if necessary

POSITIONING
- Protect face/breasts when prone
- Pad pressure points

MARKINGS (Fig. 84-3)

- Use black ink to outline areas to be treated.
- Use *X*s over areas of maximal prominence.
- Mark zones of adherence and other areas to be avoided with parallel lines.

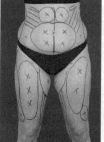
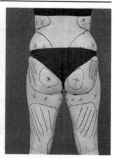

Fig. 84-3

INCISIONS (Fig. 84-4)

- Longer for ultrasound-assisted liposuction (UAL) than suction-assisted lipoplasty (SAL) (6-8 mm versus 2-3 mm)
- **Locations**
  - **Breast (male):** Lateral inframammary fold (IMF) or periareolar
  - **Lateral back:** Lateral bra line
  - **Vertical back:** Midline
  - **Flank/hip:** Lateral gluteal fold/lateral lower hip/flank
  - **Abdomen:** Lateral lower abdomen/suprapubic/umbilical
  - **Buttock:** Lateral gluteal fold
  - **Lateral thigh:** Lateral gluteal fold

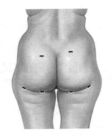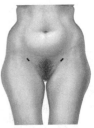

- **Posterior thigh:** Lateral gluteal fold
- **Medial thigh:** Medial gluteal crease (posterior)
- **Anterior thigh:** Inguinal crease
- **Upper arm:** Posterior radial proximal humerus (prone), distal radial humerus (supine)

Fig. 84-4

ULTRASOUND-ASSISTED LIPOSUCTION[1]

- Ultrasonic energy emulsifies subcutaneous fat.
- SAL is used for evacuation.

KEY POINTS FOR ULTRASOUND-ASSISTED LIPOSUCTION [1,2]

- Maintain a **wet environment** at all times.
- Keep the UAL cannula **in motion at all times.**

WETTING SOLUTIONS

PURPOSES

- Volume replacement
- Provide hemostasis
- Provide pain control
- Enhance cavitation (UAL)
- Dissipate heat (UAL)
- **University of Texas Southwestern Medical Center at Dallas mixture**
  - 1000 ml of lactated Ringer's at 21° C
  - 30 ml of 1% lidocaine (15 ml if large volume)
  - 1 ml of 1:1000 epinephrine
- **Klein[3]:**
  - 1000 ml normal saline solution
  - 50 ml 1% lidocaine
  - 1 ml 1:1000 epinephrine
  - 12.5 ml of 8.4% sodium bicarbonate (alkalization may decrease pain with infiltration but is not needed with general anaesthesia)

NOTE: Regardless of the anaesthetic route, large-volume liposuction (>5000 ml total aspirate) should be performed in an acute-care hospital or in a facility that is either accredited or licensed. Vital signs and urinary output should be monitored postoperatively and patients should be monitored overnight in an appropriate facility by qualified and competent staff familiar with the perioperative care of liposuction patients.[4,5]

LIDOCAINE

- Provides analgesia for up to 18 hours postoperatively
- Recommended maximum is **7 mg/kg**
- Klein[5] used up to 35 mg/kg, resulting in peak levels (12 hours) less than the toxic threshold (3 μg/ml)
- **Use of such high quantities of lidocaine is possible because of:**
  - Diluted solution
  - Slow infiltration
  - Vasoconstriction of epinephrine
  - Relative avascularity of fatty layer
  - High lipid solubility of lidocaine
  - Compression of vessels by infiltrate

NOTE: **After 20-30 minutes, wet environment may be lost.**

FLUID RESUSCITATION

- 1 liter of isotonic fluid is absorbed from the interstitium in 167 minutes.
- **25%-30%** of the infiltrate is removed during suctioning. *50 - 70 % remains after done*
  - Rest is reabsorbed over 6-12 hours postoperatively
- **Intravenous fluid (IVF) (using superwet infiltration):**
  - Crystalloid at maintenance (adjust to urine output and vital signs)
  - Replacement IVF of 0.25 ml per cc of aspirate over 5 liters
- Continue maintenance IVF until oral intake is adequate.

LIPOSUCTION STAGES

STAGE I: INFILTRATION[6]
- Infiltrate **intermediate plane** with superwet technique.
- Record delivered amount to each area.
- End point is uniform blanching and skin turgor.
- Allow 7-10 minutes for maximal vasoconstriction from epinephrine.

STAGE II: UAL TREATMENT (OMIT IF PERFORMING SAL ONLY)
- Place access incisions asymmetrically.
- Use port protector and wet towels.
- Treat posterior areas first **(can treat 70%-80% of the circumference from this position).**
- Move cannula at all times.
- Withdraw to within 3 cm of incision to redirect and minimize torque.
- Move from **superficial to deep (SAL goes deep to superficial).**
- **End points** (Table 84-1):
  - **Primary:** Loss of resistance, blood in aspirate
  - **Secondary:** Final contour, treatment time

Table 84-1 *Surgical End Points for UAL and SAL/PAL*

End Point	UAL	SAL/PAL
Primary	Loss of tissue resistance Blood aspirate	Final contour Symmetrical pinch test results
Secondary	Treatment time Treatment volume	Treatment time Treatment volume

PAL, Power-assisted liposuction.

STAGE III: EVACUATION AND FINAL CONTOURING[7]
- Set aspirator at 60%-70% of usual suction
- Begin with deep layer and move superficially

DRAINS

- Not routinely used
- Consider drains for liposuction procedures combined with resection

INCISION CLOSURE

- Massage out excess fluid
- Close with suture of choice
- Antibiotic ointment, 2- by 2-inch gauze, and paper tape
- Compression garment with TopiFoam™ (Byron Medical, Tucson, AZ): Not in buttocks, posterior flank, or back

POSTOPERATIVE CARE

- Dressing changes in 3-4 days
  - Tell patients to sit at bedside for 5 minutes after removing the garment before standing.
- No tub baths for the first week
- Compression garment at all times for 2 weeks; then at night for 2 weeks
- Foam under the garment for first 7 days

CAUTION: Make sure foam padding is flat against the patient's body to prevent potential contour deformities from rippling.

- Return to work in 3-5 days after small-volume procedures
- Large-volume procedures may need 7-10 days
- Full activities in 3-4 weeks as tolerated

HEALING COURSE

- **1-3 days:** Drainage from access incisions
- **3-5 days:** Maximal edema, drainage slows
- **7-10 days:** Resolving ecchymosis
- **4-6 weeks:** Resolving edema
- **8-10 weeks:** Induration in large-volume areas[8]
- **3-4 months:** Final contour

COMPLICATIONS

Table 84-2 *Plasma Lidocaine Levels and Symptoms of Toxicity*

Levels (mg/ml)	Symptoms
3-6	Subjective (circumoral numbness, tinnitus, drowsiness, lightheadedness, difficulty focusing)
5-9	Objective (tremors, twitching, shivering)
8-12	Seizures, cardiac depression
12-14	Unconscious, coma
20	Respiratory arrest
26	Cardiac arrest

From Matarasso A. Lidocaine in ultrasound-assisted lipoplasty. Clin Plast Surg 26:431, 1999.

Table 84-3 *Nonfatal Complications of Lipoplasty Alone and in Combination With Abdominoplasty*

Complications	Percent	Rate (Complications/Procedures)
Skin slough	0.0903	1:1107
Ultrasound-assisted lipoplasty skin burns	0.0712	1:1404
Deep venous thrombophlebitis	0.0329	1:3040
Pulmonary embolus	0.0266	1:3759
Excessive blood loss	0.0149	1:6711
Fluid overload	0.0138	1:7246
Fat emboli	0.0053	1:18,868
Cannula penetration of abdominal cavity	0.0021	1:47,619
Lidocaine toxicity	0.0021	1:47,619
Surgical shock	0.0011	1:90,909

From Hughes CE III. Reduction of lipoplasty risks and mortality: An ASAPS survey. Aesthetic Surg J 21:120, 2001.

Table 84-4 *Deaths from Lipoplasty, September 1, 1998 to August 31, 2000 (N = 94,159)*

Procedure	Percent	Rate (Death/Procedures)
Lipoplasty alone	0.0021	1:47,415
Lipoplasty with other procedures, excluding abdominoplasty	0.0137	1:7314
Lipoplasty with abdominoplasty, with or without other procedures	0.0305	1:3281

From Hughes CE III. Reduction of lipoplasty risks and mortality: An ASAPS survey. Aesthetic Surg J 21:120, 2001.

LIPOSUCTION BY AREA

HIP AND FLANKS

- **Flank (males)**
  - Begins in paraspinous area
  - Widest just above iliac crest
  - Anteriorly blends with lower abdominal adiposity of lateral rectus sheath
  - Begins at convexity below flare of rib cage; becomes convex and full over the iliac crests
  - Inferiorly defined by zone if adherence lying along the iliac crest
- **Hips (females)**
  - Similar area as the flank, only more inferior so that its bulk is centered **over the crests**
  - Ends lower than the flank
- **Gluteal depression**
  - Convexity between the hips above and the lateral thigh below
  - Also known as the *"saddlebag"*
- **Incisions**
  - Access incision on each side, either in lower hip/flank in the bikini line or in the lateral gluteal fold
  - Posteriorly may use paraspinous locations
- **Technical details**
  - Jackknife when prone
  - Average infiltration volumes: 500-800 ml in the hip

THIGHS

- Thigh should be a shallow convex arc on both anterior and posterior surfaces.
- Lateral thigh extends from the gluteal depression to the knee.
- Buttock extends from sacrum to inferior gluteal fold.
- *"Banana roll"* is the fullness from inferior gluteal fold to posterior upper thigh zone of adherence.
- There should be an unbroken curve from the iliac crest to the distal thigh.
- Medially there should be a slight convexity of the upper third of the medial thigh; middle to distal third is flat or slightly concave.
- **Ideal buttock**
  - Slightly convex
  - Nonptotic
  - Firm with a slight lateral gluteal depression

- In **women** the buttocks are **rounded,** and they flow into the lateral thigh.
- **Male** buttocks are more **angular** and almost **squared laterally;** more muscle, less fat, more firm.

KEY POINTS FOR THE THIGHS

- Do not treat the lateral buttock.
- Incise in both lateral gluteal creases.
- Four areas can be treated with the same incision: Banana roll, lateral thigh, buttock, flank.

ABDOMEN
- **Borders**
  - Xiphoid superiorly
  - Pubic ramus inferiorly
  - Laterally extends to the anterior iliac crest along the inguinal ligament
- Clearly delineated linea alba depression from top to bottom
- **Anteriorly**
  - Slight supraumbilical concavity
  - Infraumbilical convexity
- **Women**
  - Highlighted by bilateral concavities as defined by the flank from the rib to the iliac crest
- **Men**
  - Do **not** have a bilateral convexity (hourglass shape)
  - No flare at the iliac crest
  - Infraumbilical region should be flat
- **Incisions** (Fig. 84-5)
  - Suprapubic region
  - Inguinal creases
  - Umbilicus

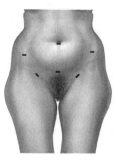

Fig. 84-5

ARMS
- Ideal arm is lean and has an anterior convexity of the deltoid merging with a convexity of the biceps.
- Posterior surface of the arm should be slightly convex from axilla to elbow.
- Patients with at least 1.5 cm of fat by the pinch test are good candidates.
- **Technical details**
  - When prone: Incision placed in posterior axillary fold and SAL incision at radial elbow
  - Long radial strokes to avoid waviness/contour deformity
  - Use full-length contoured TopiFoam

CAUTION: Perform UAL from a radial incision only to prevent ulnar nerve problems.

KEY POINTS
- ✔ Consider whether you have chosen the correct procedure: Liposuction versus skin resection.
- ✔ Mark the patient while he or she is awake; allow him or her to guide you in choosing the areas to be treated.
- ✔ Allow 7-10 minutes after infiltration before suction for maximal epinephrine effect (consider infiltration before preparation and draping to save time).
- ✔ Perform repeated assessments of progress to avoid contour deformities.
- ✔ Underresection is preferable to a difficult-to-correct contour deformity.
- ✔ Strict garment use is mandatory to prevent contour deformity and chronic seroma formation.

REFERENCES

1. Rohrich RJ, Kenkel JM, Beran SJ. Ultrasound-Assisted Liposuction. St Louis: Quality Medical Publishing, 1998.
2. Rohrich RJ, Beran SJ, Fodor PB. The role of subcutaneous infiltration in suction-assisted lipoplasty: A review. Plast Reconstr Surg 99:514, 1997.
3. Klein JA. The tumescent technique for local anesthesia improves safety in large-volume liposuction. Plast Reconstr Surg 92:1085, 1993.
4. Goodpasture JC, Bunkis J. Quantitative analysis of blood and fat in suction lipectomy aspirates. Plast Reconstr Surg 78:765, 1986.
5. Courtiss EH, Choucair RJ, Donelan MB. Large-volume suction lipectomy: An analysis of 108 patients. Plast Reconstr Surg 89:1068, 1992.
6. Klein JA. The tumescent technique: Anesthesia and modified liposuction technique. Dermatol Clin 8:425, 1990.
7. Zocchi ML. Ultrasonic assisted lipoplasty. Technical refinements and clinical evaluations. Clin Plast Surg 23:575, 1996.
8. American Society of Plastic Surgeons. Practice Advisory on Liposuction: Executive Summary, 2003, p 2.

85. Brachioplasty

Sacha I. Obaid
Jeffrey E. Janis
Jason E. Leedy

ANATOMY (Fig. 85-1)

- Subcutaneous fat in the arms tends to collect **posteriorly** and **inferiorly**; very little subcutaneous fat is found medially.
  - The upper humeral fat deposits are particularly troublesome for patients when they wear fitted blouses or jackets.
- The fat and skin of the upper arm are supported by **two fascial systems.**
  - **Superficial fascial system**
    - ▸ Encases the fat of the upper arm circumferentially from axilla to elbow
  - The **longitudinal fascial system**[1]
    - ▸ Begins at the clavicle as the clavipectoral fascia
    - ▸ Extends to the axillary fascia
    - ▸ Connects to the superficial fascial system
- With age and weight gain, the superficial fascial system and the axillary fascia loosen.
  - Creates a loose hammock-like effect
  - Results in significant ptosis of the posteromedial arm
- Muscles of the arm are enveloped by a deep investing fascia.
- All major neurovascular bundles lie deep to the deep investing fascia.

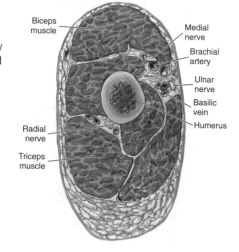

Biceps muscle
Medial nerve
Brachial artery
Ulnar nerve
Basilic vein
Humerus
Radial nerve
Triceps muscle

Fig. 85-1

NOTE: The only nerves found superficial to the deep investing fascia are small branches of the medial brachial cutaneous nerve or the intercostobrachial nerve.

TIP: The entire dissection in excisional or liposuction brachioplasty should remain superficial to the deep investing fascia. If this plane is not violated, then all of the important neurovascular structures in the upper extremity are preserved.

PATIENT EVALUATION

ASSESSMENT

- A complete history should be obtained, including weight loss/gain, tobacco use, and all other medical problems.
- Physical examination should be performed.
- General evaluation of the arms including range of motion at shoulder, elbow, and hand, and grip strength.
- Assess for excess fat, excess skin, location of any skin laxity, and overall skin quality and tone.
- **Upper arm rejuvenation** patients can be divided into **three types** (Table 85-1).[2]
  - **Type I:** Relative excess of fat in the upper arm with good skin tone and minimal laxity
    - ▸ Best treated with liposuction alone
  - **Type II:** Skin laxity that can be **horizontal, vertical,** or **both**
    - ▸ **Type IIA:** Only **proximal** arm redundancy
      - ◆ If redundancy is **strictly horizontal,** then a vertically oriented wedge or an elliptical **excision of skin** can be made that is isolated to the axillary fold (Fig. 85-2).
      - ◆ If there is **vertical and horizontal laxity,** then a **T-shaped resection** along the proximal upper arm is required (Fig. 85-3).

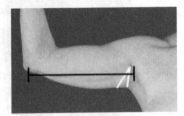

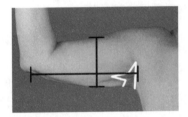

Fig. 85-2   Fig. 85-3

- ▸ **Type IIB:** Skin redundancy of the **entire upper arm** from elbow to chest wall.
  - ◆ If there is isolated **vertical** skin redundancy, a **horizontal excision** can be performed along the brachial groove (Fig. 85-4).
  - ◆ If there is **horizontal and vertical excess,** an **L-shaped excision** is made in the axilla (Fig. 85-5).
    - - Extends into the arm as far as the excess skin in the arm does.
    - - The L may extend all the way to the elbow if necessary.

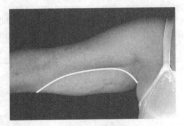

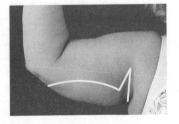

Fig. 85-4   Fig. 85-5

▶ **Type IIC:** Laxity that may extend **onto the lateral chest wall** (Fig. 85-6).
  ✦ An **extended brachioplasty** is needed that extends onto the chest wall.
  ✦ **These are typically massive-weight-loss patients.**

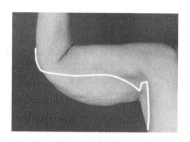

Fig. 85-6

• **Type III:** Both **significant excess fat** and **redundant skin** in the arm; several options:
  ▶ Further weight loss before surgery
  ▶ Staged treatment with liposuction first, followed by subsequent excisional brachioplasty
  ▶ Combined single-stage liposuction and excisional brachioplasty
  ▶ Subtypes A, B, and C: Specific locations of the skin excess
    ✦ A: Proximal
    ✦ B: Entire arm
    ✦ C: Arm and chest

Table 85-1 *Classification of Upper Arm Contouring*

Type	Skin Excess	Fat Excess	Location of Skin Excess
I	Minimal	Moderate	N/A
IIA	Moderate	Minimal	Proximal
IIB	Moderate	Minimal	Entire arm
IIC	Moderate	Minimal	Arm and chest
IIIA	Moderate	Moderate	Proximal
IIIB	Moderate	Moderate	Entire arm
IIIC	Moderate	Moderate	Arm and chest

From Appelt EA, Janis JE, Rohrich RJ. An algorithmic approach to upper arm contouring. Plast Reconstr Surg 118:237-246, 2006.

CONTRAINDICATIONS

■ **Absolute**
  • Neurologic or vascular disorders of the upper extremity
  • Lymphedema of the arms secondary to previous axillary lymph node dissection
  • Unrealistic patient expectations
■ **Relative[3]**
  • Symptomatic Raynaud's disease
  • Connective tissue disorders
  • Advanced rheumatoid arthritis

PATIENT EDUCATION

■ Because of their location (which is frequently exposed by everyday clothing), the scars from excisional brachioplasty *are probably the most noticeable scars in all aesthetic surgery.*
■ Given the prominence of the scars, they **must** be discussed with the patient preoperatively.

TIP: It is often helpful to draw the scars on the patient's arm during the preoperative consultation and to document this in the medical record. This may help prevent complaints postoperatively about the scars. At the same time that the scars are being demonstrated to the patient, the proposed effect of an excisional brachioplasty can be demonstrated. While the patient stands in front of a mirror with the arms out, the surgeon pinches the skin of the arm from behind to show the tightening effect a brachioplasty could have.

- Patients must also be warned of temporary areas of numbness in the upper arm secondary to transection of branches of medial brachial cutaneous nerves or intercostobrachial cutaneous nerves.

ALGORITHM FOR TREATMENT (Fig. 85-7)

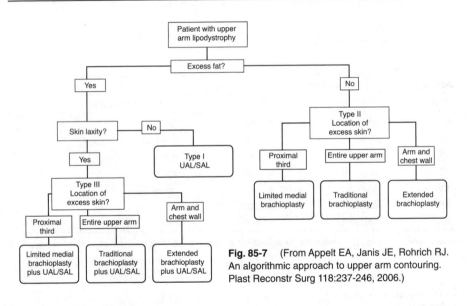

Fig. 85-7   (From Appelt EA, Janis JE, Rohrich RJ. An algorithmic approach to upper arm contouring. Plast Reconstr Surg 118:237-246, 2006.)

OPERATIVE TECHNIQUE

LIPOSUCTION
- Liposuction may be performed as a stand-alone procedure for arm rejuvenation.
- It may also be performed as the first step in excisional brachioplasty.
  - Decreases arm bulk
  - Increases the amount of skin that can be successfully resected
- Suction should be concentrated in the medial and posterior quadrants of the proximal half of the upper arm.

- Incisions should be made in posterior lateral elbow region and in superior portion of axilla anteriorly for infiltration of wetting solution and liposuction.

CAUTION: Care must be taken to keep the cannula away from the axilla and the posteromedial elbow to avoid damaging the nerves of the brachial plexus or the ulnar nerve.

- Liposuction should be performed at an intermediate depth.
- Approximately 0.5 cm of subcutaneous fat should be left on the skin to prevent contour irregularities.[3]

CIRCUMFERENTIAL PARA-AXILLARY SUPERFICIAL TUMESCENT (CAST) LIPOSUCTION

- Developed as alternative to traditional liposuction in the upper extremities[4,5]
  - Traditional liposuction of the posterolateral arm frequently left patients with sagging skin.
- Attempts to maximize skin retraction with circumferential liposuction of the arm, including superficially and in the subdermal regions
- Realistic goals to suggest when advising patients contemplating CAST liposuction:
  - Decrease in brachial fat and creation of a straighter inferior brachial border will help the patient feel better in clothes.
  - CAST liposuction **will not improve skin wrinkling.**
- **Principles**
  - Incisions are made at the olecranon, anterior axilla, posterior axilla, and middle third of the arm at the boundary of the medial and posterolateral regions.
  - Occasionally incisions are made in the dorsoradial arm and the midaxillary line at the areolar level.
  - Wetting solution is infiltrated into the arm as with traditional liposuction.
  - Wetting solution is also infiltrated superficially posterolaterally to create a **peau d'orange** appearance.
  - The arm is conceptually divided into three regions: **Anterolateral, medial,** and **posterolateral** (Fig. 85-8).
  - The **medial** region is treated by pretunneling from the olecranon and axillary sites longitudinally.
    - ▶ If the preoperative pinch test in this region is **10 mm or less,** only pretunneling is done.
    - ▶ If the preoperative pinch test is **greater than 10 mm,** superficial pretunneling and deep suctioning are performed.

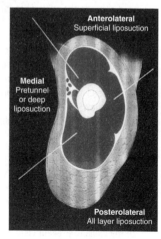

Fig. 85-8   Conceptual division of the arm into three parts. (From Strauch B, Greenspun D, Levine J, et al. A technique of brachioplasty. Plast Reconstr Surg 113:1044-1049, 2004.)

> TIP: Do not liposuction under thin anteromedial skin, especially near the axilla, because of the propensity for wrinkling in this region.

- The anterolateral arm is treated with superficial liposuction to remove superficial and dense subdermal fat.
  - Gilliland and Lyos[4,5] believe that this creates a sheet of confluent scar that will aid in skin retraction.
- The posterolateral arm is treated with deep, superficial, and subdermal liposuction to maximize skin retraction.
- In addition, a serrated cannula is used without suction to internally dermabrade the flap undersurface.
  - This theoretically creates a confluent sheet of scar extending circumferentially around the arm and onto the trunk.
  - Care must be taken not to curette more than once in a given area to prevent indentations.
  - If any indentations occur, Gilliland and Lyos advise fat grafting immediately.
- The paraaxillary region is treated with serrated cannulas.
  - Disrupts osteocutaneous ligaments
  - Allows for the most complete fat extraction possible
- Jackson-Pratt drains are placed postoperatively.
- **Outcomes**
- 84.6% of patients were satisfied or very satisfied with the results in two studies.[4,5]
- 11.5% had an excisional brachioplasty to help treat redundant skin that persisted postoperatively.
- 38.5% seroma rate occurred.
- 100% of patients develop fine skin wrinkling.

MINIBRACHIOPLASTY (Fig. 85-9)

- For patients with **mild skin laxity** and **mild-to-moderate excess fat** in the upper arm, a **minibrachioplasty** can be performed.
- Combines removal of excess fat through liposuction with removal of skin laxity through an incision limited either to the axilla or to the axilla and the proximal portion of the upper arm.
- **Preoperative markings**
- Areas of excess fat are marked as described earlier.
- Liposuction should concentrate on the excess fat found in the **posteromedial** region of the upper arm.
- After being marked, the patient should abduct the arm 90 degrees at the shoulder and flex the arm 90 degrees at the elbow.
- Use a **pinch test** to mark an ellipse of skin in the axilla that can be resected to help restore an aesthetic contour of the upper arm.
- If the proposed elliptical resection does not appear to correct the skin laxity, then a T-shaped extension of the incision can be planned, confined to the upper third of the arm.
- The elliptical excision is designed to limit the scar to the axilla to prevent visibility.

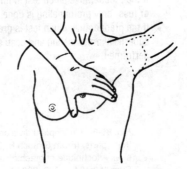

Fig. 85-9 Preoperative markings. (From Strauch B, Greenspun D, Levine J, et al. A technique of brachioplasty. Plast Reconstr Surg 113:1044-1049, 2004.)

- **Principles**
  - The first step is **liposuction** of excess upper arm fat, concentrated in the posteromedial regions, as described earlier.
  - After liposuction, an elliptical skin excision is performed transversely in the axilla.
    - ▸ The elliptical skin excision in the axilla has a **high potential for scar widening or dehiscence.**
      - ✦ Lockwood[1] advocates using permanent stitches to anchor the superficial fascial system of the arm to the dense axillary fascia and clavipectoral fascia (a tough structure firmly attached to the periosteum of the clavicle).
      - ✦ Anchoring the superficial fascial system to the axillary and clavipectoral fascia helps correct the laxity of the longitudinal fascial sling that develops with age.

TIP: The biggest key to a successful minibrachioplasty is patient selection. A minibrachioplasty with superficial fascial suspension to the axillary and clavipectoral fascia can be a highly effective operation if the patient has mild-to-moderate skin excess in addition to excess fat; however, if the patient has moderate-to-severe skin excess with or without excess fat, a standard brachioplasty should be performed to achieve the desirable contour.

STANDARD BRACHIOPLASTY

- A standard brachioplasty should be used for patients with moderate-to-severe excess skin with or without excess fat.
- If there is a significant amount of excess fat in addition to excess skin, then the procedure should begin with liposuction.
- **Preoperative markings for standard brachioplasty are as follows[3]:**
  - With the patient sitting or standing, have the patient abduct the arm 90 degrees at the shoulder and flex 90 degrees at the elbow.
  - Place a dotted line in the bicipital groove extending from the apex of the axilla down to the elbow.
    - ▸ This dotted line represents the proposed scar location.
  - Place a solid line 1 cm above and parallel to the line in the bicipital groove.
    - ▸ This line marks the proposed upper incision for the brachioplasty.
  - The surgeon should place his or her index and long fingers along the proposed upper-line incision and use the thumb to pinch the inferomedial skin up toward the upper incision.
    - ▸ This pinch test signals how much skin can be excised, and marks should be placed inferiorly to delineate the proposed lower incision.
  - Three to five vertical lines should be drawn perpendicular to the longitudinal lines.
    - ▸ This divides the proposed resection into thirds or fifths.
    - ▸ These lines assist in lining up the closure (see later).
- **Operative principles**

TIP: To help minimize edema, communicate your concerns to the anaesthesiologist preoperatively and request that the intravenous line not be placed in the upper extremity.

- Incisions should be made in the posterolateral elbow region and in the superior portion of the axilla anteriorly for the infiltration of wetting solution and for liposuction.

TIP: Even if liposuction is not going to be performed, wetting solution should be infiltrated to decrease blood loss and assist with dissection.

To prevent ulnar nerve injury, avoid placing liposuction access incisions medially at the elbow.

- Liposuction is performed leaving a **minimum of 0.5 cm of fat** on the skin.
- A No. 10 blade is used to incise through the proximal portion of the upper incision.
- Bovie electrocautery is used to dissect down to the deep investing fascia.
- Dissection is taken over the deep investing fascia toward the inferior mark.
- Towel clips are placed along the skin flap to be excised, and the flap is advanced toward the upper incision.
- Confirm that the wound will close if the proposed inferior incision is made; if not, the inferior incision is redrawn and incised.

TIP: The arm should be divided into three to five segments, and each segment should be treated sequentially, including closure. This is critical because the arm tends to become very edematous during this procedure. The edema can be severe, and it is not uncommon for surgeons to not be able to close portions of the brachioplasty incision because of it. These portions can generally be closed if performed immediately instead of closing only after dissecting the entire wound.

- Closure begins with reapproximation of the superficial fascial system, followed by closure of the deep dermal and subcuticular layers.
  - ▸ The superficial fascial system should be closed with either long-lasting absorbable sutures or permanent sutures to help relieve tension.

TIP: To avoid postoperative numbness, leave some fat on the deep investing fascia at the junction between the middle and lower third of the upper arm. This helps protect the medial antebrachial cutaneous nerve, which exits the deep investing fascia here, often with the basilic vein.[3]

- **If the wound crosses the axilla, a Z-plasty** must be performed to prevent scar retraction and axillary banding.
- Drains should be placed to prevent seroma formation.
- After skin closure, the wound is dressed and an Ace bandage is wrapped beginning distally at the hands and traveling up to the axilla to assist with edema.

BRACHIOPLASTY IN MASSIVE-WEIGHT-LOSS PATIENTS

■ Massive-weight-loss patients often develop a "bat-wing" appearance to their arms with severe skin laxity that extends from the olecranon across the axilla to the chest wall (Fig. 85-10).[6]

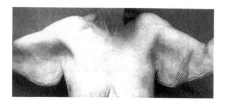

Fig. 85-10 (From Strauch B, Greenspun D, Levine J, et al. A technique of brachioplasty. Plast Reconstr Surg 113:1044-1049, 2004.)

■ A standard brachioplasty addresses skin laxity from the olecranon to the axilla.
• Does not significantly affect excess skin of the axilla or the lateral chest wall.
• To affect this skin in this zone, a brachioplasty must extend across the axilla and onto the chest wall.
■ As in a standard brachioplasty, the patient is marked with the arms abducted 90 degrees and the elbow flexed 90 degrees.
■ An elliptical incision is planned as in a standard upper arm brachioplasty.
• However, instead of terminating the incision in the axillary dome, the incision is carried further into the axilla and even down on to the chest wall as necessary.
• The incision is continued as far as the skin laxity continues.
■ To help make the scar less noticeable, a sinusoidal variation can be added to the proposed excision; this avoids the final scar lying in a straight line.
■ **An axillary Z-plasty *must* be added to the proposed skin excision to prevent contracture across the axilla and to restore the appearance of the axillary dome** (Fig. 85-11).
• Should be designed with 60-degree angles to the longitudinal incision.
• Central transverse limb of the Z should lie in transverse axis of axillary dome.
■ The intraoperative technique is similar to the standard brachioplasty described previously.
■ **Minimal undermining of the skin flaps** should be necessary given the already lax nature of the skin.
■ As with standard brachioplasty, it is critical to divide the incision into thirds, fourths, or fifths.
• Perform the operation segmentally to ensure that edema will not prevent closure of appropriately designed skin flaps.

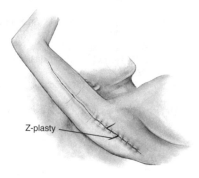

Z-plasty

Fig. 85-11

POSTOPERATIVE CONSIDERATIONS

- Postoperative complications include seroma, hematoma, infection, lymphocele, numbness, peripheral nerve pain, and wound dehiscence, especially in the axilla.
- Ace wraps should be maintained for at least 2 days postoperatively to help minimize edema.
- After 2 days, the patient may continue to use Ace wrap bandages or switch to a surgical sleeve or a long-sleeved surgical vest.
- Gabapentin, 100-300 mg/day, can be used to treat peripheral nerve pain, if needed.[3]

KEY POINTS

- ✔ Successful rejuvenation of the arm requires accurate assessment of the deformity and appropriate treatment selection.
- ✔ Patients with mild-to-moderate excess fat but good skin quality should have traditional or CAST liposuction performed.
- ✔ Patients with mild-to-moderate amounts of excess skin and fat should have a minibrachioplasty performed with skin excision confined to the axilla.
- ✔ Patients with moderate-to-severe amounts of excess skin should have a traditional brachioplasty performed with a longitudinal skin excision planned from the axilla to the elbow.
- ✔ Patients with severe excess skin, such as massive-weight-loss patients with bat-wing deformity, should have an extended brachioplasty performed with the skin excision from the elbow to the axilla and extending onto the lateral chest wall.

REFERENCES

1. Lockwood T. Brachioplasty with superficial fascial system suspension. Plast Reconstr Surg 96:912-920, 1995.
2. Appelt EA, Janis JE, Rohrich RJ. An algorithmic approach to upper arm contouring. Plast Reconstr Surg 118:237-246, 2006.
3. Nahai F. The Art of Aesthetic Surgery: Principles and Techniques. St Louis: Quality Medical Publishing, 2005.
4. Gilliland MD, Lyos AT. CAST liposuction of the arm improves aesthetic results. Aesthetic Plast Surg 21:225-229, 1997.
5. Gilliland MD, Lyos AT. CAST liposuction: An alternative to brachioplasty. Aesthetic Plast Surg 21:398-402, 1997.
6. Strauch B, Greenspun D, Levine J, et al. A technique of brachioplasty. Plast Reconstr Surg 113:1044-1049, 2004.

86. Abdominoplasty

Sacha I. Obaid
Jason E. Leedy

ANATOMY

- **The abdominal wall is composed of seven layers:**
  1. Skin
  2. Subcutaneous fat
  3. Scarpa's fascia (the superficial fascial system of the abdomen)
  4. Subscarpal fat
  5. Anterior rectus sheath
  6. Muscle
  7. Posterior rectus sheath

SKIN
- The skin of the abdominal wall receives a rich vascular supply from multiple muscle and fascial perforating vessels.
- The skin of the abdominal wall can vary in
quality depending on a person's genetics,
age, previous pregnancies, and history of
weight gain and loss.
- The skin of the abdominal wall may
feature multiple **striae**, which are
evidence of **attenuated or absent dermis**.

FAT
- The abdominal wall has **two** layers of fat,
superficial and deep, separated by
Scarpa's fascia (Fig. 86-1).
  - The **superficial layer** of fat is thicker,
denser, more durable, and has a
heartier blood supply.
  - The **deeper layer** of fat is less dense
and receives most of its blood from the
subdermal plexus and the underlying musculocutaneous perforators.

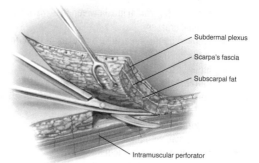

Subdermal plexus

Scarpa's fascia

Subscarpal fat

Intramuscular perforator

Fig. 86-1

TIP: Because the blood supply to the deeper fat is distinct from the blood supply to the skin, it
can be more easily excised when attempting to thin the abdominal wall flap in an abdominoplasty. By contrast, thinning the superficial layer of fat may lead to vascular compromise of
the overlying skin.

- There are **four paired muscle groups** of the abdominal wall.
  1. Rectus abdominis
  2. External oblique
  3. Internal oblique
  4. Transversalis abdominis
- The aponeurotic portions of the transversalis muscle and the two oblique muscles envelop the rectus abdominis muscles, forming the anterior and posterior rectus sheaths and meeting in the midline to form the linea alba.
- The **arcuate line** represents a transition point.
  - **Above the arcuate line,** there are distinct anterior and posterior rectus sheaths.
  - **Below the arcuate line,** contributions from the internal oblique and transversalis join contributions from the external and internal obliques to form a single anterior rectus sheath with no posterior rectus sheath.
  - The arcuate line lies roughly halfway between the umbilicus and the symphysis pubis.

VASCULARITY OF THE ABDOMINAL WALL

- Huger[1] divided the vascular supply to the abdominal wall into **three zones.**
  - **Zone I**
    - Between the lateral borders of the rectus sheath from the costal margin to a horizontal line drawn between the two anterior superior iliac spines
    - Supplied primarily by superficial branches of the **superior and inferior epigastric systems**
  - **Zone II**
    - Below the horizontal line between the two anterior superior iliac spines to the pubic and inguinal creases
    - Supplied by the superficial branches of the **circumflex iliac** and **external pudendal vessels**
  - **Zone III**
    - Superior to zone II and lateral to zone I
    - **Intercostals, subcostals,** and **lumbar** vessels
- Sensation to the abdomen is from **intercostal nerves T7-12.**
  - **Lateral cutaneous branches**
    - Perforate the intercostal muscles at the midaxillary line
    - Then travel within the subcutaneous plane
  - **Anterior cutaneous branches**
    - Travel between the transverse and internal oblique muscles to penetrate the posterior rectus sheath just lateral to the rectus
    - Eventually enter the rectus muscles and then pass to the overlying fascia and skin

UMBILICUS

- The umbilicus is located **on or near the midline at the level of the iliac crest.**
  - Only **1.7%** of patients have the umbilicus located exactly in the midline of the body.[2]
  - An **aesthetically pleasing umbilicus** has the following characteristics[3]:
    - Superior hooding
    - Inferior retraction
    - Round or ellipsoid shape
    - Shallow

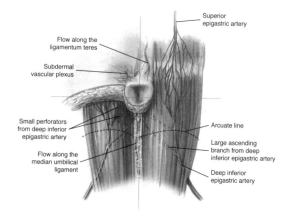

- **Blood supply to the umbilicus**
  (Fig. 86-2) **is from:**
  ▸ Subdermal plexus
  ▸ Right and left deep inferior
    epigastric artery (DIEA)
  ▸ Ligamentum teres
  ▸ Median umbilical ligament

Fig. 86-2   Blood supply to the umbilicus.

PREOPERATIVE EVALUATION

HISTORY AND PHYSICAL EXAMINATION
- **Complete history should include[3]:**
  - Number of pregnancies and children
  - Previous cesarean section or other abdominal surgery
  - Previous or current hernias
  - Exercise routine
  - Gastrointestinal history including irritable bowel syndrome or constipation
  - Respiratory history including asthma, smoking, or sleep apnea
  - History of weight loss and gain, and active diet regimen

TIP: Abdominoplasty is a huge stressor in terms of blood supply to the abdominal wall flap.
To minimize complications, avoid operating on active smokers. If a patient has a history
of smoking, the plastic surgeon should insist that the patient quit smoking before the
abdominoplasty and openly discuss the increased risk of complications. This will not only
encourage cessation of smoking but also will help discourage patients from lying about
their smoking history. A urine nicotine test may be indicated.

- Examine the skin of the abdominal wall for **striae,** which represent thinning or absent dermis.
  - The surgeon must explain to the patient that:
    ▸ Striae located inferior to the umbilicus may be removed as part of the abdominoplasty
    ▸ Most striae above the umbilicus will not be removed
    ▸ Striae above the umbilicus may become more prominent, because the abdominal wall flap is
      stretched by the abdominoplasty

- The presence of **excess skin** must be assessed.
  - The patient must be examined while standing, supine, and sitting.
  - If the patient is examined only in the standing or supine position, the surgeon may be fooled into thinking there is little or no excess skin.
  - When the patient sits, the surgeon immediately notices if there is excess abdominal skin.
- Examine for **rashes or excoriations,** especially under the abdominal pannus in obese patients and massive-weight-loss patients.
- Look for **adhesions** where the skin and fat are tethered to deeper structures.
  - There is commonly an adhesion at that level at the waist.
  - In morbidly obese or massive-weight-loss patients there may be an additional adhesion or roll of skin superiorly.
  - These adhesions may hinder the movement of the abdominoplasty skin flap.
  - Surgical release of these adhesions can pose a risk of ischemia in the overlying skin flap.
  - Options for addressing the second adhesion are discontinuous undermining with either a liposuction cannula or Lockwood dissector, a *fleur-de-lis* abdominoplasty, or a second-stage reverse abdominoplasty.
- The **presence of scars** represents alterations to the blood supply of the abdominal wall.
  - **Upper midline scars** may limit inferior movement of the abdominal skin flap.
    - ▸ They may need to be treated with release at the time of abdominoplasty.
    - ▸ In some patients consideration may be given to a *fleur-de-lis* abdominoplasty.
  - **Subcostal scars** are particularly troubling.
    - ▸ They represent an interruption of the superolateral blood supply that the abdominoplasty skin flap relies on for blood supply postoperatively.
    - ▸ **Of all those undergoing abdominoplasty, these patients are at the highest risk for postoperative wound-healing complications.**

CAUTION: To prevent wound-healing complications, the abdominal wall skin flap *must not* be undermined beneath a subcostal incision. The limitations of undermining, limited results, and high risk of complications must be discussed with these patients. Many are not candidates for an abdominoplasty.

- Musculofascial laxity must be assessed.
  - **A diver's test** can be performed with the patient first standing and then flexing at the waist.
    - ▸ Worsening of lower abdominal wall fullness indicates **musculofascial laxity.**
  - An additional test for musculofascial laxity is the **pinch test.**
    - ▸ Abdominal fullness is assessed with the patient both relaxed and actively tensing the abdominal wall.
    - ▸ If the amount of fullness that can be pinched is significantly decreased by tensing the abdominal wall, then the patient has significant musculofascial laxity.
- Midline **diastasis recti abdominis** must be examined.

TIP: Nearly all patients who have previously been pregnant have some degree of musculofascial laxity of the abdominal wall in addition to excess skin.

- Examine and document any **hernias,** including incisional, epigastric, periumbilical, and inguinal hernias, especially in patients who have had previous surgeries and massive-weight-loss patients.

NOTE: The importance of a thorough hernia examination cannot be overstated. Preoperative knowledge of hernias can help the surgeon avoid injuring the bowel during dissection. In addition, depending on the size of the hernia and the comfort level of the plastic surgeon, preoperative knowledge of a hernia may allow the plastic surgeon to coordinate with a general surgeon to assist with hernia repair at the time of the operation.

INFORMED CONSENT

- In addition to the standard risks of surgery, the plastic surgeon must discuss the location and the length of the scars with the patient.
  - The standard lower abdominal transverse scar
  - The potential need for a short vertical midline scar
    - This "T scar" may be necessary for patients with smaller amounts of excess abdominal wall skin and fat.
  - Potential for cutaneous deformities ("dog-ears") at the lateral ends of the abdominoplasty incision.
    - If these are present, revisional surgeries, including excision of this skin or liposuction of the underlying fullness, may be necessary.
- Wound-healing complications must be discussed.
  - Both the transverse incision at the waist and the umbilicus itself are at risk for poor wound healing because of poor vascularity.
- Loss or malposition of the umbilicus must be discussed.
  - Patients should be reminded preoperatively that the umbilicus is truly midline in only 1.7% of patients.[2]
- The risk of postoperative seromas must be discussed.
  - The need for and purpose of postoperative drains should be explained.
- The potential need for revisional surgeries or procedures must be discussed.
- The surgeon must discuss financial arrangements and the patient's responsibilities for these procedures.
- Patients must understand that they will not be able to walk fully erect for several days after the operation.
  - They will need a minimum of 2 weeks off from work.
  - They will not be able to do any strenuous exercise or lifting for at least 6 weeks postoperatively.
- The patient must be warned of the risk of **pulmonary embolism.**
  - Because of this risk, in addition to pneumatic devices, early ambulation is required.

PROCEDURE SELECTION

- Patients with mild fat excess, no excess skin, and good skin tone are candidates for **liposuction alone.**[4]
- Patients with mild fat excess, no excess skin, good skin tone, and rectus diastasis should have **liposuction combined with endoscopic diastasis repair.**
- Patients with skin and fat excess isolated to the infraumbilical region should have an **infraumbilical miniabdominoplasty** with liposuction and diastasis repair.
- Patients with significant amounts of skin and fat excess not limited to the infraumbilical region should have a **traditional abdominoplasty** with or without liposuction of the flank.
- Patients with significant extra skin that may extend far laterally and even around to the back should have **circumferential abdominoplasty.**
  - This is the procedure of choice for most massive-weight-loss patients.

- Patients with excess skin at the lateral abdominal area, lateral hip and thigh, pubis, and possibly anteromedial thigh are candidates for **Lockwood's high lateral tension abdominoplasty.**
- Patients with excess skin both vertically and horizontally (especially in the upper midline region) are candidates for a **fleur-de-lis abdominoplasty.**

TRADITIONAL ABDOMINOPLASTY

PREOPERATIVE MARKINGS
- Patients should be encouraged to wear their undergarments of choice the day of surgery.
  - This helps the surgeon plan the lower incision with the goal of hiding as much of it under these garments as possible.
- Preoperative markings begin with identification of the pubic bone and the anterior superior iliac spine bilaterally.
- The planned incision should be marked beginning transversely at the level of the pubic bone.
  - At least **5 cm** must be left between this incision and the top of the vulval commissure to prevent distortion of the vulvar region postoperatively.
- The transverse marks are extended laterally and superiorly toward the hips bilaterally.
  - The lateralmost points of the incision should lie inferior to the anterior superior iliac spine (ASIS) to prevent visibility of the scar postoperatively.
- The surgeon should perform a pinch test to determine how much skin can be resected from the abdomen comfortably.
  - This pinch test is used to design a proposed upper incision.
  - The surgeon should determine whether the skin and fat all the way up to and just past the umbilicus should be excised in the operating room.
  - If there is any question, the surgeon must have a discussion with the patient about the high likelihood of needing a **small vertical component** to the incision with a final "inverted T"–shaped scar, which is more noticeable than the traditional transverse abdominoplasty scar.
- Areas to be considered for concomitant liposuction are marked preoperatively.

> TIP: Most patients who present for abdominoplasty have at least some degree of fat excess in the hips, flanks, and/or thighs. These deposits frequently become more noticeable postoperatively. Both the surgeon and the patient must be aware of this and consider concomitant or staged liposuction with the abdominoplasty procedure for optimal results. Failure to recognize this and discuss it preoperatively may result in an unhappy patient with a compromised final result.

PRINCIPLES
- Before the patient enters the operating room, the surgeon and the anaesthesiologist must **test the bed** to make sure it can flex at the patient's waist to an optimal level.

> TIP: Failure to test the bed preoperatively can cause significant intraoperative difficulties.

- After induction of anaesthesia, liposuction should be performed in all planned areas.
- The abdominoplasty begins with placement of two traction sutures at 3 o'clock and 9 o'clock in the umbilicus.

TIP: Before making the circumumbilical incision, take care to place these sutures with asymmetrical tails; for instance, with one long tail and one short tail on the right and two long tails to this suture on the left to orient the umbilicus. This maneuver helps prevent twisting of the umbilical stalk during closure and subsequent poor blood flow.

- The umbilicus is incised circularly, and dissecting scissors are used to separate the umbilicus from the abdominal skin and fat all the way down to the rectus sheath.
  - Avoid skeletonizing the umbilical stalk, which leads to compromised vascularity of the umbilicus.
- The inferior incision is made bilaterally.
- Dissection is taken straight down to the fascia overlying the rectus and oblique musculature.
- The skin and fat of the abdominal wall are elevated from the underlying muscular fascia in a loose areolar plane up to the costal margins laterally and to the xiphoid process medially.
- Leave a small amount of fat on the muscular fascia in the region of the anterior superior iliac spine to prevent injury to the lateral femoral cutaneous nerve.

TIP: The importance of leaving a small amount of fat on the muscular fascia in the region of the anterior superior iliac spine cannot be overemphasized. This prevents injury to the lateral femoral cutaneous nerve, which can cause significant pain, numbness, and dysesthesia in the hip and medial thigh region postoperatively. van Uchelen et al[5] found a 10% incidence of injury to this nerve in their review of abdominoplasty procedures.

CAUTION: As dissection is taken along the muscular fascia centrally, care must be taken to identify and preserve the umbilical stalk. Failure to do so results in transection of the umbilical blood supply and likely umbilical necrosis postoperatively.

TIP: Remember that there are a number of periumbilical musculocutaneous perforating vessels. These periumbilical perforators should signal the surgeon to slow the dissection and search for the umbilical stalk to prevent transaction.

- Once the abdominal flap is elevated, the rectus diastasis is repaired.
  - A cotton-tipped applicator is used to apply methylene blue to the rectus sheath elliptically as a proposed area to be imbricated.
  - The rectus sheath is imbricated or reinforced by placing interrupted sutures along the marked repair.
  - Rectus plication helps narrow the waist and correct laxity in the abdominal wall that occurs in all women who have been pregnant.
- After a first row of interrupted permanent sutures is placed, a second reinforcing permanent suture can be run from the xiphoid to the umbilicus, and a separate reinforcing suture can be run infraumbilically to the pubis.

TIP: It is essential to begin rectus plication just inferior to the xiphoid process. Failure to do so can result in a postoperative bulge that is fairly distressing to the patient.

- **Rectus plication** must be performed using **permanent sutures.**
  - Using ultrasound imaging, van Uchelen et al[5] revealed a 40% recurrence rate for diastasis in 40 patients at 64 months when plication had been performed using absorbable sutures.
  - Nahas et al[6-8] revealed a 0% recurrence rate for diastasis in 12 patients by CT scans at 76-84 months when permanent sutures were used.

> TIP: Plication of the rectus fascia tends to be the most painful portion of the operation. Local anaesthetic delivered by continuous-infusion catheters to the region of the rectus plication can significantly reduce postoperative pain.

- If used, Jackson-Pratt drains should be brought out through the hair-bearing skin of the pubic region.
- The bed is flexed, bringing the patient to a seated position, and the amount of skin and fat that can be resected from the abdominal wall while allowing a tension-free closure is marked.
- This excess skin and fat are resected.
- The wound is copiously irrigated.
- The level of the umbilicus is transposed with a marking pen to the overlying skin of the abdominal wall.
- The umbilicus is inset.
- The superficial fascial system is closed, followed by closure of the deep dermal and subcuticular layers.
- An abdominal binder is placed postoperatively.

MINIABDOMINOPLASTY[3]

- The miniabdominoplasty is useful for patients with primarily **infraumbilical excess of skin and fat.**
- A **shorter scar** is planned than for a traditional abdominoplasty.
  - The scar should be **12-16 cm long.**
- Rather than separating the umbilicus from the abdominal wall flap, it **remains attached.**
- The umbilical stalk is transected at the level of the anterior abdominal wall fascia.
- The resulting umbilical fascial defect is repaired.
- The rectus diastasis is repaired using permanent sutures.
- A more conservative skin and fat resection is performed than for a traditional abdominoplasty.
  - The umbilicus is usually moved approximately 2 cm inferiorly with this procedure.
- Liposuction is frequently added to this procedure to further improve abdominal contour, especially in the supraumbilical region.

HIGH-LATERAL-TENSION ABDOMINOPLASTY[9]

- One basis for this procedure lies in the fact that although the excess skin infraumbilically is primarily **vertical,** the excess skin in the epigastrium is primarily **horizontal.**
  - Lockwood[9] believes that the skin of the epigastrium develops laxity horizontally because of a strong superficial fascial adherence to the linea alba, which limits vertical descent of skin and fat.
  - Therefore less skin is taken centrally and more is taken laterally.
  - This results in an **oblique vector of pull** that addresses both the infraumbilical vertical excess and the epigastric lateral pull.

- The other theory that serves as a basis for this procedure is that direct undermining to the costal margins, which is a fundamental part of traditional abdominoplasty, is actually unnecessary.
  - **Direct undermining is performed only centrally** in an area that allows for rectus plication.
  - The limited direct undermining makes liposuction safer throughout a much larger area of the abdominal flap.
  - Liposuction superolaterally creates a discontinuous undermining, allowing for advancement of the abdominal flap.[9]
- The high-lateral-tension abdominoplasty also has the advantage of performing a lift of the anterior and lateral thighs.
- It also allows for liposculpture of the abdomen, leading to a more contoured result.[9]

PREOPERATIVE MARKINGS

- Preoperative marking begins with a suprapubic mark 6.5 to 7.0 cm superior to the incisura of the vagina or the base of the penis.[3]
- The anterosuperior iliac spine is marked bilaterally, and the three marks are connected.
- The marking pen is then placed centrally at the inferior incision line, and the vertical excess of skin is pulled upward until taut. The skin that is now at the tip of the pen is marked.
- Potential excess skin is tested laterally using a pinch test.
- This excess is marked laterally and connected to the central mark.
- The resultant proposed upper incision should lie infraumbilically and superior to the umbilicus laterally.
- The proposed areas of liposuction are marked both centrally and laterally.

PRINCIPLES

- Create the lower incision and elevate the skin and fat of the rectus fascia centrally just enough to perform rectus plication.
- Rectus plication is performed.
- Laterally the abdominal skin flap remains connected to the underlying rectus fascia, but it is loosened by discontinuous undermining using vertical spreading or Mayo scissors, the surgeon's finger, an oversized suction cannula, or a Lockwood Underminer Cannula (Byron Medical, Inc, Tucson, AZ).[3]
- The amount of skin and fat that can be resected centrally and laterally is confirmed using a pinch test or a Lockwood Abdominal Demarcator (Integra NeuroSciences, Plainsboro, NJ).
  - Remember that with this technique, more skin and fat should be resected laterally than centrally.
- Depending on the amount of infraumbilical skin to be excised, the umbilicus can be left in place and pulled inferiorly, or the stalk can be transected and the umbilicus floated, or it can be excised and relocated.
- The wound is tacked closed, and liposuction is performed in both a superficial and deep plane.
- Drains are placed.
- The superficial fascial system is repaired, followed by closure of the deep dermis and the skin.

FLEUR-DE-LIS ABDOMINOPLASTY[10]

- The **fleur-de-lis** technique allows for excision of the lower abdominal excess skin and fat through a transverse incision.
- It allows for simultaneous removal of the supraumbilical horizontal skin excess through a vertical excision.

- The abdominoplasty can be taken as high as the xiphoid in the midline and as low as the mons pubis, depending on the area of skin laxity.
- The key to the skin flaps surviving is to leave them attached to the underlying fascia, except in the areas contained within the fleur-de-lis excision, to maximize vascularity.[3]
- Although this procedure can completely change the abdominal contour, the expected scars must be discussed preoperatively because they can be significant.

REVERSE ABDOMINOPLASTY

- Reverse abdominoplasty was first described in the American literature by Baroudi et al[11] in 1979.
- A transverse upper abdominal incision is made roughly at the level of the inframammary fold, and redundant superior abdominal tissue is pulled up to meet this incision and excised.
- The principal indication is for cleanup of residual redundant tissue left behind superiorly after lower abdominoplasty.
- The other indication is the rare patient who presents with excess skin and abdominal protuberance that is primarily in the upper pole of the abdomen.[3]
- The reverse abdominoplasty can be combined with a breast procedure (e.g., a Wise pattern reduction or mastopexy) because the inframammary fold incisions can be used for both procedures.

KEY POINTS

- ✔ Successful rejuvenation of the abdomen requires a thorough understanding of the anatomy of the abdominal wall and the techniques available for rejuvenation.
- ✔ The selection of a procedure is of paramount importance for obtaining a good result.
- ✔ A graduated approach should be taken for liposuction performed in patients with minimal to moderate excess fat and good skin tone or quality with little laxity. Patients with more excess skin and fat are better candidates for a traditional abdominoplasty.
- ✔ During abdominoplasty, care must be taken to preserve the lateral femoral cutaneous nerve to prevent painful postoperative neuromas.
- ✔ Permanent sutures must be used during rectus plication to prevent recurrent rectus diastasis.
- ✔ Newer techniques have been developed, including the fleur-de-lis abdominoplasty and the high-lateral-tension abdominoplasty, to address supraumbilical horizontal abdominal laxity in some patients in addition to vertical infraumbilical abdominal laxity.

REFERENCES

1. Huger WE Jr. The anatomic rationale for abdominal lipectomy. Am Surg 45:612-617, 1979.
2. Rohrich RJ, Sorokin ES, Brown SA, et al. Is the umbilicus truly midline? Clinical and medicolegal implications. Plast Reconstr Surg 112:259-265, 2003.
3. Nahai F. The Art of Aesthetic Surgery: Principles and Techniques. St Louis: Quality Medical Publishing, 2005.
4. Rohrich RJ, Beran SJ, Kenkel JM, et al. Extending the role of liposuction in body contouring with ultrasound-assisted liposuction. Plast Reconstr Surg 101:1090-1102, 1998.

5. van Uchelen JH, Kon M, Werker PM. The long-term durability of plication of the anterior rectus sheath assessed by ultrasonography. Plast Reconstr Surg 107:1578-1584, 2001.
6. Nahas FX, Augusto SM, Ghelfond C. Should diastasis recti be corrected? Aesthetic Plast Surg 21:285-289, 1997.
7. Nahas FX, Ferreira LM, Mendes Jde A. An efficient way to correct recurrent rectus diastasis. Aesthetic Plast Surg 28:189-196, 2004.
8. Nahas FX, Ferreira LM, Augusto SM, et al. Long-term follow-up of correction of rectus diastasis. Plast Reconstr Surg 115:1736-1743, 2005.
9. Lockwood T. High-lateral-tension abdominoplasty with superficial fascial system suspension. Plast Reconstr Surg 96:603-615, 1995.
10. Dellon AL. Fleur-de-lis abdominoplasty. Aesthetic Plast Surg 9:27-32, 1985.
11. Baroudi R, Keppke EM, Carvalho CG. Mammary reduction combined with reverse abdominoplasty. Ann Plast Surg 2:368-373, 1979.

87. Medial Thigh Lift

Sacha I. Obaid
Jason E. Leedy

ANATOMY

- The medial thigh has a relatively thin outer layer of epidermis and dermis.
- Beneath the dermis are two layers of fat separated by a relatively weak superficial fascial system.
- Deep to the subcutaneous fat lies the strong, thick **Colles' fascia.**[1-4]
  - Attaches to the ischiopubic rami of the bony pelvis, to Scarpa's fascia of the abdominal wall, and to the posterior border of the urogenital diaphragm
  - Has an especially strong area at the **junction of the perineum and the medial thigh**
  - Provides the **anatomic shelf** that defines the perineal thigh crease
  - Best found intraoperatively by dissecting at the origin of the adductor muscles on the ischiopubic ramus and retracting the skin and superficial fat of the vulva medially
  - Lies just at the deepest and most lateral aspect of the vulvar soft tissue[5]
- The **femoral triangle** lies lateral to the Colles' fascia dissection.
  - The surgeon must be aware of the femoral triangle and avoid entering it to prevent major vascular or nerve injury and to avoid disruption of the lymphatic channels.[5]

PATIENT EVALUATION

- Complete history and physical examination are taken.
- The skin quality and tone are assessed, along with the presence, location, and degree of skin ptosis.
- The presence or absence of extra subcutaneous fat is recorded both medially and laterally in the thighs.
  - Many women have concerns about fat collections in the trochanteric regions. These can be addressed with liposuction at the time of medial thigh lift.
  - The lower torso may require liposuction at the time of thigh lift as well.
- **Classification system:**
  - **Type I:** Lipodystrophy with no sign of skin laxity; best treated with **liposuction alone**
  - **Type II:** Lipodystrophy and skin laxity confined to the **upper third of the thigh;** treated with liposuction and a **horizontal skin excision** in the medial thigh crease
  - **Type III:** Lipodystrophy and moderate skin laxity that extends **beyond the upper one third of the thigh.** These patients require both liposuction and horizontal and vertical skin excision in the medial thigh.
  - **Type IV:** Moderate skin laxity that extends the **length of the thigh;** requires a **longer vertical resection** than type III.
  - **Type V:** Severe medial thigh skin laxity with lipodystrophy; requires a **staged procedure** with a first stage of aggressive liposuction followed by a second stage of excisional medial thigh lift.
    - These patients are often **massive-weight-loss patients.**

OPERATIVE TECHNIQUE

CLASSIC MEDIAL THIGH LIFT WITH TRANSVERSE SKIN EXCISION[5]

■ **Preoperative markings**
- Patient is marked standing with knees apart.
- Areas of excess fat are marked for liposuction.
- The femoral triangle is marked to help remind the surgeon intraoperatively to stay away from this region.
- The proposed incision line is marked in the medial thigh crease beginning at the level of the coccyx posteriorly, traveling medially along the inner surface of the buttocks fold, and proceeding anteriorly to the level of the labia majora (female).
- A pinch test determines the amount of excess skin that can be removed, and an elliptical excision is marked.
- For patients with laxity extending beyond the upper third of the medial thigh skin, a vertical ellipse is added, creating a T-shaped final proposed incision.

■ **Technique**
- A combination of the prone and supine positions with "frog legging" is used.
- The operation begins with the patient prone; liposuction is performed followed by excision of the posterior portion of skin and fat that was marked preoperatively.
  ▶ Care is taken not to violate the underlying muscular fascia.
  ▶ This wound is closed, including separate closure of the superficial fascial system, deep dermis, and subcuticular areas.
- The patient is turned supine and placed in a frog-leg position.
- The anterior portion of the incision is made with resection of skin and fat.
- Colles' fascia is carefully identified near the origin of the adductor muscles on the ischiopubic ramus.
  ▶ The skin and superficial fat of the vulva are retracted medially to aid in identification.

> TIP: Carefully preserve the soft tissue that lies between the mons pubis and the femoral triangle to prevent lymphedema.

- The superficial fascial system of the medial thigh skin is identified and anchored to Colles' fascia.
- The deep dermal and subcuticular layers are closed after drain placement.

MODIFIED MEDIAL THIGH LIFT IN MASSIVE-WEIGHT-LOSS PATIENTS[5]

■ Massive-weight-loss patients often have **severe horizontal skin laxity.**
■ This operation focuses on primary correction of horizontal laxity using a **longitudinal medial thigh incision.**
■ The transverse medial thigh crease incision is minimized and used primarily for the excision of standing cutaneous deformities (dog-ears).
■ There is no need for anchoring to the Colles' fascia.

■ **Preoperative markings**
- The patient is marked standing with the legs apart.
- The proposed line of closure is determined so that it lies medially in the thigh and is minimally visible.
- A pinch test determines how much skin and fat can be removed anteriorly and posteriorly.
- The anterior and posterior incisions are marked.

■ **Technique**
  • Intraoperatively only the supine frog-leg position is used.
  • Liposuction is performed first.
  • The anterior incision is made with dissection down to the deep fat.
  • The skin and fat to be excised are elevated as dissection is made toward the proposed posterior incision.
  • The posterior incision is made, and the wedge of skin and fat are excised.
  • It is safest to perform this operation segmentally to ensure that the wound closes with appropriate tension in each area and to minimize intraoperative edema preventing closure of the wounds.
  • Jackson-Pratt drains are placed.
  • The wounds are closed by approximating the superficial fascial system followed by the deep dermal and subcuticular layers.
  • A compression garment is placed.

FASCIO-FASCIAL SUSPENSION TECHNIQUE

■ Candiani et al[6] proposed an alternative medial thigh lift that employs a **transverse skin excision with a vertical vector of pull.**
■ Instead of relying on anchoring the Colles' fascia, this technique relies on the **strength of overlap between the gracilis and adductor longus fascia.**
■ The operation begins with a transverse incision that is made parallel to, but 6-7 cm below, the inguinal crease.
■ The skin and fat are undermined down to the fascia of the adductor longus and gracilis muscles.
■ This fascia is overlapped and closed by an amount equal to the proposed skin and fat resection.
■ The skin and fat are resected and closed under minimal tension with most of the tension borne by the gracilis and adductor longus fascia.

POSTOPERATIVE COMPLICATIONS

■ Skin irregularities and depressions
■ Hypertrophic scars
■ Flattening of the buttocks from tension of wound closure
■ Distribution of the vulva
■ Lymphedema
■ Recurrence of thigh ptosis

> **TIP:** To prevent recurrence of thigh ptosis, anchor the closures to Colles' fascia or use fasciofascial suspension of the adductor and gracilis muscles.

> **KEY POINTS**
>
> ✔ Aesthetic rejuvenation of the thigh begins with a complete history and physical examination to determine the presence, location, and severity of excess skin and fat in the thigh.
>
> ✔ Based on the degree of excess skin and fat, liposuction alone, a transverse medial thigh incision, or a vertical medial thigh incision should be made to correct the deformity.
>
> ✔ Care must be taken to preserve the soft tissue between the mons pubis and the femoral triangle to prevent postoperative lymphedema.
>
> ✔ The risk of thigh ptosis recurring is high unless a strong method of fixation is employed. This can be anchoring of Colles' fascia or fascio-fascial suspension of the adductor and gracilis muscles.

REFERENCES

1. Lockwood TE. Fascial anchoring technique in medial thigh lifts. Plast Reconstr Surg 82:299-304, 1988.
2. Lockwood TE. Transverse flank-thigh-buttock lift with superficial fascial suspension. Plast Reconstr Surg 87:1019-1027, 1991.
3. Lockwood TE. Lower body lift with superficial fascial system suspension. Plast Reconstr Surg 92:1112-1122, 1993.
4. Lockwood TE. Maximizing aesthetics in lateral-tension abdominoplasty and body lifts. Clin Plast Surg 31:523-537, 2004.
5. Mathes DW, Kenkel JM, Rohrich RJ. Current concepts in medial thigh lift. Plast Reconstr Surg (submitted for publication).
6. Candiani P, Campiglio GL, Signorini M. Fascio-fascial suspension technique in medial thigh lifts. Aesthetic Plast Surg 19:137-140, 1995.

88. Body Contouring in the Massive-Weight-Loss Patient

Rohit K. Khosla

CLASSIFICATION OF MORBID OBESITY[1,2]

- **Obesity:** BMI more than 30 kg/m^2
- **Severe Obesity:** BMI more than 35 kg/m^2
- **Morbid Obesity:** BMI more than 40 kg/m^2
  - Morbidly obese individuals exceed their ideal body weight (IBW) by more than 100 pounds or are more than 100% over their IBW.
- **Superobesity:** BMI more than 50 kg/m^2
  - Superobese individuals exceed their IBW by more than 225%.

COMORBIDITIES OF MORBID OBESITY[1,2]

- Osteoarthritis
- Obstructive sleep apnea
- Gastroesophageal reflux
- Lipid abnormalities
- Hypertension
- Diabetes mellitus
- Congestive heart failure
- Asthma

COMPLICATIONS OF SKIN REDUNDANCY

- Intertriginous infections and rashes
- Musculoskeletal pain
- Functional impairment, especially with ambulation, urination, and sexual activity
- Psychological issues such as depression and low self-esteem

BARIATRIC SURGERY TECHNIQUES[2]

- These techniques are performed through traditional **open** approaches or **laparoscopically.**
- **Laparoscopic techniques** substantially reduce the morbidity from postoperative wound infections, dehiscence, and incisional hernias.

RESTRICTIVE PROCEDURES
- Manipulate the **stomach only**
- Reduce caloric intake by decreasing the quantity of food consumed at a single time
  - **Vertical band gastroplasty (VBG)**
    - ▶ Not very effective: 50% of patients unable to maintain weight loss
  - **Laparoscopic adjustable gastric band (lap band)**
    - ▶ Achieves approximately 50% reduction of excess weight

COMBINATION RESTRICTIVE AND MALABSORPTIVE PROCEDURES
- *Superior for weight reduction*
- **Malabsorptive component**
  - Limits nutrient and calorie absorption from ingested foods by bypassing the duodenum and other specific lengths of the small intestine
- **Biliopancreatic diversion (BPD)**
  - Achieves near 75%-80% reduction of excess weight
  - Produces significant nutritional deficiencies
- **BPD with duodenal switch**
  - Approximately 73% of excess weight lost
- **Roux-en-Y gastric bypass (RYGB)**
  - **Most common** bariatric procedure performed and considered the gold standard
  - Achieves excess weight loss greater than 50%

FUNDAMENTALS OF BODY CONTOURING AFTER MASSIVE WEIGHT LOSS[1,3,5]

- Bariatric surgery is a life-altering event for patients with morbid obesity; the body contouring that follows has an equally profound impact on the patient's physical and psychological well-being.
- All areas of the body present with varying degrees of skin redundancy that can be addressed surgically.
- Deformities of tissue ptosis are typically circumferential.
- Body contouring surgery is not formulaic: Each patient provides distinct challenges of redundant skin distribution and severity.

LIPOSUCTION

- Not effective as a sole modality for massive-weight-loss patients
- Can be used in areas of mild contour irregularities as an adjunct to excisional procedures
- Can be performed after recovery from major excisional procedures for refinement of contour

SURGICAL STRATEGY

- The goals of surgery are to alleviate functional, aesthetic, and psychological impairments of skin redundancy.
- Determine the priorities of the patient; however, the general sequence should be:
  1. Trunk, abdomen, buttocks, lower thighs
  2. Upper thorax/breasts, arms

3. Medial thighs
4. Face

■ Attention to intravenous fluid (IVF) resuscitation during the perioperative period is essential for large-volume excisional surgeries (e.g., belt lipectomy).
  • Intraoperative fluid management should consist of **maintenance fluid plus 10 ml/kg/hr.**
  • Monitor urine output closely during the first 24-48 hours postoperatively with continued IVF resuscitation as needed.

> TIP: It is best to multistage body contouring surgery in individuals who require several areas of correction to minimize complications, pain, and need for blood transfusions.

TIMING OF BODY CONTOURING AFTER BARIATRIC SURGERY[1,3-5]

■ Delay surgery until patient's weight has stabilized for **at least 6 months,** which corresponds to approximately 12-18 months after gastric bypass.
  • The patient is allowed time to achieve metabolic and nutritional homeostasis.
  • The period of rapid weight loss is detrimental to wound healing.
  • The risk of surgical complications decreases significantly from approximately 80% to 33% as patients approach their IBW.
  • Aesthetic outcomes are better for patients who are near their IBW.
■ Most patients settle at a BMI of 30-35 kg/m^2 after bariatric surgery.
  • Consider an initial panniculectomy or breast reduction for motivated patients in this category to improve comfort during exercise.
    ▶ This may facilitate lifestyle changes that result in further weight loss and give better aesthetic outcomes with subsequent surgery.
■ **The best candidates for extensive body contouring after massive weight loss have a BMI of 25-30 kg/m^2.**

PREOPERATIVE EVALUATION[1,3]

■ Record greatest and presenting BMI.
■ Assess stability of medical comorbidities and psychiatric problems.
■ Determine smoking history.
■ Common nutritional deficiencies include:
  • Iron deficiency anemia
  • Vitamin B$_{12}$
  • Calcium
  • Zinc
  • Fat soluble vitamins (A, D, E, and K)
  • Protein
■ Preoperative laboratory examinations should include complete blood count (CBC), electrolytes, blood urea nitrogen (BUN), creatinine, urine analysis (UA), liver function (LFTs), glucose, calcium, ferritin, total protein, and albumin.
■ Physical examination focuses on regional fat deposition and laxity of the skin envelope. Use pinch test to estimate extent of tissue resection.

TISSUE CHARACTERISTICS AND SURGICAL TECHNIQUES

TRUNK/ABDOMEN[1,4,6]

- The abdomen usually demonstrates the greatest deformity in massive-weight-loss patients.
- Most tissue descent is along the lateral axillary lines.
- Truncal tissues take on an appearance of an "inverted cone" (Fig. 88-1).
- The mons pubis has varying degrees of ptosis.
- **Surgical goals**
  - Flatten contour.
  - Tighten abdominal wall with fascial plication.
  - Repair ventral hernia if present.
  - Elevate and widen mons pubis.
- **Surgical approach**
  - *Traditional abdominoplasty* techniques fail to maximally improve body contour because they do not address lateral tissue laxity.
  - *Vertical abdominoplasty* techniques can be performed for patients who do not have back and lateral thigh ptosis.[6] (Fig. 88-2)

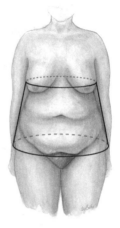

Fig. 88-1 Truncal body contour after massive weight loss. The trunk takes on the form of an inverted cone. The soft tissue is narrow at the rib cage and wider at the pelvic rim. A belt lipectomy eliminates the inferior aspect of the cone.

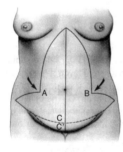

Fig. 88-2 Markings for vertical abdominoplasty. The redundant vertical tissue above the umbilicus is removed as a triangle connecting to the redundant skin in the lower abdomen, which is marked as a standard abdominoplasty. Points *A* and *B* will join as an inverted-T closure in the midline at the pubic symphysis *(C)*. In patients with significant mons ptosis, C' is marked 4-6 cm below to resect additional inferior redundancy and elevate the mons. (From Fernando da Costa L, Landecker A, Marinho Manta A. Optimizing body contour in massive weight loss patients: The modified vertical abdominoplasty. Plast Reconstr Surg 114:1917-1923, 2004.)

- *Circumferential belt lipectomy/lower body lift* addresses the circumferential nature of tissue ptosis in the trunk[4] (Fig. 88-3).
  - ► Allows resection of the entire lower section of the inverted cone deformity
  - ► Allows elevation of the buttocks and lateral thighs to produce a comprehensive lower body lift
- Patients with BMI more than 35 have a higher risk for complications after belt lipectomy/lower body lift.[1]
- **Key components of surgical technique**
  - ► Markings are as shown in Fig. 88-3.
  - ► Start prone; make superior incision first on back and dissect inferiorly.

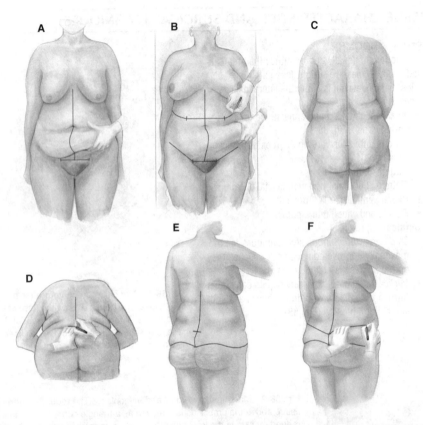

Fig. 88-3 Markings for belt lipectomy. **A,** The midline is marked initially. The horizontal pubic incision is marked below the natural hairline to allow elevation of the mons. The inferior midline of the closure should be level with the pubic symphysis. The pannus is elevated superiorly and medially to allow marking of the lateral extension of the inferior incision to just below the anterior superior iliac spine. **B,** The superior markings are made anteriorly using the pinch technique to determine the extent of resection. **C,** The midline of the back is marked with the inferior point at the coccyx. **D,** The patient is slightly bent at the waist, and the pinch test is used to estimate the superior extent of resection. **E and F,** The superior and inferior back marks are made to meet the abdominal marks laterally.

- The posterior resection should be taken down deep to the superficial fascia to maintain a layer of fat on the deep fascia and to minimize seroma formation.
- Perform liposuction on lateral thighs to release zones of adherence, which allows for lateral thigh elevation.
- Align final scars below pelvic rim (horizontal level across the superior aspect of iliac crests) to keep scars hidden under most undergarments and bikinis.
- Make inferior incision first on the abdomen, similar to traditional abdominoplasty technique.
- An umbilicoplasty is required to shorten the umbilical stalk flush with the newly contoured abdominal skin, regardless of the contouring technique used.
- Widely drain anteriorly and posteriorly to prevent seroma formation.

> TIP: Mark in the office the day before surgery for patient comfort and to avoid delays on the day
> of surgery.
>
> Minimize posterior skin resection to avoid competing anterior and posterior tension forces.
>
> Be more aggressive with lateral and anterior resections because these areas are most
> visible to the patient.

BACK[1,4,5]

- Massive weight loss can lead to upper and lower back rolls.
- Upper back rolls are typically singular and may be an extension of the lateral breast.
- Lower back rolls may be multiple and can be oriented horizontally or in an upward-sweeping direction.
- **Surgical goals**
  - Resect as many rolls as possible.
  - Create a flat contour for the back.
- **Surgical approach**
  - A circumferential belt lipectomy/lower body lift is effective for resecting lower back rolls.
  - An upper back roll requires direct excision in a staged procedure separate from the belt lipectomy.

> TIP: Align transverse and posterior scars along the bra line in women.

WAIST AND LATERAL THIGHS[1,4]

- Massive weight loss creates a contour that lacks waist and hip definition.
- Lack of definition is caused by ptosis of the abdomen, lateral thighs, and buttocks.
- Maximal vertical relaxation occurs along lateral body contours.
- Tissue excess spirals down the thigh in an anterior and posterior direction.
- **Surgical goals**
  - Narrow waist as much as possible.
  - Create a smooth natural curve from the rib cage through the waist and down onto hips.
- **Surgical approach**
  - The lateral thigh is structurally dependent on truncal tissues. It is not possible to effectively elevate the thighs if trunk remains lax.
  - Circumferential belt lipectomy/lower body lift is effective to define the waist and lateral hips in a single-stage procedure.

> TIP: Use independent leg extensions on the OR table that will allow hip abduction while prone
> and supine to eliminate tension on the lateral thigh advancement.
>
> Suture the superficial fascial system (SFS) to the deep fascia with permanent sutures on
> both skin flaps in a three-point configuration to hold the elevation of the lateral thigh, effec-
> tively establishing a new zone of adherence at the level of the final scar.

MEDIAL THIGHS[1]

- Most massive-weight-loss patients have more horizontal skin excess of the thighs relative to the vertical excess.

- A vertical medial thigh lift is more effective than a horizontal medial thigh lift.
- To reduce potential for labial spreading, avoid a horizontal scar technique.
- Medial thigh lift should be performed in a separate staged procedure after addressing the lateral thighs.
- This can be combined with liposuction of the medial, anterior, and posterior thigh as an adjunct to mild contour irregularities.
- **Contraindications**
  - Preexisting lymphedema
  - History of lower extremity deep vein thrombosis
  - Presence of varicose veins.
    - ▶ Obliterate varicosities before performing medial thigh lipectomy
- **Surgical goals**
  - Create a flat contour for the medial thigh.
  - Minimize labial spreading.
- **Surgical approach**
  - Mark the perineal crease on the inner thigh as the superior extent of the vertical ellipse.
  - Perform a pinch test in a superior-to-inferior direction to estimate the extent of resection.
  - Preserve the superficial saphenous vein during resection.
  - Avoid dissection anteriorly in the femoral triangle.
  - A superior dog-ear can be worked out along the posterior inferior buttock crease or anterior inguinal crease.

> TIP: Wait 6-12 months after lower body lift to minimize tension on the medial thigh.
>
> Resect skin only if incision is taken anteriorly to preserve inguinal lymphatics.
>
> Suture SFS of thigh to Colles' fascia with nonabsorbable sutures if horizontal medial thigh lift is performed.

BUTTOCKS[1,4,5]

- The back and buttocks tend to blend together, which gives the appearance of a long vertical buttock height.
- The central buttock crease descends, leaving minimal soft tissue coverage over the coccyx.
- The lateral inferior buttock crease lies more horizontally without a shapely curve.
- **Surgical goals**
  - Define the buttocks by creating a line of demarcation from the back to the buttocks. Align the final scar following the superior gluteal curve in a central gull-wing pattern.
  - Elevate the buttocks, including the central crease.
  - Cover coccyx with additional soft tissue if there is a deficiency.
  - Develop an upward curve of the inferior buttock crease.
- **Surgical approach**
  - The goals of buttock definition are effectively achieved with circumferential belt lipectomy/lower body lift.
  - Consider autogenous gluteal augmentation to enhance buttock contour, especially with central buttock projection.
  - Autogenous gluteal augmentation can be performed with fat grafting or dermal/fat flaps.

BREASTS[1,5]

- The volume and characteristics of breast tissue are highly variable after massive weight loss.
- **Surgical approach**
  - Reduction mammaplasty is indicated for persistent macromastia.
    - ▶ There is no single reduction technique that is superior in this patient population.
  - Mastopexy or augmentation is indicated for patients with grade I/II ptosis.
  - Mastopexy with or without augmentation is indicated for patients with grade III ptosis.

UPPER ARMS[1,7]

- The upper arms develop severely ptotic skin that extends from the olecranon across the axilla onto the chest wall.
- The excess arm skin is contiguous with the posterior axillary fold on the lateral chest.
- The ideal candidate for brachioplasty is one with deflated upper arms and a small amount of residual fat.
- **Surgical goals**
  - Eliminate horizontal upper arm excess.
  - Eliminate lateral thoracic skin excess.
  - Create a smooth transition from the lateral chest onto the upper arm.
  - Minimize scar visibility and contracture.
- **Surgical approach** (Fig. 88-4)
  - Brachioplasty techniques that place incisions posterior to the bicipital groove are less noticeable when viewed from the front.
  - A sinusoidal incision pattern decreases the possibility of linear scar contracture.
  - Resect the entire subcutaneous tissue down to the muscular aponeurosis.
  - Identify and prevent injury to the ulnar nerve and medial antebrachial cutaneous nerve during resection.
  - The incision should be carried onto the axilla with a Z-plasty to reduce axillary ptosis and restore a more natural dome shape to the axilla.

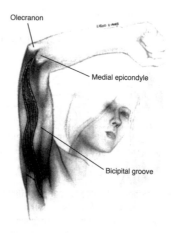

Fig. 88-4 Sinusoidal brachioplasty technique made behind the bicipital groove with Z-plasty and extension into the axilla. (From Strauch B, Greenspun D, Levine J, et al. A technique of brachioplasty. Plast Reconstr Surg 113: 1044-1048, 2004.)

Olecranon

Medial epicondyle

Bicipital groove

> TIP: Patients with significant remaining upper arm fat benefit from liposuction as a staged procedure before excisional lipectomy.

FACE AND NECK[8]

- Skin redundancy exceeds that of the superficial musculoaponeurotic system (SMAS) laxity after massive weight loss.
- Appearance of premature aging develops.
- The aged facial appearance may be more displeasing to younger patients than redundant skin elsewhere, because they are able to camouflage skin redundancy elsewhere with clothing.
- **Surgical goals**
  - Redrape the skin over the face and neck to restore a normal-appearing jawline and neck.
  - Harmonize facial appearance with the contouring of the rest of the body.

- Modify the SMAS rhytidectomy for the massive-weight-loss patient[8]
  - Correction of facial skin redundancy requires more skin undermining to produce a smooth contour relative to a typical rhytidectomy.
  - Less elevation of SMAS is required, because laxity at this tissue level is not the structural problem; normal SMAS plication is performed.
  - Platysmaplasty should be performed if platysmal banding present.
  - Perform suction-assisted or direct lipectomy of remaining fat deposits in jowls and submental triangle.
  - The skin incision can enter the temporal hairline above the helical root if the planned vector of facial elevation is posterior and superior.
  - Carry the incision around the earlobe and onto the conchal bowl posteriorly.
    - The vector of elevation on the neck can be mostly superior, which avoids an incision across the occipital hairline.
    - Use a traditional postauricular incision with occipital hairline extension if the neck has severe skin laxity.

COMPLICATIONS[1,3,5]

HEMATOMAS
- Typically occur in the immediate postoperative period
- Require operative drainage and exploration

SEROMAS
- A higher incidence is seen in patients with BMI more than 35 kg/m², primarily in the lower back after belt lipectomy/lower body lift.
- Maintain drains until output is less than 40 ml over 24 hours.
- Drain seromas early, before capsule formation.
- Aspiration can be performed in the office; may need serial aspiration.
- Large seromas can be drained by percutaneous closed suction drains.
- Inject cavity with doxycycline to sclerose walls, if necessary.

LYMPHOCELES
- Seen primarily in the inguinal region from aggressive resection into femoral triangle
- Perform serial aspiration
- Percutaneous drainage with placement of closed suction drain
- Doxycycline injection
- Requires operative exploration and ligation of leaking lymphatic channels if nonoperative management fails

DEEP VEIN THROMBOSIS AND PULMONARY EMBOLISM (DVT/PE)
- Risk is less than 0.1%.
- Truncal lipectomies create higher risk; increased intraabdominal pressure leads to decreased venous return from lower extremities.

- **Prophylaxis**
  - Administration of low-molecular-weight heparin before surgery and during hospitalization may reduce risk.
  - Epidural analgesia has been shown to decrease incidence of DVT/PE in orthopedic literature; the efficacy is unknown in body contouring.
  - Place sequential compression devices before inducing general anaesthesia and maintain postoperatively.
  - Patients should start ambulating with assistance the day of surgery.
  - Patients should perform incentive spirometry.

WOUND COMPLICATIONS

- **Dehiscence**
  - Most occur within first few days of surgery as a result of excess tension.
- **Skin necrosis**
- **Wound infection/cellulitis**
- **Factors that increase incidence of wound complications:**
  - Tobacco use
    - ▸ Patients should wait at least 1 month after cessation of smoking before undergoing surgery.
  - Diabetes
  - Active systemic steroid use
  - BMI more than 40 kg/m²

KEY POINTS

- ✔ Roux-en-Y gastric bypass is the most common reproducible and effective bariatric operation performed today.
- ✔ Start body contouring surgery when the patient's weight has stabilized for at least 6 months.
- ✔ The best aesthetic outcomes with lowest perioperative risks occur with patients near their IBW or with a BMI of 25-30 kg/m² after bariatric surgery.
- ✔ The abdomen generally demonstrates the greatest deformity, and most tissue ptosis is along the lateral axillary lines.
- ✔ Assess nutritional deficiencies before initiating body contouring surgery.
- ✔ Treat the trunk, lateral thigh, and buttocks as a single aesthetic unit.
- ✔ Circumferential belt lipectomy/lower body lift resects excess truncal tissue and elevates the buttocks and lateral thighs.
- ✔ Perform liposuction on the lateral thighs during a belt lipectomy to release the zones of adherence, which allows for more effective elevation of the lateral thigh.
- ✔ Massive-weight-loss patients may require breast reduction or mastopexy, depending on the amount of breast volume lost.
- ✔ Patients develop a prematurely aging face as a result of skin redundancy rather than SMAS laxity.
- ✔ Liposuction techniques can be used as an adjunct during or after excisional operations for additional refinement of contour.

REFERENCES

1. Aly AS. Body Contouring After Massive Weight Loss. St Louis: Quality Medical Publishing, 2006.
2. Hamad GG. The state of the art in bariatric surgery for weight loss in the morbidly obese patient. Clin Plast Surg 31:591-600, 2004.
3. Rubin JP, Nguyen V, Schwentker A. Perioperative management of the post-gastric-bypass patient presenting for body contouring surgery. Clin Plast Surg 31:601-610, 2004.
4. Aly AS, Cram AE, Heddens C. Truncal body contouring surgery in the massive weight loss patient. Clin Plast Surg 31:611-624, 2004.
5. Taylor J, Shermak M. Body contouring following massive weight loss. Obesity Surg 14:1080-1085, 2004.
6. Fernando da Costa L, Landecker A, Marinho Manta A. Optimizing body contour in massive weight loss patients: The modified vertical abdominoplasty. Plast Reconstr Surg 114:1917-1923, 2004.
7. Strauch B, Greenspun D, Levine J, et al. A technique of brachioplasty. Plast Reconstr Surg 113:1044-1048, 2004.
8. Sclafani AP. Restoration of the jawline and the neck after bariatric surgery. Facial Plast Surg 21:28-32, 2005.

Index

927